Atlas of HEAD AND NECK SURGERY

Volume 1

Atlas of HEAD AND

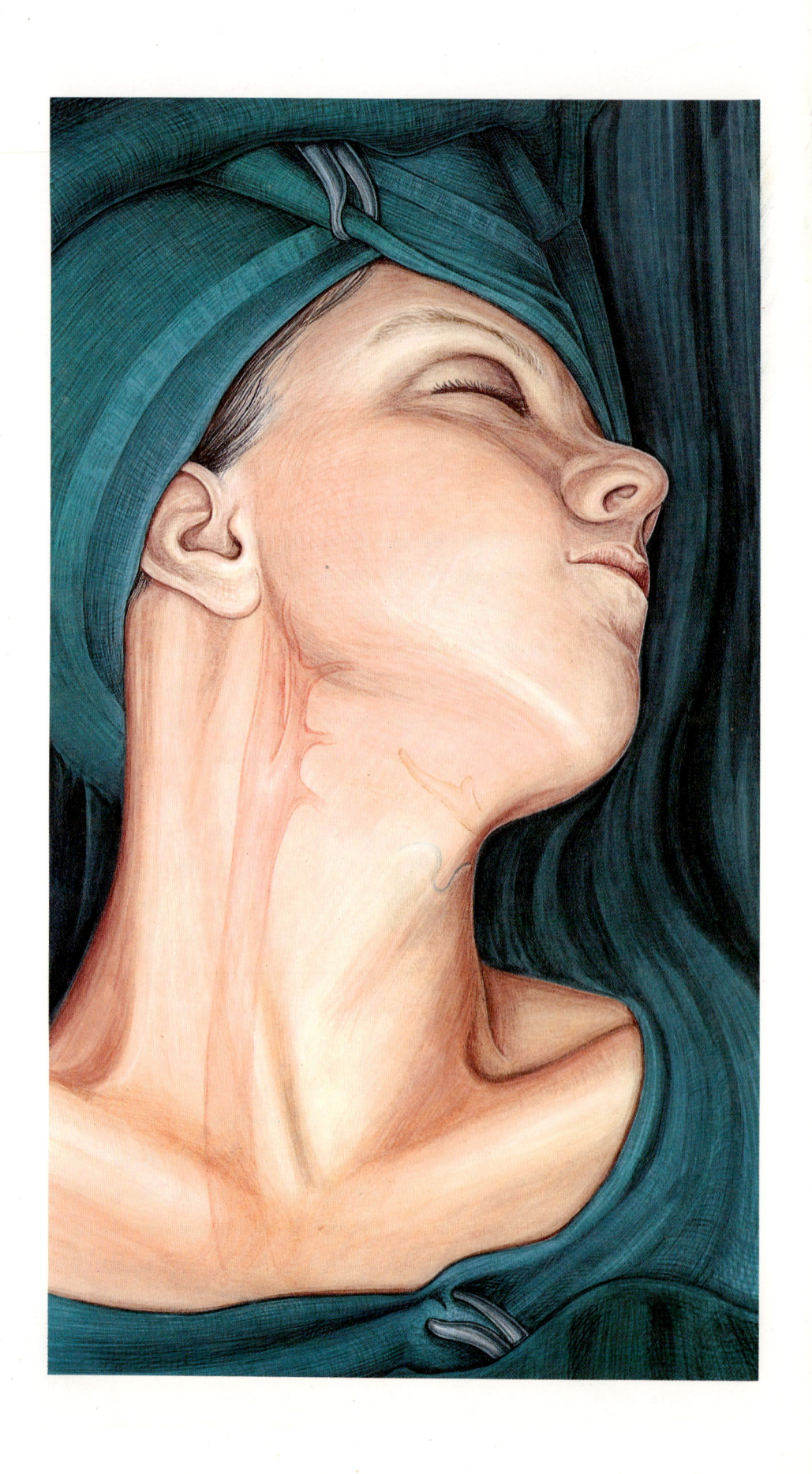

NECK SURGERY

Edited by
Michael E. Johns, M.D.   Volume 1
Andelot Professor and Director
Department of Otolaryngology–Head and Neck Surgery

John C. Price, M.D.
Associate Professor
Department of Otolaryngology–Head and Neck Surgery

Douglas E. Mattox, M.D.
Associate Professor and Deputy Director
Department of Otolaryngology–Head and Neck Surgery
Associate Professor
Department of Neurosurgery

Illustrations by
Mark M. Miller, M.A.
Instructor
Department of Art as Applied to Medicine

The Johns Hopkins University Medical Institutions
Baltimore, Maryland

B.C. DECKER, INC.   Philadelphia   Toronto

Publisher

B.C. Decker Inc
3228 South Service Road
Burlington, Ontario L7N 3H8

B.C. Decker Inc
320 Walnut Street
Suite 400
Philadelphia, Pennsylvania 19106

Sales and Distribution

United States and Puerto Rico
The C.V. Mosby Company
11830 Westline Industrial Drive
Saint Louis, Missouri 63146

Canada
McAinsh & Co. Ltd.
2760 Old Leslie Street
Willowdale, Ontario M2K 2X5

Australia
McGraw-Hill Book Company Australia Pty. Ltd.
4 Barcoo Street
Roseville East 2069
New South Wales, Australia

Brazil
Editora McGraw-Hill do Brasil, Ltda.
rua Tabapua, 1.105, Itaim-Bibi
Sao Paulo, S.P. Brasil

Colombia
Interamericana/McGraw-Hill de Colombia, S.A.
Apartado Aereo 81078
Bogota, D.E. Colombia

Europe
McGraw-Hill Book Company GmbH
Lademannbogen 136
D-2000 Hamburg 63
West Germany

France
MEDSI/McGraw-Hill
6, avenue Daniel Lesueur
75007 Paris, France

Hong Kong and China
McGraw-Hill Book Company
Suite 618, Ocean Centre
5 Canton Road
Tsimshatsui, Kowloon
Hong Kong

India
Tata McGraw-Hill Publishing Company, Ltd.
12/4 Asaf Ali Road, 3rd Floor
New Delhi 110002, India

Indonesia
P.O. Box 122/JAT
Jakarta, 1300 Indonesia

Italy
McGraw-Hill Libri Italia, s.r.l.
Piazza Emilia, 5
I-20129 Milano MI
Italy

Japan
Igaku-Shoin Ltd.
Tokyo International P.O. Box 5063
1-28-36 Hongo, Bunkyo-ku,
Tokyo 113, Japan

Korea
C.P.O. Box 10583
Seoul, Korea

Malaysia
No. 8 Jalan SS 7/6B
Kelana Jaya
47301 Petaling Jaya
Selangor, Malaysia

Mexico
Interamericana/McGraw-Hill de Mexico, S.A. de C.V.
Cedro 512, Colonia Atlampa
(Apartado Postal 26370)
06450 Mexico, D.F., Mexico

New Zealand
McGraw-Hill Book Co. New Zealand Ltd.
5 Joval Place, Wiri
Manukau City, New Zealand

Panama
Editorial McGraw-Hill Latinoamericana, S.A.
Apartado Postal 2036
Zona Libre de Colon
Colon, Republica de Panama

Portugal
Editora McGraw-Hill de Portugal, Ltda.
Rua Rosa Damasceno 11A-B
1900 Lisboa, Portugal

South Africa
Libriger Book Distributors
Warehouse Number 8
"Die Ou Looiery"
Tannery Road
Hamilton, Bloemfontein 9300

Southeast Asia
McGraw-Hill Book Co.
348 Jalan Boon Lay
Jurong, Singapore 2261

Spain
McGraw-Hill/Interamericana de Espana, S.A.
Manuel Ferrero, 13
28020 Madrid, Spain

Taiwan
P.O. Box 87-601
Taipei, Taiwan

Thailand
632/5 Phaholyothin Road
Sapan Kwai
Bangkok 10400
Thailand

United Kingdom, Middle East and Africa
McGraw-Hill Book Company (U.K.) Ltd.
Shoppenhangers Road
Maidenhead, Berkshire
SL6 2QL England

Venezuela
McGraw-Hill/Interamericana, C.A.
2da. calle Bello Monte
(entre avenida Casanova y Sabana Grande)
Apartado Aereo 50785
Caracas 1050, Venezuela

Notice

The authors and publisher have made every effort to ensure that the patient care recommended herein, including choice of drugs and drug dosages, is in accord with the accepted standards and practice at the time of publication. However, since research and regulation constantly change clinical standards, the reader is urged to check the product information sheet included in the package of each drug, which includes recommended doses, warnings, and contraindications. This is particularly important with new or infrequently used drugs.

Atlas of Head and Neck Surgery,
Volume 1

ISBN 1-55664-113-3

© 1990 by B.C. Decker Incorporated under the International Copyright Union. All rights reserved. No part of this publication may be reused or republished in any form without written permission of the publisher.

Library of Congress catalog card number:
89-51036

10 9 8 7 6 5 4 3 2 1

Printed in Hong Kong

Contributors

Maria Allo, M.D. — Clinical Associate Professor of Surgery, Stanford University School of Medicine, Stanford; Chief, General Surgery, and Chairperson, Department of Surgery, Santa Clara Valley Medical Center, San Jose, California

Manning Miles Goldsmith, M.D. — Clinical Assistant Professor of Otolaryngology, University of North Carolina at Chapel Hill, Chapel Hill, North Carolina

Michael E. Johns, M.D. — Andelot Professor and Director, Department of Otolaryngology–Head and Neck Surgery, The Johns Hopkins Medical Institutions, Baltimore, Maryland

Jordan S. Josephson, M.D. — Assistant Professor, SUNY Health Science Center at Brooklyn; Attending, Long Island College Hospital, Brooklyn, New York

Haskins K. Kashima, M.D. — Professor of Otolaryngology–Head and Neck Surgery, The Johns Hopkins Medical Institutions, Baltimore, Maryland

David W. Kennedy, M.D. — Associate Professor, Departments of Otolaryngology–Head and Neck Surgery and Neurosurgery, The Johns Hopkins Medical Institutions, Baltimore, Maryland

Wayne M. Koch, M.D. — Assistant Professor, Department of Otolaryngology–Head and Neck Surgery, The Johns Hopkins Medical Institutions, Baltimore, Maryland

Donlin M. Long, M.D., Ph.D. — Professor and Director, Department of Neurosurgery, The Johns Hopkins Medical Institutions, Baltimore, Maryland

Bernard R. Marsh, M.D. — Associate Professor, Department of Otolaryngology–Head and Neck Surgery, The Johns Hopkins Medical Institutions, Baltimore, Maryland

Contributors

Douglas E. Mattox, M.D. — Associate Professor and Deputy Director, Department of Otolaryngology–Head and Neck Surgery, and Associate Professor, Department of Neurosurgery, The Johns Hopkins Medical Institutions, Baltimore, Maryland

Mark M. Miller, M.A. — Director of Facial Prosthetics, Art as Applied to Medicine, The Johns Hopkins University School of Medicine, Baltimore, Maryland

Robert M. Naclerio, M.D. — Associate Professor, Department of Otolaryngology–Head and Neck Surgery, The Johns Hopkins Medical Institutions, Baltimore, Maryland

Peter W. Orobello, Jr., M.D. — Director of Pediatric Otolaryngology–Head and Neck Surgery, All Children's Hospital, St. Petersburg, Florida

Ira D. Papel, M.D. — Assistant Professor and Director, Division of Facial Plastic and Reconstructive Surgery, Department of Otolaryngology–Head and Neck Surgery, The Johns Hopkins Medical Institutions, Baltimore, Maryland

Glenn E. Peters, M.D. — Assistant Professor, University of Alabama at Birmingham School of Medicine, Birmingham, Alabama

Rafael R. Portela, M.D. — Former Instructor, Department of Otolaryngology–Head and Neck Surgery, The Johns Hopkins Medical Institutions, Baltimore, Maryland

Loring W. Pratt, M.D. — Visiting Professor 1986-1987, The Johns Hopkins University School of Medicine, Baltimore, Maryland; Honorary Staff and Former Chief of Otolaryngology, Mid-Maine Medical Center, Fairfield, Maine

John C. Price, M.D. — Associate Professor, Department of Otolaryngology–Head and Neck Surgery, The Johns Hopkins Medical Institutions, Baltimore, Maryland

William J. Richtsmeier, M.D., Ph.D. — Associate Professor and Director, Division of Head and Neck Oncology, The Johns Hopkins Medical Institutions, Baltimore, Maryland

Preface

The specialty of Otolaryngology–Head and Neck Surgery has experienced unprecedented growth and development over the last decade. Advances in instrumentation and techniques of nasal and tracheobronchial endoscopy, tissue transposition and microvascular transfer, biocompatible implants, and sensory stimulators have increased the scope and depth of the specialty. In this atlas we have compiled the experience and techniques of prominent subspecialists in Otolaryngology–Head and Neck Surgery that reflect the current management and philosophy at The Johns Hopkins Hospital.

The authors, all faculty at The Johns Hopkins University School of Medicine at the time this volume was written, have presented their most useful techniques and alternatives. Although we have made no attempt to catalogue all the variations of each procedure, the reader will note some variation in the methods and approaches used to manage similar problems. Our faculty, like most others, does not have unanimity on the best techniques to solve all problems. The editors, however, have chosen methods that should be useful to both the generalist and the subspecialist.

All of us have been fortunate to collaborate with our medical illustrator, Mark Miller. The quality of his full-color illustrations is the product of hours in the operating room with us and his persistent attention to detail. We all have respect and admiration for his work.

Michael E. Johns
John C. Price
Douglas E. Mattox

This book is dedicated in memory of L. Stefan Levin, D.D.S., M.S.D. (1939-1989), Associate Professor of Otolaryngology–Head and Neck Surgery at The Johns Hopkins University. He was an oral pathologist and geneticist, and a world-renowned clinician, teacher, and research scientist. Most important, Steve was a warm, caring human being who was a dear friend.

Contents

Volume 1

Chapter I		ENDOSCOPY 1
	Haskins K. Kashima	Diagnostic Laryngoscopy 2
		Operative Laryngoscopy 14
		CO_2 Laser Excision of Polyps, Cysts, and Nodules 20
		CO_2 Laser Excision of Benign Lesions 25
		CO_2 Laser Excision of Malignant Lesions 35
		CO_2 Laser Arytenoidectomy and Transverse Cordotomy 41
		CO_2 Laser Excision of Laryngeal Web 46
		T-Tube Insertion 49
	Bernard R. Marsh	Diagnostic Bronchoscopy 53
		Removal of Bronchial Foreign Bodies 60
		Bronchial Laser Use 65
		Diagnostic Esophagoscopy 68
		Removal of Esophageal Foreign Bodies 72
		Treatment of Esophageal Caustic Burns 75
Chapter II		FUNCTIONAL ENDOSCOPIC SINUS SURGERY 79
	David W. Kennedy & Jordan S. Josephson	Diagnostic Nasal Endoscopy 80
		Maxillary and Sphenoid Sinuscopy 84
		Endoscopic Sphenoethmoidectomy 88
		Special Problems 98
Chapter III		THE NOSE 103
	Ira D. Papel	Nasal Polypectomy 104
	John C. Price	Septoplasty 109
	Douglas E. Mattox & Donlin M. Long	Transseptal Transsphenoidal Hypophysectomy 121
	Ira D. Papel	Septal Dermoplasty 135
	Manning Miles Goldsmith	Closure of Nasal Septal Perforations 141
	Rafael R. Portela & Robert M. Naclerio	Choanal Atresia 150
	Ira D. Papel & John C. Price	Nasal Reconstruction 160

John C. Price	Rhinectomy	187
Mark M. Miller	Fabrication of a Nasal Prosthesis	193

Chapter IV PARANASAL SINUSES 201

Douglas E. Mattox	Caldwell-Luc with Transantral Ethmoidectomy	202
	Transantral Maxillary Artery Ligation	209
	Ligation of Ethmoidal Arteries	215
	External Ethmoidectomy	218
Loring W. Pratt	Frontal Sinus Trephination	223
W. J. Richtsmeier	Frontoethmoidectomy	229
Loring W. Pratt	Osteoplastic Frontal Sinusectomy	237
John C. Price	Midfacial Degloving Approach to the Sinuses	251
John C. Price & Wayne M. Koch	Medial Maxillectomy	264
Wayne M. Koch & John C. Price	Lateral Rhinotomy Approach to the Sinuses	270
	Medial Maxillectomy with En Bloc Ethmoidectomy	273
	Maxillectomy	276
	Radical Maxillectomy	289
John C. Price & Wayne M. Koch	Orbital Exenteration	292
Mark M. Miller	Fabrication of an Orbital Prosthesis	297

Chapter V THYROID AND PARATHYROIDS 303

Maria Allo	Thyroidectomy	304
	Parathyroidectomy	317

Chapter VI SALIVARY GLANDS 323

Michael E. Johns & Wayne M. Koch	Submandibular Gland Excision	324
Michael E. Johns	Parotidectomy	331
Peter W. Orobello, Jr.	Excision of First Branchial Cleft Cyst	343
Douglas E. Mattox	Excision of Parapharyngeal Space Tumors	347

Chapter VII   THE NECK   357

Glenn E. Peters
- Excision of Second and Third Branchial Cleft Cysts   358
- Excision of Thyroglossal Duct Cyst   364
- Fine Needle Aspiration Biopsy   374

Glenn E. Peters, John C. Price, & Michael E. Johns
- Cervical Lymphadenectomy   378

Index   413

Atlas of HEAD AND NECK SURGERY

Volume 1

Chapter I

ENDOSCOPY

Haskins K. Kashima, M.D.

DIAGNOSTIC LARYNGOSCOPY

Indirect Laryngoscopy

Indications

The purpose of laryngoscopy, or visual inspection of the larynx, is to evaluate the structural and functional status of the larynx, hypopharynx, and base of tongue. The structural parts of the larynx include specific anatomic sites, their investing epithelium, and deeper structures (Fig. 1A, coronal section of the larynx). The functional evaluation assesses movement of the vocal cords. The examination should *detect* anatomic abnormalities and define their extent and uncover functional disorders and their severity; points of uncertainty are identified and require clarification by further diagnostic studies.

Preparation for Examination

A complete history of the throat is the essential preliminary step for the laryngeal examination. The *"competent throat"* concept recognizes that safe and adequate *airway, swallowing,* and *vocalization* are integrated and overlapping functions. In the healthy throat, all three functions are performed to perfection; a significant impairment in any single function is accompanied by a corresponding disturbance in the remaining two functions. The laryngologic history inquires into the function-dysfunction of airway, swallowing, and voice production. An unhurried and thorough history-taking serves the twin purposes of focusing the examination on specific anatomic or functional disturbances and of putting the patient at ease so that he or she is able to cooperate optimally during the examination.

Examination Technique

First and foremost, both the examiner and examinee must be comfortable; the examinee's feet should be firmly placed on the floor or supporting platform, hips snug against the back of the examining chair and the upper torso bent forward; the neck is flexed on the chest and the head is extended on the neck, achieving the so-called rose-sniffing position. The ideal vertical positioning is adjusted so that the illumination source—the examiner's head mirror—and the patient's oropharynx are at the same horizontal plane (Fig. 1B). The examiner may stand or be seated but must be comfortable.

Preliminary to mirror laryngoscopy, a thorough examination of the oral cavity is performed to determine the status of the teeth and dentures, and to evaluate the patient's ability to open the mouth widely to permit placement of the laryngeal mirror. Correct wording of instructions to the patient is important; it is preferable to state that the tongue will be "steadied" rather than "pulled forward." A gauze strip is grasped by the index finger and thumb and placed on the patient's tongue, which is gently steadied in the forward position; this flattens the tongue dorsum and removes the tongue base from the line of vision to the larynx. The middle finger is placed on the upper teeth (or gums), and the patient is guided into position until the reflected light is focused at the uvula. A prewarmed mirror is placed under the uvula and elevated until a clear

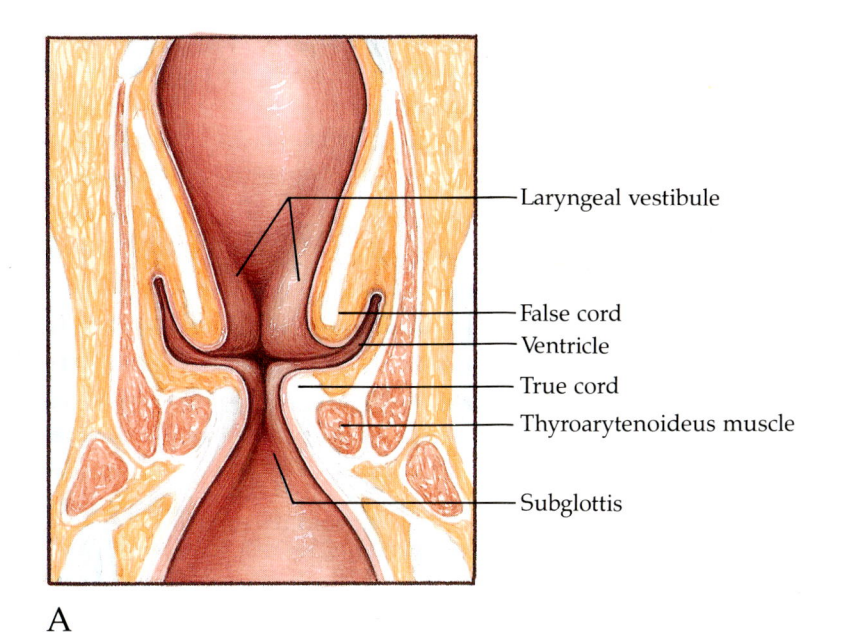

Plate 1

A

- Laryngeal vestibule
- False cord
- Ventricle
- True cord
- Thyroarytenoideus muscle
- Subglottis

B

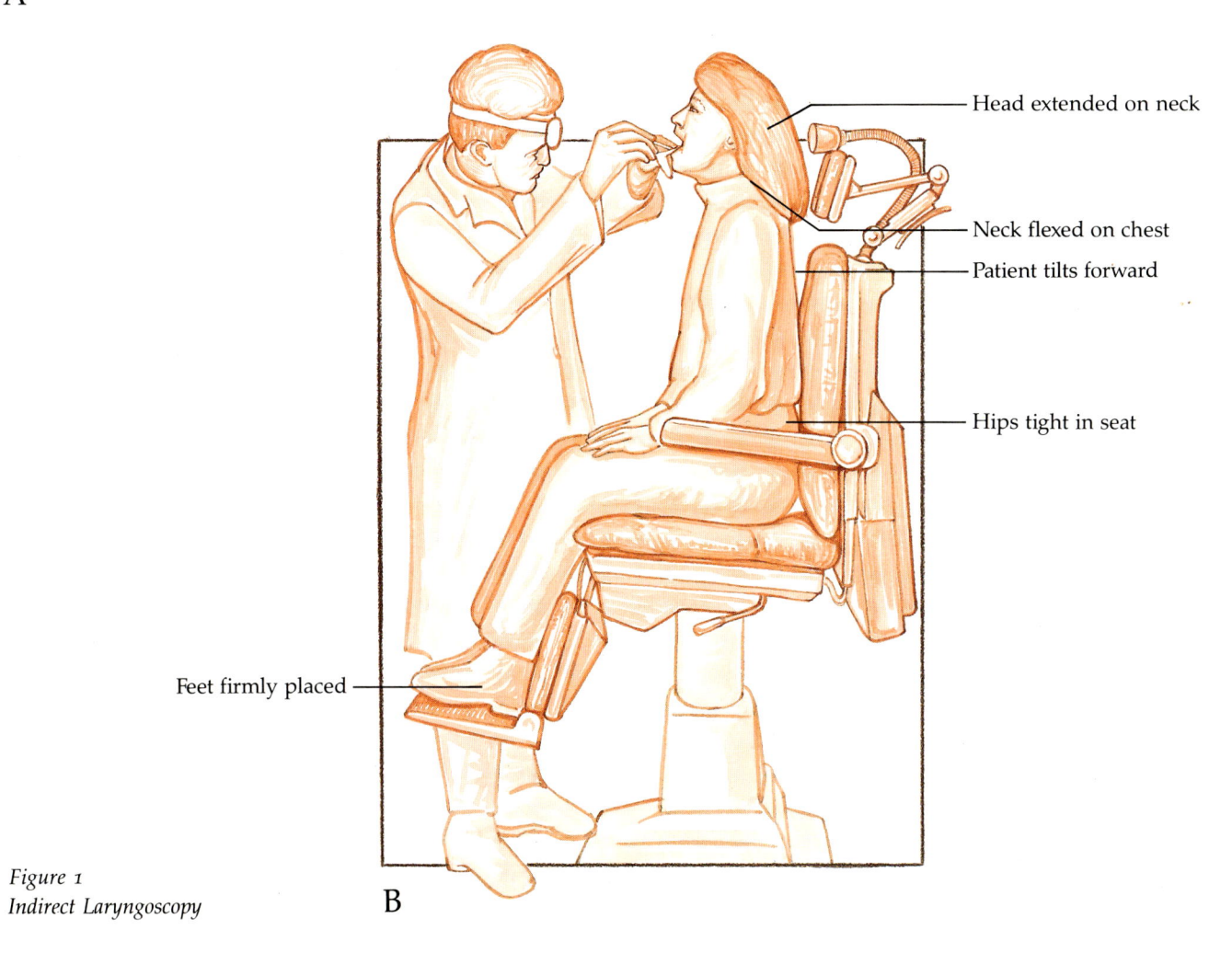

- Head extended on neck
- Neck flexed on chest
- Patient tilts forward
- Hips tight in seat
- Feet firmly placed

Figure 1
Indirect Laryngoscopy

3

image of the larynx is achieved. The largest possible laryngeal mirror is utilized to obtain an optimal panoramic view of the hypopharynx and larynx (Fig. 1C).

The laryngeal image is centered on the mirror so the examiner may note the symmetry of the larynx and surrounding structures. Quiet breathing or panting respirations on the part of the patient help to attain full visualization of the laryngeal inlet, true and false cords, arytenoids, and aryepiglottic folds. Attention is also directed to the base of the tongue, the vallecula, the piriform sinuses, and the esophageal inlet. Notation should include symmetry of the foregoing structures and the normally pink and glistening epithelium, with the exception of the true cords, which appear translucent white. When the vocal cords are fully abducted, a satisfactory view of the anterior trachea as far as the upper border of the cricoid mucoperichondrium is achieved.

The epiglottis, a delicately thinned structure, has a characteristic curved contour. On its laryngeal surface, a peaked prominence, the petiole, is seen. Unusual prominence of the petiole and epiglottic base may indicate expansion in the pre-epiglottic space by tumor, hematoma, or other space-occupying lesion; palpable fullness of the thyrohyoid membrane also indicates pre-epiglottic space expansion.

The supraglottis consists of the false cords, bordered medially by the free margin and laterally by the thin aryepiglottic fold. The vestibular surface has a supple concave surface; a convex or fixed appearance suggests a possible space-occupying lesion in the upper paraglottic space arising from the ventricle or saccule; a bulge of the medial wall of the piriform sinus reinforces this concern.

The false cords oppose tightly during a gag or forced cough and in dysphonia plicae ventricularis, although this may not be a constant finding in the last condition.

THE ARYTENOIDS

The arytenoids provide important information regarding vocal cord motion; they appear as symmetric, paired prominences in the posterior larynx. The posterior and lateral cricoarytenoid muscles rotate the arytenoids, and the interarytenoid muscles cause them to glide to the midline (adduction) position. Interarytenoid mucosa corrugates during vocal cord adduction and is smoothed on abduction (see Figs. 1D and 1E). The absence of corrugation occurs in scarring due to trauma or infiltrative disorders and limits vocal cord abduction.

TRUE CORDS

The true cords normally appear translucent white; their free borders are sharp, vocal cord motion is crisp and symmetric, and the free borders meet cleanly in the midline during phonation. When the patient is hoarse, laryngeal examination endeavors to discover the cause of imperfect vocal cord apposition during phonation, due either to paralysis or to a space-occupying lesion.

Vocal cord adduction results in precise apposition of the vocal cords during phonation of a high-pitched E (see Fig. 1D). Imperfect vocal cord apposition results from impaired vocal cord motion or from space-occu-

Plate 2

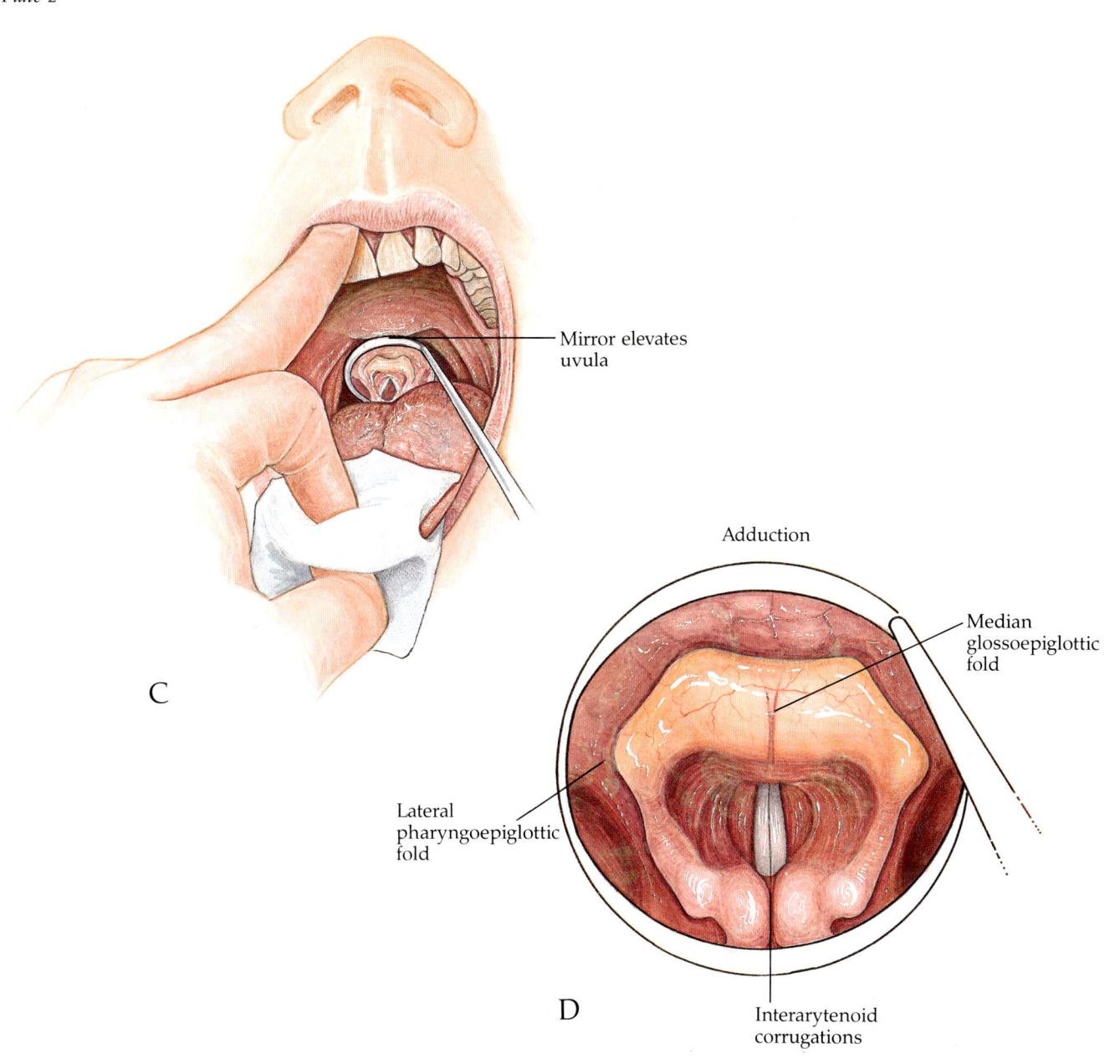

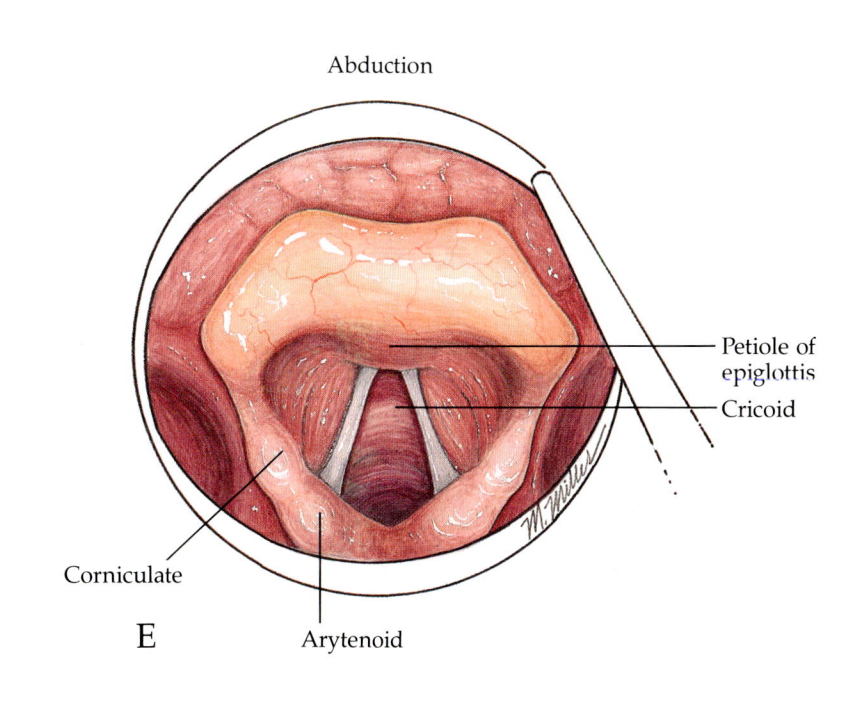

C — Mirror elevates uvula

D — Adduction
- Median glossoepiglottic fold
- Lateral pharyngoepiglottic fold
- Interarytenoid corrugations

E — Abduction
- Petiole of epiglottis
- Cricoid
- Corniculate
- Arytenoid

Figure 1 (Continued)
Indirect Laryngoscopy

pying lesions such as cysts, reactive swelling or tumors, and less commonly, vocal cord atrophy. The false cords remain separated during phonation; tight approximation and hyperemic change along the free border may occur in plicae ventricularis.

Vocal cord abduction occurs during voluntary inspiratory effort, and the symmetric lateral movement permits a view of the subglottic larynx (see Fig. 1E). Visualization of a pink swelling located inferomedial to the free border of the true cords indicates soft tissue swelling in the subglottis caused either by inflammatory reactive swelling or by infiltrative disorder; it occurs in sarcoidosis or amyloidosis and, most important, in croup. The subglottis is also visualized in atrophy of the vocal cords, as occurs after paralysis.

Unilateral and bilateral vocal cord motion impairment is frequently difficult to evaluate accurately. The causes of abnormal vocal cord motion are impaired innervation by the recurrent laryngeal nerve(s), cricoarytenoid joint arthrodesis, infiltrative disorders of the vocal cord, and restraining mucosal web or scar formation. The initial task in the laryngeal examination is to determine that vocal cord motion is imperfect; determination of the precise underlying cause may require additional examinations such as palpation and passive displacement at *operative* laryngoscopy (see page 16).

Focal erythema over the arytenoids and posterior larynx may occur in septic cricoarytenoid arthritis, in rheumatoid arthritis, and in reactive inflammation due to gastroesophageal reflux.

The commonest space-occupying vocal cord lesion is reactive swelling resulting from overuse or abuse of the voice. This swelling occurs at the midportion of the membranous vocal cords where the impaction force is greatest. Inasmuch as the posterior one-third of the vocal cords is occupied by the arytenoid, the midmembranous point corresponds to the junction of the anterior and middle thirds of the vocal cord. Although the vocal cord lesion may appear to be unilateral, a companion (often inconspicuous) paired lesion is usually present on the contralateral cord.

The terms *nodule* and *polyp* are used interchangeably, and both describe the inflammatory reactive lesion resulting from vocal abuse. The initial changes after vocal abuse result in epithelial or stromal reaction; the former results in epithelial thickening, the latter in subepidermal swelling with or without hyperemia (due to extravasation). The *nodule*, or epithelial thickening, results from the cumulative effect of long-standing vocal abuse, whereas the polyp can occur after a single episode of voice strain. Cessation of vocal abuse is accompanied by lesion regression but, when the aggravating forces continue, the stromal swelling *polyp* progresses until the entire vocal cord becomes swollen (polypoid degeneration); the fluid component in the vocal cord swelling may become mucoid and is unlikely to regress even after voice restraint. Advanced polypoid lesions may be accompanied by reactive epithelial change of variable severity. Rarely, the epithelial change is the primary lesion and the polypoid swelling is secondary; lesions of different pathogenesis may be indistinguishable on clinical examination.

Epithelial change due to reactive or neoplastic growth can appear as a plaque-like thickening when the outer cells fail to shed, become macerated, and appear white, i.e., leukoplakia. Persistent leukoplakia requires excisional biopsy to exclude the possibility of an early neoplasm. Continued epithelial proliferation produces infiltration manifested by *stiffness*, an important clinical finding best demonstrated by stroboscopic examination or by palpation at operative endoscopy. Exophytic proliferation or endophytic infiltration interferes with precise vocal cord apposition and produces hoarseness. Deeper infiltration into the vocalis muscle upstages a T_1 to T_3 cancer with important prognostic and therapeutic consequences. The degree of vocal cord infiltration is detected by an increase in vocal cord mass, the extent of vocal cord fixation, or stiffness on stroboscopic examination. Other features, such as disturbance of supraglottic or subglottic symmetry, arytenoid fixation, and expansion of the medial wall of the piriform sinus, are observations needing confirmation by appropriate radiographic studies *prior to* endoscopic instrumentation so that accurate assessment of the extent of the lesion can be made.

Among the specific benign lesions, the *papilloma* has a characteristic multibosselated appearance with a central vascular tuft in each nodule; papilloma lesions tend to be multiple but can be solitary and in this form may be indistinguishable from a squamous cell carcinoma.

Granular cell myoblastoma is usually single and exophytic and is located in the posterior larynx; its surface resembles peau d'orange.

The *contact granuloma* (or less frequently, *ulcer*) occurs on the medial facette or vocal process of the arytenoid. It may be alarmingly large but rarely causes hoarseness. Not infrequently, the presenting symptom is referred ear pain. The combination of otalgia and a posterior glottic lesion without hoarseness has a high probability of being a contact granuloma. The contralateral cord may have a companion saucerized deformity, and, together with the granuloma nodule, it forms the characteristic "cup-and-saucer" deformity.

Laryngeal asymmetry may be due to a swelling, such as a subepithelial cyst or tumor, or to atrophy. Accentuation of the fine reticulated vascular pattern or a granular texture indicates zones of irritation; sites exhibiting these features are described as *erythroplakic*. A focal zone of thickened whiteness is termed *leukoplakia*. Coexisting erythroplakia and leukoplakia are regarded as suspicious for epithelial dysmaturation and possible neoplasia.

The lymphoepithelial tissues in the base of the tongue may be conspicuously prominent in otherwise asymptomatic individuals. Sites of localized erythema or abnormal vessel pattern should be examined by digital and bimanual palpation for possible infection or neoplasia.

Optimal visualization of the vallecula is achieved during inspiratory effort. Vallecular landmarks include the median glossoepiglottic fold and the lateral pharyngoepiglottic folds; the latter demarcates the tongue base from the upper limits of the piriform sinus. The piriform sinuses are best visualized during a forced inspiratory phonation effort; the medial and lateral walls as well as the piriform sinus apex should be identified.

Pooled secretions in the vallecula, piriform sinuses, or the distal hypopharynx indicate imperfect swallowing performance due to obstruction or impaired muscle action. Pooled secretions are frequently present in odynophagia due to inflammatory, traumatic, or neoplastic disorders. Foamy secretions indicate imperfect swallowing due to a distal obstructive lesion. Cricovertebral crepitus is present normally and is absent when soft tissue swelling separates the cricoid lamina from the vertebral bodies.

Pearls and Pitfalls

With rare exception, mirror laryngoscopy is practical in patients as young as 3 years of age. When local anesthesia is necessary, topical lidocaine by spray or by application with a cotton-soaked pledget to the base of the uvula is used. Alternatively, sips of several milliliters of 2 percent lidocaine solution will provide the desired level of hypoesthesia. Patients should be cautioned to take nothing by mouth for 1 or 2 hours following this anesthesia, so as to prevent aspiration.

When the patient indicates pain or dysfunction in specific neck positions, the mirror examination is repeated with the patient positioned to duplicate the pain or dysfunction. These maneuvers are particularly useful in patients with unilateral cord motion impairment; a stronger voice is often produced with the head turned toward the side of paralysis. In patients suspected of having a subglottic lesion, gentle external pressure to the ipsilateral subglottis facilitates visualization of this compartment.

Evaluation of cord motion impairment may be particularly difficult in some patients. The laryngeal mirror is centered on one arytenoid, and adduction (phonation) and/or abduction (inspiration) effort will lead to identification of the paretic or paralyzed vocal cord. The determination as to whether a vocal cord is restrained in its motion because of arthrodesis or synechia (web) requires direct palpation at the time of operative laryngoscopy (see Direct Laryngoscopy, later in this chapter).

The cause of unexplained cough may be clarified by use of methylene blue solution, which normally stains hypopharyngeal mucosa but spares the laryngeal vestibule. Staining of the laryngeal vestibule or frank entry of blue dye into the trachea detects penetration or aspiration as the inciter of cough.

Diagnostic Laryngoscopy

Rigid Telescopic Technique

Indications

The magnified image provided by the *rigid telescope* (70, 90, or 110 degrees) provides detailed and precise visualization of mucosal changes in the hypopharynx and larynx and permits photographic and video documentation. With experience, this technique of examination can be used routinely and only rarely requires topical anesthesia.

Examination Technique

The preliminary history and patient positioning are identical to those used in the mirror laryngoscopy examinations. The tongue is steadied in the manner identical to that used for mirror examination, and the telescope is introduced by firm pressure along the tongue dorsum until a clear image of the larynx is obtained (Fig. 1F). This examination is particularly suitable for individuals with limitation of temporomandibular joint motion, which prohibits the mirror examination.

Pearls and Pitfalls

One hundred eighty degree rotation of the 90 degree telescope provides a superb panoramic view of the nasopharynx. As with the mirror examination, topical anesthesia has rarely been necessary. The telescopic examination has been equally applicable in pediatric patients (as young as 3 years of age).

Plate 3
Figure 1 (Continued)
Rigid Telescopic Technique

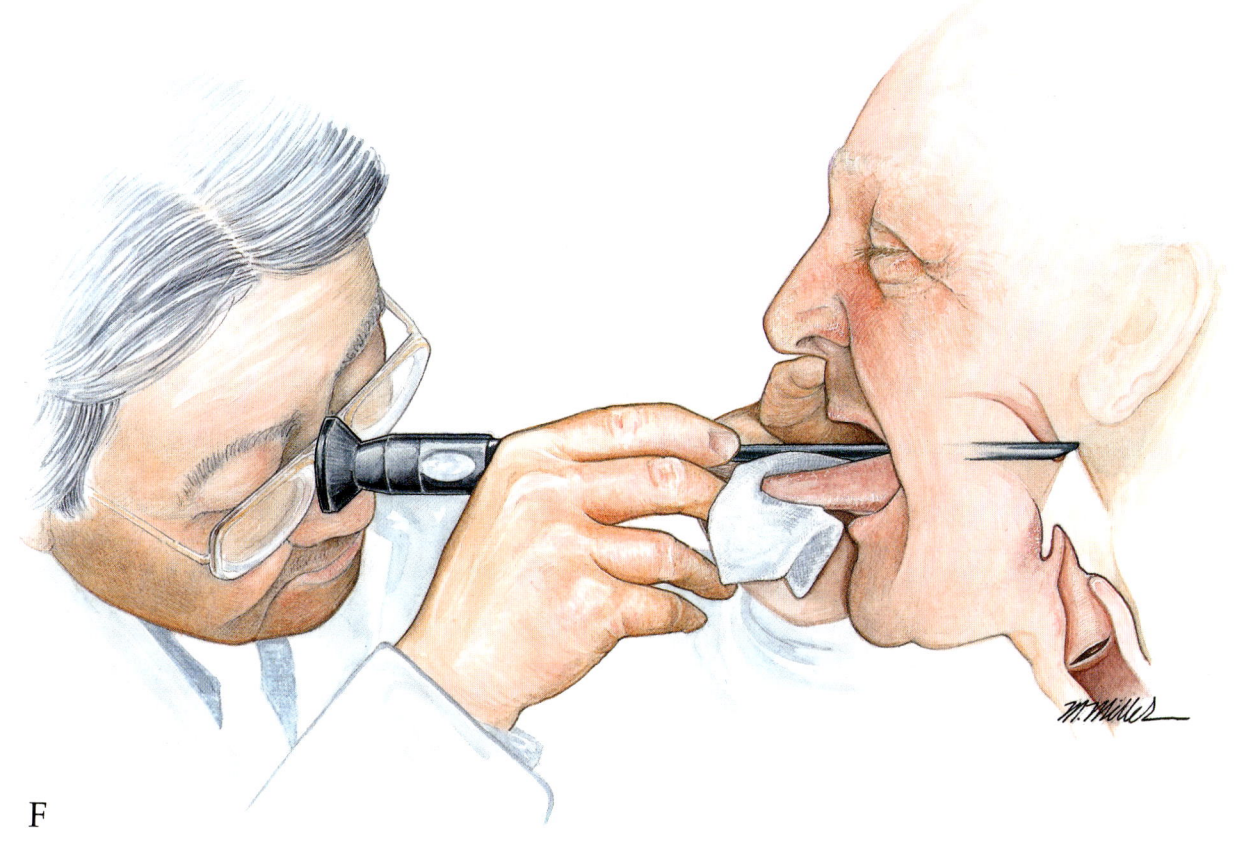

F

Fiberoptic Laryngoscopic Examination

Indications

The indications for this examination are the same as for the mirror and telescopic examinations. The fiberoptic technique is used in patients who are unsuitable for mirror or rigid telescopic examination, and it is especially useful in patients in whom laryngeal evaluation during swallowing is desirable or in bedridden patients. It is particularly indicated in the office evaluation of patients with upper airway obstruction in that comprehensive tracheal and bronchoscopic examination can be performed at a single sitting.

Technique of Examination

The preliminary evaluation should include anterior rhinoscopy, preferably by telescope, to determine a preferred side of instrument passage on the basis of nasal patency. A topical decongestant such as phenylephrine hydrochloride (Neo-Synephrine) is applied first, followed by a topical anesthetic solution (lidocaine or cocaine). When close-up views of the anterior larynx are desirable, the laryngeal vestibule is additionally anesthetized by spray or by direct placement of the solution.

The fiberoptic laryngoscope is passed through the nose and positioned just above the epiglottis or into the laryngeal vestibule, as necessary. Direction of the fiberoptic instrument tip is controlled by the thumb to achieve optimal viewing of specific laryngeal parts (Fig. 1G). The fiberoptic laryngoscope (or bronchoscope) can be passed through an indwelling endotracheal tube to evaluate the laryngotracheal region prior to extubation after prolonged intubation. In these instances, safe and atraumatic reintubation is achieved by advancing the endotracheal tube over the fiberscope when extubation is not possible.

As with the telescopic examination, fiberoptic laryngoscopy is well suited for still photographic or video recording. The image size is smaller than that obtained by mirror examination and considerably smaller than that obtained by rigid telescopic examination.

Pearls and Pitfalls

The fiberoptic laryngoscopic examination is particularly well suited to the examination of bedridden, comatose, or intubated patients. The instrument can be taken to the patient's bedside and the examination performed in the manner previously described, with the exception that the patient is usually recumbent. In patients who are unable to clear throat secretions, a suction catheter placed in the hypopharynx is helpful to remove the accumulated secretions so that a satisfactory view of the larynx can be obtained. In intubated patients, the fiberoptic laryngoscope can be placed through the endotracheal tube, which is withdrawn so that a view of the larynx can be obtained to evaluate for cord motion or inflammatory reactive changes attributable to intubation or pre-existing injury or disease. The fiberoptic laryngoscope can be reintroduced into the trachea and the endotracheal tube advanced to restore an adequate airway safely and atraumatically.

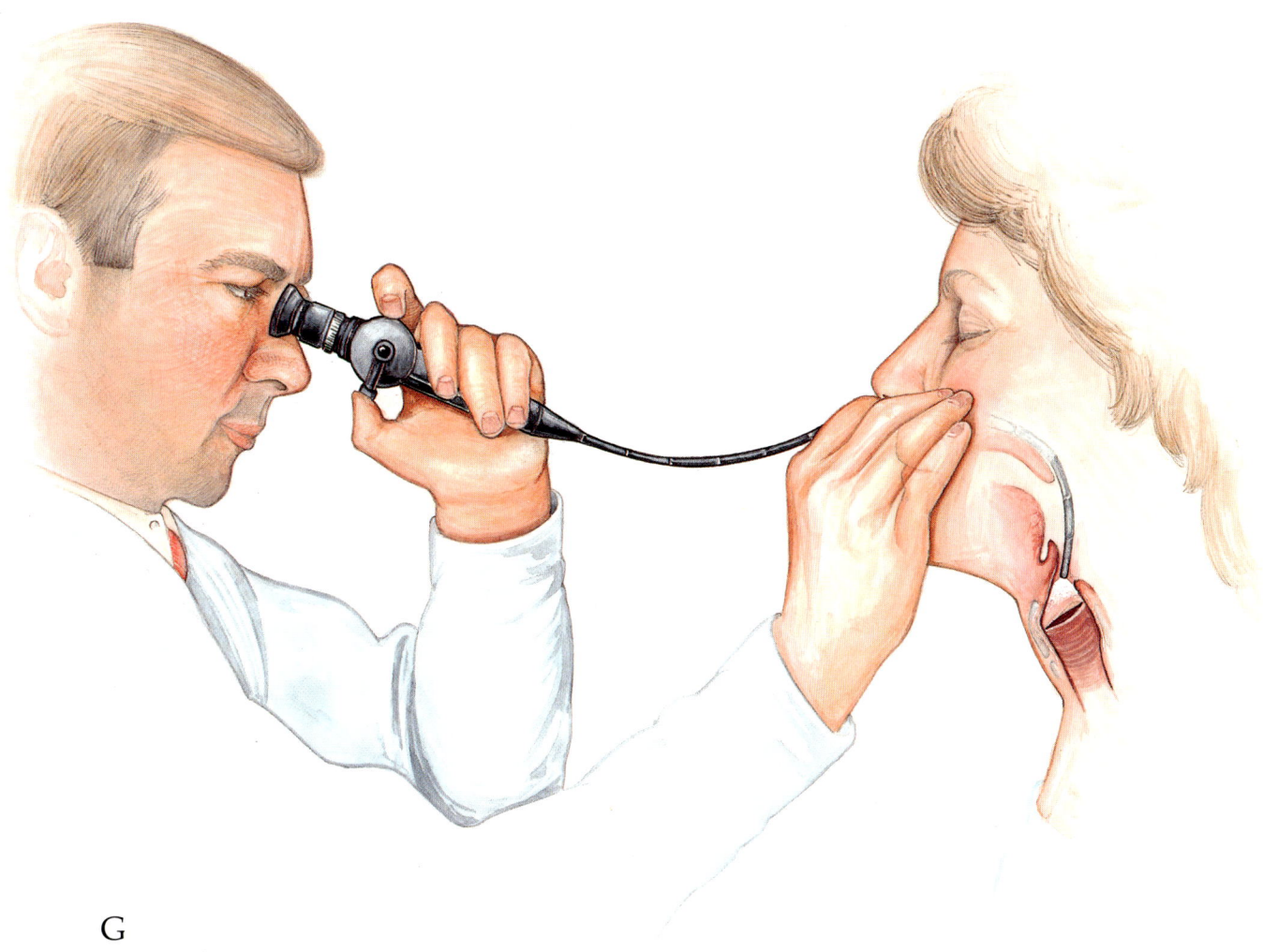

G
Figure 1 (Continued)
Fiberoptic Laryngoscopic Examination

Retrograde Tracheoscopic Examination

Indications

This examination is used in patients who have a tracheostomy. It visualizes the subglottic larynx and cervical trachea, proximal and distal to the tracheostome. Questions of cord motion impairment, subglottic web, and space-occupying lesions such as inflammatory reactive lesions (granuloma, tumor) are evaluated by this technique. When cord motion cannot be evaluated by the peroral and fiberoptic techniques, retrograde tracheoscopy is a useful alternative. Moreover, subglottic synechiae and webs cannot be visualized by any other technique.

The tracheoscopic examination is particularly useful in patients with blunt (external) trauma, postintubation sequelae, and subglottic and primary tracheal tumors.

Technique of Examination

Anesthetic solution is introduced through the indwelling tracheotomy tube and the anesthetic is dispersed through the trachea and accessible larynx by the patient's coughing against the occluded tracheotomy tube. The tracheotomy tube is removed, and a small 90-degree telescope is inserted to visualize the subglottic larynx and cervical trachea (Fig. 1H). The vocal cord motion, its range of excursion, and the presence of webs or other restricting scars, granulomas, or tumors and of extra- or transmural masses causing displacement of the tracheal wall can be evaluated as to location, severity, and nature of the lesion.

Examination of the distal trachea is performed to evaluate changes resulting from the indwelling tracheotomy tube (granuloma or stenosis).

Plate 5

H

Undersurface of vocal cord

Cricoid

Figure 1 (Continued)
Retrograde Tracheoscopic Examination

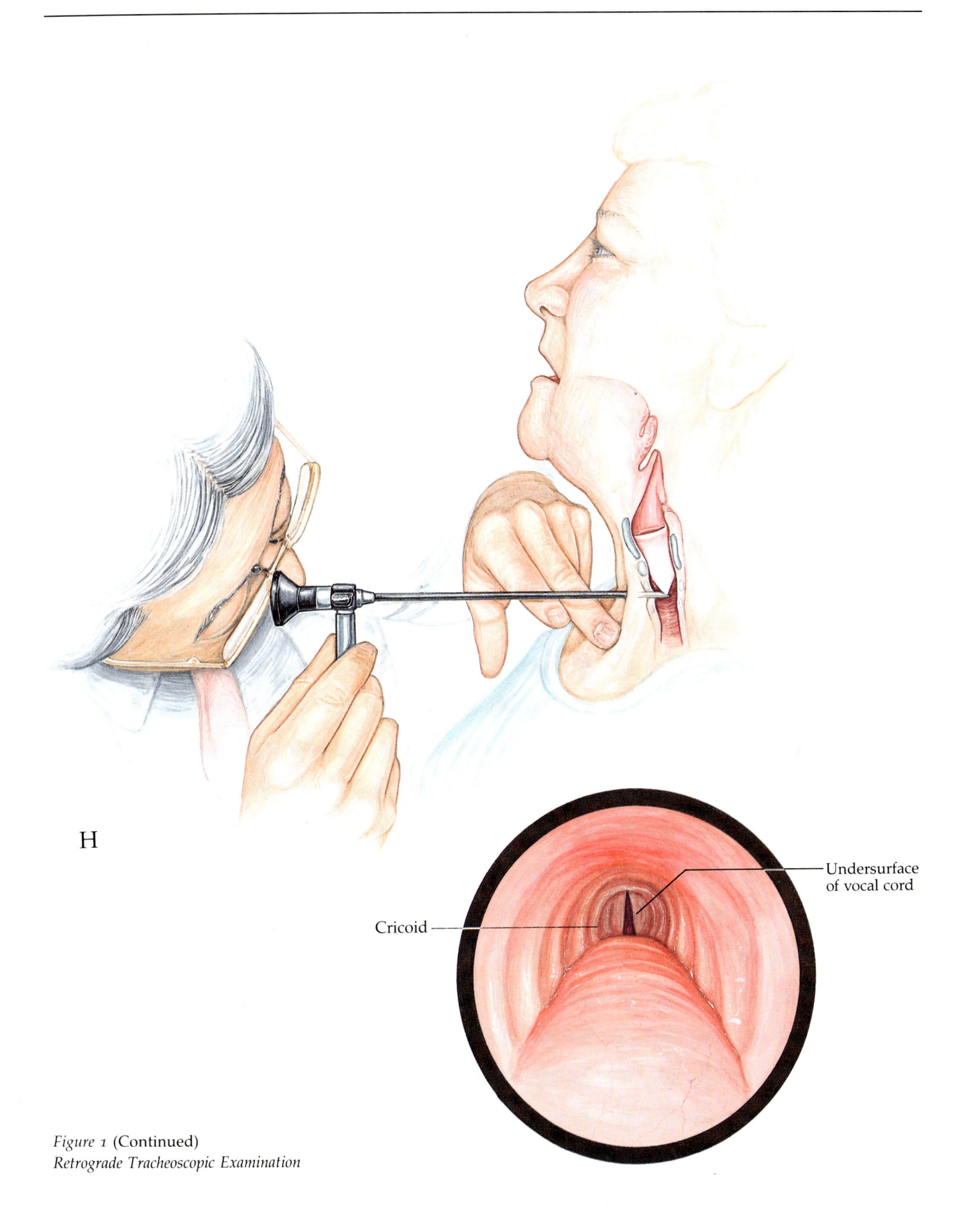

13

Haskins K. Kashima, M.D.

OPERATIVE LARYNGOSCOPY

Indications

This examination should be preceded by mirror, telescopic, or fiberoptic laryngoscopy in order to identify unresolved questions to be clarified by operative laryngoscopy. Operative laryngoscopy is performed for diagnostic and/or therapeutic purposes; it can be carried out under topical or general anesthesia suitable for examination under microscopic magnification, instrumentation, and biopsy for histologic examination.

Diagnostic laryngoscopy clarifies uncertainties regarding impaired vocal cord motion, whether due to paralysis, cricoarytenoid arthrodesis, or synechial or interstitial induration. Unresolved issues such as paraglottic and subglottic extension of tumor are precisely evaluated by operative endoscopic examination and documented by precise biopsy.

Preoperative Considerations

Preoperative preparations include the patient history and preliminary evaluation by mirror, telescopic, or fiberoptic examination. In instances of suspected tumor, appropriate radiographic studies such as soft tissue examination, contrast laryngography, computed tomography, or magnetic resonance imaging scans are obtained in the proper orientation. The patient should be given nothing by mouth for a minimum of 6 hours prior to elective examinations so that the risks of regurgitation and possible aspiration can be eliminated or minimized. Appropriate sedation and, when indicated, anticholinergics are administered to suppress oropharyngeal secretions.

Operative Steps

The patient is positioned on the operating table with an adjustable-head platform so that the C7 to T1 intervertebral space rests at the junction of the head platform; this assures maximal mobility for optimal surgical exposure.

The initial view of the larynx should be obtained prior to intubation whenever feasible. Placement of the endotracheal tube obscures the posterior glottis, and exophytic growths and fragile mucosa are at risk of detachment or injury at the time of intubation.

After the patient is adequately oxygenated and the level of anesthesia is suitable for the instrumentation achieved, the laryngoscope is inserted and positioned. The left middle finger is placed against the patient's palate, with the upper teeth and upper lips protected by a moistened gauze or tooth protector; the left index finger is placed in the mandibular gingivobuccal sulcus to protect the lower lip, and the laryngoscope is introduced over the tongue dorsum (Fig. 2A). Introduction of the laryngoscope at the (right) commissure and along the lateral tongue avoids undue pressure to the bulky body and base of tongue (Fig. 2B). The posterior pharyngeal wall is visualized, and the patient's head is extended on the neck until the tip of the epiglottis is visualized (Fig. 2C). The epiglottis is elevated with the tip of the laryngoscope until the arytenoids are seen. The neck is flexed on the chest and the laryngoscope advanced until the level of the vocal cords is reached; then the head is extended still farther on the neck until a clear view of the anterior commissure and of the entire glottis is achieved. During this maneuver, the thumb elevates the shaft of the laryngoscope so that excessive pressure on the upper teeth and lips is avoided.

Plate 6

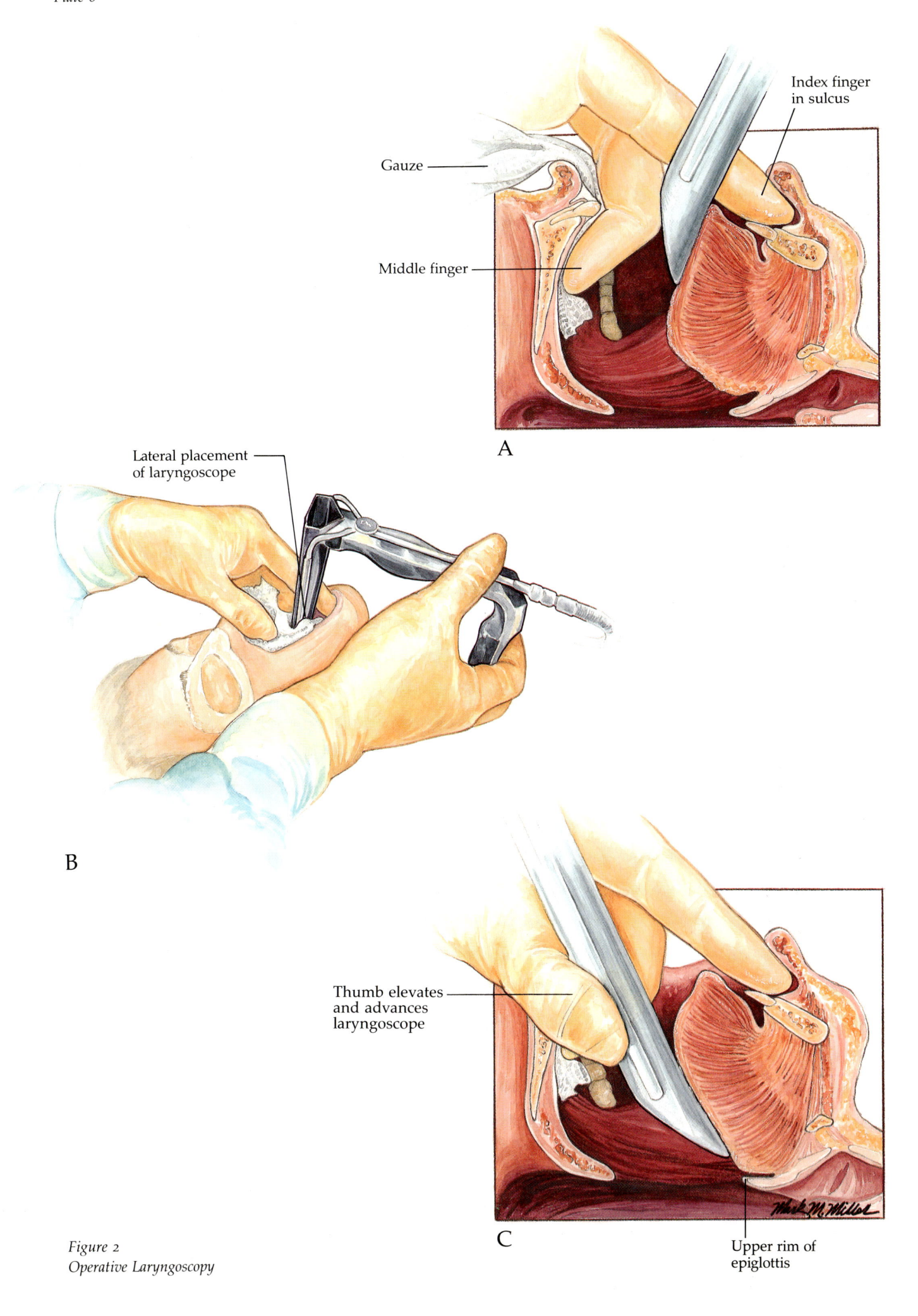

Gauze

Index finger in sulcus

Middle finger

A

Lateral placement of laryngoscope

B

Thumb elevates and advances laryngoscope

Upper rim of epiglottis

C

Figure 2
Operative Laryngoscopy

When satisfactory exposure of the larynx has been achieved, the laryngoscope is stabilized using a Lewy or similar suspension apparatus. The latter is on a platform previously mounted to the operating table with a vertical adjustment that prohibits interference with chest excursion during respiration (Fig. 2D; see also Fig. 4B).

Oxygenation and anesthesia are maintained utilizing either jet ventilation or the apnea technique. Under the apnea technique, the endotracheal tube is passed through the lumen of the operating laryngoscope during oxygenation and withdrawn during the surgical phase so that unimpeded visual and instrumental access is possible. The blood oxygen saturation levels and end-expiratory CO_2 levels are closely monitored so that a safe and smooth level of anesthesia can be maintained. Oxygen saturation levels in the mid-90s and CO_2 levels of less than 50 can be maintained by alternating 2- to 3-minute intervals of operating and oxygenation.

When evaluating vocal cord motion disorders, the cords are palpated to determine the presence or absence of interstitial induration or fibrosis and arytenoid fixation due to arthrodesis, synechial bands, or webs. Lateral pressure against the vocal process or body of the arytenoid is the test maneuver and is performed after withdrawal of the endotracheal tube.

Plate 7

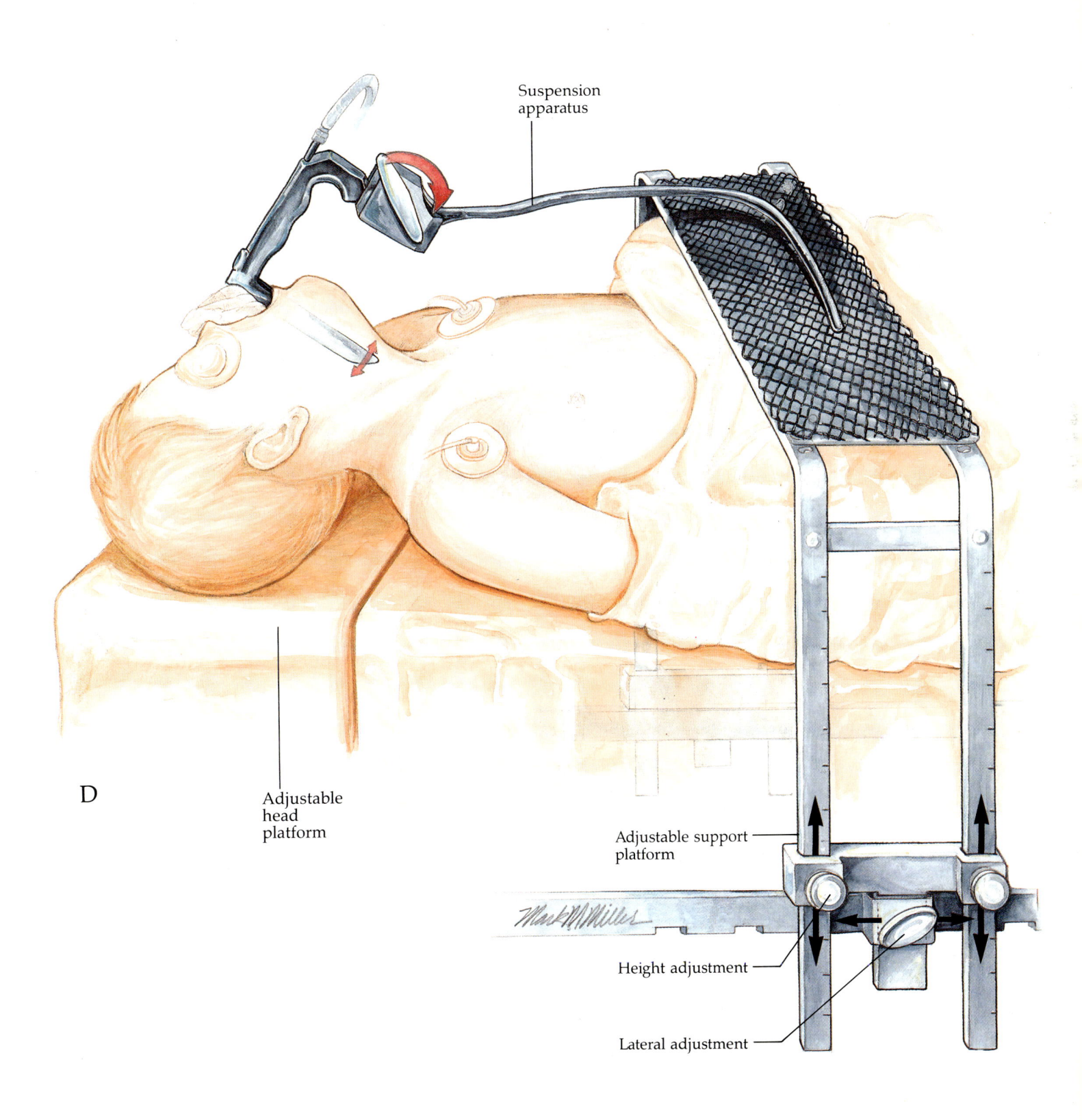

D

Figure 2 (Continued)
Operative Laryngoscopy; Suspension Apparatus

External pressure applied to the lower border of the cricoid produces unimpeded visualization of the subglottic larynx laterally and anteriorly ("the third hand technique") (Fig. 2E). The posterior subglottis is evaluated by releasing the extension on the suspension apparatus, which changes the axis for line of vision so that the anterior face of the cricoid lamina is viewed en face (Fig. 2F).

The upper surface of the true cords and the lateral extent of the floor of the ventricle are evaluated by rotation and displacement of the larynx using external pressure or by rotating the laryngoscope toward the ventricle under examination. Alternatively, 30- and 90-degree telescopes are utilized to evaluate the ventricular recess and subglottis and a 0-degree telescope is introduced through the laryngoscope to inspect the trachea as far as the level of the carina and main stem bronchi.

The remainder of the hypopharyngeal examination is completed after intubation of the larynx; the lateral and medial walls of the piriform sinuses, the pharyngoepiglottic fold, and the piriform sinus apex as well as the base of the tongue and the vallecula are evaluated.

Pearls and Pitfalls— Biopsies at Laryngoscopies

Each biopsy should be decisive for histologic diagnosis, clinical staging, and therapeutic planning. As a rule, biopsies are obtained *after completion of the preliminary inspection*; distal lesions are biopsied first so that obscuration by blood is avoided. Biopsies from the paraglottic tissues are decisively important in cancer and infiltrative disorders. These biopsies are accurately obtained through a laser incision along the aryepiglottic fold, laryngeal vestibule, or floor of the ventricle in order to access the supraglottic, glottic, and subglottic compartments.

A separate forceps is used for each specimen so that tissue fragments remaining from a prior biopsy will not introduce any uncertainty in histologic interpretation.

Figure 2 (Continued)
Operative Laryngoscopy; "Third Hand Technique"

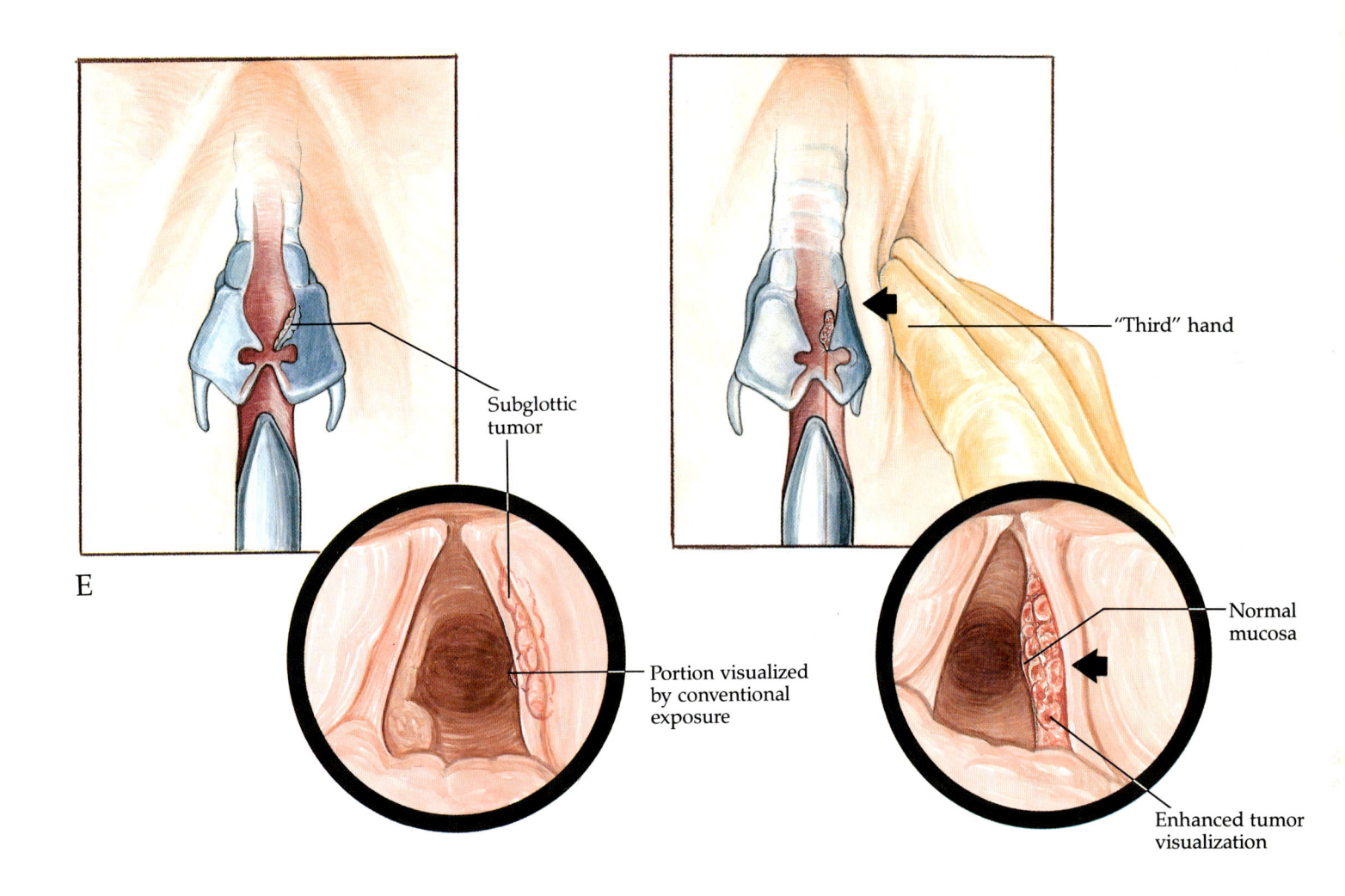

Plate 8

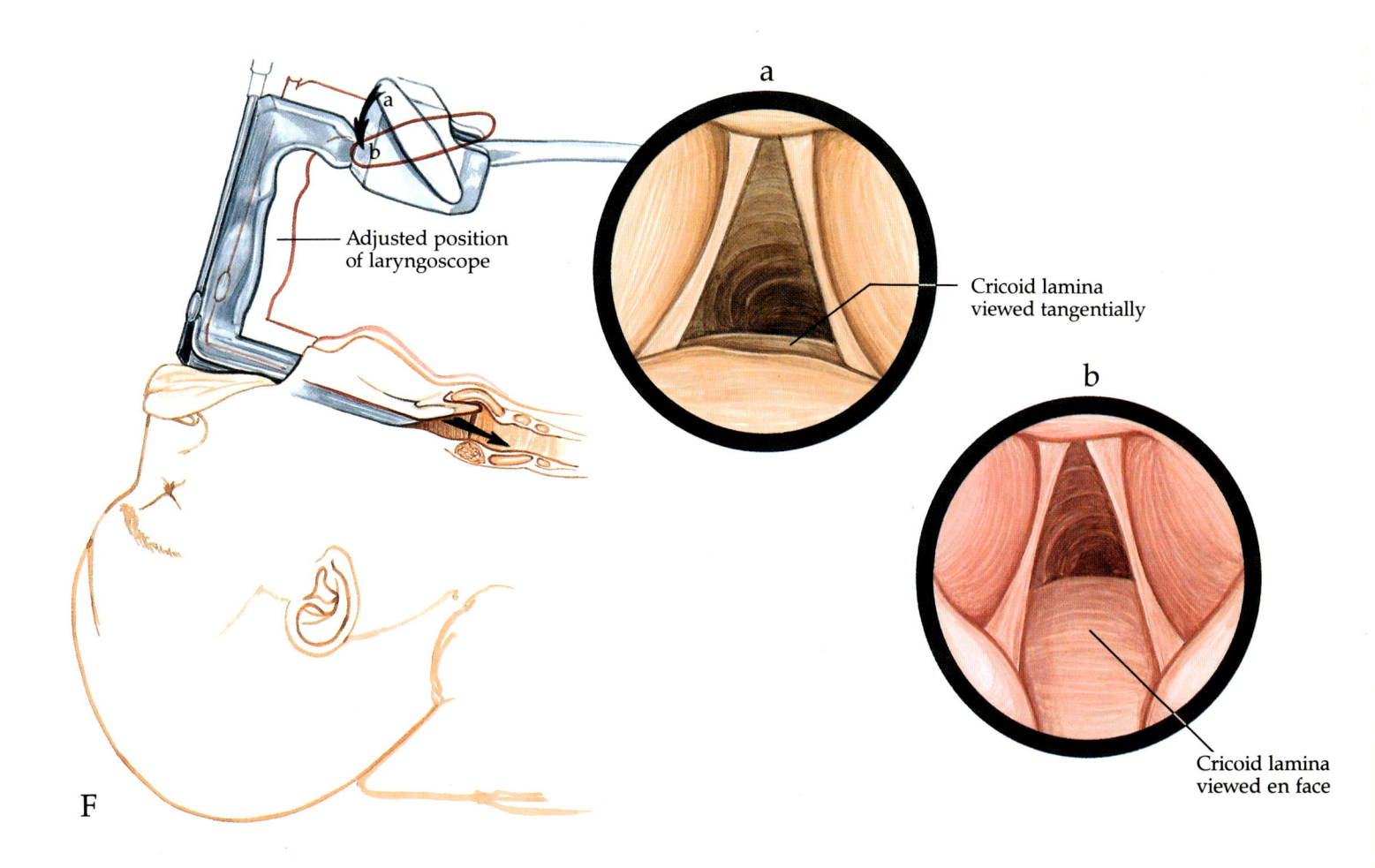

E — Subglottic tumor / Portion visualized by conventional exposure

"Third" hand / Normal mucosa / Enhanced tumor visualization

F — Adjusted position of laryngoscope

a — Cricoid lamina viewed tangentially

b — Cricoid lamina viewed en face

Haskins K. Kashima, M.D.

CO_2 LASER EXCISION OF POLYPS, CYSTS, AND NODULES

Indications

Space-occupying lesions of the true cords are clinically manifested by hoarseness. Cystic and polypoid swellings occurring elsewhere (false cords, epiglottis, aryepiglottic folds, valleculae, median glossoepiglottic fold, or lateral pharyngoepiglottic folds) may be asymptomatic, cause a foreign body sensation, or, rarely, manifest as a swelling in the neck (pre-epiglottic cyst, external or combined ventriculocele).

The vocal cord swelling (*polyp*) is typically located in the midmembranous segment of the vocal cords. The early lesion is pink or blood-tinged and fusiform, reflecting its traumatic origin due to vocal abuse. Persistent aggravation by cough or throat clearing causes enlargement of the swelling; bilateral vocal cord swelling is not uncommon. An advanced state of swelling occupying much of the membranous segment of the true vocal cords is termed polypoid degeneration; this impressive swelling may appear to obliterate the laryngeal opening but dyspnea is rare. Air flow rate studies are usually within the normal range.

Epithelium overlying the vocal cyst, nodule, or polyp is normal on clinical and histologic examination; in long-standing cases epithelial hyperplasia and subepidermal inflammation may occur. In the habitual throat abuser, these secondary changes may assume a worrisome clinical appearance, but spontaneous rupture of a cyst or polyp is rare.

Preoperative Considerations

Inasmuch as the initiating and perpetuating cause of the polyp and/or nodule is vocal abuse, consultation and advice from a speech pathologist are essential; this voice use inventory and evaluation are integral to the therapy plan. The patient is examined jointly with the speech pathologist so that understanding of the probable causes of the voice and laryngeal dysfunction is achieved and insight is gained into the importance of reversing abusive voice and throat habits. The regression of inflammation and hyperemia during the period of counseling and rehabilitation is important in that inflammatory changes compromise the desired objective of endoscopic instrumentation. During this period of voice use rehabilitation, polypoid swellings may undergo regression and voice improvement may occur. The majority of patients presenting with benign reactive swellings can be successfully managed with voice counseling alone, without resorting to surgical instrumentation or excision.

The indications for endoscopic excision biopsy of vocal cord lesions are (1) persistence of the clinical lesion in spite of earnest voice therapy, and (2) lesions with features suggestive of neoplastic or infectious disease.

Operative Steps

Suspension microlaryngoscopy is performed according to the manner previously described (see Operative Laryngoscopy). Evaluation of the vocal cord lesions preferably is performed without encumbrance of an endotracheal tube. Topical anesthesia or general anesthesia with jet ventilation or apnea technique is utilized during examination of the laryngeal mucosa under the operating microscope at 6, 10, and 16 power magnifications. Dimensions of the polypoid swelling in anteroposterior and mediolateral dimensions are altered, depending upon the tension of the suspension technique; ideally, this tension should be minimized so that precise limits of the polypoid swelling can be accurately assessed. Palpation of the vocal cord determines the presence or absence of infiltrating or indurative change, and ballottement of the polyp establishes the limits of the lesion. The free border and undersurface of the vocal cord and lesion should be inspected prior to instrumentation to ascertain that epithelial abnormality or lesion extension is not overlooked.

The objective during polyp removal is maximal preservation of vocal cord epithelium. The CO_2 laser at 5 to 10 W setting is focused to its sharpest spot size and outlines the incision site on the upper surface of the vocal cord, close to the limits of the lesion (Figs. 3A,B). The incision

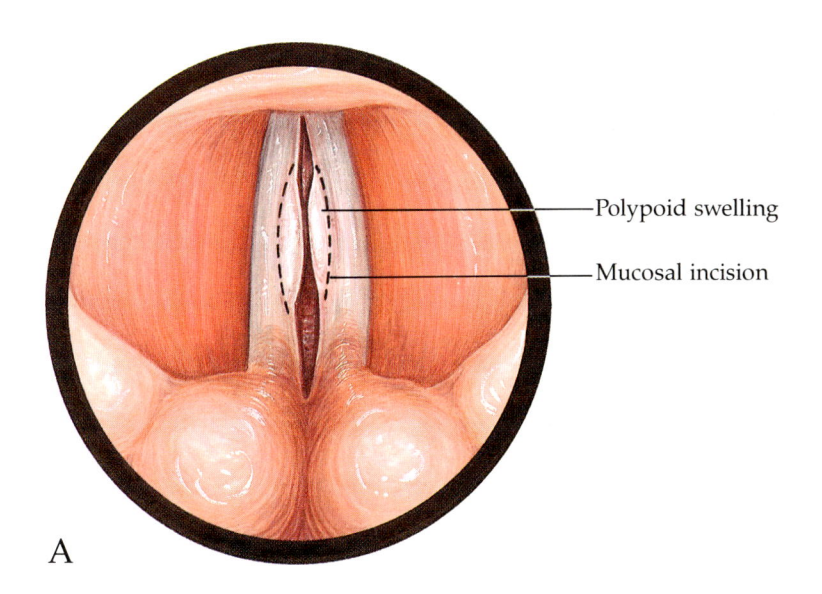

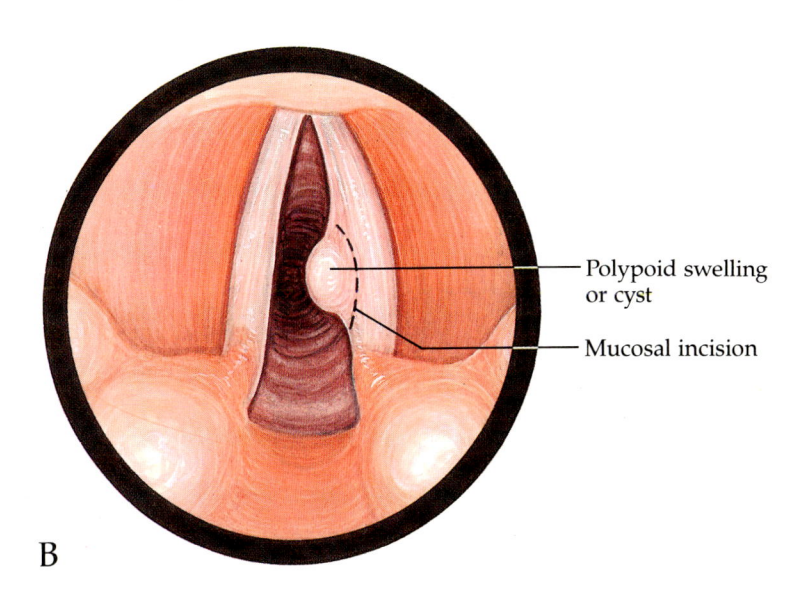

Plate 9
Figure 3
Laser Excision of Polyps, Cysts, and Nodules

is made with the laser at a power setting sufficient to coagulate the epithelium and achieve hemostasis while the cyst is exposed (Fig. 3C). When the lesion is well defined, the overlying epithelium is displaced medially by a suction tip or blunt-ended spatula of suitable size and the pearl-like lesion is enucleated. In some cases the cyst lining is ruptured, yielding an amber-colored or opalescent white fluid that is removed by aspiration (Fig. 3D). Pressure with a spatula along the free border and undersurface of the cord obliterates the swelling and approximates mucosa at the incision line; some advocate sealing the incision with the laser (Fig. 3E).

A similar technique of incision over the cyst and dissection with low-powered laser is used for lesions of the false cord, aryepiglottic fold, median glossoepiglottic and lateral pharyngoepiglottic folds, and the vallecula. Epithelial preservation is not as important as in sites away from the free border of the true cords. Cysts at these latter locations are likely to be of minor salivary gland origin, and cyst contents are more viscid. Some supraglottic cysts extend into the paraglottic or pre-epiglottic spaces. External pressure using the third hand technique delivers the lesion into the surgical field, and laser excision is achieved.

An alternative method for centrally placed lesions of the false cord is wide excision of the laryngeal vestibule; this technique of *vestibulectomy* is identical to that described elsewhere (see Vestibulectomy). When the

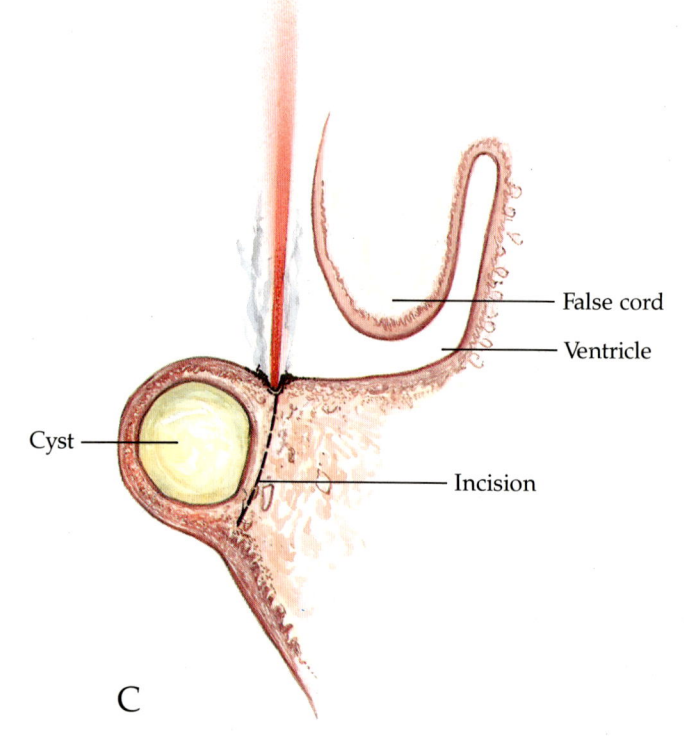

C

Plate 10
Figure 3 (Continued)
Laser Excision of Polyps, Cysts, and Nodules

Plate 11

Suction

D

Reattached epithelium

Figure 3 (Continued)
Laser Excision of Polyps, Cysts, and Nodules

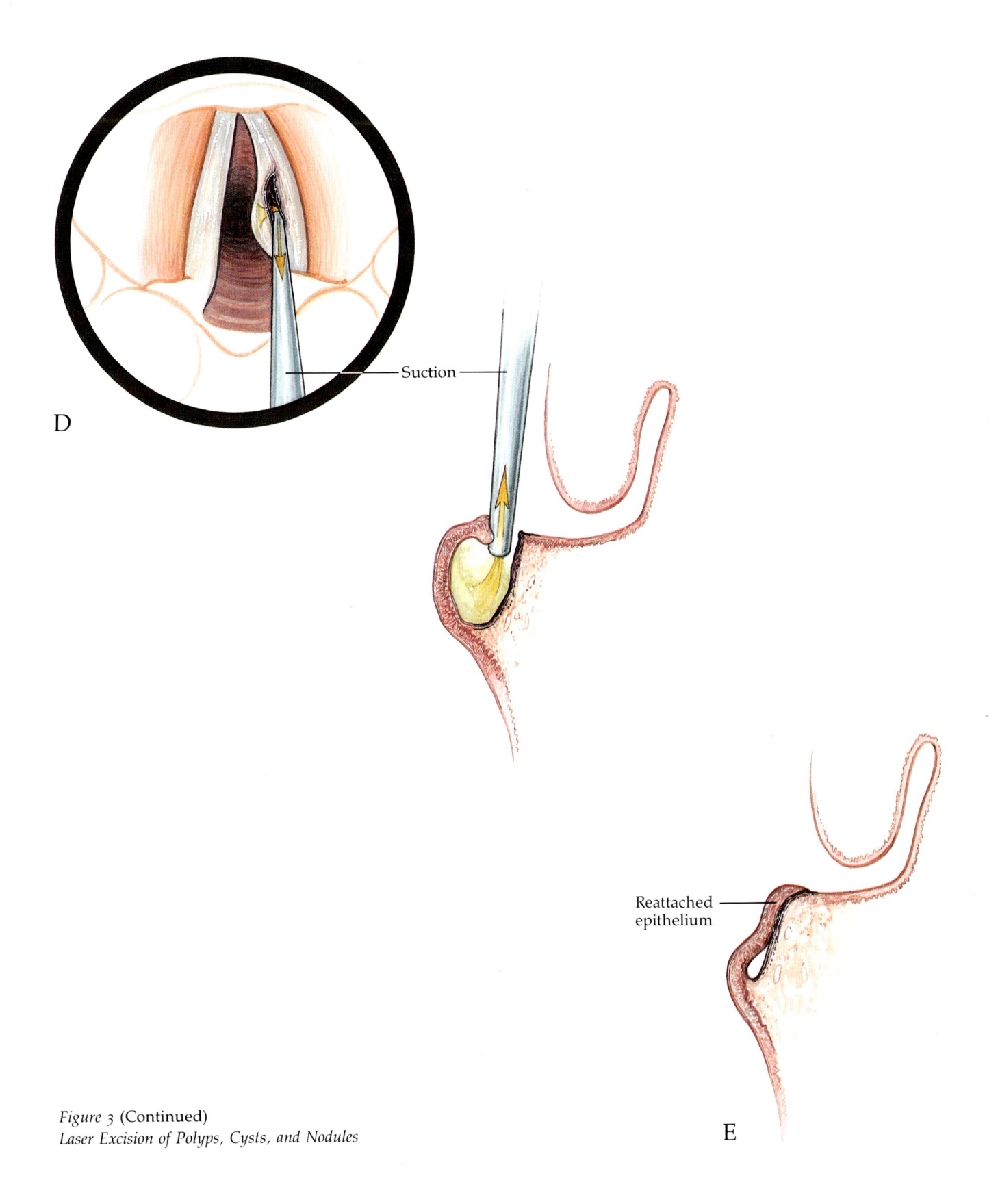

E

lesion is within or deep to the aryepiglottic fold, a laser incision along the aryepiglottic fold or perpendicular to its axis provides satisfactory exposure and access for laser excision. Deeply seated larger supraglottic lesions may be derived from glands of the laryngeal ventricle (internal ventriculocele), and total cyst excision unroofs the ventricle. These defects heal uneventfully, and the final clinical appearance is deceptively normal.

Postoperative care for excisions from the true cord requires minimal trauma from excessive, prolonged, or exaggerated voice effort. Coughing is suppressed, and habitual throat clearing is discouraged. Respiratory irritants such as tobacco smoke, gasoline fumes, and chemicals should be avoided. Essential voice use in quiet ambient settings is permitted. Ideally, the patient is seen at a joint appointment with the speech therapist to monitor the postoperative course and offer counseling.

Complications

An unfortunate outcome from endoscopic excision of benign true cord lesions is worsening of voice quality. This is usually due to *excessive* excision of vocal cord epithelium or stroma or functional dysphonia in an apprehensive patient.

Vocal cord "stripping" is the technique wherein the polyp and overlying epithelium are removed from the free border of the cord in a single motion. Although immediate inspection reveals an impressively sharp free border of vocal cord, unexpected excessive tissue removal results in dysphonia due to imperfect apposition of the vocal cords.

Pearls and Pitfalls

Risk of excessive removal of tissue is equal with the CO_2 laser and other microsurgical techniques. Wherever possible, the epithelium is preserved unless it is clinically diseased. Redundant mucosa will redrape over underlying muscle or can be secondarily excised. After removal of the lesion, it is useful to release the tension of the suspension apparatus and to palpate the cord, examining for residual mucosal tags that may become the nidus of a new polyp. Overzealous removal is exceedingly difficult to correct; it is preferable to re-excise redundant tissue at a later operation.

All of the foregoing complications and undesirable outcomes are more likely to occur when the lesion is instrumented while it is actively inflamed or when the patient is unable (or unwilling) to be a partner in the postoperative care.

Lesions of the vocal cord that interfere with normal voice production are treated according to the principles of maximal epithelial preservation and excision of the subepithelial soft tissue swelling. An exception to this principle is the nodule that has undergone organization. The terms polyp, cyst, and nodule indicate progression from edematous polyp to a circumscribed cyst and finally to an organized nodule. The well-formed nodule may be alternatively treated by exposing the free border en face and vaporizing only the epithelial thickening, using a sharply focused laser. The technique of laser "shaving" of an imperfectly exposed nodule carries risks of excessive tissue ablation and permanent voice impairment.

Haskins K. Kashima, M.D.

CO₂ LASER EXCISION OF BENIGN LESIONS

Recurrent Respiratory Papillomatosis

Recurrent respiratory papillomatosis (RRP) defines a subset of disorder of histologically benign growths occurring in the upper aerodigestive tract. Papillomas commonly occur in the oral cavity and larynx but also in the nose, nasopharynx, tracheobronchial tree, and rarely in the lung. The laryngeal lesion is recognized as the commonest neoplasm in children (juvenile onset RRP). A histologically identical lesion occurs in adults (adult onset RRP).

Endoscopic excision is the conventional standard treatment. Papilloma regrowth and recurrence, frequently with disease extension to previously normal epithelium, creates a major dilemma for both the patient and the physician.

Human papillomavirus types 6 and 11 are recognized as the etiologic agents. The same virus types are associated with genital warts (condyloma acuminatum). The epidemiology and transmission of human papillomavirus disorders are under intensive study, but effective control of the papillomatous growths remains an unsolved problem.

Meticulous excision of all detectable papillomas is the goal of endoscopic operations. In spite of thorough microsurgical excision utilizing the CO_2 laser, papilloma regrowth frequently occurs at the precise site from which it had been previously removed. Viral DNA has been demonstrated in clinically normal epithelium, and papilloma regrowth or "reseeding" is attributed to virus present.

One concept of respiratory papillomatosis is that the widespread presence of human papillomavirus in the respiratory tract epithelium serves as the reservoir of infection. The strategy for surgical management is removal of exophytic lesions that cause hoarseness, airway obstruction, or other symptoms. It is generally recognized that the total elimination of the infectious viral agent requires systemic treatment with antiviral or antiproliferative agents or intervention in the host immunoregulatory system, producing a "spontaneous regression."

The rarity of occurrence of respiratory papillomatosis has prohibited determination of the proportion of cases that yield to a single or limited number of endoscopic excisions. Experience in management of a large number of cases occurs at medical centers where the most difficult cases are referred. Although aggressive expression of disease may occur in only a small proportion of papillomatosis cases, the principles of treatment and surgical technique are uniformly applicable to all cases.

Principles of Treatment

ATRAUMATIC TECHNIQUE
All instrumentation from intubation, laryngoscopic exposure, excision of lesions, or use of suction is performed with utmost care to avoid inadvertent dislodging of potentially infectious lesions or viruses and causing unintentional mucosal injury, introducing a potential site for papilloma seeding.

HISTOLOGIC CONFIRMATION
The typical papilloma is multilobulated and exophytic. The surface may be pink and glistening or may be finely fuzzy and white (see Fig. 4C). The large lesion often arises from a narrow base, causing the growth to

have excessive mobility, leading to exaggerated breathing effort and thereby causing stridor. When it is solitary, a broad sessile pattern of growth can be mistaken for a benign polyp or reactive swelling. When they are examined under 16-power magnification, virtually all lesions exhibit a pinpoint pink or blue discoloration due to subepithelial capillary tufts. Representative lesions are biopsied to verify histopathology and to establish the precise extent of disease.

PRINCIPLES AND TECHNIQUE OF LASER VAPORIZATION OF PAPILLOMA
The CO_2 laser is used at 5 to 10 W at 0.1 or 0.2 sec in an interrupted or pulsed mode. Rarely is the laser used in a continuous mode. The laser vaporizes residual papilloma after prior forceps removal of the exophytic portions, achieves hemostasis, and treats the lesion base. Neither clinical papilloma nor viral presence has been demonstrated in subepithelial tissues, and therefore laser application is not directed to these tissues, thereby minimizing thermal injury and resultant scarring.

The technique of laser excision of papilloma consists of forceps removal of the exophytic portions and the laser vaporization of minimal residual disease. Hence, large exophytic lesions are almost always debulked with standard cup forceps technique initially, and laser is reserved for the treatment of the stalk or base. The sessile growths, particularly those on the anterior membranous segment at or close to the anterior commissure and overlying the arytenoid or epiglottis, are ill suited for forceps removal and are treated entirely with the laser. In the latter circumstances the exposure is optimized so that the aiming beam can be focused en face (rather than tangentially), and the lesion center is treated with low wattage. This causes a shallow crater, and the lesion is caused to involute in a manner that reverses the growth sequence (see Fig. 4F).

Operative Steps

Safe anesthesia induction requires carefully planned coordination on the part of the anesthesiologist and the surgeon. Proper oxygenation is achieved by mask, and relaxant is administered. Exposure by suspension laryngoscopy prior to intubation permits global assessment of disease extent in the larynx and subglottis. Tracheal lesions are assessed by a narrow-caliber operating telescope. Initial intubation is performed by the surgeon through the operating laryngoscope, taking particular care not to dislodge exophytic growths. Rarely, obstructing papilloma may require removal prior to intubation so that unintentional dislodgment of papillomatous growths can be avoided. The preferred endotracheal tube for laser operations of the larynx is a red rubber endotracheal tube that is protectively wrapped with an adhesive aluminum tape (Fig. 4A). The rubber tube is least likely to be ignited by laser impaction, and the aluminum tape diffusely reflects an errant laser beam impaction. A moistened fenestrated towel is draped over the operative field, exposing only the laryngoscope (Fig. 4B). This towel is periodically moistened to absorb any unintentional laser impaction.

The laryngeal papillomas are treated from the vocal cords, ventricles, false cords, and epiglottis, in the order named (Fig. 4C). Exophytic papillomas are debulked with cup forceps (Fig. 4D), and hemostasis is achieved

Plate 12

A — Red rubber endotracheal tube (Rusch)
Aluminized protective tape

B — "Third" hand

C — Laryngeal papilloma

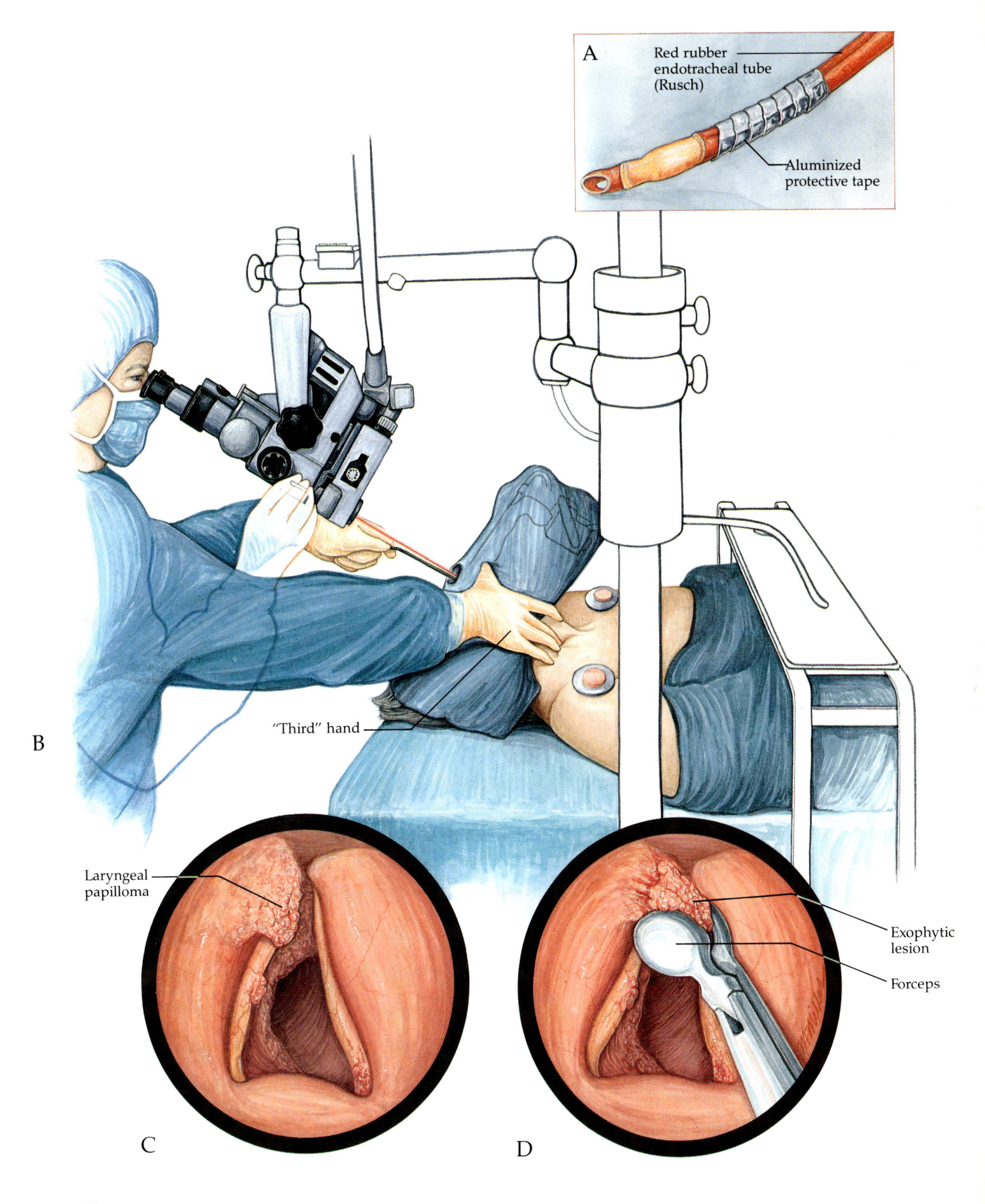

D — Exophytic lesion
Forceps

Figure 4
Laser Therapy of Recurrent Respiratory Papillomatosis

with the application of vasoconstrictive solutions or laser. Optimal exposure of lesions in the ventricle is achieved by applying external pressure to the neck (so-called third hand technique) (see Fig. 4B and Operative Laryngoscopy, Figs. 2F and H) to incline the larynx and bring the lesion into the preferred position for forceps removal or CO_2 laser application. Lesions of the supraglottic larynx are exposed by withdrawing the laryngoscope and applying external pressure to the neck, as needed. Lesions of the epiglottis can be optimally exposed by applying direct pressure posteriorly from the anterior midline of the neck. Papillomas are rarely present on the lingual surface of the epiglottis.

Lesion ablation is achieved by microsurgical instrumentation (cup forceps) and CO_2 laser. Cup forceps removal permits securing a tissue specimen for histologic and other diagnostic studies and also serves to debulk the tumor. The stalk or base of the lesion is treated with a finely focused laser at 5 to 10 W, using interrupted bursts of 0.1 to 0.2 sec. Whenever possible, the lesions are exposed in a manner permitting en face application of the laser. Moistened cottonoid pads are packed behind the targeted lesion or around the endotracheal tube for protection against inadvertent laser injury (Fig. 4E).

Following the initial pass, the laryngoscope is reintroduced to the level of the anterior commissure and the previously operated zone is reinspected to ensure that all detectable papillomas have been excised and each lesion base has been adequately treated. The endotracheal tube obscures lesions in the posterior laryngeal aperture and commissure. Lesions at these sites can be optimally exposed by displacing the endotracheal tube anteriorly or by removal of the endotracheal tube and utilization of the apnea technique of anesthesia (Fig. 4F).

Lesions of the anterior and lateral subglottic compartment are optimally exposed by endotracheal tube removal, and optimal exposure is achieved using the third hand technique (see Fig. 2E, Operative Laryngoscopy). Lesions of the posterior subglottic compartment are best exposed by relaxing the tension of the suspension apparatus (see Fig. 2F, Operative Laryngoscopy).

Plate 13

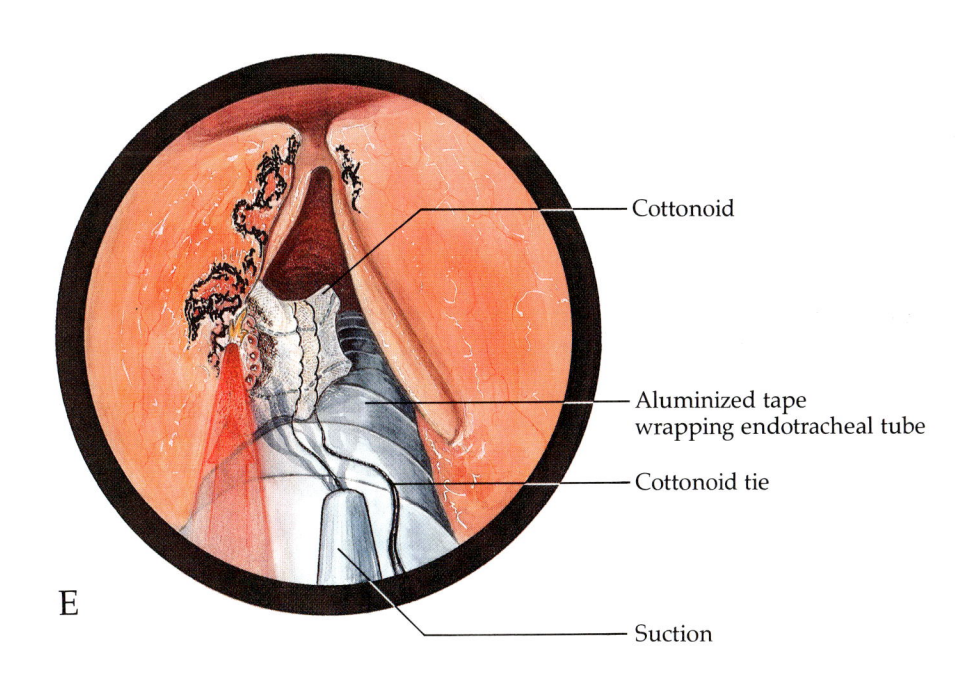

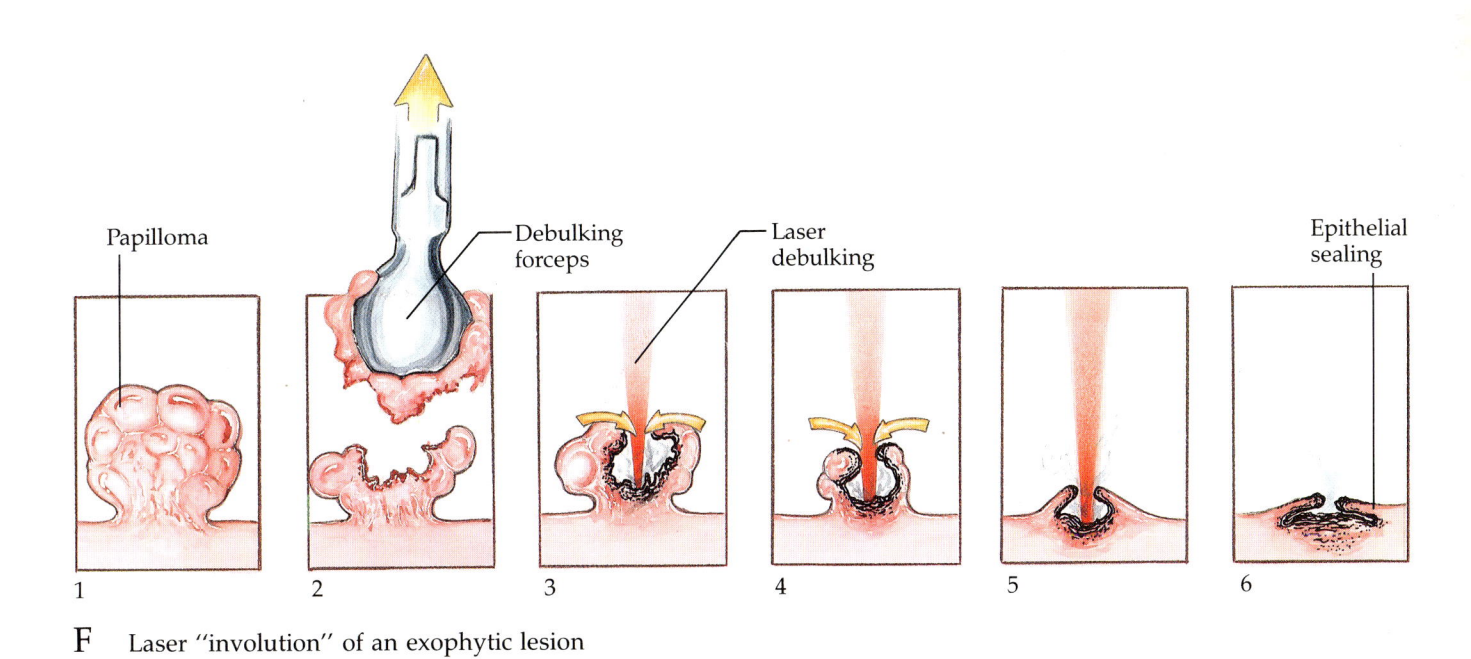

- Cottonoid
- Aluminized tape wrapping endotracheal tube
- Cottonoid tie
- Suction

E

Papilloma — Debulking forceps — Laser debulking — Epithelial sealing

1   2   3   4   5   6

F   Laser "involution" of an exophytic lesion

Figure 4 (Continued)
Laser Therapy of Recurrent Respiratory Papillomatosis

The ventilating bronchoscope is utilized for CO_2 laser excision of tracheobronchial lesions (Fig. 4G). The bronchoscopic attachments permit sharp focusing of the laser beam at variable distances. A Mylar attachment protects the reflecting surfaces within the control unit, and the vapors resulting from laser application are evacuated by the flushing system and by the flow of the anesthetic gases. The Mylar lens separating the bronchoscope from the control unit should be inspected and cleaned of any other particles. Whenever possible, the distalmost lesions are addressed first and the bronchoscope is progressively withdrawn to expose and treat the more proximal lesions (Fig. 4H). This sequence avoids the obscuring effects of bleeding from prior treatment of papillomas in the upper thoracic and cervical trachea. Whenever practical, exophytic papillomas are removed with forceps and the base of the lesions are treated with laser. The combined treatment with forceps removal and laser minimizes the thermal effect of the laser. Papillomas as far distally as the main stem bronchi can be accessed in this manner.

When papillomas are present in the tracheostomal tract, the ventilating bronchoscope is left in place. The laser is transferred to the operating microscope, and the tracheostomal tract is exposed with a nasal speculum or other suitable instrument; papillomatous growths within the stomal tract are managed in a manner identical to that described for the larynx and trachea.

In patients who have had repeated endoscopic treatment for papillomatosis, the likelihood of laryngeal webs is high. The subglottic space under the anterior glottic web may be the site of papilloma deposit. A 90-degree telescope can be passed through the glottic aperture to examine this compartment prior to dividing the web to gain access to these lesions. Similarly, the subglottic compartment underlying the posterior horizontal web should be examined for papilloma deposits with the telescope. Lesions on the upper surface of a posterior glottic web are accessible without web division, but treatment should be judicious inasmuch as vigorous application of laser predisposes to aggravation of the web, resulting in airway narrowing.

Extralaryngotracheal Sites

Following treatment of papillomas in the larynx and trachea, the endotracheal tube is reinserted and attention is directed to the oral cavity and nasopharynx. The nasopharynx is examined with a right-angled telescope with the palate retracted for optimal exposure. The placement of rubber catheters intranasally is avoided because of the potential risks of mucosal injury and papilloma seeding. The common sites of asymptomatic papilloma deposits are at the nasopharyngeal surface of the soft palate and, less commonly, along the posterior and superior walls of the nasopharynx. Lesions at these sites may be unexpectedly large and remain asymptomatic. The superior and lateral margins of the limen vestibulae are common sites where asymptomatic lesions may occur. All of the foregoing sites can be exposed and treated using direct (nasal vestibule) or reflecting polished metal platform (nasopharynx) techniques.

In summary, the surgical objective in papillomatosis is to excise papillomatous lesions causing airway obstructive symptoms or hoarseness. All normal structures are protected from intentional or unintentional injury so that full recovery of function can be assured.

Plate 14

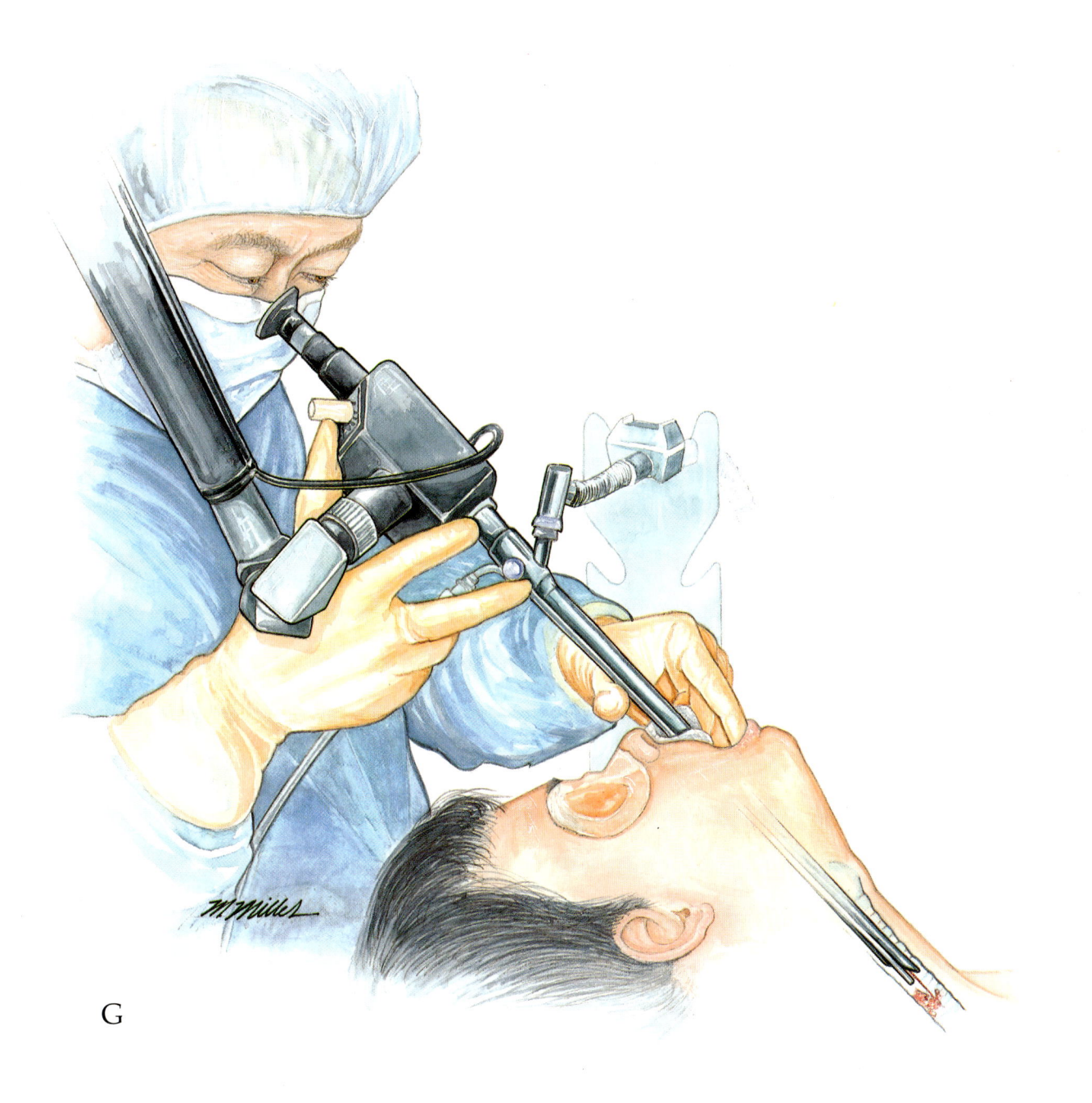

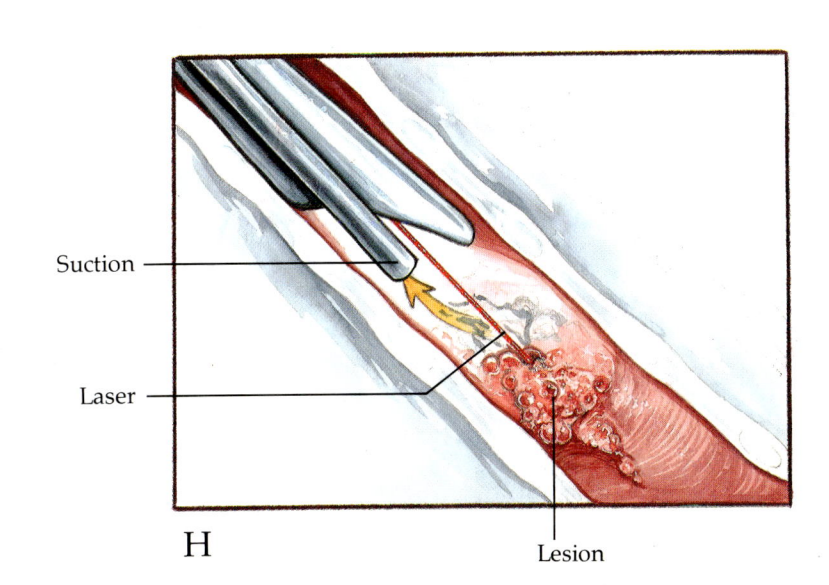

G

H

Suction

Laser

Lesion

Figure 4 (Continued)
Benign Lesions; Bronchoscopic Laser Techniques

Contact Granuloma

This lesion of typical clinical appearance and histopathology has been associated with a pattern of vocal abuse and a driving personality trait, and it is thought to be aggravated by gastroesophageal reflux or regurgitation. The lesions characteristically appear at the posterior glottis on the vocal process and medial aspect of the arytenoids. A contact or companion lesion occurs on the contralateral vocal process. Hoarseness is unusual as a symptom, and the lesion is often discovered during the course of examination for unexplained otalgia; surgical excision is successful in a small percentage of cases only. Voice therapy is crucial in the treatment and rehabilitation plan, and proper voice production patterns can cause complete disappearance of the lesions.

Persistence of the granuloma may be attributable to microtrauma to the arytenoid perichondrium and may be aggravated by surgical instrumentation. Inasmuch as CO_2 laser application results in thermal effect to the nonvaporized tissue, surgical excision of the polypoid lesion with a laryngeal sickle blade may be least traumatic to the underlying tissues at the point of granuloma origin. The residual tissue at the base of the granuloma is treated with low wattage (5 W) interrupted application with frequent swabbing to minimize heat build-up. Speech therapy is resumed postoperatively, and joint examination by the otolaryngologist and the speech therapist is important.

Surgical intervention for the typical contact granuloma or postintubation granuloma is undertaken only *after* thorough orientation of the patient to voice therapy, which is continued postoperatively. Not infrequently the granuloma reappears, indicating return to prior voice abuse patterns or failure to eliminate the presumed primary pathology in the subperichondral space.

Nonmalignant Cysts

A wide variety of cystic lesions occur in the larynx in patients of all age groups. In the newborn, cystic lesions may be related to epithelial rests, whereas in the adult cystic swelling represents obstruction in subepithelial glands and occurs on the lingual surface of the epiglottis, false cord, or ventricle. Rarely, cystic lesions may represent specific histopathologic entities such as oncocytoma, neurofibroma, or minor salivary gland neoplasms.

Nonlaser operations are largely "uncapping" procedures resulting in marsupialization that is curative in the majority of instances. Complete excision is rarely achieved, and bleeding accompanying such interventions prohibits definitive and total excision.

The CO_2 laser is well suited to the total excision of cystic lesions; maximal patience and precision are required. Low to moderate wattage (5 to 10 W) in interrupted application, coupled with optimal exposure using moistened cottonoids, is necessary. Even in large lesions, the accompanying bleeding can be controlled by laser or application of astringent solution–soaked pledgets. Rarely, more vigorous bleeding is encountered from larger terminal branches of the superior laryngeal artery, and laser application or injection with vasoconstrictive solutions may be necessary. The end result of a normal-appearing larynx with a normal voice should be the goal in treating cystic lesions.

Infiltrative Lesions

Lesions fitting this category are superficially spreading or infiltrating lesions, often associated with systemic disease such as sarcoidosis, proteinosis, amyloidosis, or related disorders. Surgical objectives are to obtain tissue for precise histopathologic diagnosis and to maximally restore or preserve laryngeal function. The advantages of the CO_2 laser are its precision and hemostatic properties, which can excise or debulk diseased tissues endoscopically and preserve essential normal structures. When the infiltrative lesion causes an obstruction, the cordotomy operation restores patency.

An uncommon lesion occurring in the newborn is the subglottic hemangioma. Although spontaneous regression usually occurs, the CO_2 laser is ideally suited to achieving hemostasis after biopsy and vaporization of the lesion. Rarely, an extensive lesion with cavernous channels may be encountered, and this should be managed by tracheotomy until spontaneous involution occurs. The equally uncommon endocricoid chondroma resembles the hemangioma and should be biopsied and can be treated with the CO_2 laser.

Pearls and Pitfalls

The CO_2 laser is an effective and unique surgical alternative in the management of laryngeal disorders. The ablation of exophytic, superficially spreading, and infiltrative disorders can each be addressed using this treatment modality. The objectives in all instances are, first, to obtain adequate and representative tissue specimens for histologic diagnosis, and second, to ablate diseased tissues adequately while preserving laryngeal anatomy and function as much as possible. Although the targeted tissue effects stem from thermal energy derived from direct laser application, two additional dimensions of residual tissue effects also occur. The first is thermal build-up in tissues in the excision bed. Injudicious application of high wattage or of prolonged (continuous) application may cause irreversible thermal injury and delayed healing and produce unwanted scarring. In the larynx and trachea, these effects translate into stenosis and web formation.

A second source of potential thermal injury derives from vapors resulting from laser vaporization. Failure to evacuate vapors may result in heat build-up and cause subclinical thermal injuries resembling inhalation injuries. Without doubt some indurated scars and webs are caused or aggravated by thermal effects from laser vapors permitted to remain at the operation site.

Haskins K. Kashima, M.D.

CO$_2$ LASER EXCISION OF MALIGNANT LESIONS

The CO$_2$ laser is ideally suited for endoscopic management of early laryngeal cancers. Under current conventional management of laryngeal cancer, the extent of disease is determined by physical examination, radiographic studies, and biopsy findings confirmed at operative endoscopy; on the basis of select critical biopsies, the appropriate management options are considered and selected.

The CO$_2$ laser has a useful role in the endoscopic staging as well as in primary and adjunctive treatment of laryngeal cancer. The following section describes utilization of the laser in each of these roles.

Laryngeal cancer occurs initially as an epithelial abnormality, either solitary or multifocal. Clinical examination discloses patchy epithelial thickening, termed leukoplakia. Leukoplakia is a descriptive term and does not specify microscopic histologic appearance. Varying degrees of disturbance in keratinization and epithelial hyperplasia with and without disturbed maturation pattern (dysplasia) may be present and are regarded as precancerous. Carcinoma in situ and microinvasive and superficially invasive cancers also present with leukoplakia. Clinical leukoplakia often is present adjacent to invasive cancer as well as at sites far removed from the dominant lesion. Moreover, subclinical epithelial dysplasia often has an unsuspected wide distribution. Visualization under magnification and utilization of topical toluidine blue or 5 percent acetic acid solution identify these lesions as well as the peripheral extent of the primary tumor or of satellite lesions.

Staging of Laryngeal Cancer

Clinical staging, according to the tumor, nodes, and metastasis (TNM) classification, is relevant to predicting the clinical course and, therefore, to deciding on a treatment modality. The precise extent of tumor invasion is determined by the clinical, radiographic, and endoscopic examinations. In addition, access to deeper subepithelial tissues is facilitated by the CO$_2$ laser, which provides bloodless exposure through mucosal incisions or tissue excisions (see Ventriculectomy). Critical biopsies from the lateral ventricle, paraglottic space, and subglottic sites can thus be obtained. The depth of tumor invasion, thus determined, has critical importance in the ultimate treatment choice.

Treatment

The dual objectives of endoscopic operation are diagnostic and therapeutic. The *diagnostic* objective is to obtain tissue samples for establishing the histopathology and extent and limits of the tumor. The *therapeutic* objective is to achieve total excision whenever possible. In lesions limited to the epithelium, endoscopic excision by conventional microsurgical technique is complemented by laser application to the excision bed, assuring total destruction of abnormal epithelium. This method of *laser decortication* is appropriate for leukoplakic lesions exhibiting atypia, carcinoma in situ, and superficial microinvasion. Decortication is performed using a defocused 5 to 10 W beam at 0.1 sec interrupted mode to minimize thermal effect in the wound bed and nondiseased tissue (Fig. 5A). Carbonized particles are removed to lessen thermal injury and thereby to avoid excessive scarring. In all lesions other than those that are superficial and have distinct and easily visualized margins, a *vestibulectomy* is performed to ensure full exposure and accurate assessment (Figs. 5B and 5C). The excision site is reinspected during office and operative endoscopy.

Plate 15
Figure 5
Laser Ablation of Leukoplakia

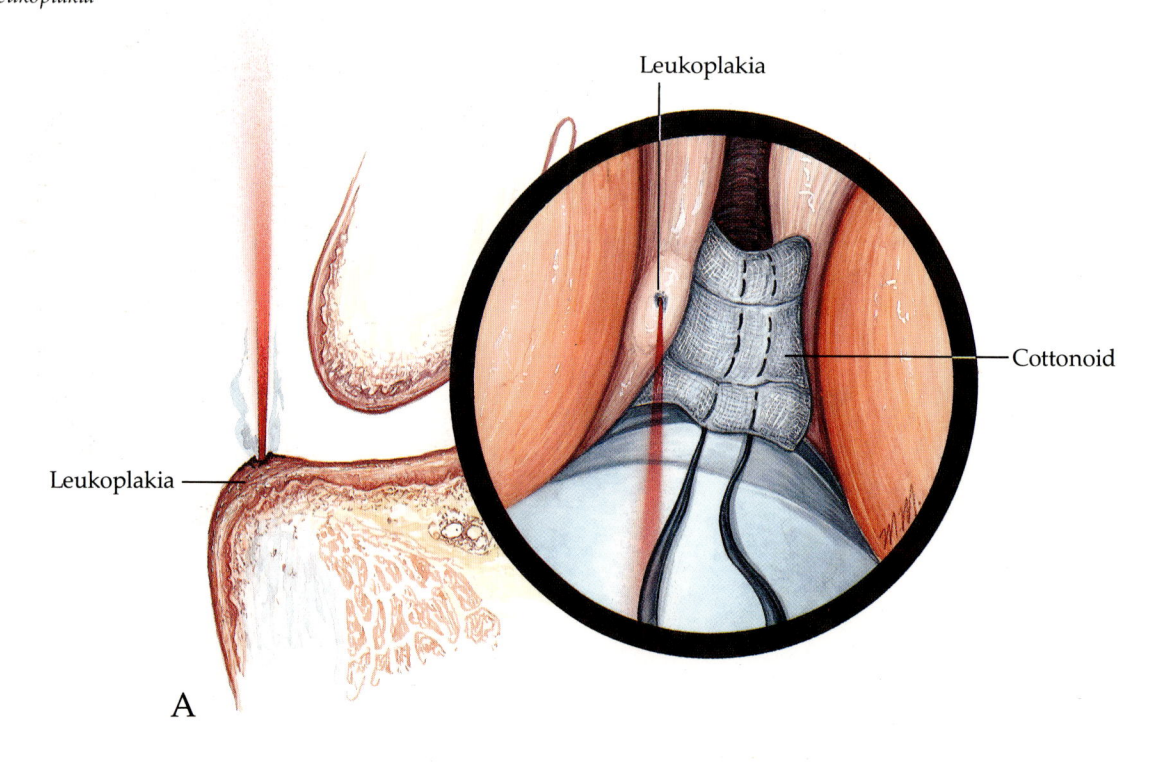

Plate 16

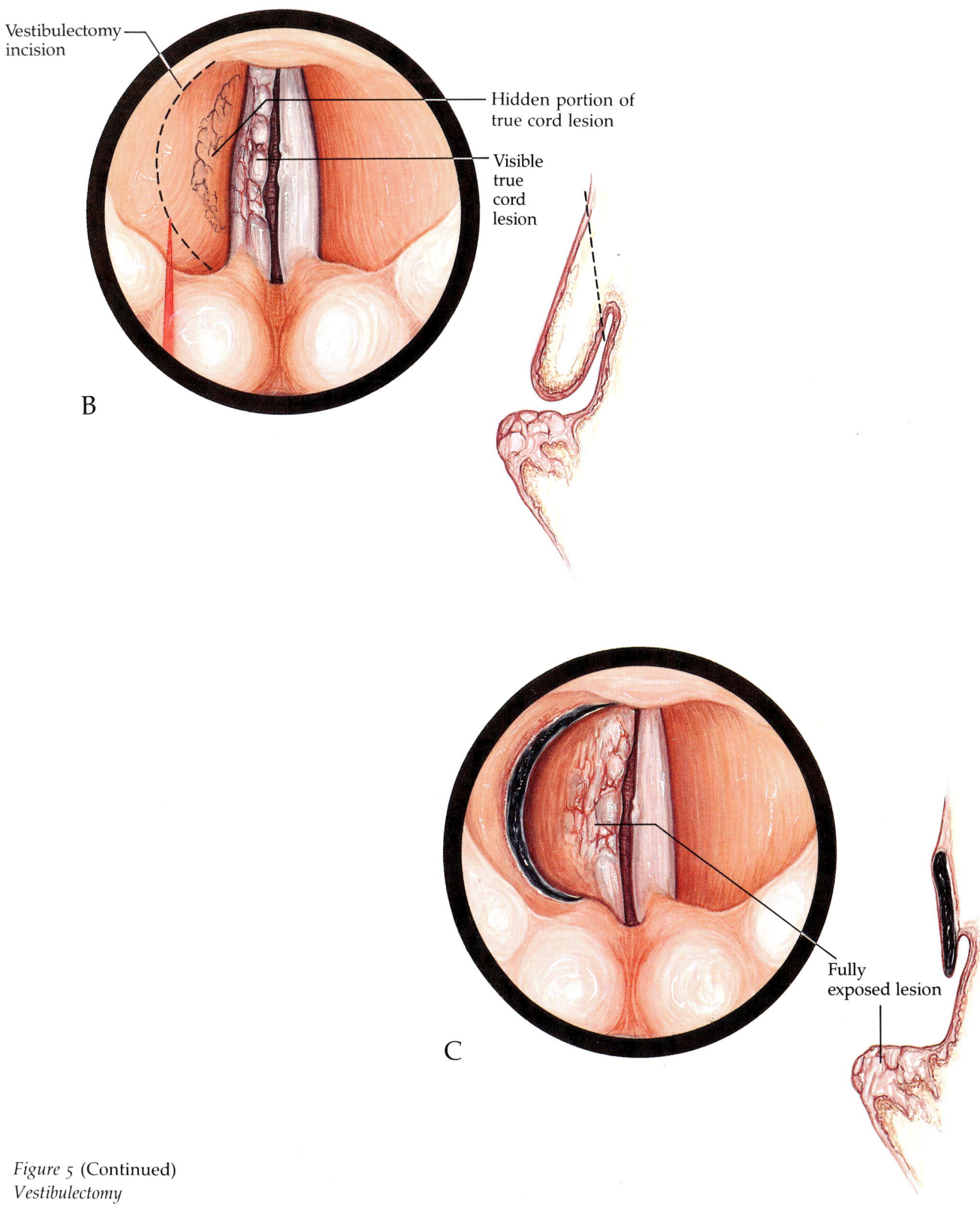

B
- Vestibulectomy incision
- Hidden portion of true cord lesion
- Visible true cord lesion

C
- Fully exposed lesion

Figure 5 (Continued)
Vestibulectomy

37

All suspicious areas are rebiopsied and retreated with laser.

In infiltrating lesions, as indicated by stiffness on stroboscopic examination or induration on palpation, a subtotal cordectomy (lesionectomy) (Fig. 5D) or total cordectomy (Fig. 5E) is performed. The margin of excision is defined by retracting the lesion medially to expose the lateralmost margin, and the proposed incision line is marked by spot evaporization using the laser. The anterior and posterior excision limits are also determined by palpation and marked by spot laser application. The actual excision is performed using a sharply focused laser beam at 10 to 15 W in interrupted or continuous mode, and it connects the previously placed spot marks. The sharply focused laser beam is moved at a rate consistent with accuracy; the specimen for excision is retracted at all times so that the focused aiming beam is targeted to a flat surface and not in the depths of a trough. In supraglottic excisions, branches of the superior laryngeal artery are regularly encountered posterolaterally, and these require hemostasis by tamponade, additional lasering or, rarely, injections of vasoconstrictive solutions. Excisions can be carried to the inner perichondrium of the thyroid cartilage, which is identified by the intense white afterburn. Laser applications at this site are done with caution inasmuch as chondritis and chondronecrosis follow excessive cartilage exposure or perichondral damage. *Lesionectomy* designates excision of limited lesions, and *cordectomy* designates excision of the entire membranous cord to the inner perichondrium.

The precise specimen is oriented so that histopathologic examination will identify tumor-free margins and specify sites requiring subsequent reinspection and biopsy. The excision margins of specimens are altered by thermal injury resulting from laser therapy and are of limited reliability for determining adequacy of tumor excision unless the tumor-free margin is wide. Evaluation of the excision margin is, therefore, determined by *separate* biopsies obtained from the excision bed, precisely identified as to site. Patients who have had the foregoing laser decortication for dysplasia, carcinoma in situ, or microinvasive cancer generally return to a nearly normal-appearing larynx with minimally altered voice. After laboratory review of permanent histologic sections, these patients are recalled for a "second-look" endoscopy, at which time the steps described for the initial laser endoscopy are repeated. Patients with carcinoma in situ are followed indefinitely, and repeat endoscopy is performed if clinical leukoplakia or other abnormalities occur.

Patients who have undergone lesionectomy (partial cordectomy) or total cordectomy are examined at weekly intervals until full re-epithelialization of the excision bed has been achieved; 2 to 3 weeks are required for full epithelialization, and 6 to 8 weeks may be needed in patients who have had prior radiation therapy or multiple endoscopic excisions. A second-look endoscopy is performed, and targeted biopsy specimens are obtained from sites at high risk for tumor persistence, as judged from the initial or preceding operation.

Externally applied pressure (the third-hand technique) allows optimal exposure of the subglottic compartment.

Bulky exophytic tumors, particularly those in patients who have had hoarseness of long duration, are often well-differentiated supraglottic

Plate 17

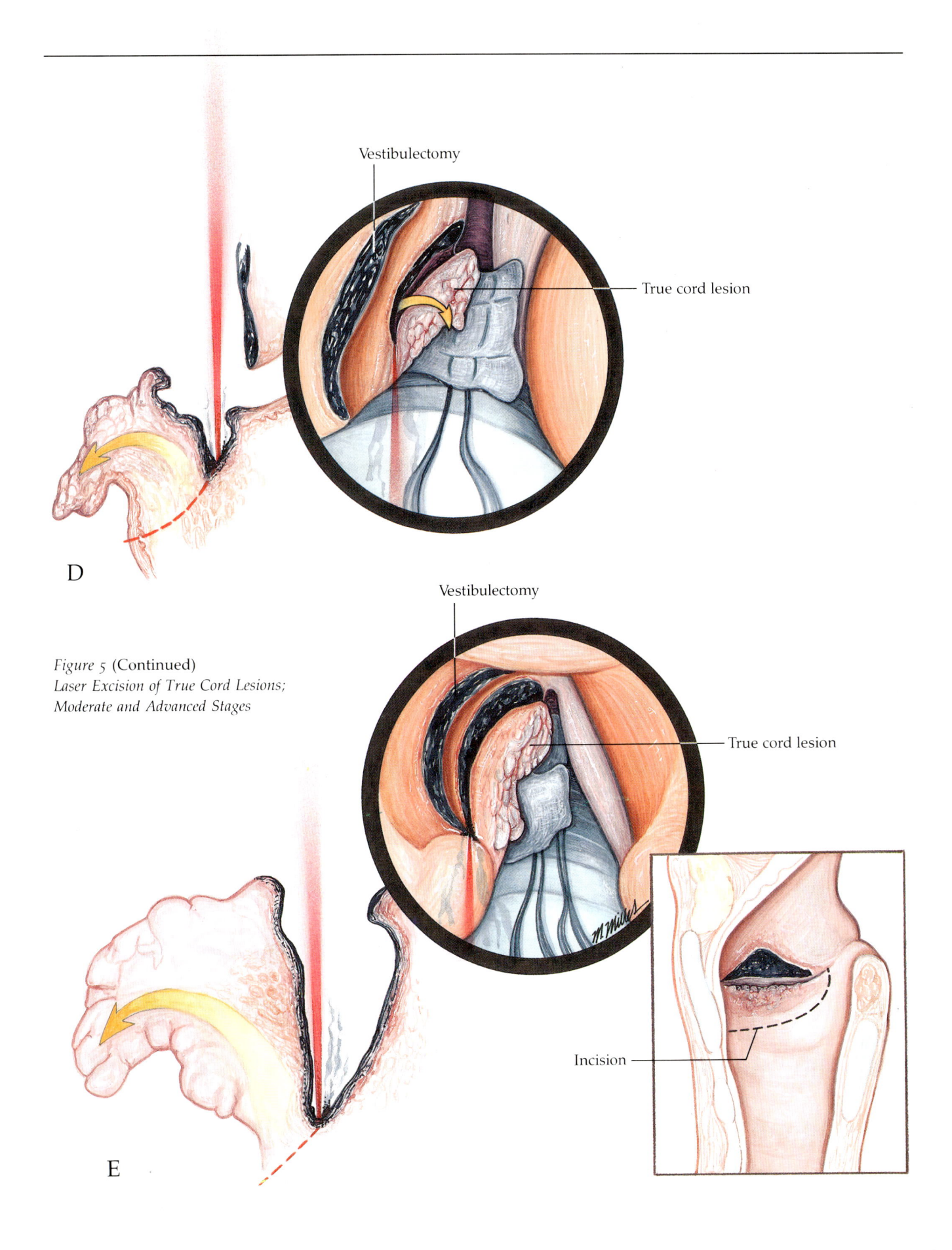

Vestibulectomy

True cord lesion

D

Figure 5 (Continued)
*Laser Excision of True Cord Lesions;
Moderate and Advanced Stages*

Vestibulectomy

True cord lesion

Incision

E

39

tumors arising from the laryngeal surface of the epiglottis or the aryepiglottic folds. Clinical inspection may indicate unilateral or bilateral vocal cord motion impairment due to tumor mass rather than infiltration into the musculus vocalis. In this setting, the CO_2 laser fulfills two important functions: (1) debulking of the large tumor mass obviates the need for tracheotomy, and (2) it permits accurate assessment as to the precise tumor extent. This tumor debulking is not performed with curative intent but to improve the accuracy of examination for possible horizontal partial (supraglottic) laryngectomy. In many instances, the tumor bulk reduction restores vocal cord motion and improves the voice.

Debulking the massively exophytic tumor restores a safe and adequate breathing space so that medical stabilization and diagnostic studies can be pursued without the encumbrance and handicap of a tracheotomy.

Indications

The special features of the CO_2 laser are well suited to the management of laryngeal cancer from the earliest precancerous lesions to noninvasive, microinvasive, and certain deeply invasive cancers. The laser is uniquely useful in managing large exophytic tumors as well. Moreover, the versatility of the laser is suited for obtaining precise biopsies, improving the precision of clinical staging, and for treatment itself, whether by laser decortication or subtotal or total cordectomy. In the advanced obstructive cancers the tumor bulk is reduced, thereby restoring a safe and adequate airway, obviating tracheotomy, and, at the same time, identifying cases suitable for larynx preservation operations.

Pearls and Pitfalls

The menu for treatment alternatives in laryngeal cancer has included irradiation and partial and total laryngectomy. In the past, laryngeal cancers that persisted or occurred after primary irradiation therapy were managed by total laryngectomy and, only rarely, by subtotal laryngectomy operations. The CO_2 laser introduces an important therapeutic alternative in the form of "extended excisional biopsy"—a realistic alternative to irradiation therapy in early and select advanced cancers. Preservation of irradiation therapy as a second line of treatment is especially important for the increasingly younger patient with laryngeal cancer. The young adult with many years of life expectancy faces the potential risk of an irradiation-induced cancer; CO_2 laser excision emerges as an equally effective cancer treatment and is particularly preferred in the young adult patient. Irradiation therapy applied as the first line of treatment in this younger patient group expends a treatment modality that should be held in reserve.

Haskins K. Kashima, M.D.

CO₂ LASER ARYTENOIDECTOMY AND TRANSVERSE CORDOTOMY

Indications

Bilateral vocal cord paralysis caused by dysfunction of both recurrent laryngeal nerves is an uncommon disorder; it occurs most commonly after thyroidectomy. It has been described in Arnold-Chiari syndrome and in other disorders of the midbrain. Bilateral vocal cord motion impairment occurs after blunt trauma to the neck or following traumatic or prolonged endotracheal intubation.

Bilateral vocal cord paralysis, or more accurately impaired vocal cord mobility, is frequently accompanied by one or more of the following: cricoarytenoid arthrodesis, web formation (posterior glottic), or vocal cord induration-fibrosis. Arytenoidectomy is the most frequently performed operation to relieve upper airway obstruction due to bilateral vocal cord motion impairment.

Historical Background

The concept that arytenoidectomy relieves airway obstruction caused by bilateral vocal cord paralysis derives from the report of its successful use in veterinary upper airway obstruction. King proposed lateral arytenoid-*opexy*; Kelly and Woodman described external approaches for arytenoid-*ectomy* and, in Woodman's procedure, the vocal process was ligated to the thyroid ala to stabilize vocal cord repositioning. Arytenoidectomy via the endoscopic route was successfully performed by Thornell. Following the introduction of surgical lasers, arytenoidectomy using the CO₂ laser has been reported by Ossoff, Lim, and others.

The objective in arytenoidectomy is repositioning of the vocal cords laterally by the combined effects of favorable scarring and re-epithelialization after total or subtotal arytenoid excision (see Fig. 6E). Centripetal epithelial migration results in resurfacing of the defect, and lateralward repositioning of the posterior glottis is achieved.

Operative Steps

Arytenoidectomy begins with optimal endoscopic exposure of the targeted arytenoid; the more mobile arytenoid, as determined by endoscopic palpation, is selected. The mucosa over the body of the arytenoid is incised, taking particular care to preserve epithelium at the glottic free border and to minimize thermal injury to the interarytenoid mucosa (Fig. 6A). The arytenoid is released from its muscular attachments, which are excised by sharp instrumental or laser excision (Fig. 6B). Total arytenoidectomy is rarely achieved. The defect remaining after arytenoid excision is lasered for hemostasis (Fig. 6C). This defect is epithelialized by centripetal epithelial ingrowth, and the posterior cord is retracted laterally to improve the laryngeal airway (Figs. 6D, 6E, and 6F).

Arytenoidectomy, by the Woodman procedure or by laser, is the most commonly utilized technique for relief of upper airway obstruction due to bilateral vocal cord motion impairment. The operative outcomes are variable due in part to the underlying pathophysiology—recurrent laryngeal denervation, cricoarytenoid arthrodesis, vocal cord fibrosis, and mucosal webs—and due also to variations in surgical technique. Wedge cordectomy, originally used as an adjuvant to arytenoidectomy, has been modified to a transverse cordotomy and has been a reliable and effective operation of wide applicability. At present we are using the transverse cordotomy as an independent procedure of choice.

Vaporization of the arytenoid results in thermal injury and promotes scarring, contracture, and lateral repositioning of the posterior glottis, provided that the free border of epithelium has been preserved. Epithelial injury to the free border promotes web formation and vocal cord fixation. Vaporization or unrecognized thermal injury to the interarytenoid fold causes contracture and draws the contralateral arytenoid toward the midline, thereby counteracting the intent of arytenoidectomy.

Dennis has described a technique of wedge (partial) cordectomy in which a transverse division of the posterior vocal cords creates a de-epithelialized cleft that is transformed into a larger defect as a result of the contraction of the residual vocalis muscle. Epithelialization of the cut surface forms a boot-shaped glottic aperture that effectively triples or quadruples the previous cross-sectional area at the glottic lumen.

Plate 18

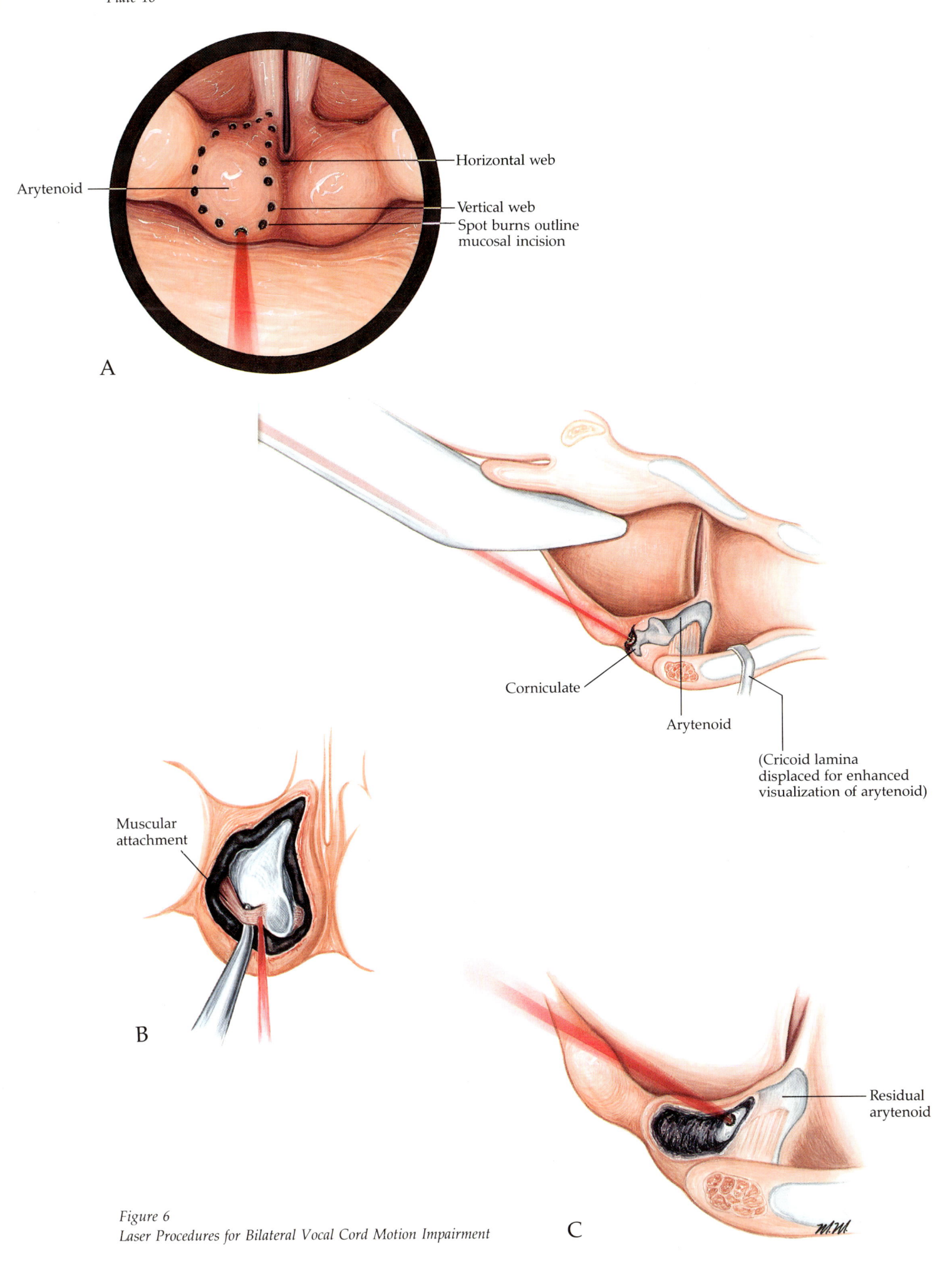

Arytenoid

Horizontal web
Vertical web
Spot burns outline mucosal incision

A

Corniculate

Arytenoid

(Cricoid lamina displaced for enhanced visualization of arytenoid)

Muscular attachment

B

Residual arytenoid

C

Figure 6
Laser Procedures for Bilateral Vocal Cord Motion Impairment

43

The technique of wedge resection of the thyroarytenoid muscle, proposed by Kirchner, has been modified as follows: first, vestibulectomy is performed to expose the vocal cord widely, including its lateralmost extent (refer to Vestibulectomy). A highly focused CO_2 laser transversely incises the vocal cord at the tip of the vocal process (Fig. 6E); the incision is extended laterally until a yellow-white afterburn indicates arrival at the inner perichondrium of the thyroid cartilage. Contraction of the thyroarytenoid muscle creates a triangular defect at the lasered vocal cord site (Fig. 6E). The final L-shaped laryngeal aperture consists of an enlarged space at the posterior glottis (Fig. 6F*) for the airway and a thin, tapered aperture anteriorly (Fig. 6F**) where the membranous vocal cords appose to produce voice.

The foregoing technique has been successfully utilized in patients who have failed prior arytenoidectomy as well as in patients with laryngeal stenosis after blunt trauma (external and intubation), partial laryngectomy, and irradiation therapy.

Arytenoidectomy by CO_2 laser is accompanied by a variable degree of postoperative edema due to trauma; hence, most surgeons performing arytenoidectomy advise tracheotomy in order to avoid an airway emergency in the postoperative period. The transverse cordotomy results in minimal reactive edema; therefore this operation can be safely performed without preliminary tracheotomy. The cordotomy operation is suitable in cases of vocal cord motion impairment with or without cricoarytenoid joint fixation, posterior glottic web, or vocal cord induration-fibrosis.

Pearls and Pitfalls

Inasmuch as thermal injury is an inescapable consequence after laser application to the larynx, the laser should be maximally focused and used in the interrupted mode at low power (10 to 15 W). Nonlaser instrumentation is minimized, and trauma to the mucosa at the posterior commissure and interarytenoid region must be avoided.

At the conclusion of the operation, a nasogastric tube is passed into the stomach to evacuate its contents and reduce the risks of aspiration. Ranitidine or a similar medication is prescribed in patients with a history of reflux or regurgitation. The flow volume loop spirogram is utilized for sequential and objective monitoring of upper airway patency. Antibiotics and anti-inflammatory agents are used, as indicated, based on findings from frequent and repeated endoscopic examinations.

Plate 19

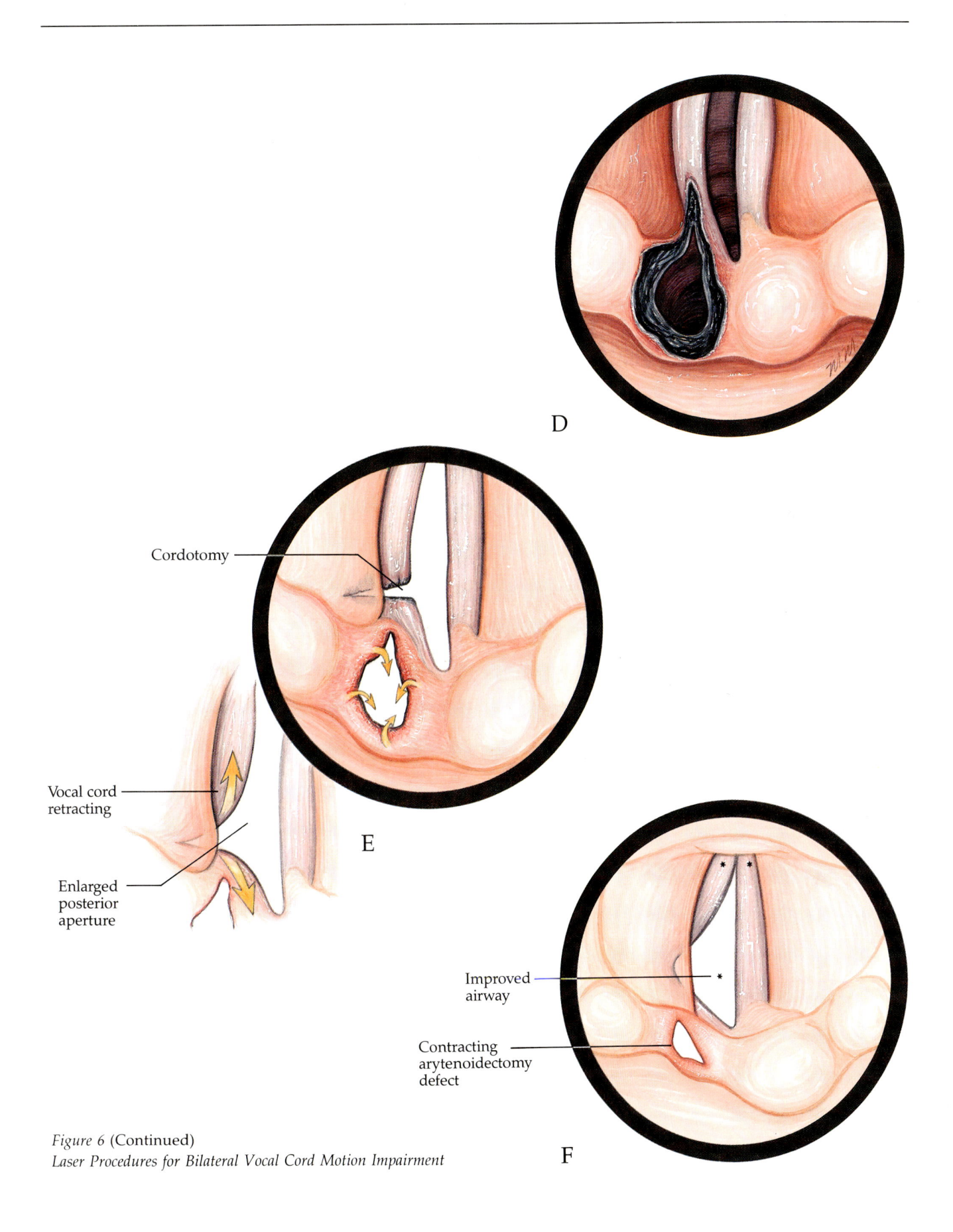

Cordotomy

Vocal cord retracting

Enlarged posterior aperture

D

E

Improved airway

Contracting arytenoidectomy defect

F

Figure 6 (Continued)
Laser Procedures for Bilateral Vocal Cord Motion Impairment

45

Haskins K. Kashima, M.D.

CO₂ LASER EXCISION OF LARYNGEAL WEB

The laryngeal web denotes a membranous adhesion causing limitation of vocal cord motion, subtle change in voice, and, uncommonly, airway obstruction. There are three distinct types of glottic webs located at (1) the anterior commissure, (2) the posterior commissure, and (3) the interarytenoid fold. The *anterior* glottic web fuses the free margins of the membranous vocal cords and obliterates the anterior laryngeal aperture (Fig. 7A). This lesion may be present at birth as a gossamer-thin membrane, but more often it is a lesion of variable thickness resulting from the trauma of forced or prolonged intubation or after vocal cord instrumentation. The *horizontal posterior* glottic web is a U-shaped band joining the arytenoids at the posterior commissure and immobilizing the vocal cords. This lesion is a sequela to de-epithelialization after prolonged endotracheal intubation, granulomatous inflammations, ill-advised instrumentation, or laser application at the posterior commissure. The *vertical posterior* web occurs either as a deep cicatrix within the interarytenoid fold or as epithelial scarring, either of which effectively binds the arytenoids together. The horizontal and vertical posterior webs mimic bilateral vocal cord paralysis in that the voice is deceptively normal, and the inspiratory airway is variably compromised. A fourth lesion, a thread-like *synechial glottic band,* bridges one vocal process to the other; it is an uncommon lesion usually resulting from fusion of postintubation granulomas.

These lesions share the common pathogenesis of inflamed de-epithelialized surfaces adhering to one another by exudative reaction and bound together by epithelial ingrowth. Juxtaposition of the denuded surfaces is facilitated by vocal cord inflammation, swelling, or paralysis.

Operative Steps

The endoscopic treatment of laryngeal webs is exasperatingly difficult except for management of the thin membranous anterior glottic web, which can be "laceration-repaired" by dilatation of an endotracheal tube. However, even meticulous microendoscopic division of the web is usually followed by reappearance of the lesion. An *open* surgical division of the anterior glottic web via anterior thyrotomy and use of a tantalum (more recently, silicone) keel was introduced by McNaught and became the gold standard for this condition. The principal drawbacks have been the tracheotomy (although not performed in McNaught's original operation) and the secondary operation for removal of the keel.

Although initial expectations that laryngeal webs would yield to the surgical laser have not been met, interest in laser endoscopy was rekindled by the availability of more finely focused beams and a surgical strategy based on converting an unfavorable (or difficult) web to a more favorable (or easier) lesion to correct. The fundamental requisite for successful web repair is to achieve epithelial continuity across the free border of the divided web, thereby preventing horizontal bridging of the freshly exposed tissues. Surgical division of the web should maximally preserve epithelium and reduce subepithelial stroma, thereby effectively converting the thick web into a more easily repaired gossamer thin web.

Surgical Technique

The larynx is exposed by suspension microlaryngoscopy under apnea or jet ventilation anesthesia. The laryngeal aperture is dilated using graduated Jackson laryngeal dilators so that the web is both thinned and stretched taut. A highly focused low wattage (3 to 5 W) laser is applied in short bursts (0.1 to 0.2 sec) to divide the upper epithelium at the midline. The divided epithelium separates laterally, exposing the subepithelial tissues (Fig. 7B); successively larger dilators displace the divided epithelium farther laterally and, simultaneously, improve exposure to the stroma for additional lasering. These steps of progressive dilation and lasering are repeated, layer by layer, until the undersurface epithelium of the web is exposed, dilated, and divided by laser (Fig. 7C). This step-by-step division of the thick web effectively debulks the web and maximally preserves the epithelium so that epithelial continuity can be re-established at the freshly created free border of the true vocal cords. The surplus (undersurface) epithelium is pulled over the cut surface and, in some cases, the upper and lower epithelial free borders can be sealed by low wattage laser welding.

The stomach contents are evacuated by passage of a nasogastric tube, and the patient is awakened. Postoperatively, minimal voice use is permitted and throat clearing is discouraged. The larynx is examined on a daily basis and newly forming adhesions are gently divided under suspension microlaryngoscopy.

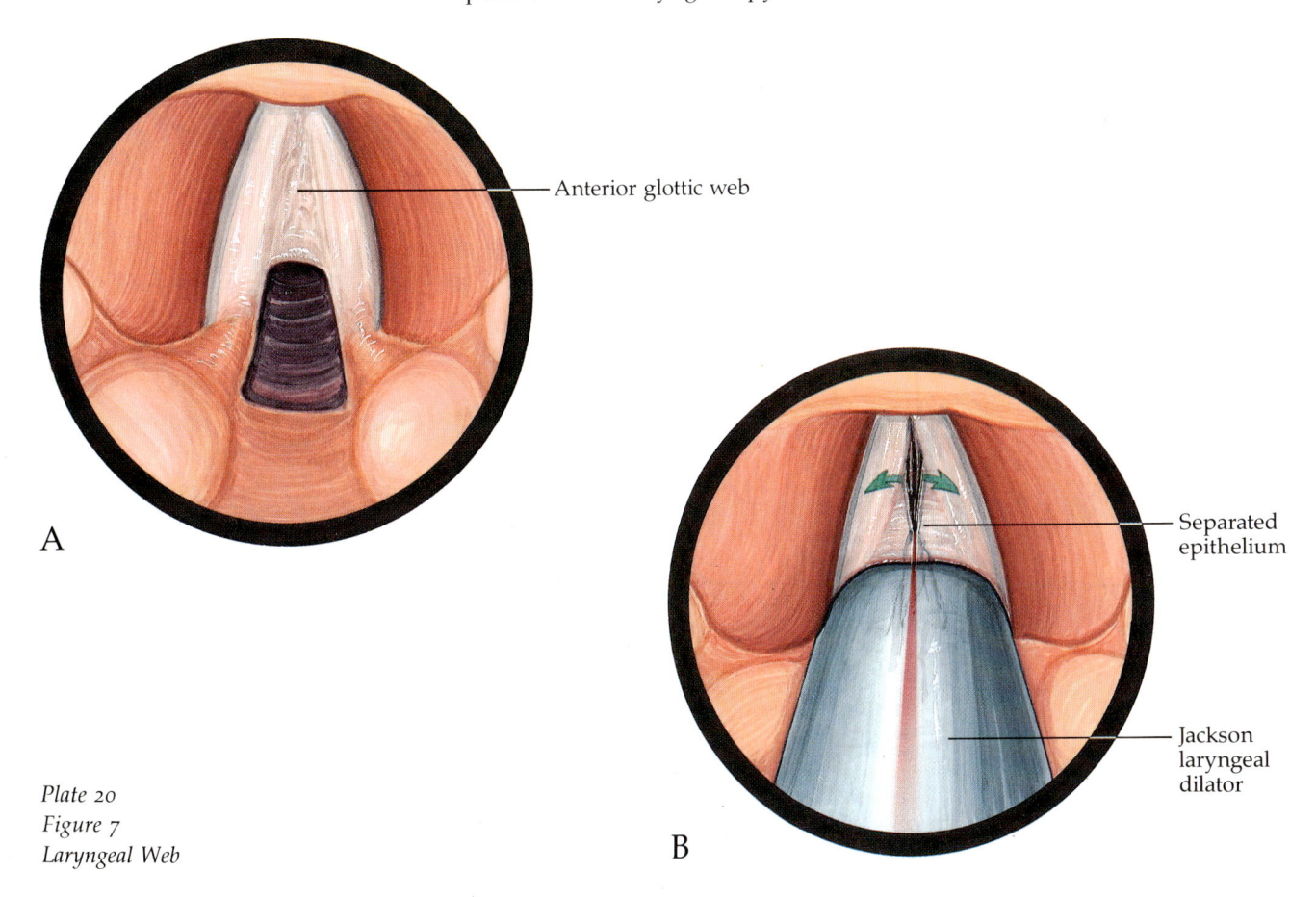

Plate 20
Figure 7
Laryngeal Web

Plate 21
Figure 7 (Continued)
Laryngeal Web

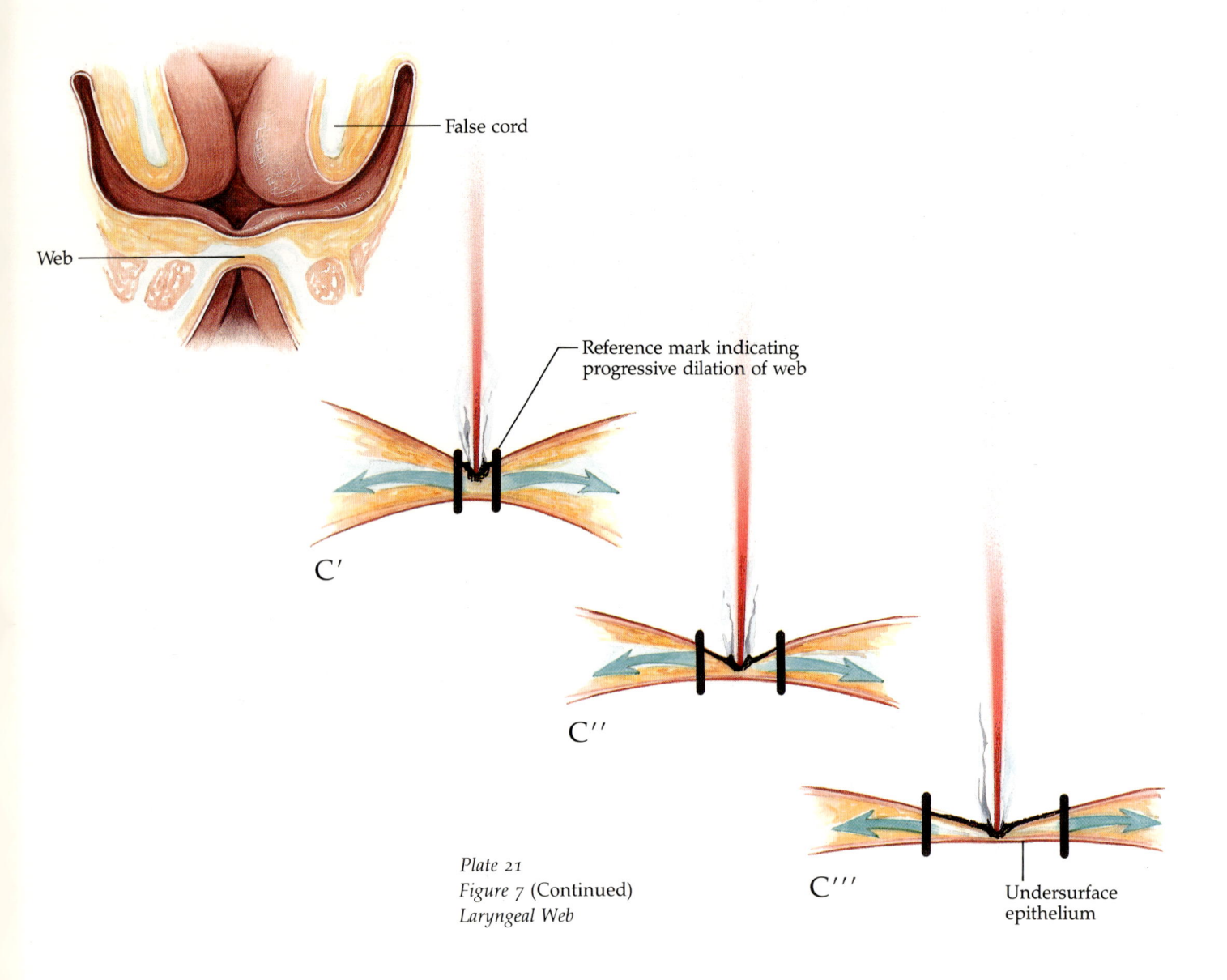

Postoperative Care

The principles outlined in the section on polyps and cysts are equally appropriate for the preoperative evaluation and the aftercare of laryngeal webs.

Pearls and Pitfalls

The anterior glottic web may contribute to voice perturbation of varying severity but rarely interferes with airway performance. The decision to proceed with surgical web division is predicated on voice improvement; it follows, therefore, that a speech pathologist should be actively involved from the outset and should participate in the decision to proceed with an operation. The speech pathologist's input and insight are invaluable in maximizing voice improvement.

The posterior glottic webs (horizontal and vertical) are treated by cordotomy (see section on Arytenoidectomy). The synechial band is managed by laser excision and, when there is vocal cord motion impairment, by cordotomy.

Haskins K. Kashima, M.D.

T-TUBE INSERTION

Indications

The use of a prosthetic stent after surgical reconstruction of the larynx or of the trachea has a long history of imaginative designs and improvisations. Intraluminal support is intended to *stabilize the repair* and *facilitate re-epithelialization;* the stent maintains a desirable lumen size by inhibition of cicatricial scarring, by facilitating re-epithelialization by a graft, or from centripetal ingrowth of surrounding epithelium.

Use of the prefabricated rubber Silastic T-tube in the trachea has had widespread acceptance and reliable performance. It is utilized after surgical repair of acute laceration or avulsion injuries and after tracheal reconstructive restoration for chronic stenosis.

Preoperative Considerations

The patient with airway obstructive symptoms requires a thorough history and endoscopic evaluation. The flow-volume loop spirogram is a noninvasive study ideally suited for evaluating the nature and quantitating the severity of the obstruction; it is particularly useful in monitoring the clinical course of patients during the follow-up period to verify the subjective assessment of airway patency.

Preoperative assessment establishes (1) the *severity* and *extent* of the stenotic segment, and (2) the *anatomic composition* of the stenotic segment. The severity of the stenosis is clinically determined by measurement of cross-sectional dimensions of the lumen by axial and coronal thin-section CT scans; the extent of the stenosis is measured on longitudinal X-ray films in the coronal and/or sagittal planes. Axial scans demonstrate the state of the skeletal rings—whether they are intact, comminuted, or otherwise distorted—and the position and thickness of the subepithelial fibrosis. The choice of repair technique is determined after review of these and other coexisting factors and the surgeon's preference based on personal experience.

Tube Design

The hollow rubber Silastic T-tube is pliable and consists of two portions: (1) the vertical portion for support of the tracheal lumen, and (2) the horizontal portion, a right-angled extension that serves as the tracheotomy vent. A full selection of T-tubes of varying diameters and lengths is available so that a precisely appropriate tube can be selected for each patient.

The following description is of the T-tube use in correcting chronic stenosis of the cervical trachea. Dimensions of the stenotic segment are measured, and an appropriate T-tube is selected for use.

Operative Steps

General anesthesia is delivered via the pre-existing tracheotomy opening, and suspension laryngoscopy is performed. The zone of stenosis is examined with a 0-degree telescope to exclude the presence of any companion lesions, such as a granuloma, exposed cartilage, or an occult infection focus. Saline-moistened Jackson laryngeal dilators are passed through the stenotic segment until an unforced maximal lumen size has been achieved. In significant subepithelial fibrosis, as determined by axial CT findings, vertical mucosal incisions are placed where soft tissue thickness is greatest. Further dilations to a larger caliber and additional mucosal incisions are made if preoperative CT studies are supportive. Mucosal incisions rarely exceed three or four, and as much epithelium as possible should be preserved inasmuch as this is the source for re-epithelialization. The greatest lumen diameter as measured from the final dilator determines T-tube size.

Precise placement of the T-tube begins with retrograde passage and (repeat) dilation of the stenotic segment using serially linked Tucker esophageal bougies. The dilators are withdrawn retrograde through the laryngoscope by the surgeon (Fig. 8A). These dilations are interrupted whenever necessary by reintroducing the endotracheal tube at the linking loops connecting the bougies; in this manner, proper oxygenation can be maintained. The T-tube is mounted onto the leading end of the bougie matching the final Tucker dilator caliber (Fig. 8B). The bougie carrying the T-tube is linked to the preceding bougie by a discardable silk ligature, in turn shielded by a segment of nasogastric tube; this silk is cut to permit bougie recovery after proper T-tube positioning. The T-tube is guided into the tracheotomy opening by the assistant (Fig. 8C) while the surgeon continues withdrawal of the serially connected bougies through the laryngoscope until the lower limb of the T-tube slips through the tracheotomy opening and falls into position in the distal trachea (Fig. 8D). The bougie carrying the T-tube is withdrawn and disengaged from the T-tube, and the discardable silk suture is cut. All bougies are withdrawn.

The interior of the sealed T-tube is inspected with a 0-degree telescope to assure that it is properly unfolded and correctly positioned to stent the stenotic segment. Anesthesia is continued by occluding the horizontal limb of the T-tube and passing an uncuffed endotracheal tube via the larynx or by occluding the upper limb of the T-tube (Fig. 8E) and delivering the anesthetic mixture through the horizontal limb. The stomach is evacuated of its contents and the patient is awakened, preferably with the horizontal limb of the T-tube corked.

The T-tube can also be placed at the time of open tracheoplasty. The appropriately proportioned T-tube is placed in the reconstructed segment, and a tracheal window is created for the horizontal limb. An endotracheal tube passed from above engages the T-tube, the horizontal limb is sealed, and anesthesia is continued until completion of the surgical closure.

Postoperative Care

The patient is reinstructed in tube care; emphasizing meticulous cleansing of the interior and suctioning technique. The T-tube interior is moistened with saline to prevent any crusting or desiccation of secretions. The patient and family members should be particularly instructed regarding emergency removal of the T-tube in case of acute obstruction and replacement with a standard tracheotomy tube, which should be carried by the patient at all times.

Ideally, the horizontal limb remains continuously sealed except for suctioning; this prevents secretion desiccation and tube obstruction. The interior of the T-tube should be carefully inspected at each return appointment; a thin 90-degree telescope is passed as in retrograde tracheoscopy (q.v.). The tracheal lumen immediately beyond the T-tube should also be assessed for patency and to exclude granuloma or polyp formation.

Plate 22

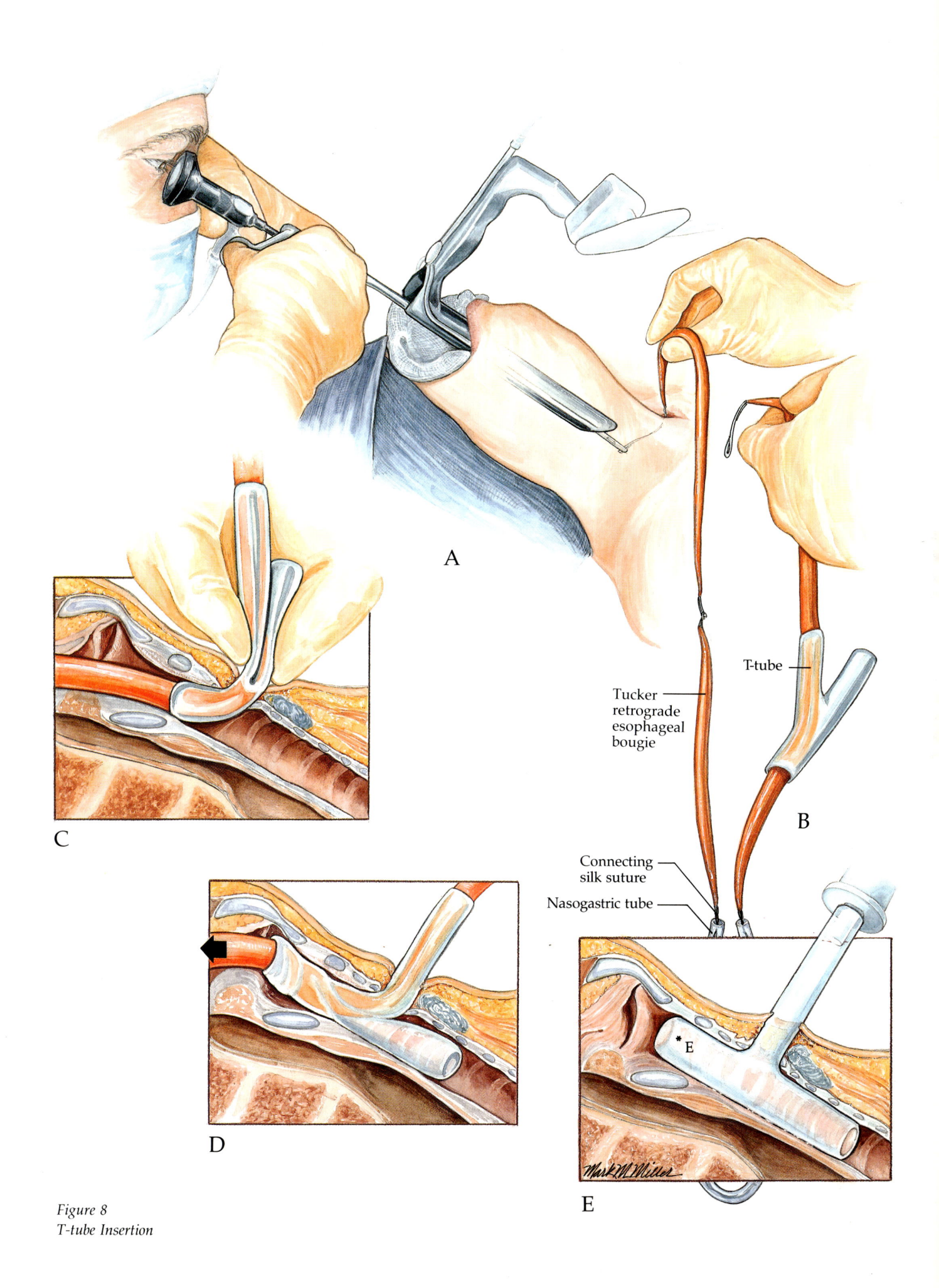

A

B

T-tube

Tucker retrograde esophageal bougie

C

D

Connecting silk suture

Nasogastric tube

E

Figure 8
T-tube Insertion

The T-tube is not necessary to support an uncomplicated tracheal anastomosis. When used to support a complex reconstruction or after a dilation, the T-tube is left in place for at least 3 and preferably 6 months or longer. In adult females a No. 14 tube and in adult males a No. 16 tube provides an airway adequate for moderate physical activity. At successive endoscopies the size of the T-tube can be advanced and the airway objectively evaluated using the flow-volume loop spirogram. Final decannulation is managed in a manner identical to that used with the standard tracheotomy tube.

CT scan through the T-tube verifies that the stent is functioning to support the repair area. Air space surrounding the T-tube indicates regression of the reactive swelling and assists in the decision to replace the indwelling tube with one of a larger size when necessary.

Pearls and Pitfalls

The hollow T-tube stent is a useful and appropriate adjunct for tracheal stenosis repair. Complex laryngotracheal stenosis requires separate management of the laryngeal and tracheal aspects. T-tube abutment against the subglottis and larynx results in granulomatous reaction and may lead to permanent impairment of vocal cord motion, voice quality, or both. The T-tube can be tailored to size at the operating table, but its sharp edges promote inflammatory swelling in the host tissue and may lead to bleeding and obstruction. The customized T-tube can be prepared in a machine shop from dimensions measured in preoperative x-ray films; the sanding belt gives the most acceptable smooth surface at the revised T-tube tip.

In summary, the T-tube is an invaluable prosthesis which, when properly used, is reliable and effective. The patient, the family, and the hospital attendants must have an adequate understanding and the manual dexterity necessary for its safe management.

Bernard R. Marsh, M.D.

DIAGNOSTIC BRONCHOSCOPY

Examination of the tracheobronchial tree is now performed almost exclusively with flexible fiberscopes. Only in small children is there a continuing need to use open tube instruments for *diagnostic* bronchoscopy.

Indications

Diagnostic bronchoscopy is indicated when there is any unexplained bronchopulmonary condition or as part of a complete evaluation for upper respiratory tract malignancy to rule out a second primary tumor.

Preoperative Considerations

Review the patient's history, perform a physical examination, and obtain current x-ray studies and laboratory test results. Be sure you understand the specific question to be answered. (Selection from among the many different types of specimen retrieval now available requires a clear understanding of the issues to be addressed.)

Operative Steps

Position the patient in the supine or semireclining position. Attach a pulse oximeter and an electrocardiographic monitor. Intravenous sedation should be administered. Give supplemental oxygen by nasal cannula. Check the fiberscope and lubricate with viscous lidocaine. Anesthetize the patient's nose with lidocaine or cocaine by cotton applicator or spray (Fig. 9A). If general anesthesia is used, the fiberscope can be passed through a T-adapter into the endotracheal tube (Fig. 9B). A bite block should be used to prevent instrument damage in case of light anesthesia (Fig. 9C).

Plate 23

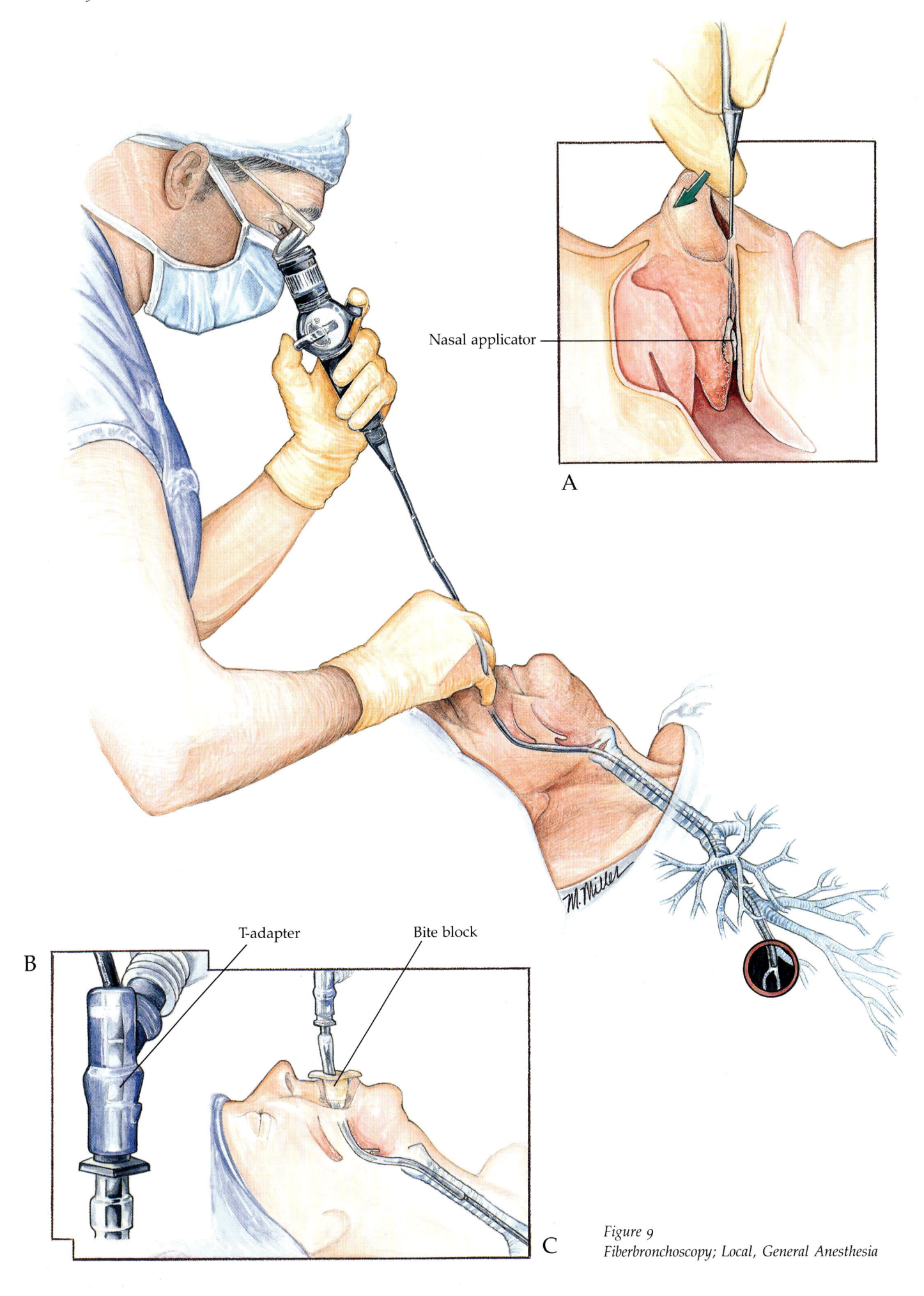

Nasal applicator

A

T-adapter　　Bite block

B

C

Figure 9
Fiberbronchoscopy; Local, General Anesthesia

Pass the fiberscope gently along the nasal floor into the pharynx to expose the larynx (Fig. 9D). (The fiberscope may be passed through the mouth if desired.) Instill lidocaine 2 percent (the syringe contains 2 cc of lidocaine and 2 cc of air to permit the solution to be fully expelled) and repeat two or three times until the larynx is anesthetized (Fig. 9E). Pass the scope into the trachea and instill anesthetic in the left main bronchus and both upper lobe bronchi. Examine each lobe and segment in serial fashion, noting any abnormalities. Obtain biopsy and brush specimens for histologic and cytologic study of bronchial lesions (Figs. 9F and 9G). An assistant should aid the surgeon in forceps and brush manipulation (Fig. 9H). Use fluoroscopy to obtain biopsies of peripheral lesions. Obtain a transtracheal needle specimen for diagnosis of paratracheal nodes. Use bronchoalveolar lavage (BAL) for immunosuppressed patients with pulmonary complications. (Wedge the scope in a segment and obtain several sequential 20-cc lavage specimens for cytologic evidence of opportunistic infection and for cultures.)

Postoperative Care

Give oxygen by nasal cannula. Administer intravenous fluids until the patient recovers from anesthesia. Monitor the patient for 4 to 6 hours. A postoperative chest radiograph may be indicated if a lung biopsy or needle aspiration specimen has been obtained. Permit the patient to leave the hospital after full recovery and accompanied by an adult who can do the driving.

Figure 9 (Continued)
Fiberbronchoscopy; Anesthesia and Biopsy

Plate 24

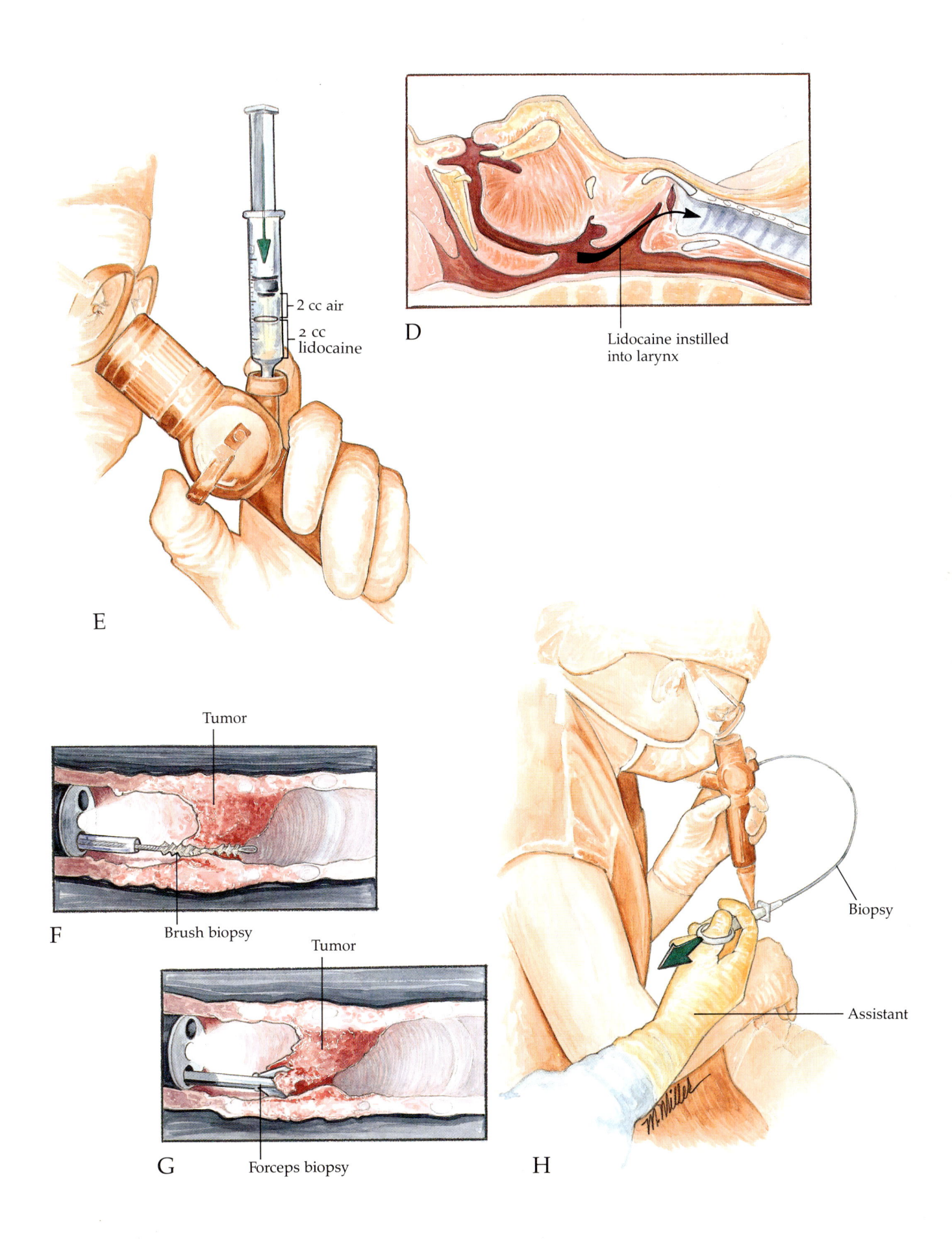

D Lidocaine instilled into larynx

E 2 cc air / 2 cc lidocaine

F Tumor / Brush biopsy

G Tumor / Forceps biopsy

H Biopsy / Assistant

Risks, Complications, and Sequelae

1. In those patients with compromised pulmonary function, hypoxia must be anticipated and prevented.
2. Excessive bleeding or pneumothorax from biopsy is rarely encountered but should be anticipated and a plan of management prepared in advance.
3. Anesthetic complications are mostly preventable if careful attention is given to dose and rate of administration.
4. Postoperative fever may be encountered.
5. Severe bronchospasm may be anticipated in asthmatic patients.
6. A foreign body from a broken instrument (e.g., brush or Fogarty catheter tip) may be found postoperatively.

Pearls and Pitfalls

Make sure instrument optics and controls are fully satisfactory before you begin.

Know the maximum safe dose of the anesthetic used and do not exceed it.

If oral insertion of the fiberscope is used, *be sure to provide a bite block* for the patient. One misadventure will destroy a fiberscope.

Check the nasopharynx and larynx for lesions or evidence of paralysis.

Monitor oxygen saturation to avoid hypoxia and arrhythmia.

If stridor develops, consider vocal cord paralysis resulting from anesthesia (a rare but possible complication).

Move along expeditiously, and go straight to the area of concern before checking out the remainder of the lung. A good visual inspection before cough or instrument trauma occurs is vital.

Additional topical anesthesia after cough returns is frequently useless. (Salivary aspiration and bronchial secretions may obscure visualization.)

Never perform bilateral lung biopsy because of the risk of bilateral pneumothorax.

If a lesion is found, determine the bronchial margins for possible later thoracotomy.

Obtain both tissue biopsies and cytologic specimens for laboratory verification of a suspected malignancy.

A cloudy image can usually be cleared by instilling saline and suctioning against the bronchus wall to create a wiping effect.

Insert the biopsy forceps through a relatively straight tip and then deflect the instrument to reach an upper lobe lesion.

If the fiberscope is used through an endotracheal tube, effective lubrication is essential. Lidocaine ointment, silicone spray, soap solution, and water-soluble jelly have all been used.

Have a back-up light source, biopsy forceps, brushes, and so forth readily available.

Use fluoroscopy if you plan lung biopsy, since the risk of pneumothorax is reduced.

If you are performing this procedure on children, be sure you have smaller fiberscopes and open tubes appropriate for the patient's age.

Leave any discovered foreign bodies alone unless you are fully equipped and prepared to remove them.

Have an assistant monitor vital signs for you.

Suggested Reading

Marsh B, Ravich W. Laryngoscopy, bronchoscopy and esophagoscopy. In: Johns ME, ed. Complications in otolaryngology—head and neck surgery. Vol 2: Head and Neck. Toronto: BC Decker, 1986:83–92.

Marsh B, Wang K. Bronchoscopy. In: Straus MJ, ed. Lung cancer—clinical diagnosis and treatment. Orlando, FL: Grune & Stratton, 1983.

Oho K, Amemiya R. Practical fiberoptic bronchoscopy. 2nd ed. Tokyo, New York: Igaku-Shoin, 1984.

Wang K, Gupta P, Haponik E, Erozan Y. Flexible transbronchial needle aspiration: Technical considerations. Ann Otol Rhinol Laryngol 1984; 93:233–236.

Wang K, Terry P. Transbronchial needle aspiration in the diagnosis and staging of bronchogenic carcinoma. Am Rev Respir Dis 1983; 127: 344–347.

Zavala DC. Flexible fiberoptic bronchoscopy, a training handbook. Iowa City: University of Iowa, 1978.

Bernard R. Marsh, M.D.

REMOVAL OF BRONCHIAL FOREIGN BODIES

One of the first and still important applications of bronchoscopy is the removal of foreign material lodged in the airways. The basic principles and techniques were developed to a high degree of perfection by Chevalier Jackson during the early part of this century. Refinements of instrumentation and anesthesia have occurred in recent years, but the fundamental concepts and guidelines for safe, efficient, and effective foreign body bronchoscopy remain as valid today as when published 50 years ago. Those engaged in this activity would benefit from reading the classic works in this field.

Indications

The suspicion of bronchial foreign body is the only necessary indication. A careful history is of the utmost importance. The physical examination may be quite normal or reveal a localized wheeze. The chest radiograph may show air trapping but often proves inconclusive. The procedure itself is often required to establish the presence or absence of a foreign body. Experience in this field shows the validity of the adage, "You bronchoscope not for the foreign body but for the suspicion of foreign body." The risks of the procedure performed by an experienced operator are far less than the risk of complications resulting from a retained foreign body.

Preoperative Considerations

Discuss the procedure with the patient and/or the parents. Obtain a chest radiograph in two planes immediately preoperatively. Review the proposed technique and the airway management plan with the anesthesiologist. Obtain a duplicate foreign body if such is available. Select assorted foreign body forceps, bronchoscopes, telescopes, laryngoscopes, light sources, cables, and all ancillary equipment in appropriate sizes and assure not only their satisfactory working condition but also their compatibility with one another. Always prepare the bronchoscope and related instruments not only in the size anticipated but also in a size smaller should you encounter a problem passing the instrument through the subglottis.

Operative Steps

Anesthesia induction should commence only after the equipment has been set up, the monitors have been attached, and the surgeon is thoroughly prepared. The bronchoscope may be introduced either with the aid of an anesthesia laryngoscope or directly. An indwelling telescope positioned so as to reveal the distal end of the bronchoscope greatly assists in safe passage through the infant larynx and in efficient identification of the foreign body. A connector permits anesthesia and ventilation through the bronchoscope. After the foreign body has been identified, the appropriate forceps may be selected. Two general types are available, but the greatest selection is provided by the traditional Jackson-style instrument (Fig. 10A). A somewhat newer double-action forceps is available in a limited assortment and is popular even though it lacks the facility for adjustment to meet special needs (Fig. 10B). Its simplicity, reliability, and ease of maintenance and use make it a favorite for most vegetable objects. The optical forceps is a telescope-forceps combination permitting a magnified view of the foreign body retrieval. This instrument is available in

Plate 25

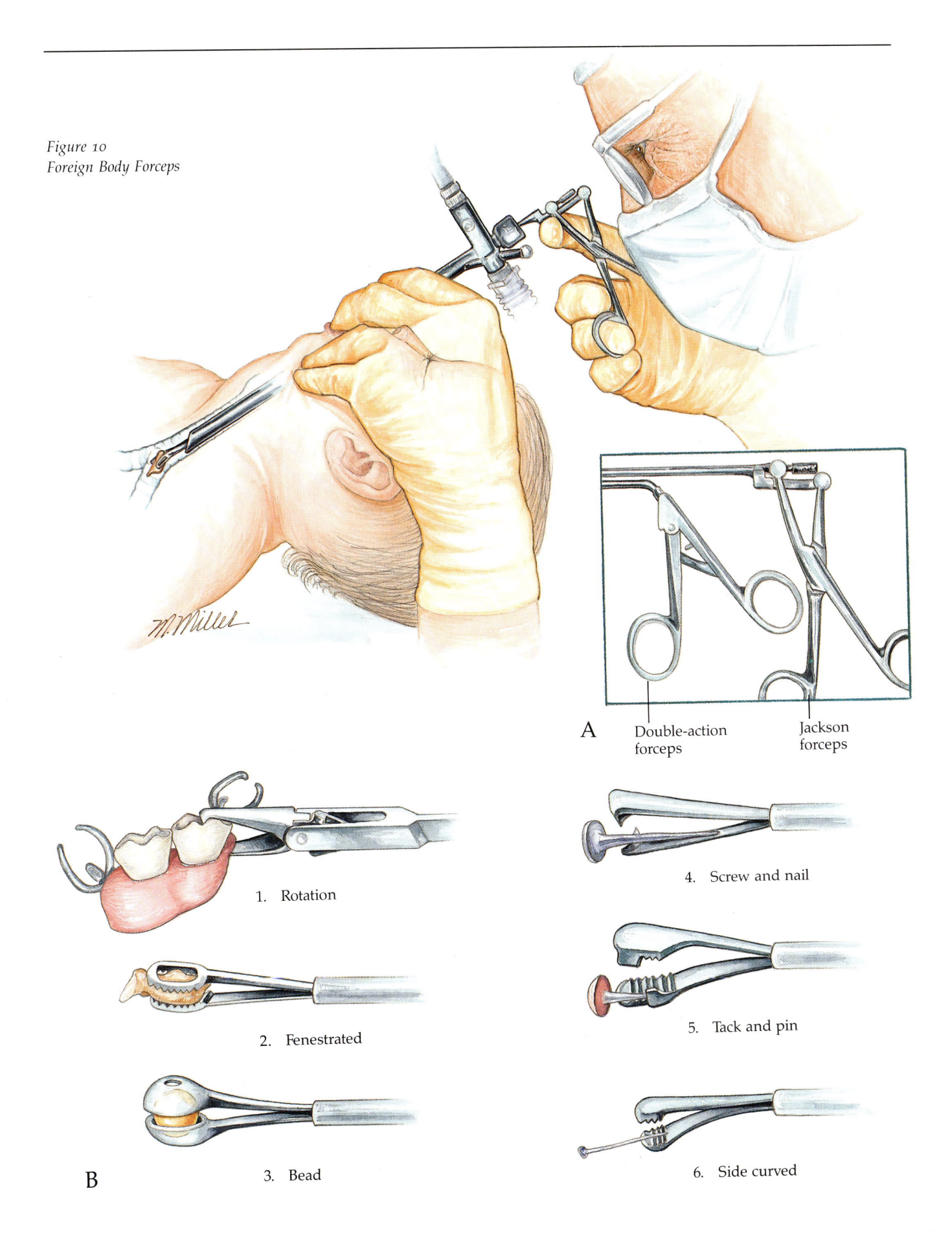

Figure 10
Foreign Body Forceps

A Double-action forceps   Jackson forceps

1. Rotation
2. Fenestrated
3. Bead

4. Screw and nail
5. Tack and pin
6. Side curved

B

61

a very limited selection, but it greatly aids in proper forceps placement in selected cases (Fig. 10C). The prismatic light deflector must be slightly withdrawn to permit passage of the instrument through the bronchoscope. A microforceps designed for passage through the auxiliary channel and alongside the telescope also provides a magnified view of the forceps application (Fig. 10D). This has a very limited role, but it becomes especially important in the removal of a small fragment in a distal bronchus of a small child. The very small jaws may crush a nut fragment unless used with great care, but they do permit withdrawal of the foreign body into a larger bronchus where a fenestrated forceps may be applied for its safe removal.

Under most circumstances the foreign body must be removed along with the bronchoscope and a second look taken to assure that no fragments remain.

The fiberoptic bronchoscope has mostly been used to remove some foreign bodies in older children and adults. The four-pronged and the basket forceps are generally available, but frequently they prove less satisfactory than might be anticipated (Fig. 10E).

Postoperative Care

Perform careful monitoring for respiratory distress, and obtain a chest radiograph.

Risks, Complications, and Sequelae

1. Laryngeal edema may result from rough handling, use of too large a bronchoscope, or improper retrieval of the foreign body.
2. Dental injury may occur if the patient is not properly protected by a tooth guard.
3. The procedure may not succeed because of inappropriate equipment or inadequate training.
4. The foreign body may slip into the opposite lung, become fragmented, or be pushed into a more distal bronchus.

Pearls and Pitfalls

No one should think of attempting bronchial foreign body removal without extensive laboratory practice and demonstrated skill. Minimum experience includes competence in use of the following forceps (see Fig. 10A): (1) rotation, (2) fenestrated forward grasping, (3) bead, (4) screw nail, (5) tack and pin, and (6) side curved forward grasping.

After an initial choking episode, most foreign bodies remain symptomatically silent for a period of time ("the silent interval").

Always have a back-up light source.

When using the optical forceps, always have an extra telescope available for initial evaluation.

When using the microforceps, place the forceps part way through the bronchoscope, then insert the telescope.

Plate 26

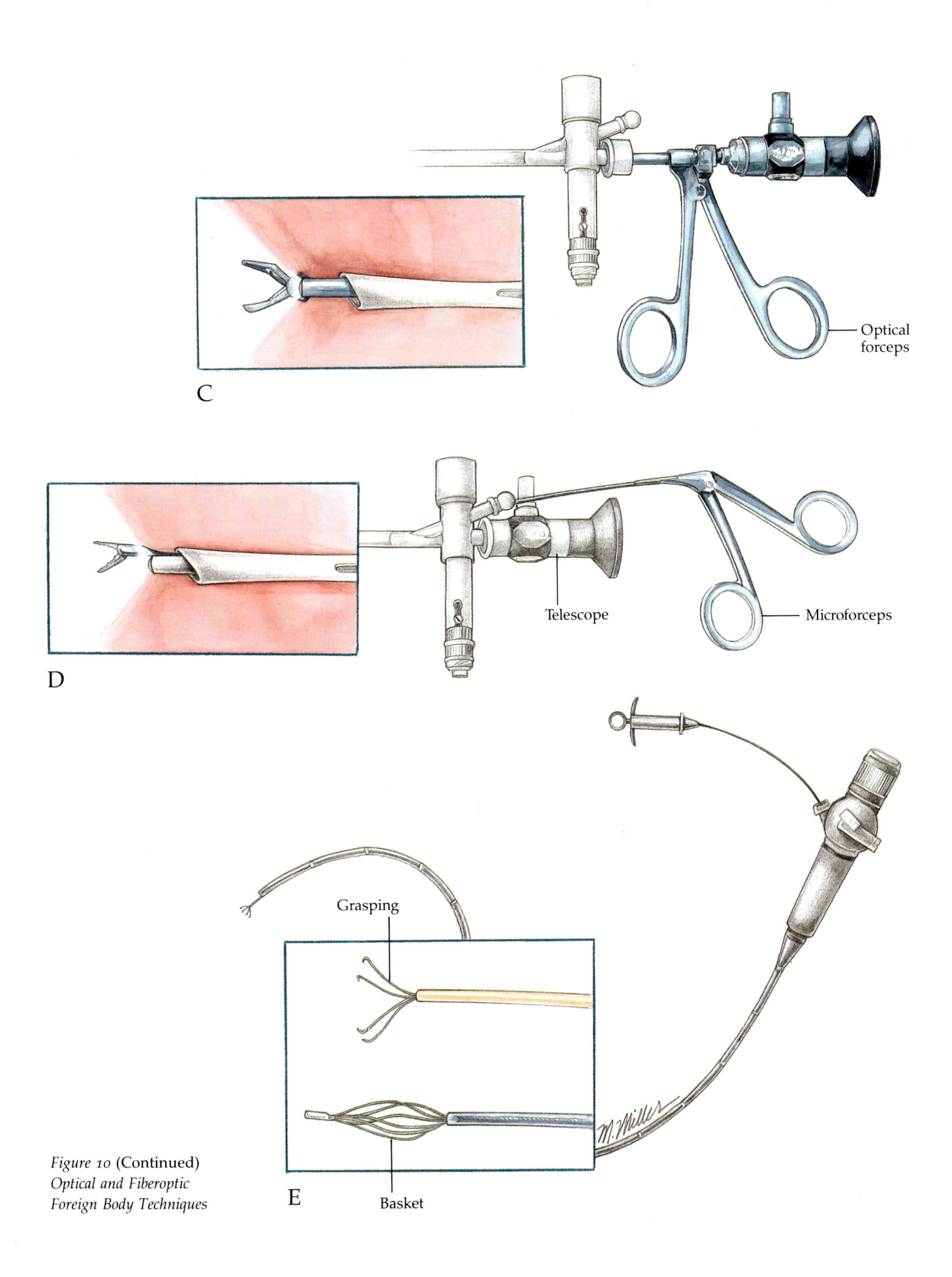

C

D

Optical forceps

Telescope — Microforceps

Grasping

E   Basket

Figure 10 (Continued)
Optical and Fiberoptic
Foreign Body Techniques

63

Always have a trained assistant who can pass instruments correctly.

Do not forget that an esophageal foreign body may be manifested by respiratory symptoms in the small child.

Remember that bilateral foreign bodies may be present.

Most foreign bodies are not true emergencies and require careful though expeditious work-up and treatment.

Sharp points on the foreign body must either be converted to a trailing orientation or be protected by the forceps and bronchoscope.

Fluoroscopy is sometimes essential and should always be available for use on radiopaque objects.

Peanut fragments are notorious for creating a marked bronchial reaction, sometimes obscuring the foreign body by granulation tissue.
Approach the object carefully so as not to override or displace it distally.

Suggested Reading

Ballenger JJ. Diseases of the nose, throat, ear, head, and neck. Philadelphia: Lea & Febiger, 1985:1293–1385.

Jackson C, Jackson CL. Bronchoesophagology. 2nd ed. Philadelphia, WB Saunders, 1950.

Marsh B. Foreign bodies of the aerodigestive tract. In: Gates GA, ed. Current therapy in otolaryngology—head and neck surgery. 3rd ed. Toronto: BC Decker, 1987:358–361.

Bernard R. Marsh, M.D.

BRONCHIAL LASER USE

Several types of lasers are currently being used for treatment of assorted tracheobronchial lesions. The CO_2 and Nd:YAG instruments are in common use, whereas the argon-dye, KTP, and other lasers have more selective application. The Nd:YAG laser is probably the most efficient and versatile instrument for use in the adult with obstructing airway tumors. We describe this instrument below.

Indications

Indications include intraluminal tracheobronchial tumor obstruction and localized short stenosis.

Preoperative Considerations

Review the chest x-ray study and check the position and degree of obstruction. Obtain pulmonary function tests, blood gas values, and other routine laboratory studies. Discuss the anesthesia technique with the anesthesiologist. Position the patient in the supine position with the head over a head rest. Test fire the laser instrument. Be sure that everyone, including the patient, is wearing protective goggles.

Operative Steps

A special laser bronchoscope should be used that will accommodate ventilation, a laser fiber, suction tubing, and a telescope (Fig. 11A). After induction of general anesthesia, the bronchoscope may be introduced. To reduce the anesthetic gas leak, a wet pharyngeal gauze pack may be placed. If the obstruction is within the trachea, ventilation may be difficult and it may be necessary to force the bronchoscope beyond the tumor and to begin treatment at the distal tumor margin. The suction tubing and laser fiber should be positioned within view of the telescope near the distal end of the bronchoscope (Fig. 11B). The laser should be set for the desired effect, either coagulation or resection. Friable tumor should first be coagulated (low power—30 W) with long (1 to 1.5 sec) shots. The laser fiber is passed just distal to the tip of the bronchoscope, and treatment is begun in the center of the lesion. Care is taken to keep the firing angle as nearly parallel as possible to the tracheal wall, especially posteriorly, where there is no cartilage to protect against esophageal injury. Fragments of coagulated tumor are then mechanically shaved off by the lip of the bronchoscope and removed by suction or forceps. The base of the tumor can then be resected by short bursts of the laser (0.5 to 0.8 sec) at high power (40 to 50 W). Hemostasis can be provided by thorough coagulation at low power. Great care must be exercised to prevent blood from reaching the tip of the laser fiber. The slightest suspicion of blood requires fiber removal and cleaning. Otherwise the tip of the fiber may be ruined by heat. Skillful use of the suction tube and bronchoscope will minimize this hazard. Finally, the field should be suctioned or lavaged free of any debris. The fiberoptic bronchoscope may be useful at this point.

Postoperative Care

Give the patient oxygen by face mask in the recovery room. Hypoxemia is the main hazard, and intubation and positive pressure ventilation are sometimes required. Overnight hospitalization is frequently advisable.

Plate 27

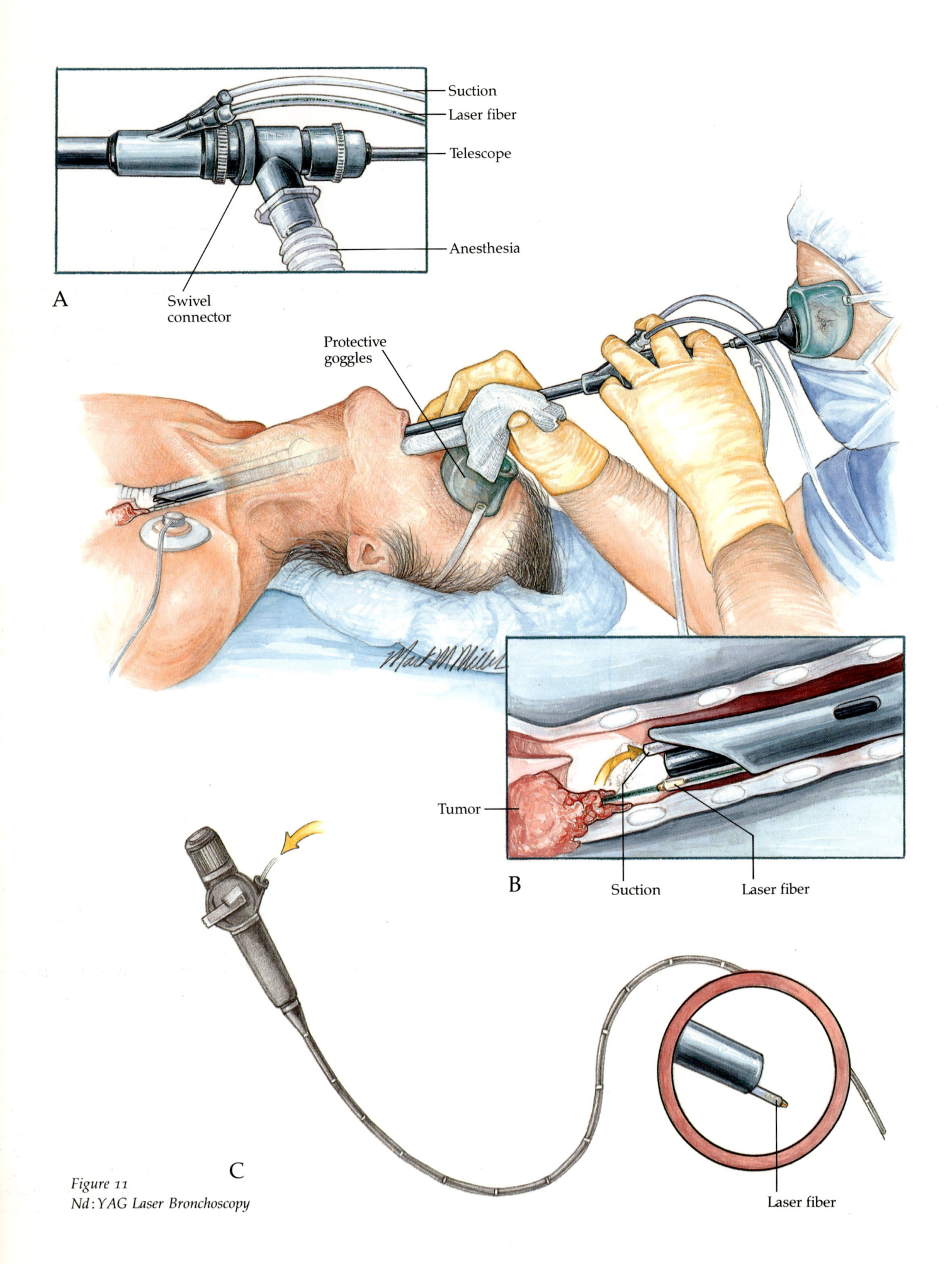

- Suction
- Laser fiber
- Telescope
- Anesthesia

A

Swivel connector

Protective goggles

Tumor

B

Suction   Laser fiber

C

Laser fiber

Figure 11
Nd:YAG Laser Bronchoscopy

66

Risks, Complications, and Sequelae

1. Bleeding can become life-threatening. Use of a rigid bronchoscope permits tamponade, good suction, and ventilation. When possible, the suction tube can be placed on the bleeding site while laser coagulation is begun around the periphery of the bleeding site, gradually closing in on the center.
2. Perforation of the airway is usually prevented by avoiding firing the laser perpendicular to the wall and by avoiding using power settings higher than 50 W. Continuous laser mode should not be used in the airway.
3. Flammable materials in the laser path, especially in the presence of increased oxygen concentrations, create a risk of fire. This is of great concern when using the fiberscope with the laser.
4. In order to avoid eye injury, strict controls must be enforced on all personnel concerning proper use of goggles. Unauthorized entry into the laser treatment area must be prevented.

Pearls and Pitfalls

Never attempt to treat airway tumors causing extrinsic compression, only tumors of the lumen with a patent distal airway.

Avoid treating tumors of the segmental bronchi. Risks of perforation are high and potential benefits are minimal in most patients.

The fiberscope may be used to treat smaller lesions under local anesthesia, but oxygen concentrations must be kept below 30 percent and great care taken to ensure that the laser fiber is well outside the channel when the laser is fired. Power levels should be kept low, and repeated treatments may be necessary to accomplish a satisfactory result (Fig. 11C).

Always have a spare fiber available for use in case one becomes inoperative during the course of treatment.

Suggested Reading

Brutinel WM, McDougall JC, Cortese DA. Bronchoscopic therapy with neodymium yttrium-aluminum-garnet laser during intravenous anesthesia. Chest 1983; 84:518–521.

Casey KR, Fairfax WR, Smith SJ, Dixon JA. Intratracheal fire ignited by the Nd-YAG laser during treatment of tracheal stenosis. Chest 1983; 84:295–296.

Dumon JF. YAG laser bronchoscopy. Vol. 5. Surgical science series. New York: Praeger, 1985.

Ossoff R, Davis O, Vrabec J. Laser surgery. In: Johns ME, ed. Complications in otolaryngology—head and neck surgery. 2nd ed. Toronto: BC Decker, 1986:93–101.

Shapshay SM. Laser applications in the trachea and bronchi; a comparative study of the soft tissue effects using contact and noncontact delivery systems. Laryngoscope 1987; 97(Suppl 41):1–26.

Shapshay SM, Dumon JF, Beamis JF. Endoscopic treatment of tracheobronchial malignancy—experience with Nd-YAG and CO_2 lasers in 506 operations. Otolaryngol Head Neck Surg 1985; 93:205–210.

Bernard R. Marsh, M.D.

DIAGNOSTIC ESOPHAGOSCOPY

Most diagnostic esophagoscopy is performed by gastroenterologists who use flexible fiberoptic panendoscopes almost exclusively. Even in children, these instruments are being used increasingly for study of the upper gastrointestinal tract. The otolaryngologist–head and neck surgeon finds that some patients are best served by use of the open tube esophagoscope. This instrument is quite commonly needed in therapeutic esophagoscopy and in diagnostic procedures, especially in the cricopharyngeal area. The otolaryngologist–head and neck surgeon must have facility in the use of both types of instruments.

Indications

Esophagoscopy is performed following a careful history, physical examination, detailed radiologic studies, and sometimes measurements of esophageal function. It is frequently used to enhance the evaluation in dysphagia, hematemesis, suspected foreign body, suspected tumor, caustic ingestion, suspicion of anatomic defects causing aspiration, vascular anomalies, tracheoesophageal fistulas, esophageal diverticula, esophagitis, and trauma.

Preoperative Considerations

Special attention is given to dental and oral structures as well as to the mobility of the jaw and cervical spine. Are there large anterior osteophytes that might create an additional risk? The patient should be positioned in the supine position and as close to the head of the table as possible for use of rigid scopes. General anesthesia for open tube technique should be provided by means of a relatively small endotracheal tube secured to the left side of the face. Local anesthesia and sedation with the patient in a left lateral decubitus position are preferred for flexible esophagoscopy. The head should be elevated on a small pillow, the eyes covered, and a head towel applied. All instruments should be checked by the surgeon.

Operative Steps

The cervical spine should be flexed by a small pillow and the head extended. A gauze sponge or other protection should be placed over the upper teeth and the esophagoscope lubricated as desired. The esophagoscope is then placed almost vertically in the right side of the mouth using the fingers of the left hand to protect the upper lip and the thumb to limit pressure on the upper teeth. The right hand is used to stabilize the proximal end of the esophagoscope. The surgeon's right eye (with a right-handed surgeon) is used for viewing through the scope. Both of the operator's eyes are kept open. The tip of the epiglottis should be raised by the lip of the scope to expose the right arytenoid and piriform sinus. The neck is extended further to allow the scope to pass to the right lateral side of the right arytenoid and into the piriform sinus. Maximum extension of the head on the spine is now provided by pressure of the right hand over the occiput (the head is still on a pillow). The scope is angled further forward by simultaneous lowering of the right hand and greater anterior thrust with the left thumb. This maneuver permits exposure of the cricopharyngeal sphincter. Great care must be taken at this point to avoid perforation. Gentle technique and patience are required. The only advancing force is provided by the left thumb. Direct vision of the lumen must be maintained at all times. If there is uncertainty as to orientation, a filiform bougie may be gently inserted to confirm the correct axis but *not* to act as a stent over which the scope can be forced. This part of the procedure can be difficult in the aged, arthritic patient with a thick neck and a full set of teeth. When these features are present, you may want to consider using a flexible scope.

As the esophagoscope is advanced, the cricopharyngeus opens to permit a view of the now open esophagus. If one is using an instrument permitting air insufflation, a greater area can be seen, making for easier comparison between proximal and more distal mucosal changes. When the examination reaches the thoracic esophagus, the patient's head is moved from the high position to a low position (Fig. 12A). In the lower esophagus, not only the head but also the shoulders may need to be lowered below the table level to straighten the thoracic spine and keep the instrument off the posterior wall. The head may be moved to the right to allow passage to the left and anteriorly into the gastroesophageal junction and stomach. Here again, gentle technique and a clear lumen ahead are essential to avoid perforation. Many congenital and acquired abnor-

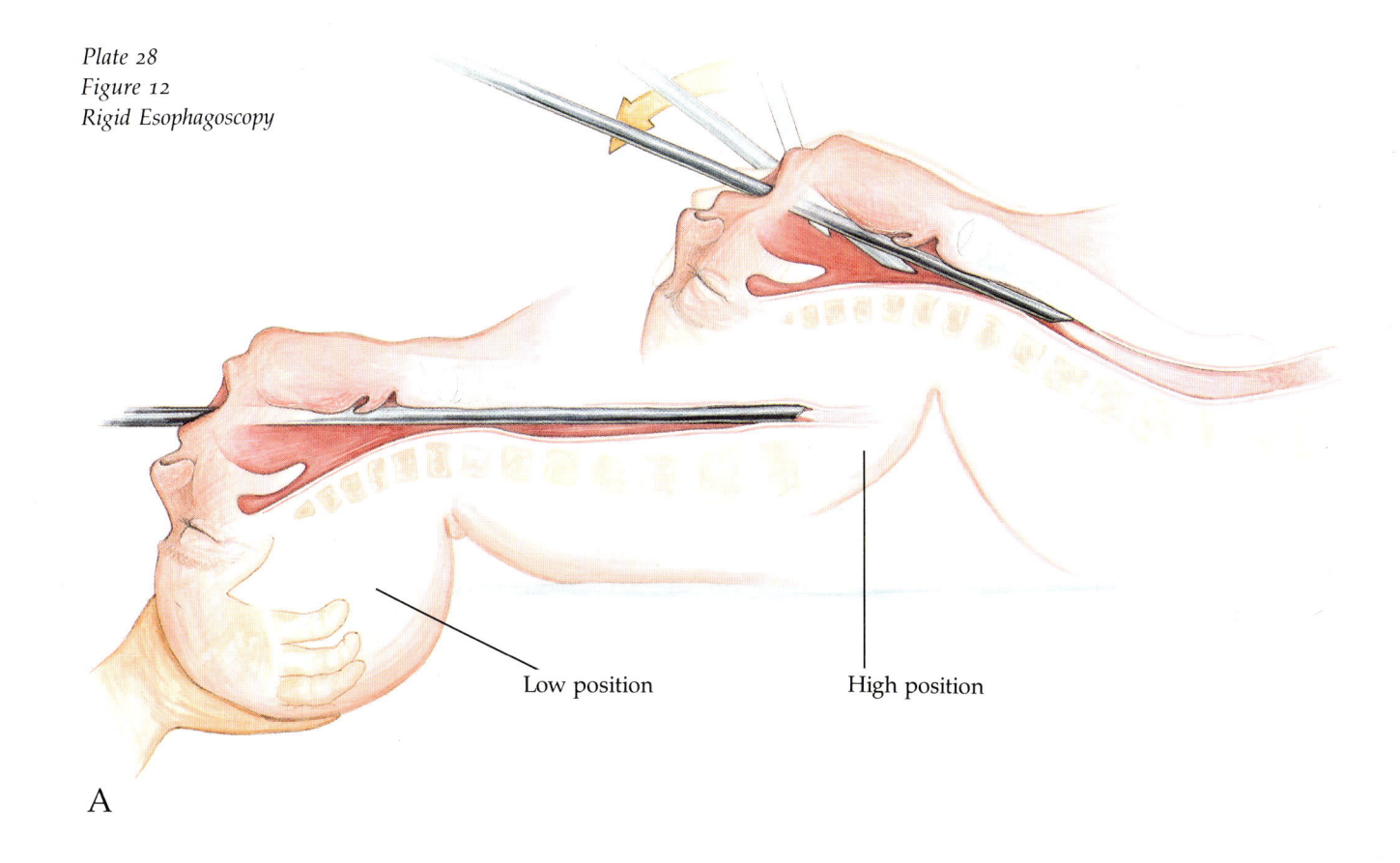

Plate 28
Figure 12
Rigid Esophagoscopy

Low position   High position

A

malities occur in this area, and a thorough understanding of the x-ray studies is a prerequisite to this study. It is not always possible or necessary to see the gastric mucosa with a rigid esophagoscope, but this can usually be achieved if it is indicated. A telescope is often helpful in the recognition of less apparent mucosal changes (Fig. 12B).

As the instrument is withdrawn, a second look should be made for previously unrecognized pathology. The head and neck positioning are reversed from that of insertion. Cytology and appropriate biopsy specimens or samples for cultures may be obtained as appropriate.

Postoperative Care

Check the mouth for any dental injuries, and obtain a chest radiograph. When the patient is recovered, instruct him or her to report any chest or back pain.

Plate 29
Figure 12 (Continued)
Rigid Esophagoscopy

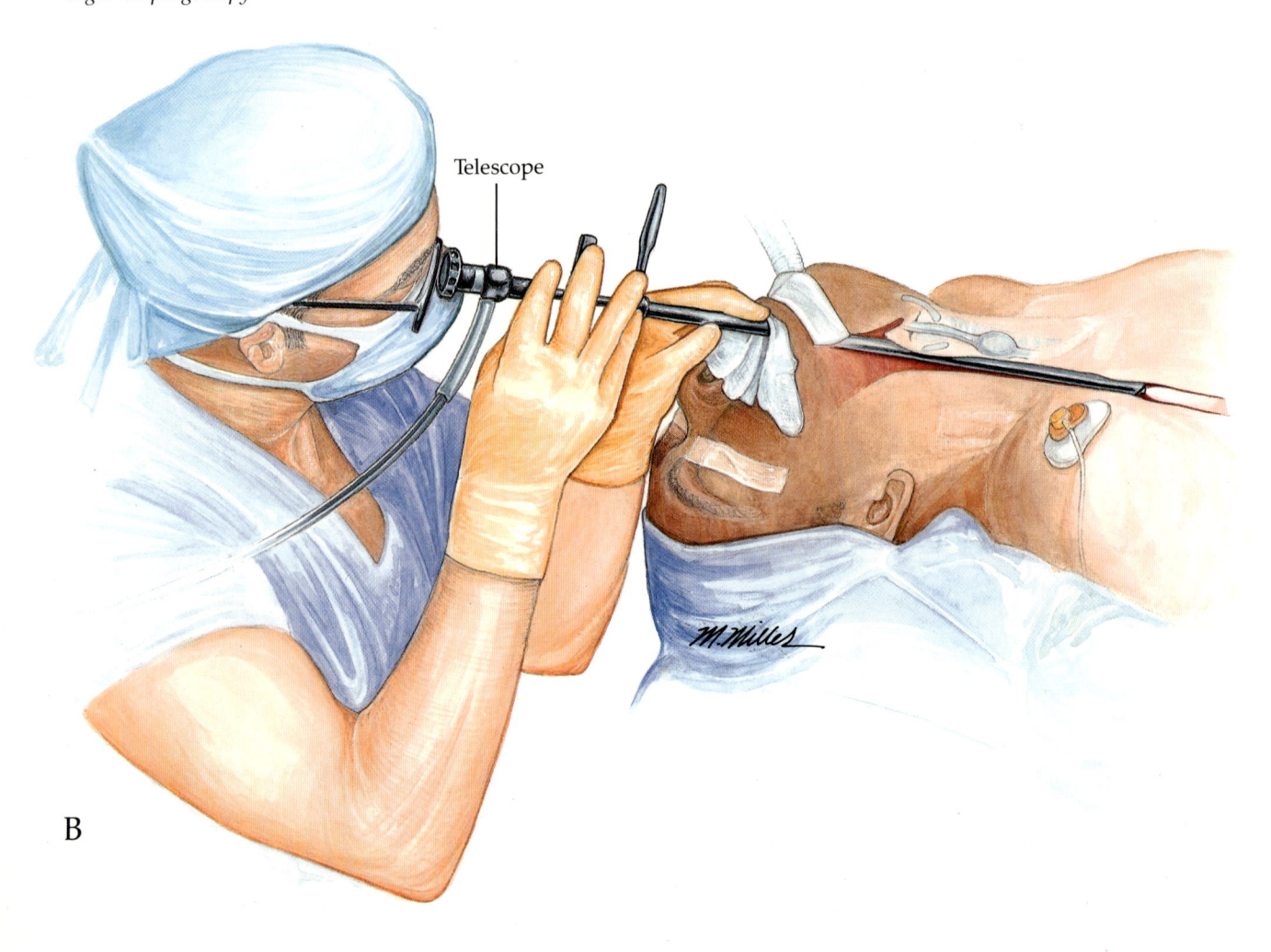

B

Risks, Complications, and Sequelae

Problems resulting from diagnostic esophagoscopy include esophageal perforation, dental injury, bleeding, and an overlooked lesion or foreign body.

Pearls and Pitfalls

If difficulty is encountered, terminate the procedure. It is not a disgrace if you fail to complete the study; it is far more important to avoid the risk of a catastrophic perforation.

If anything unusual occurs to create concern about a possible perforation, obtain a contrast x-ray study as soon as possible and request thoracic surgical consultation.

Have a flexible scope available in case your planned approach does not work out.

Discovery of an upper or midesophageal tumor should be followed immediately by bronchoscopy to determine whether extension has occurred.

Remember that esophageal tumors extend submucosally a considerable distance from the visible lesion. A biopsy performed proximal to the lesion may help in planning treatment.

Suggested Reading

Ballenger J. Diseases of the nose, throat, ear, head and neck. 13th ed. Philadelphia: Lea & Febiger, 1985;1354–1381.

Blackstone M. Endoscopic interpretation. New York: Raven Press, 1984.

Jackson C, Jackson CL. Bronchoesophagology. Philadelphia: WB Saunders, 1950.

Bernard R. Marsh, M.D.

REMOVAL OF ESOPHAGEAL FOREIGN BODIES

Foreign bodies of the esophagus are common in children who put inedible objects into their mouths. The edentulous adult is also not infrequently a victim of bones and other inedible objects whose transit through the mouth may be unrecognized until they are already within the pharyngeal constrictors. Most of these objects lodge just below the relatively powerful cricopharyngeus within the weaker upper esophagus. The next most common location is just above the gastroesophageal junction. Other locations include the sites of crossing the aortic arch and the left main bronchus. Pre-existing esophageal disease may also predispose to lodgment of a foreign body.

Indications

Suspicion of an esophageal foreign body with or without radiographic confirmation.

Preoperative Considerations

Good quality plain radiographs should be obtained to include posteroanterior and lateral chest as well as posteroanterior and lateral neck views. Rarely, a computed tomographic or an esophageal contrast study may be required. If a radiopaque foreign body is present, fluoroscopy should be available. The anesthesiology staff should be consulted about endotracheal tube size and placement as well as risk of regurgitation and aspiration during induction. If the foreign body is a metallic object such as an open safety pin, a duplicate should be obtained and forceps tested on the table before the patient is anesthetized. A chest radiograph must be taken immediately before induction of anesthesia to determine whether a radiopaque object has passed into the stomach.

Operative Steps

I prefer a Jesberg esophagoscope for most esophageal foreign bodies, but flexible instruments play a useful role in selected cases. The proper size instrument and appropriate forceps should be selected and tested. A laryngoscope and bronchoscope should also be made ready. Under general endotracheal anesthesia, the patient is positioned with the cervical spine flexed and the head extended. The upper teeth or gingivae should be protected by a tooth guard or moist sponge. The esophagoscope should be carefully introduced, as described in the section Diagnostic Esophagoscopy (Fig. 13). A foreign body at the cricopharyngeus can sometimes be exposed more easily with a laryngoscope. This is often the case with a coin.

Care should be taken not to displace the object distally, but the tip of the esophagoscope should be positioned close enough to the foreign body to provide good exposure and proper forceps application. Sharp objects, such as an open safety pin, must be removed either by endogastric version or by sheathing the point to prevent perforation. Other techniques have been described, but all require extensive practice and proficiency before attempting a clinical case. Unless the foreign body can be removed through the lumen of the instrument, extraction should proceed with the foreign body held as close as possible to the tip of the scope, and both should be rotated so as to bring the largest diameter of the object into the transverse plane. Following extraction, the scope should be replaced to determine whether or not any other pathologic condition remains.

Postoperative Care

In the case of sharp foreign bodies, difficult extractions, and whenever there is any suspicion of perforation or residual disease, a postoperative contrast x-ray study is recommended before resumption of eating by the patient. Instructions should be given for the patient to return to the hospital immediately if chest, back pain, fever, or dyspnea develops.

Risks, Complications, and Sequelae

Problems resulting from these procedures include esophageal perforation, unrecognized foreign body, dental injury, loss of the foreign body into the stomach, and airway obstruction.

Pearls and Pitfalls

The Foley catheter technique of foreign body removal is potentially dangerous and not recommended.

Occasionally a fiberoptic technique may prove useful in passing a large tube over a sharp foreign body in order to protect against injury during extraction.

Plate 30
Figure 13
Esophagoscopy for Foreign Body

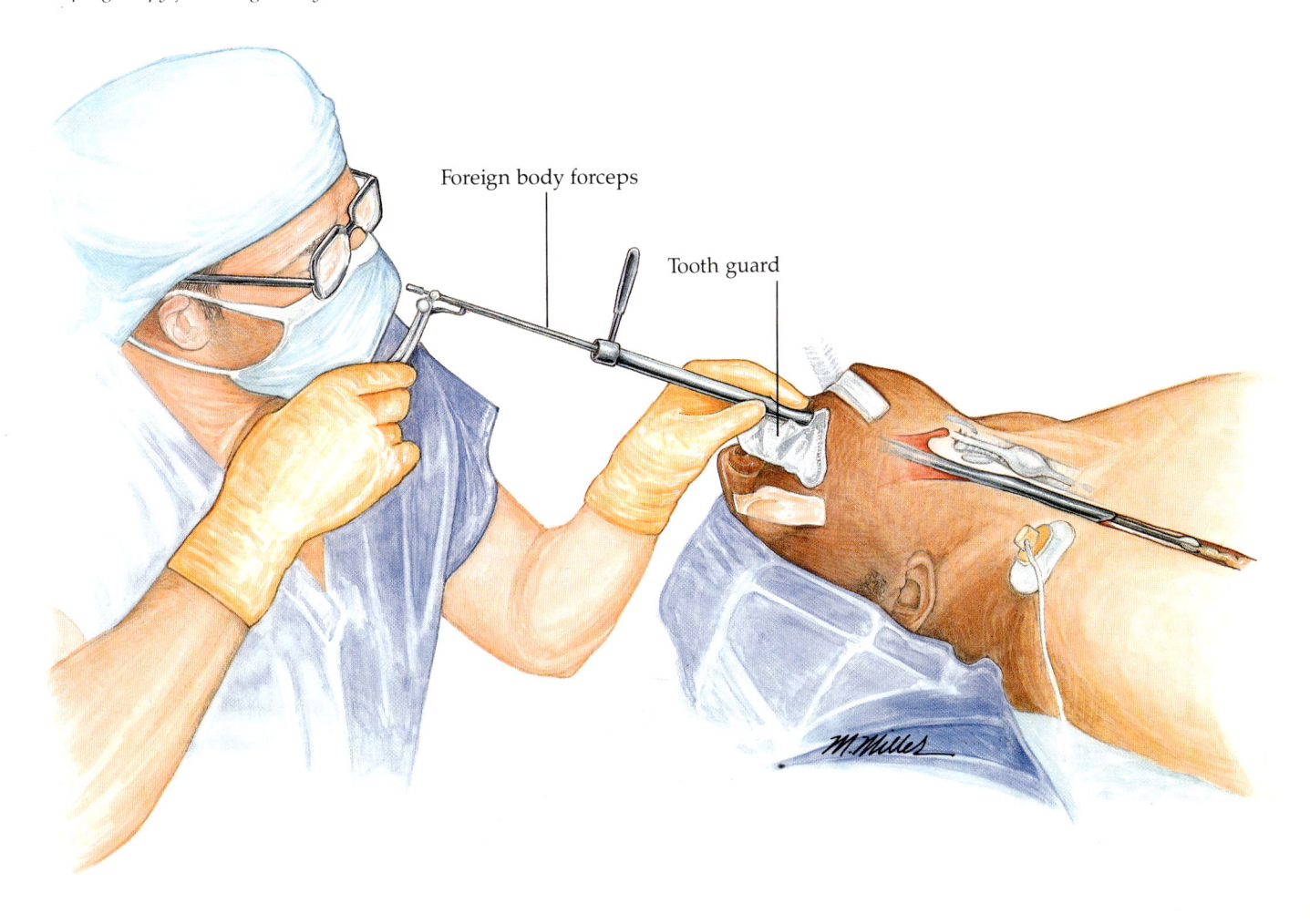

When appropriate, do not hesitate to displace an esophageal foreign body into the stomach rather than risk potential perforation.

Always have fluoroscopy available for radiopaque objects, especially when attempting endogastric version and extraction.

Be careful to avoid catching mucosa within the forceps.

Endogastric version and extraction with a fiberscope is my preference for removing most open safety pins.

Suggested Reading

Jackson C, Jackson CL. Bronchoesophagology. Philadelphia: WB Saunders, 1950.

Bernard R. Marsh, M.D.

TREATMENT OF ESOPHAGEAL CAUSTIC BURNS

Children usually ingest caustic substances by accident, whereas adults occasionally attempt suicide by this means. Sodium hydroxide, as found in various household cleaning agents, is notorious for causing severe burns, but many other chemical bases and acids also are potentially injurious. Basic substances penetrate tissue deeply by liquefaction necrosis that may perforate the esophagus. Acids produce a coagulation necrosis that tends to limit penetration; nevertheless, severe complications including gastric perforation may result. The severity of the injury is probably most dependent upon (1) the agent, (2) the quantity and concentration ingested, and (3) the duration time the substance is in contact with tissue. Management remains controversial.

Indications

The history of ingestion of a potentially dangerous caustic substance requires immediate investigation.

Preoperative Considerations

An accurate determination of the agent and amount ingested should be found out if possible. Perform a complete physical examination of the patient, with special attention given to the airway (mouth, pharynx, and larynx) and to evidence of complications. Perform a chest radiograph and order a cineradiologic contrast study to include the stomach and duodenum if a severe burn is suspected. Replace fluid, electrolytes, and blood, as necessary. Perform endoscopy promptly.

Operative Steps

Administer general anesthesia. Carefully evaluate the hypopharynx, larynx, and piriform sinuses (Fig. 14A). Pass the Jesberg esophagoscope; stop at the first significant burn, which is usually seen at locations of anatomic narrowing (Figs. 14B and 14C). In experienced hands a small-caliber flexible gastroscope may be safer than a rigid instrument and permits passage through minimally burned areas to provide a more complete assessment of the extent of the burn, including the stomach and duodenum. Perform a tracheotomy if necessary for a compromised airway.

Postoperative Care

Give antibiotics and steroids for a significant burn. Perform a cineradiologic barium study to further assess the extent of the burn if it was not obtained preoperatively. Feed liquids and a soft diet when the patient's condition permits.

Repeat the cineradiologic barium study in 3 weeks. If stricture is developing, stop the steroids and begin dilation with great care. Severe strictures may require gastrostomy and retrograde dilation with Tucker bougies. Multiple strictures are usually refractory to dilation, and esophageal replacement should be considered early. Obtain thoracic surgical consultation for severe burns.

Plate 31

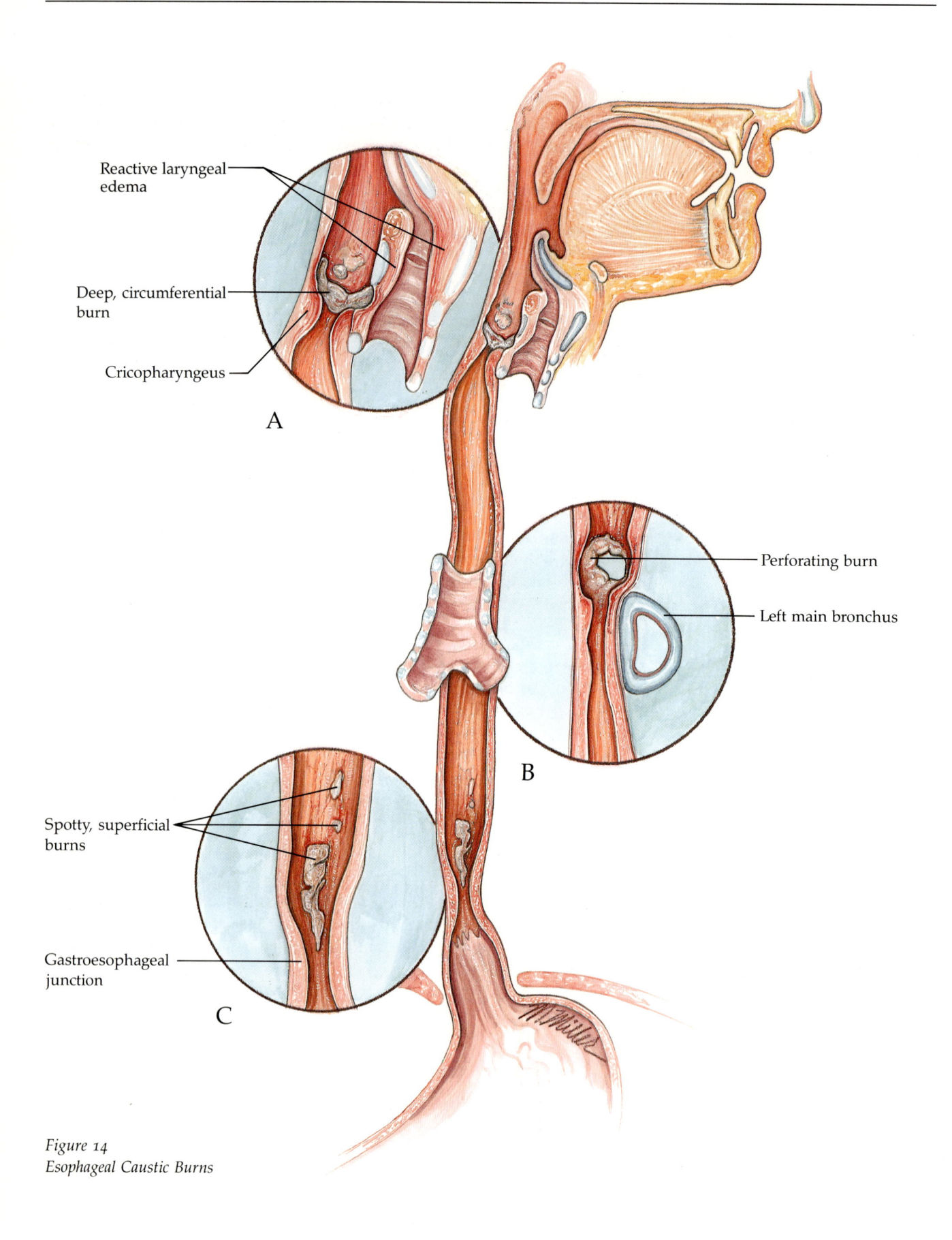

Reactive laryngeal edema

Deep, circumferential burn

Cricopharyngeus

A

Perforating burn

Left main bronchus

B

Spotty, superficial burns

Gastroesophageal junction

C

Figure 14
Esophageal Caustic Burns

Risks, Complications, and Sequelae

Problems resulting from treatment of esophageal caustic burns include esophageal or gastric perforation, failure to appreciate the full extent of the burn, airway obstruction, and fistulas, abscesses, and strictures later on.

Pearls and Pitfalls

Do not pass the instrument beyond the first severe burn.

Sodium hypochlorite (household bleach) rarely, if ever, causes significant esophageal injury.

Radiographic studies with water-soluble contrast agent should be used to evaluate the extent of injury beyond the safe limit of endoscopy.

Steroids are unnecessary in superficial burns and are contraindicated in severe burns.

The risk of developing esophageal carcinoma 24 years after lye ingestion is increased 1,000-fold.

Early esophagectomy or gastrectomy may be a necessary lifesaving measure in some severe burns.

Suggested Reading

Appleqvist P, Salmo M. Lye corrosion carcinoma of the esophagus; A review of 63 cases. Cancer 1980; 45:2655–2658.

Goldman L, Weigert J. Corrosive substance ingestion: A review. Am J Gastroenterol 1984; 79:85–90.

Hawkins D, Demeter M, Barnett T. Caustic ingestion; controversies in management. A review of 214 cases. Laryngoscope 1980; 90:98–109.

Moazam F, Talbert J, Miller D, Mollitt D. Caustic ingestion and its sequelae in children. South Med J 1987; 80:187–190.

Oakes D, Sherck J, Mark J. Lye ingestion—clinical patterns and therapeutic implications. J Thorac Cardiovasc Surg 1982; 83:194–204.

Postlethwait R. Chemical burns of the esophagus. Surg Clin North Am 1983; 63:915–924.

Thompson J. Corrosive esophageal injuries; A study of nine cases of concurrent accidental caustic ingestion. Laryngoscope 1987; 97:1060–1068.

Thompson J. Corrosive esophageal injuries; II, An investigation of treatment methods and histochemical analysis of esophageal structures in a new animal model. Laryngoscope 1987; 97:1191–1202.

Chapter II
FUNCTIONAL ENDOSCOPIC SINUS SURGERY

David W. Kennedy, M.D.
Jordan S. Josephson, M.D.

DIAGNOSTIC NASAL ENDOSCOPY

The principles of the functional approach to sinus disease were appreciated by early otolaryngologists, and the rationale for considering the anterior ethmoid–middle meatal area (ostiomeatal unit) as the key to sinus disease has also been recognized for some time. However, it was not until 1978 that the first systematic and detailed work documenting endoscopic findings was published in the English literature by Messerklinger.

The term functional endoscopic sinus surgery denotes an approach in which the major objective is the re-establishment of sinus ventilation and mucociliary clearance. The surgery is tailored to the individual pathology. The most significant advance in the functional endoscopic sinus approach is the advantage gained from more accurate diagnosis. The other important advantages are the ability to preserve normal structures, the decreased need for wide exposure during surgery, and the ability to provide direct and meticulous postoperative care to the diseased areas.

The key to the functional endoscopic technique is accurate diagnosis of areas of mucociliary or ventilatory obstruction. The importance of the well-defined patterns of mucociliary clearance has been shown by Messerklinger. The role of impaired ventilation in the pathogenesis of acute, recurrent, and chronic sinusitis has been well documented by Carenfeldt, Aust, and Drettner. Based on these principles, particular care must be taken to search for areas of localized inflammation or anatomic deformities within the ostiomeatal complex that may cause secondary infection, either chronic or recurrent acute sinusitis (Fig. 1A).

Indications

Comprehensive nasal endoscopy not only identifies patients requiring surgical intervention but also provides objective information about response to medical therapy. When necessary, it allows for accurate culture and tissue biopsy. The response to steroid and/or antibiotic therapy may be visualized with greater accuracy than with anterior rhinoscopy. Cases that are selected for surgery are those that have failed to resolve with medical therapy and those that have anatomic abnormalities requiring surgical correction. Following surgery, endoscopy allows early treatment of residual or recurrent disease within the ostiomeatal complex.

Despite the superb optical quality of rigid endonasal telescopes, there are important limitations to endoscopic examination. These include a frequent inability to visualize the maxillary ostium, as it is typically hidden behind the uncinate process, and a limited view of the ethmoidal infundibulum. Deeper ethmoid sinus involvement cannot be evaluated, and disease within a severely constricted or scarred middle meatus may not be visualized. Thus adjunctive computed tomographic (CT) studies are frequently required. On the other hand, endoscopy provides more accurate information than CT about areas that can be seen, and CT frequently demonstrates incidental asymptomatic areas of mucosal thickening. The additional valuable information provided by performing routine endoscopic nasal examination in addition to anterior rhinoscopy suggests that the former will soon become a standard of care for patients with nasal complaints.

Plate 32

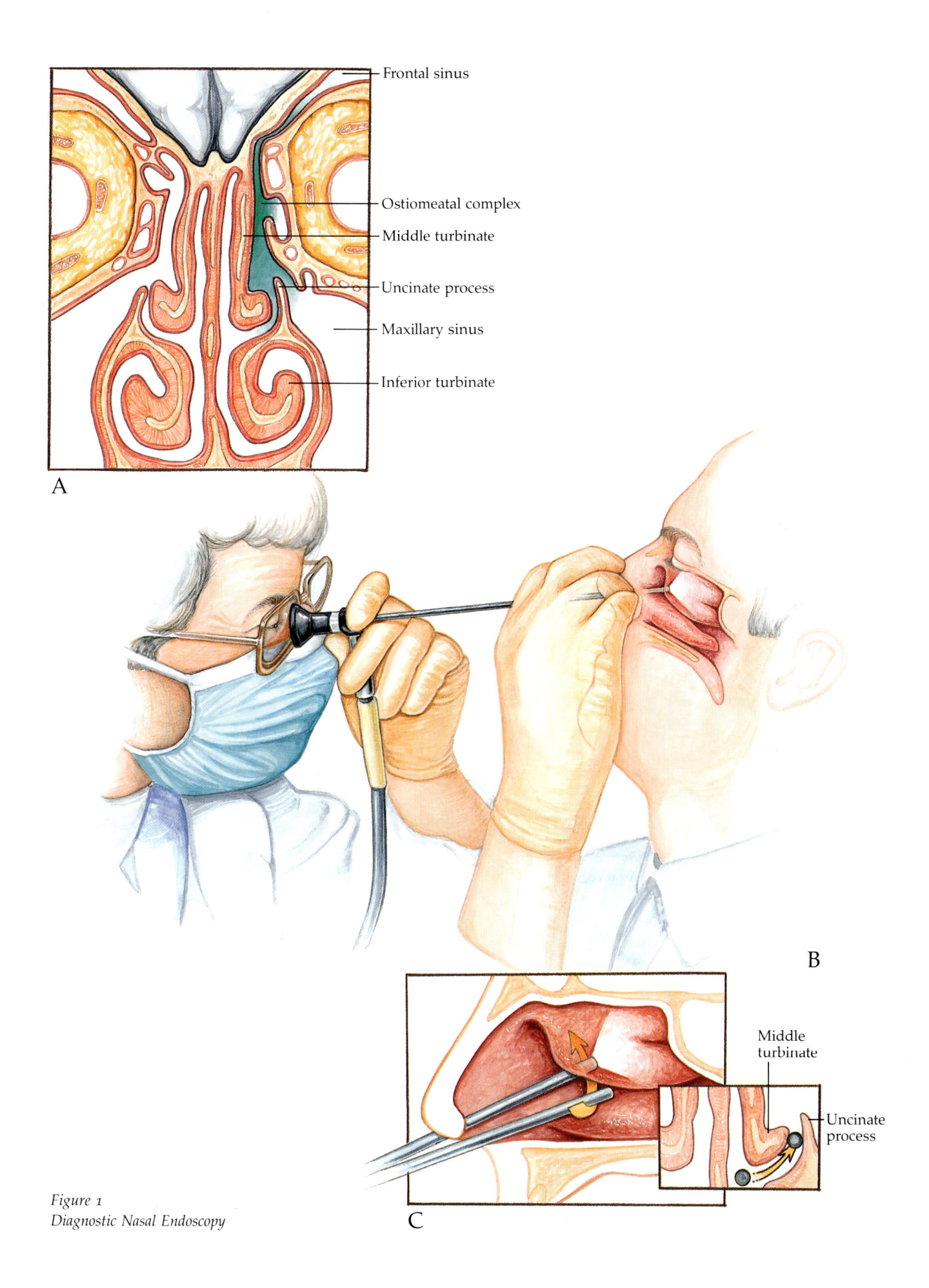

- Frontal sinus
- Ostiomeatal complex
- Middle turbinate
- Uncinate process
- Maxillary sinus
- Inferior turbinate

A

B

C

Middle turbinate
Uncinate process

Figure 1
Diagnostic Nasal Endoscopy

Technique

Systemic nasal endoscopy may be performed with the patient in the sitting or supine position using rigid Hopkins* telescopes (Fig. 1B). These are preferred over the flexible scopes because of their superior optical resolution and varied angles of view and because it is easier to introduce other instrumentation concurrently. The endoscopes are available with 0-, 30-, 70-, and 120-degree deflected angles and in 2.7-mm and 4.0-mm sizes, with the exception of the 120-degree scope (4.0 mm only). The examiner should always take appropriate precautions when dealing with secretions and blood. Gloves, a mask and gown, and eye protection are recommended. The patient's nose is decongested and anesthetized using sprays (tetracaine [Pontocaine] 2.0 percent and xylometazoline [Otrivin] 0.5 percent). Topical cocaine 5 percent on nasal applicators may also be used in areas where the scopes may exert pressure, such as the inferior aspect of the middle turbinate. A complete examination can be successfully accomplished in an organized manner with three passes of the endoscope.

The 4.0-mm 30-degree telescope is selected first and is passed posteriorly along the floor of the nose. Overall nasal anatomy should be evaluated and the presence of pathologic secretions and the condition of the nasal mucosa observed. Examination of the inferior meatus allows identification of the nasolacrimal duct orifice. Localization may be aided by digital pressure over the lacrimal sac. Inflammation here suggests agger nasi cell infection. A patent antrostomy allows visualization of the antral mucosa, and the sinus may be further evaluated by changing to a 70-degree endoscope. As the endoscope is passed into the nasopharynx, any secretions on the lateral nasal wall can be identified. The tubal orifice and its dynamic action during swallowing may also be visualized.

A second pass of the telescope is performed below the middle turbinate and then into the sphenoethmoidal recess. Anteriorly, the uncinate process and anterior middle meatus are seen. More posteriorly, the fontanelles and inferior aspect of the hiatus semilunaris can be visualized. From the sphenoethmoidal recess, the sphenoid sinus ostium and posterior ethmoid cells can be studied.

The third pass is made as the telescope is withdrawn. The middle meatus is rarely wide enough to permit endoscopic entry and examination from the anterior aspect. The telescope is inserted into the posterior aspect of the middle meatus by rolling the endoscope inferiorly under the middle turbinate and into the middle meatus (Fig. 1C). A 2.7-mm 30- or 70-degree telescope with or without gentle subluxation of the middle turbinate may be required, and occasionally the middle meatus is so constricted that no visualization is possible. Middle meatal endoscopy permits inspection of the ethmoidal bulla, the hiatus semilunaris, the infundibular opening, and occasionally the maxillary sinus ostium.

*Karl Storz Endoscopy America Inc., Culver City, California.

Significant endoscopic findings that do not resolve with medical therapy or a well-documented history of chronic or recurrent acute sinusitis requires adjunctive CT. This is needed to evaluate properly deeper pathology not visualized with the telescopes, and when surgery is indicated, to detail the anatomy and extent of disease. The study is most beneficial if performed after the acute episode has resolved.

Suggested Reading

Aust R, Drettner B. Oxygen tension in the human maxillary sinus under normal and pathological conditions. Acta Otolaryngol (Stockh) 1974; 78:264–269.

Carenfeldt C. Pathogenesis of sinus empyema. Ann Otol 1979; 88:16–20.

Draf W. Endoscopy of the paranasal sinuses. New York: Springer Verlag, 1983.

Drettner B. The permeability of the maxillary ostium. Acta Otolaryngol (Stockh) 1965; 60:304–314.

Kennedy DW. Functional endoscopic sinus surgery: Technique. Arch Otolaryngol 1985; 111:643–649.

Messerklinger W. On the drainage of the normal frontal sinus of man. Acta Otolaryngol (Stockh) 1967; 63:176–181.

David W. Kennedy, M.D.
Jordan S. Josephson, M.D.

MAXILLARY AND SPHENOID SINUSCOPY

Indications

Maxillary sinus endoscopy is of diagnostic benefit in the case in which an unusual radiographic finding is present or if medical therapy fails to resolve maxillary sinus opacification. Endoscopy of the maxillary sinus can contribute to the early diagnosis of antral tumors or be helpful in the search for an unknown primary tumor. However, maxillary sinus endoscopy is not a routine part of nasal endoscopy. In cases of suspected malignancy, an inferior meatal entrance may be preferable to prevent the risk of sublabial seeding.

Operative Steps

In adults a 5.00-mm trocar and cannula are typically used with a 30- or a 70-degree 4.00-mm endoscope. A 3.3-mm trocar and cannula with a 2.7-mm telescope are substituted in children. The sublabial approach provides the best visualization of the area of the ostium and the greatest arc of rotation for inspection of the sinus; therefore it is generally preferred. Therapeutic intervention for more diffuse disease is more typically performed by access through a widened middle meatal antrostomy at the end of a procedure on the ostiomeatal complex.

A topical anesthetic applied to the sublabial mucosa, followed by sublabial injection of 1 percent lidocaine with 1:100,000 epinephrine into the area adjacent to the infraorbital nerve, provides excellent anesthesia. The canine fossa is identified digitally, and the trocar is inserted into the upper lateral part so as to avoid the infraorbital nerve. The nerve should also be digitally palpated prior to trocar insertion (Fig. 2A). The trocar is then inserted using gentle pressure and a to-and-fro rotation until the sinus is entered. A prewarmed and antifogged 4.0-mm endoscope is inserted through the trocar (Fig. 2B). Masses, cysts, fluid, or other pathologic conditions are identified. Following traces of blood allows examination of the flow of mucociliary clearance. Purulent or mucoid material may be removed through the trocar with a No. 10 tracheal suction. If a cyst is present, a sharpened No. 10 tracheal catheter may be used to puncture the cyst and aspirate the contents. Puncturing a small cyst may be therapeutic, but removal is recommended for larger cysts. Removal may be performed by aiming the trocar at the lesion with a 0-degree telescope and then exchanging the endoscope for the straight biting forceps. An entire lesion may thus be removed, re-aiming the trocar from time to time by alternating the telescope and forceps. Biopsies or removal of the last remnants of disease may also be performed under direct vision utilizing the rigid or flexible optical biopsy forceps. No sutures are required following maxillary sinus endoscopy. The patient is instructed not to blow his or her nose for several days in order to avoid subcutaneous emphysema.

Disease of the sphenoid sinus is less frequent than disease of the other paranasal sinuses. Endoscopy of the sphenoid sinus should be reserved for unusual diagnostic dilemmas, as in the case of a possible tumor. The examination may be performed after a transnasal sphenoidotomy following insertion of a trocar. Because of the many vital structures (including the optic nerve and the carotid artery) that surround the sphenoid, placement of a trocar in this area is not a procedure for the novice

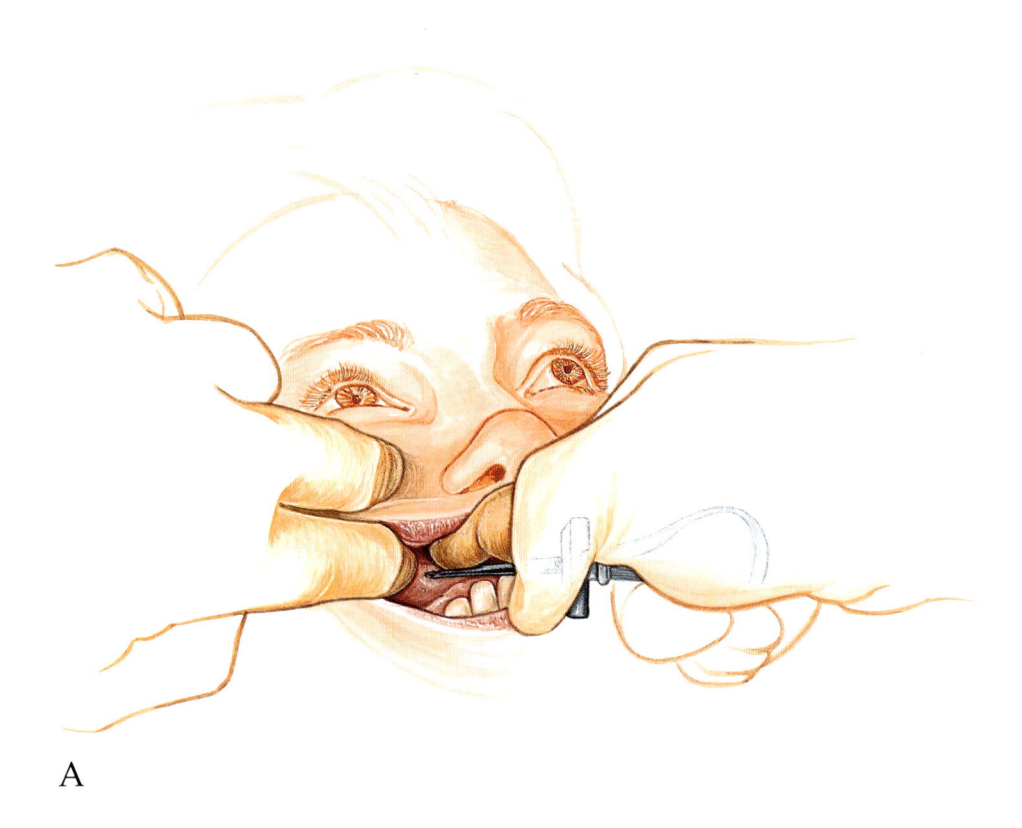

Plate 33

A

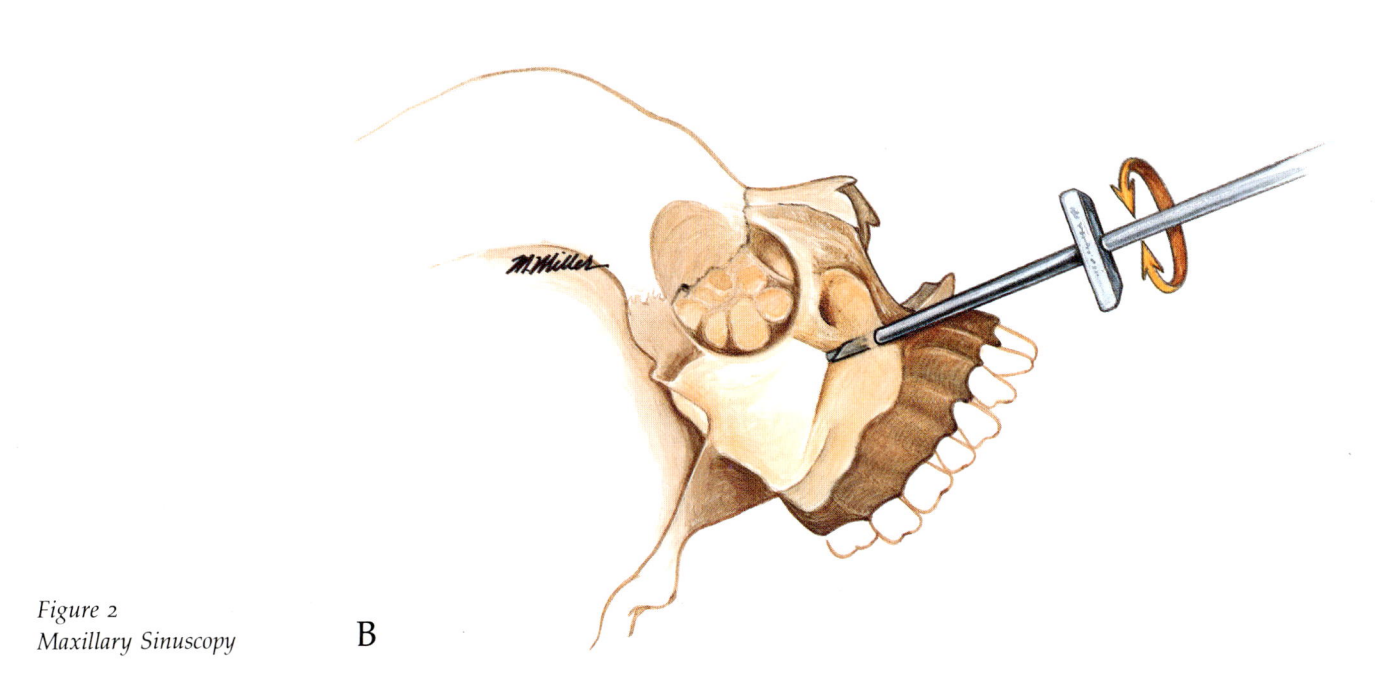

Figure 2
Maxillary Sinuscopy

B

85

endoscopist. A CT scan is essential for definition of the anatomy so that the relationship of the intersinus septa, the walls of the carotid artery, and the optic nerve can be carefully analyzed.

Local anesthesia is provided by cocaine on nasal applicators applied to the nose and the anterior wall of the sphenoid sinus. Infiltration of the anterior wall of the sphenoid sinus may be performed with 1 percent lidocaine and 1:100,000 epinephrine administered by a tonsil needle.

The surgeon first identifies the sphenoid sinus ostium with the 30-degree telescope and then places the trocar and cannula onto the anterior wall just inferior to the ostium (Figs. 2C and D). The telescope is removed and the trocar inserted, with the operator using both hands for control of the depth of entry. The trocar then serves as a guide for the 30-degree or a 70-degree endoscope. The optic nerve and carotid bulge should be identified (Fig. 2E). If the ostium is not visualized or there is associated ethmoid disease, standard transethmoidal sphenoidotomy may be preferable. In the case of an extremely small sinus or when maximal exposure is required, a trans-septal route remains the approach of choice.

Suggested Reading

Messerklinger W. Endoscopy of the nose. Baltimore: Urban & Schwarzenberg, 1978.

Draf W. Endoscopy of the paranasal sinuses. New York: Springer Verlag, 1983.

Plate 34

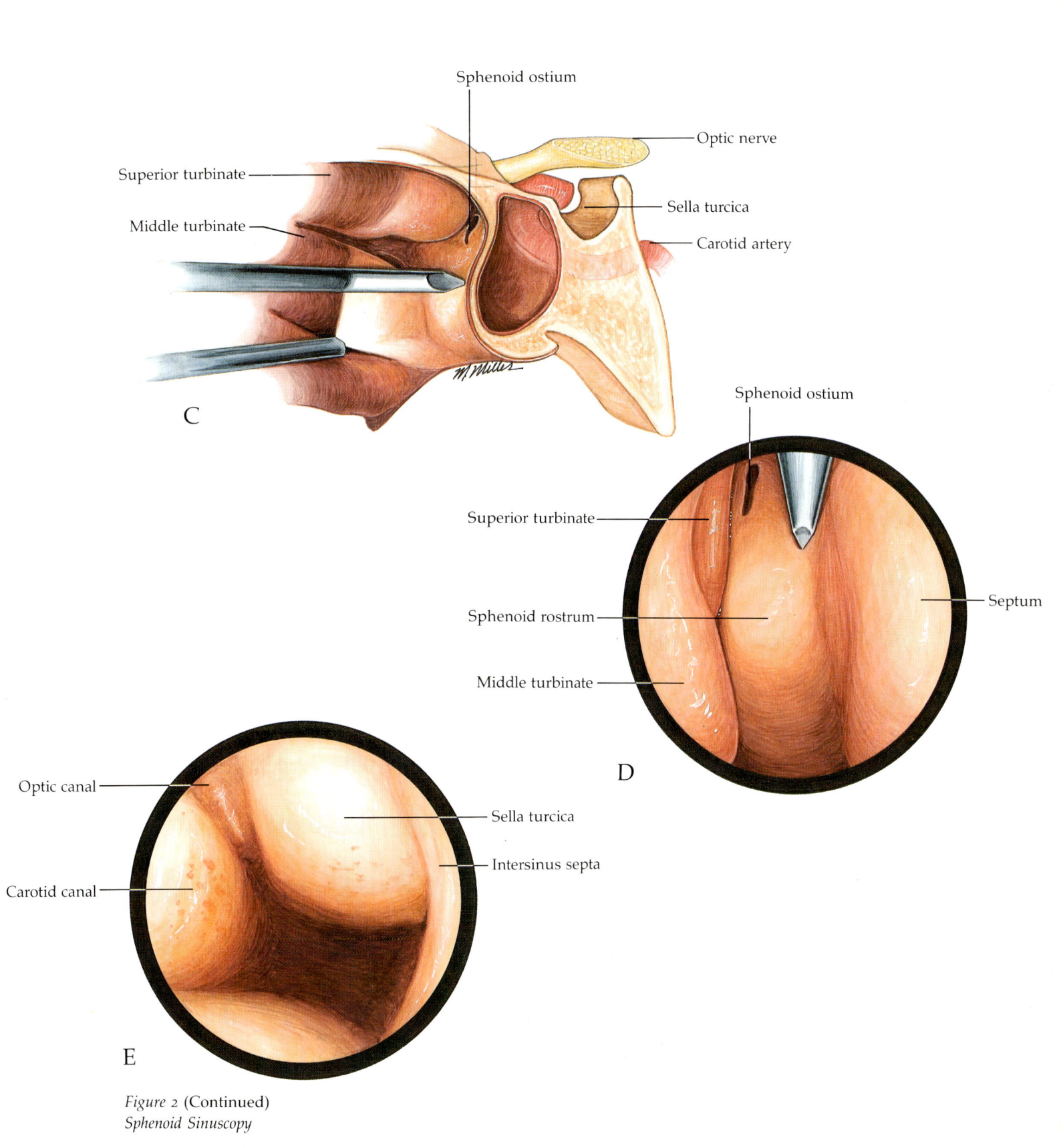

Figure 2 (Continued)
Sphenoid Sinuscopy

David W. Kennedy, M.D.
Jordan S. Josephson, M.D.

ENDOSCOPIC SPHENOETHMOIDECTOMY

Indications

Messerklinger stressed the restoration of mucociliary clearance and surgery tailored to the extent of the disease, an approach the senior author has termed functional endoscopic surgery. By far the greatest advantage of functional endoscopic technique is when accurate diagnostic evaluation reveals a localized underlying ostiomeatal etiology of frontal or maxillary sinusitis. In this situation a minor surgical procedure may be substituted for a more extensive external approach, providing a dramatic reduction in surgical morbidity. This does not imply, however, that functional endoscopic techniques are useful only for limited disease, and the same technique is used to perform a complete sphenoethmoidectomy for nasal polyposis.

Preoperative Considerations

The surgery is usually performed under local anesthesia with sedation. The 0-degree 4.0-mm telescope is selected as the primary endoscope during surgery. The straight-ahead view increases safety and simplifies instrument manipulation. Deflected angle endoscopes are only used after landmarks have been identified, and the use of such scopes is restricted to portions of the procedure when access to a recess is required. Topical anesthesia and vasoconstriction are obtained first by placing nasal applicators with cocaine in the nose (Fig. 3A). The applicators are placed in the area of the anterior ethmoidal artery, the sphenopalatine artery, the posterior end of the inferior turbinate, and the middle meatus. Atraumatic technique is of the utmost importance, as bleeding secondary to traumatized tissue may cause difficulty with visualization during the remainder of the procedure, possibly even necessitating its termination.

Operative Steps

Using a tonsillectomy needle, under direct endoscopic vision (4.0-mm 0-degree endoscope), infiltration of the lateral nasal wall with a lidocaine-epinephrine solution is performed (Fig. 3B). The lateral wall anterior and inferior to the uncinate process, the inferior middle turbinate, and if visible the ethmoidal bulla are injected. The presence of slight bleeding from an injection site in the area where the endoscope will be passed may obstruct vision. Thus it is best to locate the injection sites as far away as possible from areas where the endoscope will be passed, to maximize each injection, and to minimize the number of sites. Occasionally, injection in the area of the septum may be helpful when the mucosa is reactive and boggy and access is limited.

Following injection, the middle turbinate may be subluxed medially if necessary in order to allow adequate visualization of the middle meatus. The patient is instructed to breathe through his or her mouth to avoid droplets of blood being blown onto the telescope lens. Occasionally it may be desirable to place a small temporary pack into the posterior choana.

Plate 35

A

Septum

Middle turbinate

- Injection site

Uncinate process

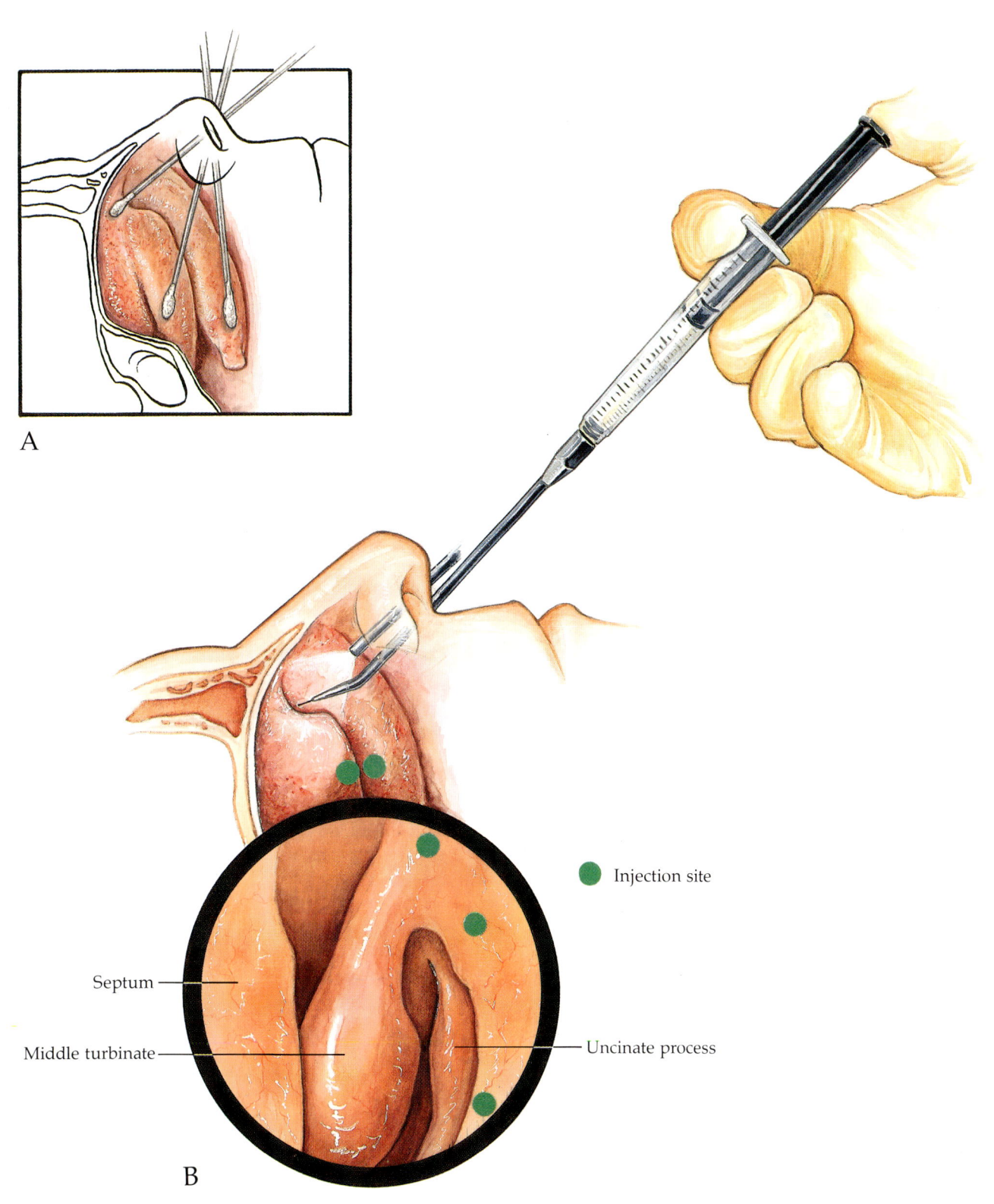

B

Figure 3
Anesthesia for
Endoscopic Sphenoethmoidectomy

The surgery is performed by introducing the instruments below the telescope. The tip of the telescope is kept as far away from the operative site as is compatible with good visualization during the surgery. Because even small traces of blood in the region of the telescope lens may lead to fogging during the surgery, the anterior part of the nose is meticulously cleaned of blood from time to time during the surgery. Using a 4.0-mm 0-degree telescope, the surgery is begun by incising the uncinate process just posterior to its attachment (Fig. 3C). The incision begins at the anterior insertion of the middle turbinate and parallels its free border going posteriorly at the inferior aspect of the incision. If the incision is too far anterior, the bone will be too hard to incise and mucosal bleeding will be increased. If it is too far posterior, a portion of the uncinate process will be left, and ethmoid access will be narrowed. However, this residual uncinate may be resected secondarily. Some debulking of polyps may be necessary prior to infundibulotomy, but this should be minimized to whatever is needed to identify the area, and the polyp removal should be performed as atraumatically as possible under endoscopic visualization. Those polyps attached to the uncinate may be removed with minimal bleeding at infundibulotomy. The KTP 532 laser or a small RF probe is helpful in removing large masses of intranasal polyps bloodlessly. After incising the uncinate process, it is removed with the Blakesley forceps, thus completing the infundibulotomy. This exposes the ethmoidal infundibulum, the area most frequently involved in inflammatory sinus disease (Fig. 3D). From this point on, the procedure is variable and must be custom-tailored to the patient's disease. A complete sphenoethmoidectomy is frequently not required, but the full procedure is described.

The ethmoidal bulla is first removed by in-fracturing it in its medial aspect and then removing it with forceps (Fig. 3E). The medial orbital wall should be cleaned and identified. Using a 30-degree telescope and upbiting forceps, the roof of the ethmoid sinus and the anterior ethmoidal artery may be recognized and dissection of the frontal recess performed. The bone of the roof of the ethmoid is slightly different in color from the intersinus septa and, in the area of the anterior and posterior ethmoid neurovascular bundles, is substantially more sensitive to pain than the bone of the bony labyrinth. Unless the anterior skull base is easily identified at this time, it is safer to defer surgery in the area of the frontal recess and ethmoidal dome until the posterior ethmoid cells have been entered and the roof has been clearly identified. In-fracture of the basal

Plate 36

C — Infundibulotomy incision / Middle turbinate

Middle turbinate

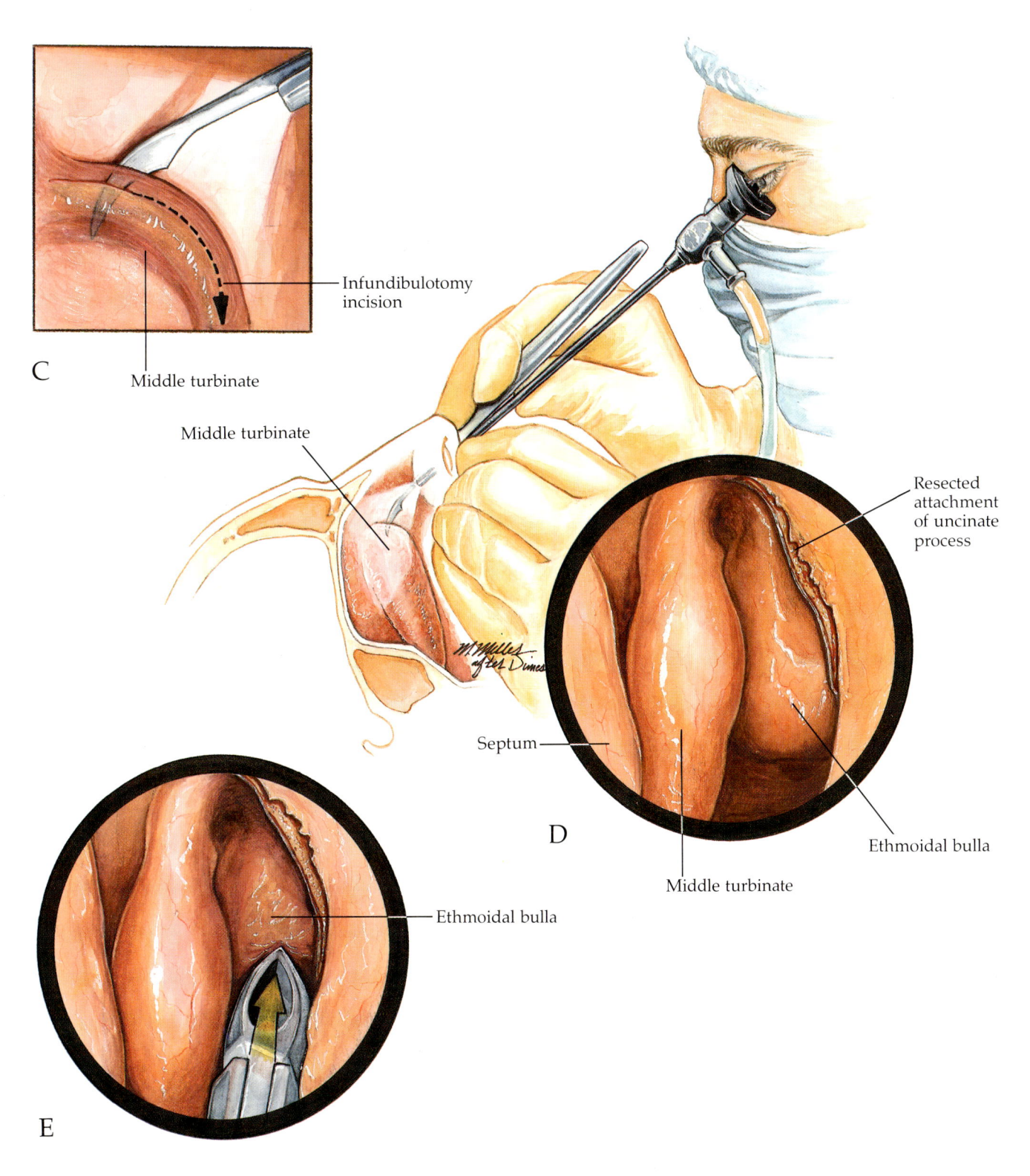

D — Resected attachment of uncinate process / Septum / Middle turbinate / Ethmoidal bulla

E — Ethmoidal bulla

Figure 3 (Continued)
Infundibulotomy

or ground lamella of the middle turbinate provides access to the posterior ethmoid cells (Fig. 3F). The ground lamella is entered inferiorly slightly above the inferior border of the middle turbinate, so as to stay well away from the skull base. Before the ground lamella is in-fractured, the telescope should be withdrawn slightly in order to check the position of the forceps in relation to the middle turbinate. The ground lamella is then removed and the medial orbital wall further skeletonized to maximize access to the posterior ethmoid cells. Like the skull base, the medial orbital wall is more sensitive to pain than the surrounding ethmoid cell partitions. It is usually possible to identify and begin skeletonization of the skull base at this time. If the roof still cannot be identified, further dissection superiorly is deferred until the sphenoid sinus has been entered or, occasionally, until further frontal recess dissection has been performed. The most posterior ethmoid cell typically has a pyramidal shape with the apex toward the anterior clinoid process, and the optic nerve may occasionally be seen passing posteromedially as a convexity in the lateral wall of this cell.

Dissection of the frontal recess is accomplished with the 30-degree telescope and upbiting forceps and in general is best performed after the skull base has been identified. It is important to remember that anteriorly the roof slopes down medially and is thinnest in this area. The forceps should thus be kept pointing slightly laterally. The anterior ethmoidal artery usually passes immediately below the skull base slightly posterior to the ethmoidal dome and, when seen, may be used as a superior landmark. The posterior ethmoidal artery frequently lies within the roof of the ethmoid, somewhat anterior to the optic nerve. Both arteries are typically encased in bony canals. The use of Kennedy-Blakesley suction forceps improves visualization during the ethmoid dissection when mucosal oozing is present and reduces the need to alternate forceps with suction. If arterial bleeding occurs, it is controlled with microfibrillar collagen or suction cautery.

As dissection of the frontal recess is performed, the internal os of the frontal sinus os usually becomes evident toward the medial aspect of the cavity. A second opening slightly more posterior and lateral typically represents the opening of a supraorbital ethmoid cell. Frontal sinus access may be reduced by the presence of the roof of an agger nasi cell anterior to the internal os. In this situation the roof of the cell is removed with forceps or an angled spoon after first rechecking its position relative to the skull base (Fig. 3G).

Plate 37

Dome of ethmoid

Anterior ethmoidal a.

Middle turbinate

Ground lamella

F

Posterior ethmoid cell

Frontal sinus

Agger nasi cell

Frontal sinus

Dome of ethmoid

Middle turbinate

G

Internal os of frontal sinus

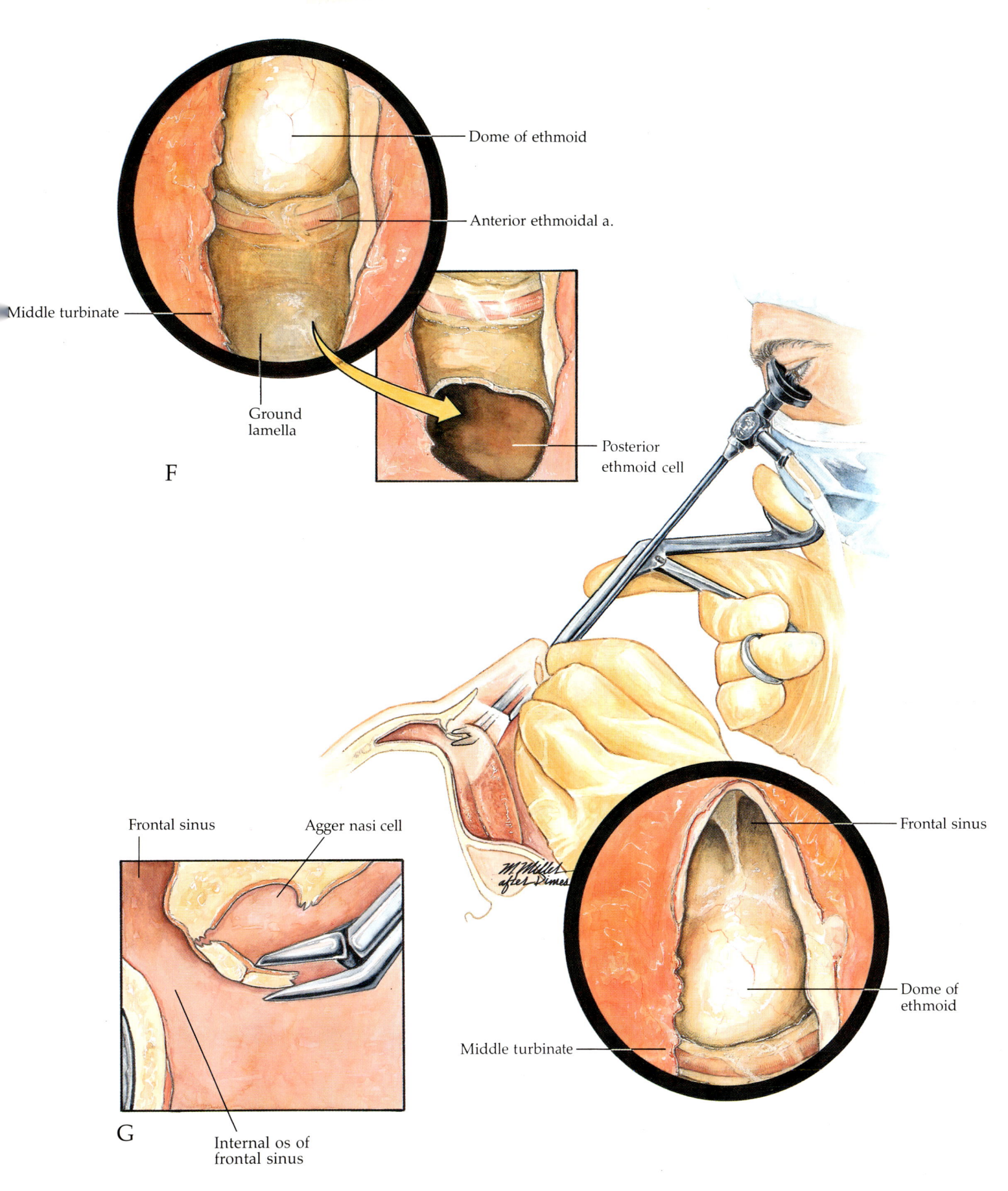

Figure 3 (Continued)
Entry into Posterior
Ethmoid and Frontal Sinuses

93

Endoscopic Sphenoethmoidectomy

The sphenoid sinus is entered through the inferomedial wall of the most posterior ethmoid cell, where the anterior wall can usually be appreciated as a bulge (Fig. 3H). The sinus always lies more inferiorly than expected by less experienced surgeons. The importance of reviewing the CT scan at this time is re-emphasized. If the bulge of the sphenoid sinus is not readily appreciated, the natural sphenoid ostium may be identified medial to the superior turbinate and the sinus entered in this area.

Widening of the natural ostium of the maxillary sinus is only performed when the ostium is stenotic or closed. Middle meatal osteoplasty is always performed after the sphenoethmoid part of the procedure. A 30-degree telescope and curved suction or a fine-angled oblong curet is used to identify the opening. The inferior aspect of the anterior one-third of the middle turbinate provides a useful landmark for the site of the ostium (Fig. 3I).

When widening of the ostium is indicated, the initial opening is created with an angled spoon (Fig. 3J). If the mucosa of the posterior fontanelle is still intact, scissors or a sickle knife may be used to divide it horizontally (Fig. 3K), and reflection of the flaps will extend the ostium

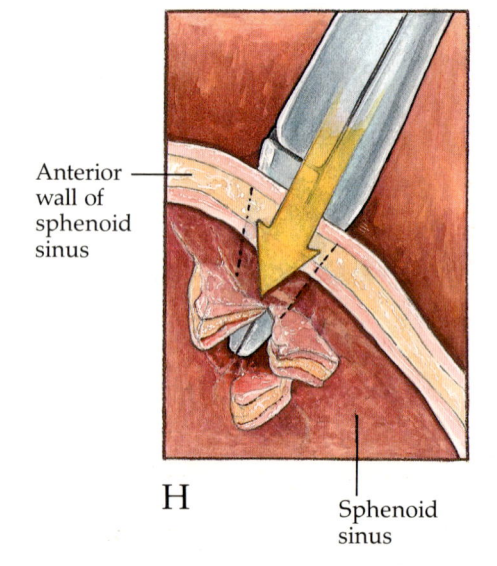

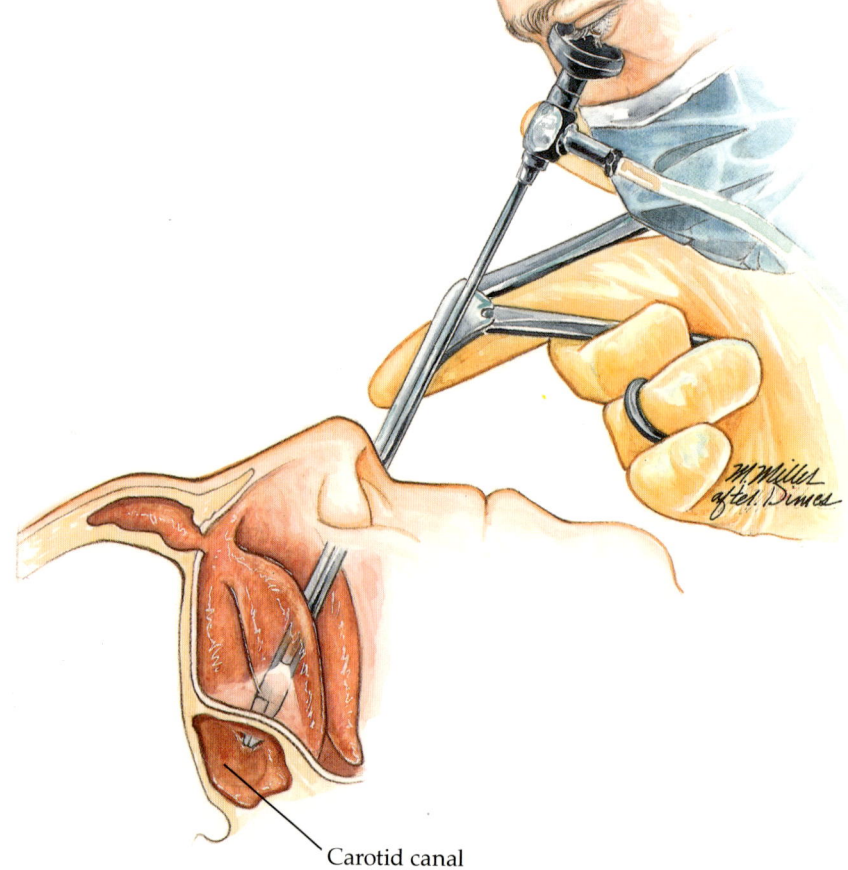

Plate 38
Figure 3 (Continued)
Entering the Sphenoid Sinus

Plate 39

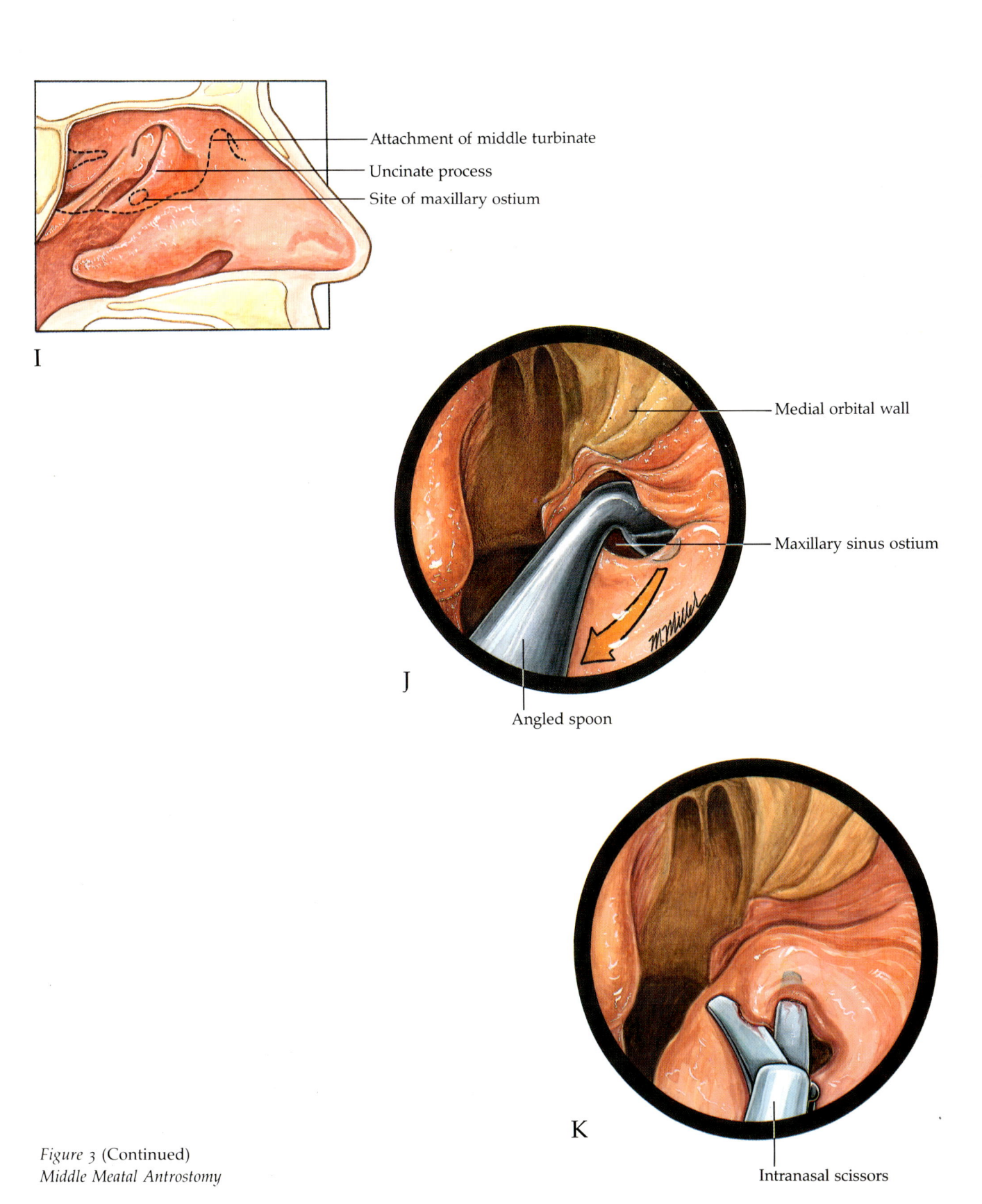

- Attachment of middle turbinate
- Uncinate process
- Site of maxillary ostium

I

- Medial orbital wall
- Maxillary sinus ostium
- Angled spoon

J

- Intranasal scissors

K

Figure 3 (Continued)
Middle Meatal Antrostomy

95

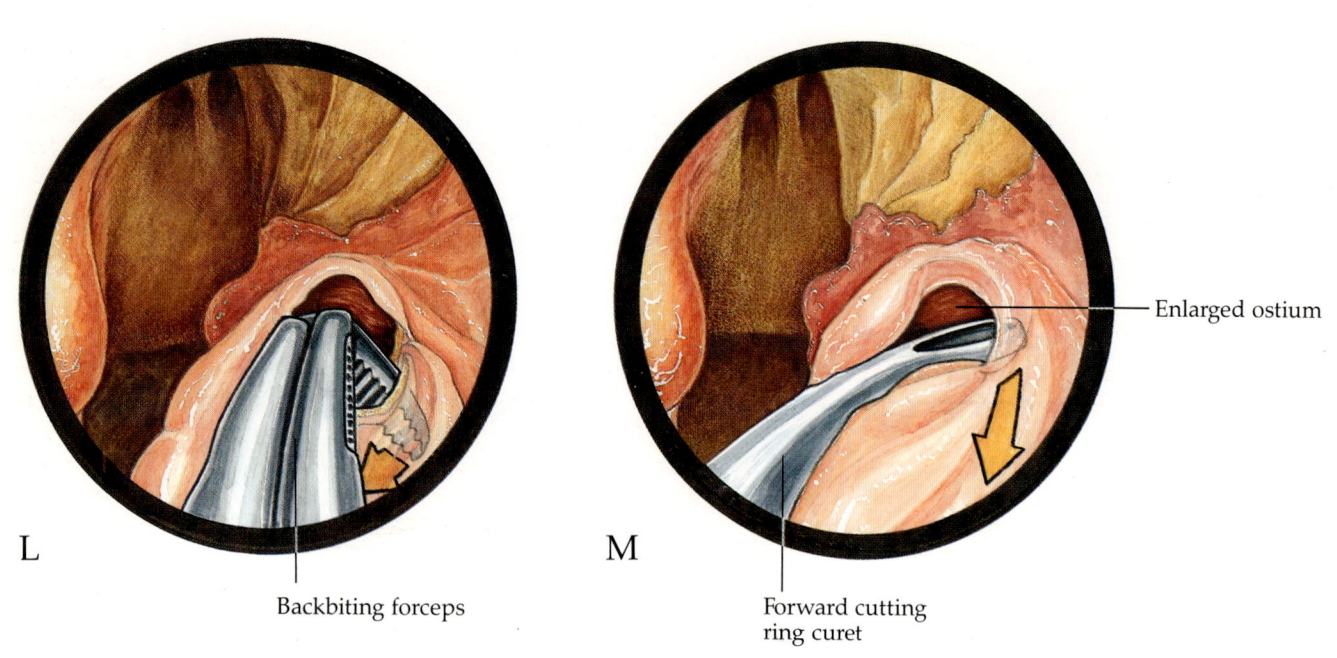

Plate 40

L — Backbiting forceps

M — Enlarged ostium; Forward cutting ring curet

Figure 3 (Continued)
Middle Meatal Antrostomy;
Postoperative Sponge Placement

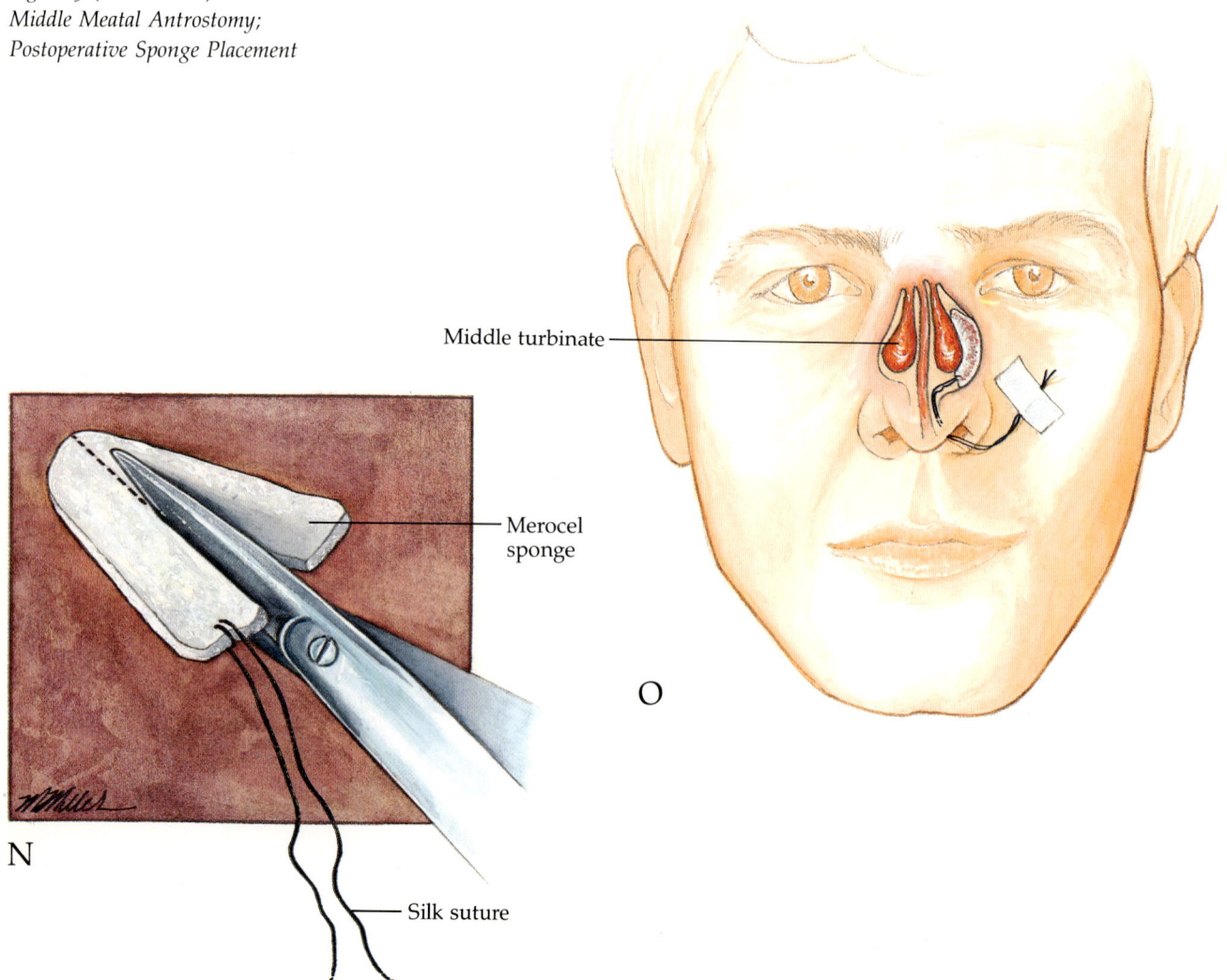

N — Merocel sponge; Silk suture

O — Middle turbinate

posteriorly. Backbiting forceps (Fig. 3L) are used to widen the ostium inferiorly while at the same time draping the sinus mucosa over the inferior edge of the bone (Fig. 3M). Frequently when the natural ostium is obstructed, the initial opening occurs in the area of the posterior fontanelle. In this situation it is extremely important that the antrostomy be brought sufficiently anterior to connect with the natural ostium if persistence of disease is to be avoided. When using the backbiting forceps, care must be taken to avoid trauma to the nasolacrimal duct, which lies anterior to the ostium.

If the patient is bleeding significantly at the end of the procedure or if the surgeon is worried about bloody postnasal discharge causing bronchospasm in the asthmatic patient, a sponge may be placed lateral to the middle turbinate. A sponge may also be helpful in reducing scarring in the presence of tight anatomy or very reactive nasal mucosa. A Merocel sponge with a silk suture at one end is cut to size and coated with antibiotic ointment (Fig. 3N). The sponge is placed lateral to the middle turbinate under direct visualization and removed within 24 hours (Fig. 3O). If it is anticipated that leaving the sponge for a longer period of time may be desirable, it is placed in an antibiotic-coated finger cot prior to insertion. The silk suture is taped to the patient's cheek for easy removal.

Suggested Reading

Kennedy DW, Zinreich SJ. The functional endoscopic approach to inflammatory sinus disease: Current perspectives and technique modifications. Am J Rhinol 1988; 2:89–96.

Stammberger H. Endoscopic endonasal surgery—concepts in treatment of recurring rhinosinusitis. Part I. Anatomic and pathophysiologic considerations. Otolaryngol Head Neck Surg 1986; 94:143–146.

Stammberger H. Endoscopic endonasal surgery—concepts in treatment of recurring rhinosinusitis. Part II. Surgical technique. Otolaryngol Head Neck Surg 1986; 94:147–156.

David W. Kennedy, M.D.
Jordan S. Josephson, M.D.

SPECIAL PROBLEMS

Concha bullosa, fungal disease, and frontal sinus mucocele are three important entities that require special discussion. If the concha bullosa is large and is causing ostiomeatal compromise or airway obstruction, excision may be necessary. A sickle knife is used to make an incision in the inferior conchal mucosa and bone (Fig. 4A). The incision runs along the length of the middle turbinate and is completed anteriorly and posteriorly with scissors (Fig. 4B). The KTP 532 laser may also be used. The lateral portion is then removed with forceps, thus increasing the middle meatal space (Fig. 4C).

Fungal disease in the maxillary sinus (e.g., aspergilloma), may be radiographically diagnosed by the appearance of a metallic-like density on plain film or diffuse areas of increased density on CT scan. Magnetic resonance imaging will show a reduced T2-weighted signal intensity. The diagnosis may be confirmed by performing sublabial maxillary sinus endoscopy. The cannula is left in place in the canine fossa, and a wide middle meatal antrostomy is made after all associated ethmoid disease has been removed intranasally. The maxillary sinus cannula may then be used to manipulate the fungal ball toward the superior part of the sinus, where it can be removed with angled forceps through the widened middle meatal antrostomy. The mucosa is always biopsied to rule out mucosal invasion, and long-term follow-up is always required. A Caldwell-Luc opening is still required if all the fungal material cannot be removed through the antrostomy.

The majority of frontal sinus mucoceles extend down into the frontal recess and are thus accessible intranasally. A limited anterior ethmoidectomy is first performed, and the skull base is then identified. The upbiting or long-angled forceps may be used to open the frontal recess widely, and the mucocele is evacuated with a curved suction. All surrounding bony septa are meticulously removed, but every attempt is made to preserve the duct mucosa of the internal os. Careful postoperative cleaning and evacuation of the mucoid discharge are imperative until the mucosa has returned to normal.

Postoperative Care

The importance of postoperative care in endoscopic surgery cannot be overemphasized. Postoperative care requires meticulous cleaning of blood and fibrin clots in the operative cavity. This is usually performed the day after surgery, 3 to 4 days later, 1 week later, and then weekly for approximately 1 month, the exact period depending upon the severity of disease and the postoperative appearance. Under topical anesthesia and direct endoscopic visualization, blood and mucus are aspirated from the maxillary sinus via the widened natural ostium using a curved suction. Any residual diseased air cells are opened and any diseased mucosa or synechiae are removed under topical anesthesia. Meticulous care is of paramount importance in order to avoid adhesions between the middle turbinate and the lateral nasal wall and the possibility of renewed stenosis and recurrent disease. It is therefore extremely important that the patient be closely followed and the area cleaned until the cavity is fully re-epithelialized.

Plate 41

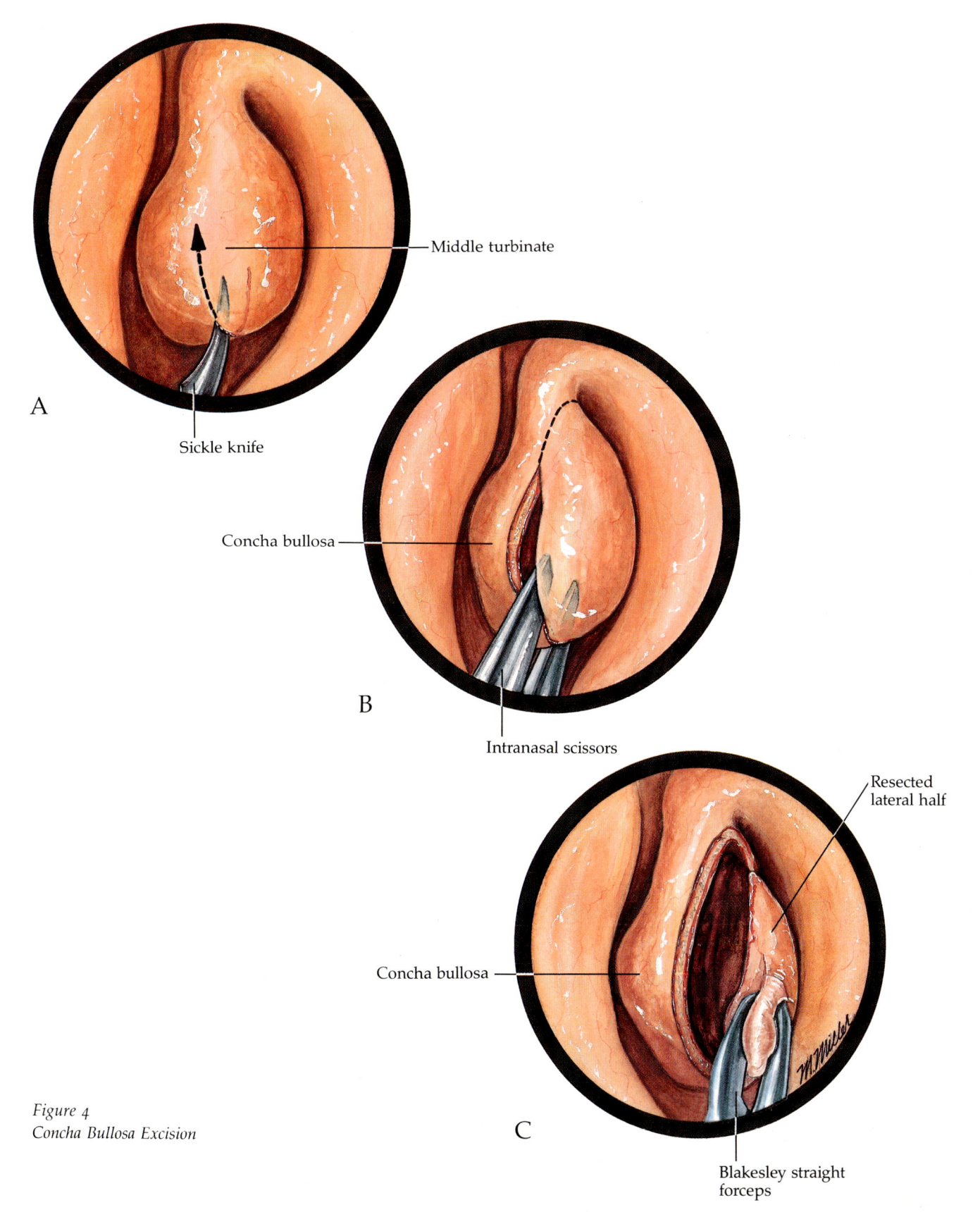

Figure 4
Concha Bullosa Excision

A — Middle turbinate; Sickle knife

B — Concha bullosa; Intranasal scissors

C — Resected lateral half; Concha bullosa; Blakesley straight forceps

Risks, Complications, and Sequelae

The necessity for an in-depth knowledge of the anatomy of the area and extensive experience with instrument handling and atraumatic technique on the part of the surgeon cannot be overemphasized. The excellent view provided by endoscopes improves diagnostic accuracy and allows thorough and more accurate surgical obliteration of the disease and improved local care of the cavity postoperatively. However, potential complications of intranasal ethmoidectomy can be serious and even fatal. Although intraoperative visualization is improved, a surgeon unfamiliar with the endoscopic technique may become disoriented or develop a false sense of security and traumatize the critical adjacent anatomy. Therefore we must stress the importance of repeated cadaver dissections, meticulous technique, and frequent reorientation during the surgery. Careful evaluation of the anatomy on coronal CT scan should be completed before each procedure because of the wide individual variability. Although the diagnostic and postoperative use of endoscopes would benefit all patients with sinus disease irrespective of the surgical technique used, endoscopic sphenoethmoidectomy is a difficult technique that demands rigorous training.

The most common problem is bleeding of mucosal origin. Although this is best avoided by meticulous technique, a slurry consisting of normal saline and microfibrillar collagen absorbed onto a temporary pack has been found efficacious in dealing with the problem when it occurs. This provides excellent hemostasis, and the problem of removing excess collagen after hemostasis is avoided. Arterial bleeding may occur as a result of damage to the anterior and/or posterior ethmoidal arteries. Violation of either the anterior or the posterior ethmoidal artery can be treated with a ball of microfibrillar collagen applied to the bleeding site. A wet cottonball is then applied over this area for approximately 5 minutes. When the bleeding has stopped, the cottonball and the excess collagen are removed. An expanding orbital hematoma with progressive proptosis may occur, with damage to the ethmoidal arteries, and this is an indication for an immediate orbital decompression if the patient's vision is threatened. If bleeding occurs during the procedure and the surgeon's view becomes obstructed, the surgery should be terminated and, if necessary, the procedure completed at a later date through either a repeat endoscopic or an external approach.

Maxillary sinus endoscopy may produce dysesthesia or anesthesia in the region of the incisor and canine teeth. Typically, this resolves within a few days, but occasionally complaints may be more persistent. It is important to tell the patient to refrain from nose blowing. Damage to the tooth roots may occur in the pediatric age group.

If superior ethmoid dissection is required, intracranial entry is best avoided by careful identification and skeletonization of the skull base. Similarly, the medial orbital wall is identified over a wide area and used as a crucial landmark. During surgery of the sphenoid sinus, the surgeon must keep the surrounding vital structures in mind. Small bony dehiscences in the area of the carotid artery are common, and occasionally dehiscences may ocur in the bony optic canal. However, loss of vision appears to be more commonly associated with retro-orbital hematoma than with direct trauma to the nerve.

Special Problems

Pearls and Pitfalls

It is essential for the surgeon to have an in-depth knowledge of the anatomy and to be familiar with the instruments and to have practiced with them. The key to the procedure is meticulous atraumatic techinque.

Careful preoperative study of the coronal CT scan and intraoperative correlation with the patient's anatomy are imperative because of the anatomic variability of the area.

The surgery is best performed under local anesthesia. The occurrence of pain during the surgery can provide important information for the surgeon, and bleeding is generally minimized.

It is imperative to avoid local trauma to the anterior nose and to suction meticulously any traces of blood from this area. If bleeding obstructs the surgeon's view, the procedure should be terminated, as the operation must be performed under direct vision.

Keep the telescope as far anterior as possible to increase the visualization of the operative field and to avoid contamination of the endoscope lens with blood.

The technique and the procedure should be custom-tailored to the patient's disease.

Identification and skeletonization of the medial orbital wall and skull base improve safety when more than minimal surgery is being done. Once the critical landmarks are defined, the remainder of the procedure is relatively simple.

The sphenoid sinus typically lies more inferiorly and medially than expected.

A middle meatal antrostomy per se is not sufficient for the resolution of maxillary sinus disease. It must communicate with the natural ostium.

Meticulous postoperative care is imperative for the success of intranasal ethmoidectomy.

Suggested Reading

Kennedy DW, Josephson JS, Zinreich SJ, Mattox DE, Goldsmith MM. Endoscopic sinus surgery for mucoceles: A viable alternative. Laryngoscope 1989; in press.

Kennedy DW, Zinreich SJ. The functional endoscopic approach to inflammatory sinus disease. Am J Rhinol 1988; 2:89–96.

Zinreich SJ, Kennedy DW. Fungal sinusitis: Diagnosis with CT and MR imaging. Radiology 1988; 169:439–444.

Chapter III

THE NOSE

Ira D. Papel, M.D.

NASAL POLYPECTOMY

Nasal polypectomy was described as early as 1000 BC, when curettage was the technique used. These and other early descriptions are found in Vancil's historical survey of polypectomy procedures. In the fourth century BC, Hippocrates employed methods such as "a sponge method" and a snare with cautery technique for hemostasis. Fabricius, in the 16th century, used a hot cannula for the treatment of nasal polyps. Not until the 19th century did Jarvis describe the use of a metal snare for polypectomy, a method still commonly employed today. Over the centuries many other herbal, folk, and surgical techniques have been used to treat this most common of all intranasal tumors.

Indications

Nasal polyps represent prolapsed respiratory mucosa arising from the nasal cavity. The cause of this prolapse is not well understood, but it may be due to increased interstitial fluid pressure and edema, excacerbated by chronic and recurrent inflammation, abnormal vasomotor responses, or allergic etiologies. The usual sites of origin are on the lateral wall of the nasal cavity, generally the middle meatal area, or the inferior borders of the middle and superior turbinates. These polyps may be asymptomatic or cause total nasal obstruction. Indications for surgery are airway obstruction, rhinorrhea, chronic sinusitis, and possibly the relief of chronic asthma. Medical therapy such as systemic or topical steroids, allergy desensitization, antihistamines, decongestants, and elimination diets has been used with variable success.

Preoperative Considerations

Nasal polyps must always be differentiated from more dangerous nasal masses, especially when the polyps appear to be unilateral. Inverted papilloma, carcinoma, and polypoid degeneration of the middle turbinate must be considered. The presence of an antrochoanal polyp must be assessed on preoperative examination, as this may change the surgical approach. If possible, maximal control of chronic sinusitis and/or allergic conditions should be achieved prior to surgery.

Preoperative imaging studies should include at least a full set of sinus radiographs. The condition of the paranasal sinsuses is important, as drainage of these areas may be necessary at the same time as the polypectomy. Computed tomography has helped to evaluate the paranasal sinuses in great detail. The information obtained about the anterior ethmoid region and the ostiomeatal complex has helped to plan polyp and sinus surgery, especially when endoscopic techniques are employed.

Operative Steps

The removal of nasal polyps is usually performed under local anesthesia. This can be accomplished as an office procedure under some circumstances, but more often it is performed in an operating room setting. Intravenous sedation may be added for the comfort of the nervous patient. In certain situations, a general anesthetic may be indicated.

Four percent cocaine solution is applied topically with cotton applicators. The entire nasal cavity should be treated, with special attention to the sphenopalatine ganglion, ethmoidal nerves, and middle meatal area. It may be necessary to slide the applicators in and around mobile polyps in order to apply the cocaine solution to the appropriate locations. A careful and slow application of anesthetic will help to assure the comfort of the patient and to create a more controlled situation in which the surgeon can work more effectively. After adequate topical anesthesia has been obtained, the uncinate process is injected with a 1 percent lidocaine and 1:100,000 epinephrine solution by using a tonsil needle. This helps to provide vasoconstriction and anesthesia in the middle meatal area, where much of the surgery is concentrated (Fig. 1A). Medialization of the middle turbinate with a Freer elevator may improve the exposure in the middle meatus.

The wire snare is then used to excise the large polyps. The snare is introduced into the nasal cavity with a vertical orientation and manipulated over the polyp as it is turned horizontally. The snare is then maneuvered up toward the pedicle of the polyp as the snare is closed just enough to follow the pedicle into the middle meatus, where most polyps originate (Fig. 1B). When the snare is maximally advanced, it is slowly closed until the pedicle is transected. The polyp is then removed from the nasal cavity with forceps, and the process is repeated until the larger polyps have been removed. Hemostasis can be improved during the procedure by the use of packing soaked in local anesthetic on the alternate

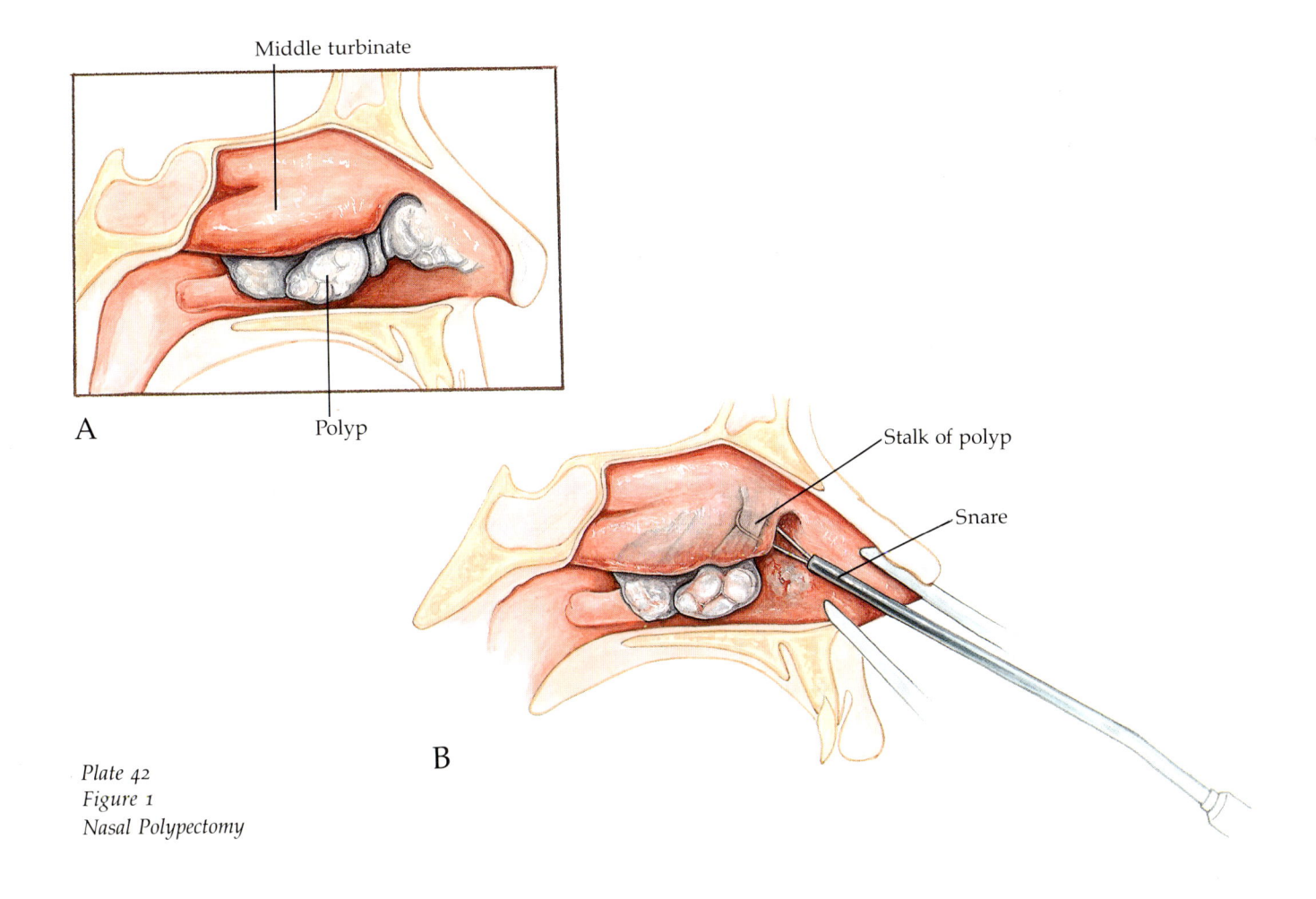

Plate 42
Figure 1
Nasal Polypectomy

side of the nose while surgery is being performed on the other side. The smaller polyps can be removed by using Blakesley or Takahashi forceps (Fig. 1C). Caution should be exercised with the forceps not to use force in the superior meatal area, as the cribriform plate may be vulnerable. All tissues removed should be sent to the laboratory for pathologic examination, as on occasion malignancies have been discovered unexpectedly. After polypectomy has been completed, concomitant sinus surgery may proceed as necessary. At the conclusion of surgery, a layered ½-inch gauze packing is placed and removed after 1 to 2 days (Fig. 1D). Antistaphylococcal oral antibiotics are prescribed for the duration of the packing.

Recently the KTP 532 laser has been used for the excision of some nasal polyps. This technique has the advantage of hemostasis with cutting and can be used with endoscopic nasal instruments to provide a finer degree of control than can be expected with traditional transnasal surgery.

Antrochoanal polyps may require a modification of the above technique. The antral portion of the polyp may require a widening of the natural maxillary ostia by either transnasal or endoscopic techniques. A Caldwell-Luc approach may also be considered. Care must be taken not to allow the choanal portion of the polyp to be aspirated when its pedicle is transected.

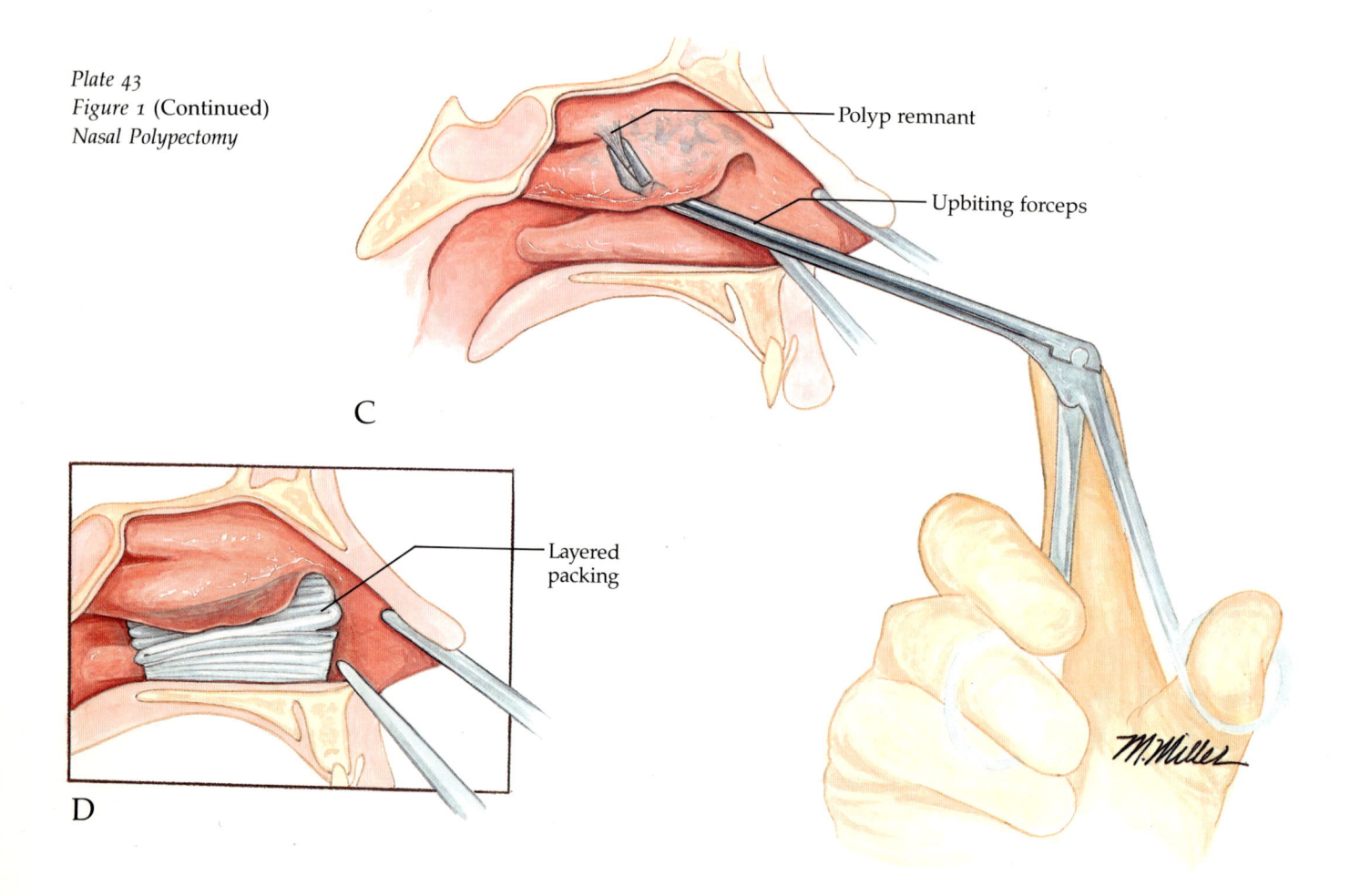

Plate 43
Figure 1 (Continued)
Nasal Polypectomy

Postoperative Care

The intranasal packing is left in place for 1 to 2 days, depending on the extent of surgery and the hemostasis during the operative procedure. Postoperative hemorrhage is rare after isolated polypectomy; it may be caused by incomplete excision of a polyp or trauma to the middle turbinate. This may be controlled by either completion of the polypectomy or replacement of the packing. Crusting and dried blood are removed after the packing has been withdrawn, and the patient is encouraged to use nasal saline spray and a humidifier in the home until healing is complete.

Topical steroid preparations are also started after 1 week in order to slow the formation of new polyps. Some surgeons may also employ systemic steroids in the early postoperative period.

Risks, Complications, and Sequelae

The most common sequela of nasal polypectomy is recurrence. Even with seemingly complete removal of disease, the underlying pathology has not been corrected. Concomitant therapy with topical and oral steroids, allergic desensitization, and avoidance of allergens may help control polyps but rarely cure the patient.

Hemorrhage, cerebrospinal fluid leak, orbital injury, and ozena are potential complications of nasal polypectomy.

Pearls and Pitfalls

The most common pitfall in polypectomy is partial removal of the polyps. This may lead to increased bleeding and difficulty in completing the procedure effectively because of decreased visibility and increased patient discomfort. Care should be taken to remove all polyps as high on their pedicles as possible. If bleeding does occur during a procedure, pack that area with gauze containing a dilute epinephrine solution, and work on the other side of the nose until hemostasis has been established.

Careful and meticulous application of the local anesthetic is essential for patient cooperation and also helps with local hemostasis. It is difficult to establish effective anesthesia after the operative procedure has been initiated and the field is bloody.

Undue force should never be applied to either the snare or the forceps when removing polyps from the superior portion of the nasal cavity or deep in the middle meatus. Traction on mucosa that is firmly attached to the cribriform plate may cause injury leading to cerebrospinal fluid rhinorrhea and further complications. Trauma to the ethmoid area poses a risk to the anterior cranial fossa and orbit.

A rare encephalocele may be mistaken for a polyp. Unusual pain, headache, cerebrospinal fluid rhinorrhea, or coma is an indication for emergency hospitalization, computed tomographic scan of the skull base, and neurosurgical consultation.

Suggested Reading

English GM. Nasal polypectomy and sinus surgery in patients with asthma and aspirin idiosyncrasy. Laryngoscope 1986; 96:374–380.

Kennedy DW, Zinreich SJ, Rosenbaum A, Johns ME. Functional endoscopic sinus surgery: Theory and diagnosis. Arch Otolaryngol 1985; 111:576–582.

Mygind N. Nasal allergy. Oxford: Blackwell Scientific Publications, 1979:235.

Vancil ME. A historical survey of treatments for nasal polyposis. Laryngoscope 1969; 79:435.

John C. Price, M.D.

SEPTOPLASTY

Indications

Septoplasty is performed primarily for nasal septal deviation with associated airway obstruction. Other nasal airway disease contributing to obstruction should be ruled out, minimized, or corrected. Acute, recurrent sinusitis or refractory chronic sinusitis also may constitute indications for correction of anatomic nasal septal deviations. Disruption of nasal air flow patterns, alteration of normal mucociliary transport, and overt obstruction of sinus drainage can result from such deformities. Septoplasty may also be effective in the relief of epistaxis when specific bleeding sites can be correlated with septal deformities or spurs. Cosmetic correction of the deviated or twisted nose may require septoplasty in conjunction with rhinoplasty. The efficaciousness of septal surgery in the management of atypical facial pain and nasal headache is questionable. Certainly thorough neurologic and radiologic evaluation should be done in this circumstance. There should be an identifiable specific septal spur contacting the turbinate or lateral nasal wall, and the pain should be able to be relieved by topical anesthetic applied to the contact point. All other potential sources of infection, neoplasm, or neuralgia should be ruled out.

Preoperative Considerations

The skin of the face should be free of suppurative process. Any active lesions should be controlled by appropriate dermatologic consultation and management. The nasal cavity should likewise be free of infection. Comprehensive nasal endoscopy with the rigid telescopes and standard paranasal sinus radiography are routine screening procedures. It is preferable to clear up active sinusitis prior to septoplasty. Occasionally this is not possible, and septoplasty must be done in conjunction with sinus surgery. Significant septal deformities may need correcting before endoscopic instrumentation of the ethmoids is possible. In this circumstance, culture-specific antibiotic therapy is recommended. Antibiotic prophylaxis is not otherwise employed. The patient should be carefully questioned regarding a history of bleeding and clotting disorders, cardiac arrhythmias, and drug allergies. Topical and local anesthetics with intravenous sedation are preferred. General anesthesia is indicated when a communication or language barrier exists between patient and physician, total patient cooperation cannot be relied upon, the patient has an unusually high level of anxiety regarding the surgery, or a prolonged, difficult procedure is anticipated. The surgery is done on an outpatient basis, and the patient is seen the following morning in the physician's office. Unscheduled hospital admissions following surgery are unusual but may arise in cases of postanesthetic nausea and vomiting, significant postoperative bleeding, or when the patient is alone and has no one to assist with postoperative care and management.

Operative Steps

The face is cleaned with a standard surgical skin preparation. The surgeon may choose between chlor-hexidine 4 percent scrub, povidone-iodine paint, or isopropyl alcohol 70 percent. Care must be taken to prevent the toxic materials from entering the eyes or mucosal surface.

Illumination of the operative area with a brilliant light is critical. A headlamp with a fiberoptic source is desirable. A parabolic reflector is ideal, as light converging to a focal point reduces problems with shadows of surgical instruments.

Intranasal anesthesia is initiated by applying topical cocaine to the mucous membranes. Crystals may be painted directly onto the septum and turbinates and the mucous blanket allowed to carry the anesthetic back to the remainder of the nasal cavity. Cocaine solution 4 to 5 percent may be applied by cotton tip applicator method or by insertion of cottonoid strips into the superior, middle, and inferior meatuses. In either case, anesthetic should be applied to the anterior ethmoidal and sphenopalatine regions. Applications of more than 200 mg of cocaine should be avoided. Our preference of local anesthetic agent has been 1 percent lidocaine with 1:100,000 epinephrine. This provides rapid onset of deep anesthesia with intense vasoconstriction and a duration of action of 1.5 to 2 hours, permitting completion of most septal surgery. Other anesthetics may produce sustained pain relief in the immediate postoperative period and have significant merits. The 3-cc plastic "three-ring" syringe and 1.5-inch 25-gauge needle are preferred for injection. The anesthetic is first infiltrated at the base of the columella. The remainder of the membranous septum is then injected. The septum is then infiltrated, taking care to insert the needle tip between the cartilage and mucoperichondrium. Successful application produces a white wheal and is accompanied by a substantial hydrodissection of the perichondrium from the cartilage (Fig. 2A). This process is continued until the posterior limit of the septum is reached bilaterally. The needle is then inserted into the piriform aperture near the nasal floor and passed laterally to the infraorbital foramen. The surgeon's fingers inserted along the inferior orbital rim protect the eye from entry of the needle. Infiltration of the infraorbital foramen and piriform aperture allows for a substantial field block and facilitates the surgeon's ability to dilate the nares effectively. Approximately 0.5 ml of anesthetic agent is then injected into the anterior tips of the middle and inferior turbinates. This substantially reduces the discomfort with further instrumentation of the nose (Fig. 2B).

Most nasal septal corrections can be accomplished through a hemitransfixion incision and development of one anterior mucoperiosteal tunnel (Fig. 2C). This is done on the concave side of the septum. The severely comminuted nasal septum requires more thorough exposure and the elevation of bilateral mucoperichondrial flaps. In this circumstance the columellar transfixion incision (Fig. 2D) is advantageous. Identification of the appropriate plane is critical to the success of the operation and to

Plate 44

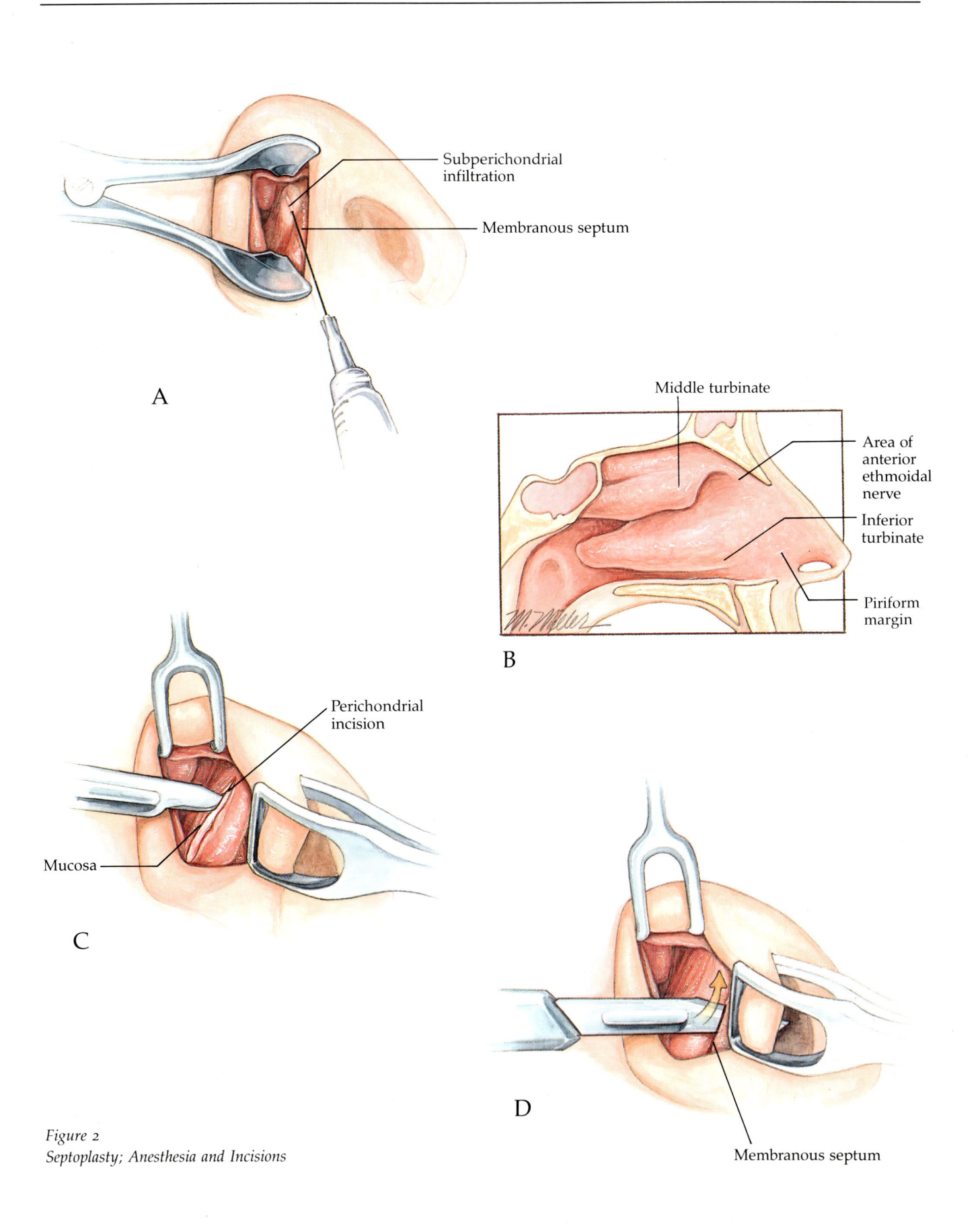

Figure 2
Septoplasty; Anesthesia and Incisions

avoidance of postoperative complications. The accurate separation of perichondrium from cartilage (Fig. 2E) establishes a relatively bloodless plane, which greatly reduces the incidence of troublesome bleeding, postoperative hemorrhage, hematoma, and septal perforations. Successful preservation of the perichondrium may also allow for partial regeneration of the cartilage. Incision of the tissue down to and even slightly into the cartilage of the anterior septal margin facilitates this maneuver. If the plane has been accurately identified, little resistance should be encountered in developing the anterior mucoperichondrial tunnel (Figs. 2E and 2F). This is carried along the surface of the quadrangular cartilage to its junction with the perpendicular plate of the ethmoid bone. The adherent fibers at this point are sharply lysed, and dissection is carried between the mucoperiosteum and the bony septum to develop the posterior nasal tunnel (Fig. 2F). This exposure may be carried to within 1 cm of the cribriform plate and to the sphenoid rostrum and margin of the choana, as necessary. The soft tissue and the periosteum overlying the base of the nasal spine are stripped away and their juncture with the piriform margin identified by direct vision. This maneuver is facilitated by use of the Cottle speculum to hold the soft tissues apart. The nasal floor elevator is then passed over the piriform margin, separating the mucoperiosteum from the nasal surface of the hard palate immediately adjacent to the junction with the maxillary crest and vomer. This inferior tunnel is completed by sweeping the elevator in a curving fashion up onto the inferior bony septum and working from posterior to anterior direction (Fig. 2F). The Cottle speculum is then positioned with one blade in the inferior tunnel and the superior blade in the anterior tunnel, thus exposing the decussating fibers between the quadrangular cartilage and maxillary crest that adhere tightly to the mucoperiosteum (Figs. 2F and 2G). These fibers are carefully lysed with a knife and intranasal scissors while exercising care to avoid laceration of the mucosal flap (Fig. 2G).

Plate 45

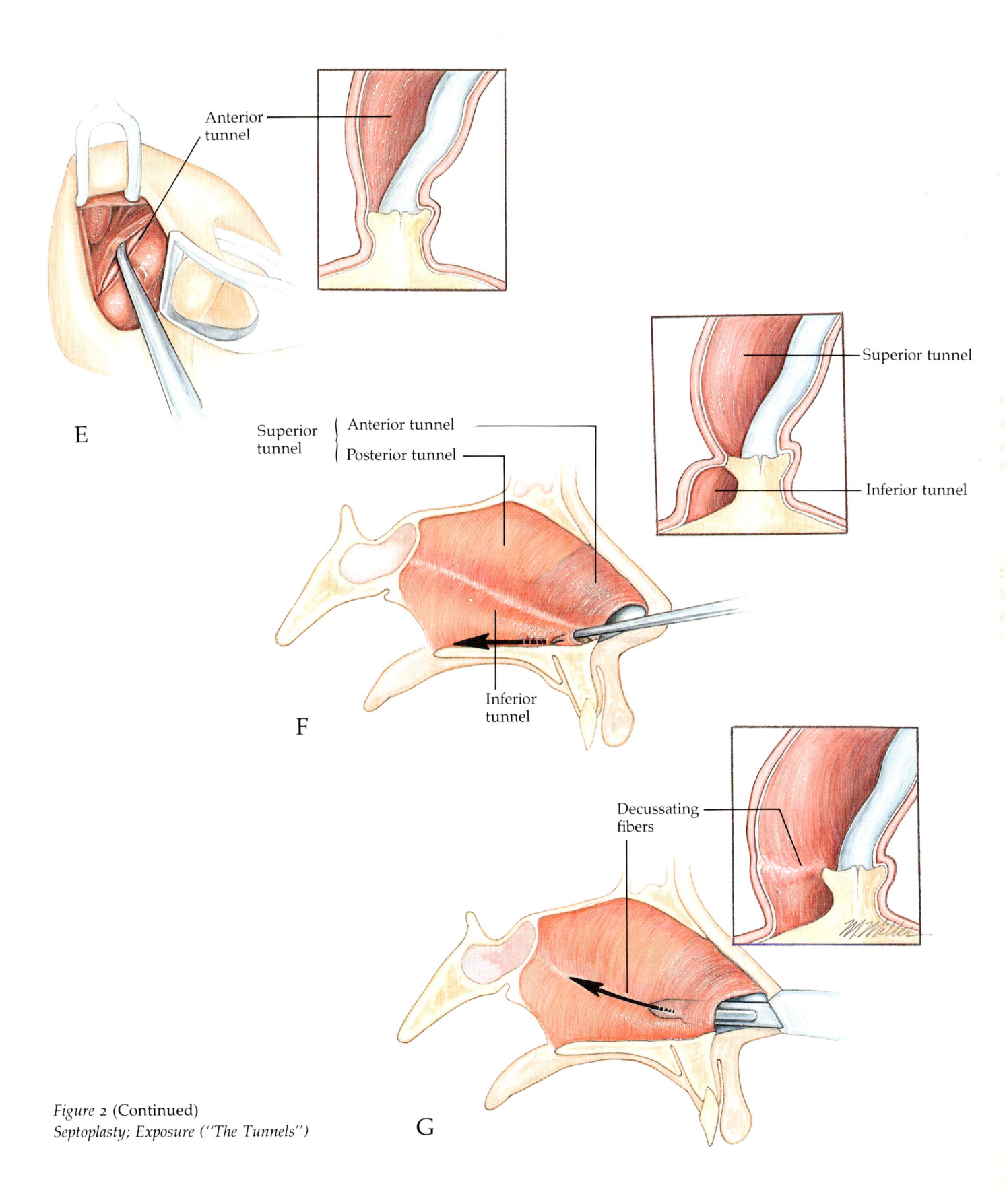

E

F

Anterior tunnel

Superior tunnel { Anterior tunnel
Posterior tunnel

Inferior tunnel

Superior tunnel

Inferior tunnel

Decussating fibers

G

Figure 2 (Continued)
Septoplasty; Exposure ("The Tunnels")

113

The juncture of the quadrangular cartilage and perpendicular plate of the ethmoid bone is usually heralded by a thickening of the cartilage and bone. Location of this juncture can be confirmed by palpation with a semisharp elevator. An angled cartilage knife or elevator (Woodson) is used to release the cartilage immediately in front of the juncture with the bone. This cut is carried to within 1 cm of the nasal bone. It is important to retain this attachment to the nasal bone in all but the most severe nasal septal deformities (Fig. 2H). A periosteal elevator is then inserted through this cartilaginous incision and a posterior mucoperiosteal flap elevated on the contralateral side of the perpendicular plate of the ethmoid bone. The quadrangular cartilage is released from the maxillary crest in a similar fashion (Fig. 2I). A strip of cartilage is removed from its inferior border. Adequate resection allows room for the cartilage to unfurl and for repositioning to the middle (Fig. 2J). The inferior septal spur (Fig. 2J) is usually composed of deformities of both the maxillary crest and septal cartilage. This is removed or remodeled with a small osteotome (Fig. 2K). Elevation of the contralateral inferior tunnel may be necessary to achieve adequate exposure for this step. (It is desirable to maintain attachment or at least contact of the caudal septum with the nasal spine to minimize

Plate 46

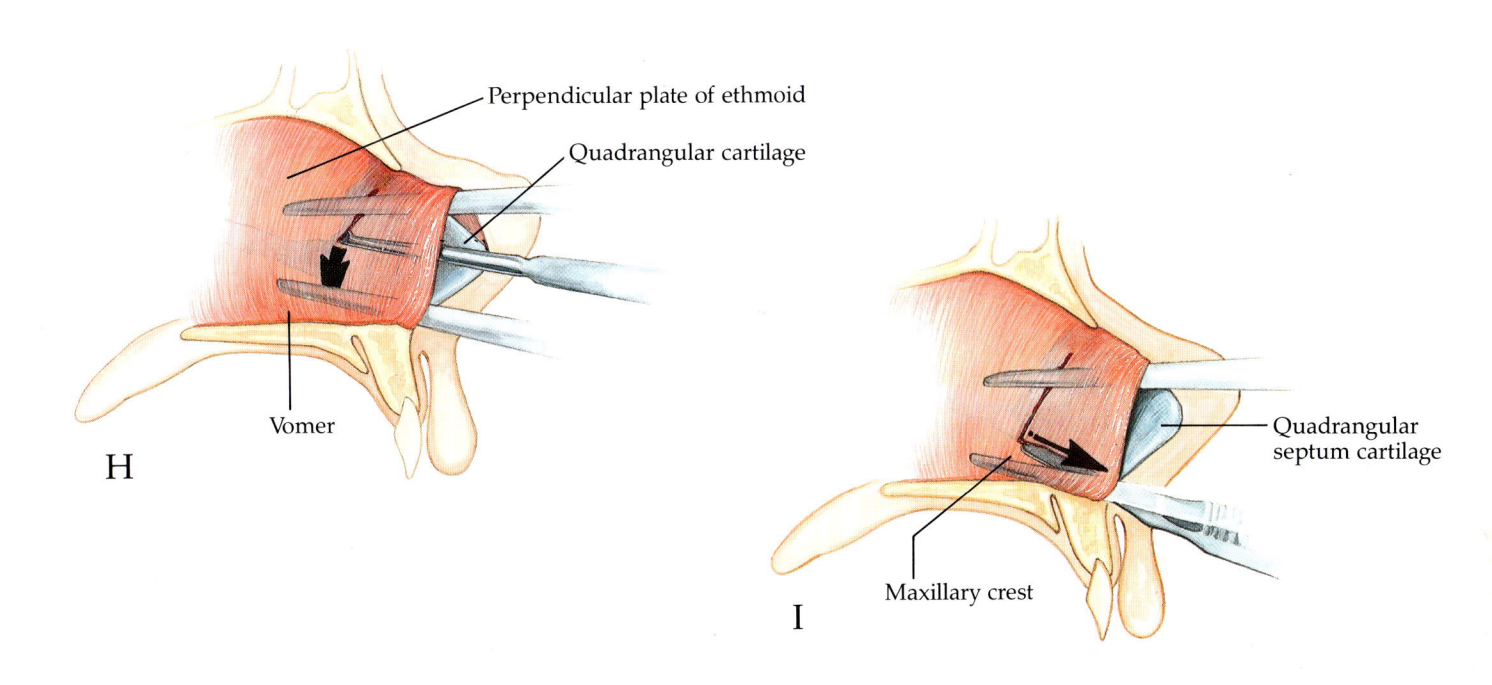

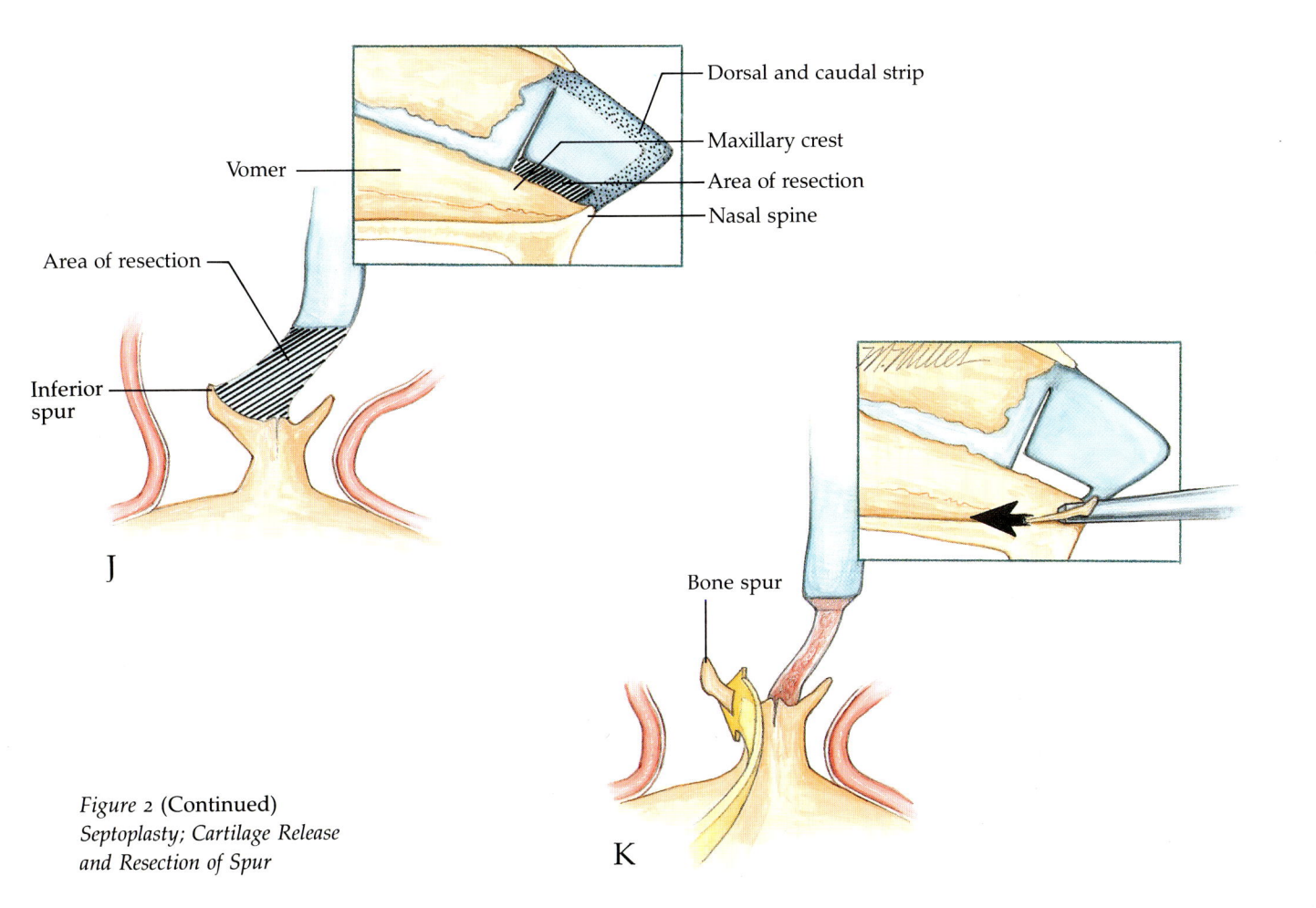

Figure 2 (Continued)
Septoplasty; Cartilage Release and Resection of Spur

115

Septoplasty

the possibility of columellar retraction.) The septal cartilage is displaced laterally with a Killian speculum of intermediate length (Fig. 2L). This reveals any significant deformity of the posterior septum, which may be removed with the Jansen-Middleton fenestrated rongeurs (Fig. 2M).

The septal cartilage is examined and an attempt made to position it in the midline. If it assumes a normal shape and position, no further work needs to be done. It is likely, however, that recontouring of the cartilage will be necessary. Deep incisions should be made nearly through the cartilage along the axis of greatest curvature of the concave side (Fig. 2N). With time, the intracartilaginous elasticity of the residual intact cartilage will allow the cartilage to assume a straight contour. The quadrangular cartilage is positioned in the midline, the septal flaps are returned to their natural positions, and the nasal airway is inspected bilaterally. If there is residual deformity with compromise of the airway, the point of maximal deformity is held with an elevator while the flaps are opened with the speculum, thereby delineating the point of deformity. This is resected or remodeled as necessary until adequate airway is established, as determined by the ability to visualize the nasopharynx through the anterior nares.

Management of the severely comminuted cartilaginous deformity requires a more aggressive disassembly of the septum. Columellar transfixion incision is preferred. Anterior and inferior nasal tunnels are developed bilaterally. An inferior cartilaginous strip is resected as previously described. The septal cartilage morsalizer is inserted with its diamond cutting blades on both sides of the cartilage. The blades are closed firmly along all major deformities (Fig. 2O). The resultant expansion of the cartilage may require additional trimming of the inferior border to accommodate the nasal septum along the maxillary crest.

Final inspection of the mucosal flaps for lacerations is carried out. Any triangular or opposing tears should be carefully approximated with 4–0 absorbable sutures. If a "perfect" flap has persisted throughout the procedure, a controlled drainage site should be produced by making a

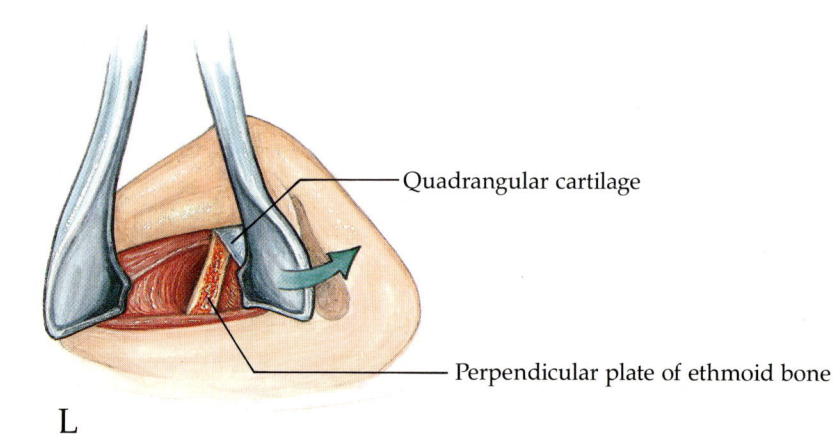

Plate 47
Figure 2 (Continued)
Septoplasty; Posterior Septal Resection

L

— Quadrangular cartilage

— Perpendicular plate of ethmoid bone

Plate 48

M — Cribriform plate, Sphenoid rostrum, Vomer

N — Concave surface of septal deviation, Intracartilaginous elasticity

O — Severe comminuted deformity, Area of resection, Septal morsalizer

Figure 2 (Continued)
Septoplasty; Posterior Septal Resection; Management of Cartilaginous Deformity

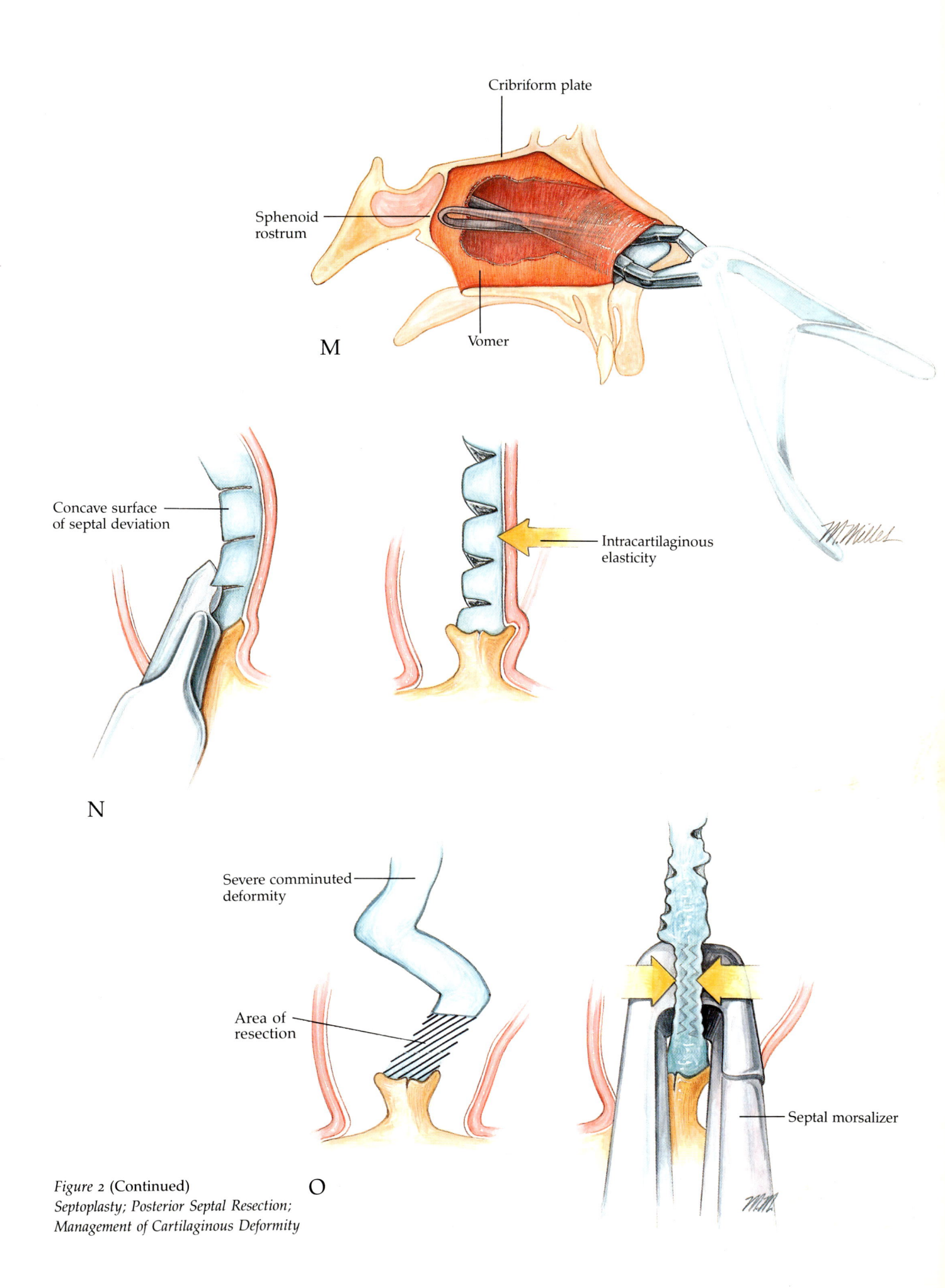

stab wound in the flap along its inferior border. The incision is closed with 4–0 absorbable sutures (Fig. 2P). The full transfixion incision is initially anchored with 3–0 absorbable sutures placed as "transfixion" stitches near the nasal tip and columellar base. Coaptation of the mucosal flaps to the septum is achieved with Silastic splints trimmed to the contour of the nasal septum. The posterior border of the splints is placed between the septum and middle turbinates. These splints may be fashioned out of 0.60 Silastic sheeting or plastic coffee can lid material, or may be commercially prepared items (Doyle splints) (Fig. 2Q). A 2–0 monofilament mattress suture is positioned through both splints, both perichondrial flaps, and septal cartilage, and it is tied securely but not tightly (Fig. 2R). The use of septal splints may be eliminated if a series of mattress sutures is passed through the septal mucosal flaps (Fig. 2R, inset). It is important to start this process in the center of the septum. Continuous full-thickness mattress sutures are passed in the indicated fashion around the perimeter of the septum. The last stitch should return the 4–0 absorbable suture to the initial side, and the stitch is then tied in the center of the septum. A light antibiotic–impregnated Vaseline gauze pack is then inserted into the nasal cavity and nasal tip dressing applied.

Postoperative Care

The patient is placed in a semisitting position and observed in the recovery room. He or she may be discharged when sufficiently aroused from sedation if no significant epistaxis or nausea is present. Perioperative antibiotics are employed when surgery is done in the face of a persistent sinus infection or when retention of the nasal packing for several days is anticipated. The packing and splints should be removed and the septum investigated if brisk bleeding develops or if severe pain occurs.

The patient is seen the following morning in the physician's office, and the nasal packing is removed. The septum is carefully inspected for signs of active bleeding and hematoma formation. The patient and the family are carefully questioned about pain, fever, nausea, vomiting, dehydration, and nutritional status. Hospital admission should be considered if progress is not satisfactory.

Normal saline drops and antibiotic ointment are applied to the nostrils three times daily for 1 week. The septal splints are removed 7 to 10 days postoperatively.

Risks, Complications, and Sequelae

Postoperative bleeding is unusual, although epistaxis and septal hematoma are by far the most common complications resulting from septoplasty. Hematoma must be detected and evacuated promptly; otherwise infection, abscess, dissolution of septal cartilage, and saddle nose deformity may result. Septal abscess also presents the threat of extension of infection intracranially or intraorbitally. Brain abscess, encephalitis, meningitis, epidural abscess, orbital subperiosteal abscess, orbital abscess, or orbital cellulitis may occur. Injuries to the eyes or central nervous system may result. Rough handling of the instruments and tissue is to be avoided. The superior portion of the perpendicular plate of the ethmoid bone must be carefully identified and released 1 or 2 cm below the crib-

Plate 49

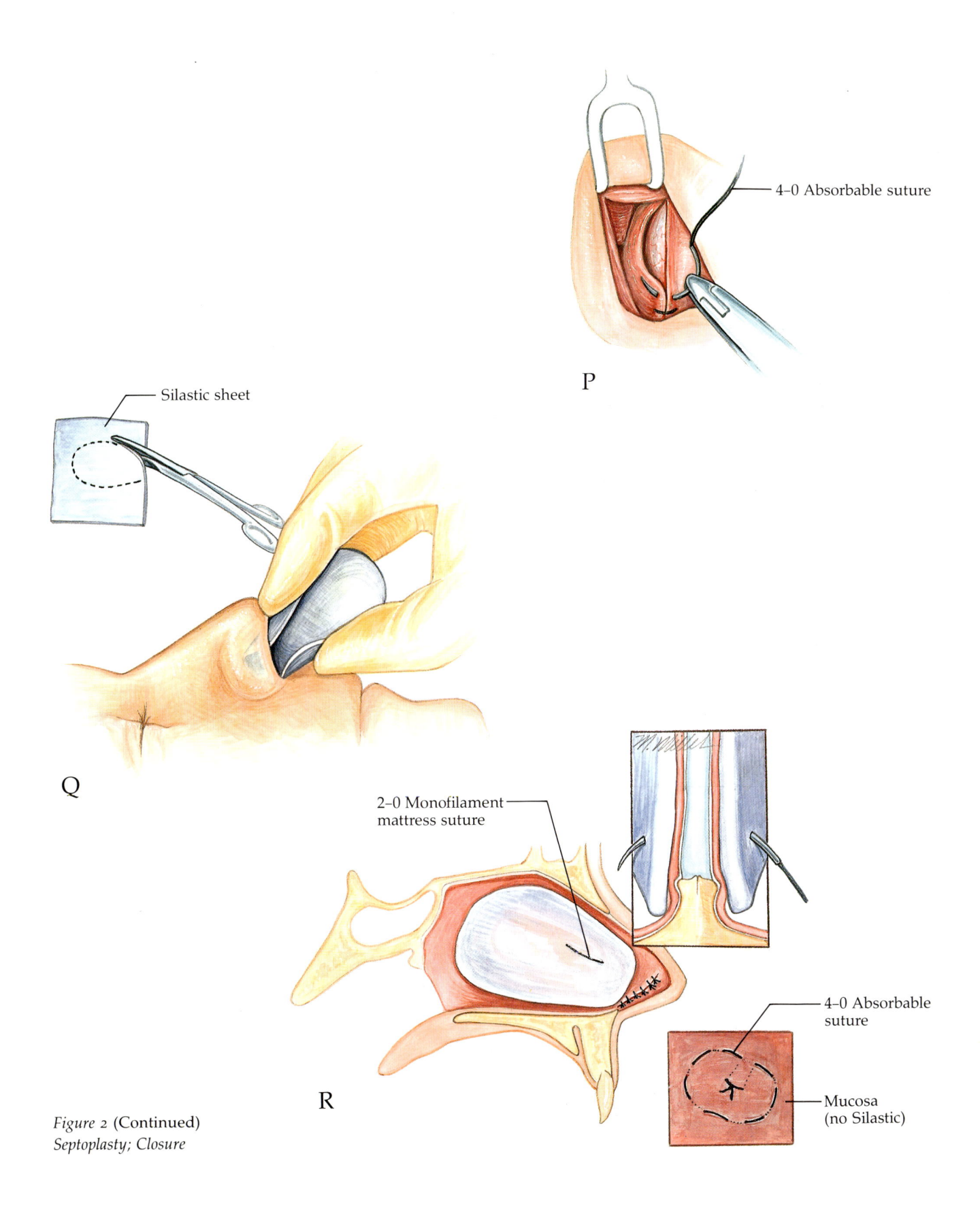

4-0 Absorbable suture

P

Silastic sheet

Q

2-0 Monofilament mattress suture

4-0 Absorbable suture

Mucosa (no Silastic)

R

Figure 2 (Continued)
Septoplasty; Closure

riform attachment with sharp, precision, bone-cutting rongeurs. The bone of the posterior septum should never be chiseled, twisted, deflected, or pulled if complete release of the superior attachment has not been accomplished.

Numbness of the lip or dentition may result. Columellar traction and nasal tip collapse may be associated with full transfixion incision and/or excessive resection of the inferior or caudal septum. Opposing septal mucosal lacerations that have been inadequately repaired seem to be the cause of septal perforations from this procedure. Failure to repair the septal deviation and relieve airway obstruction may be due to incomplete correction of the septum, delayed return of the "memory" of the septal cartilage, or an unappreciated external nasal deviation, asymmetric face, or associated sinus or turbinate disease.

Pearls and Pitfalls

Subperichondrial infiltration of local anesthetic greatly facilitates elevation of the mucoperichondrial flaps.

Precise identification and elevation of the perichondrium is essential to successful uncomplicated septal surgery.

The resection of septal cartilage should be limited.

Preserve a 1 cm dorsal and caudal strut of septal cartilage and its attachments if at all possible. Adherence to this rule must not compromise adequate straightening of the septum. If release or removal is unavoidable, adequate reconstructive techniques must be employed to ensure re-establishment of contour, support, and anchorage.

Never twist or chisel the bony septum until after it has been sharply released from the cribriform area.

Application of the septal splints greatly facilitates coaptation of the septal mucosa and alignment of minor tears. Triangular-shaped, major, or opposing tears must be repaired prior to inserting the septal splints.

Any nasal packing should be saturated with antibiotic ointment. Prophylaxis for *Staphylococcus aureus* must be administered if packing is to be retained beyond the first postoperative night in order to guard against the development of toxic shock syndrome.

Adequate airway restoration may be impossible with septoplasty alone if there is an associated major external nasal deformity, as seen in the "twisted" and "tension" noses. These circumstances require concomitant rhinoplasty in order to achieve an optimal result.

Turbinate or sinus surgery in combination with septoplasty may be essential to optimize the breathing result.

Septoplasty may be required to allow endoscopic access to the sinuses.

Douglas E. Mattox, M.D.
Donlin M. Long, M.D.

TRANSSEPTAL TRANSSPHENOIDAL HYPOPHYSECTOMY

Transseptal transsphenoidal hypophysectomy is the approach of choice for pituitary adenomas confined to the sella turcica and those with moderate suprasellar extension. The procedure has minimal morbidity, and were it not for the need for postoperative observation of fluid and electrolyte balance and endocrine status, most patients would be ready for discharge on the first or second postoperative day. Cosmetic nasal deformity and postoperative disturbance of breathing pattern are extremely uncommon. There is no comparison between the morbidity of this procedure and that of a frontal craniotomy.

Indications

The transseptal approach through the sphenoid sinus is indicated for micro- and macroadenomas of the pituitary gland. It can also be used for inflammatory disease of the sphenoid sinus (acute sinusitis, fungal sinusitis, mucoceles).

Preoperative Considerations

The patient is given general anesthesia via an oral endotracheal tube. He or she is positioned flat on the operating table, with the head slightly hyperextended to allow a perpendicular view of the rostrum of the sphenoid sinus. The skin of the face is prepared with antiseptic solution, and a standard head drape is applied. Towel clips should not be placed on the side of the head in case an intraoperative lateral x-ray film is needed. The suprapubic area or left lower quadrant is prepared for a fat graft. Fat is not harvested until it is needed in order to preserve its sterility. The operating scope is prepared with angle-eye pieces so that the surgeon can stand comfortably at the head of the table and look directly down or slightly retrograde (toward his or her feet). An f300 lens is used to provide adequate working distance for the long pituitary instruments.

Operative Steps

The initial exposure is performed using a headlight. The nose is decongested with topical cocaine. Additional vasoconstriction is obtained with 1 percent lidocaine with epinephrine 1:100,000, which is injected into the sublabial area, around the premaxillary spine, the nasal septum, and the floor of the nose. Adequate time is allowed for the vasoconstrictor to work before an incision is made.

The incision is made from the first premolar on one side to the first premolar on the opposite side (Fig. 3A). An adequate cuff of loose gingival tissue must be left above the teeth to allow closure. However, the incision must lie over the maxillary bone; if it crosses the gingival sulcus, contraction and discomfort of the lip may follow. The mucosal incision is usually made with a No. 15 blade and continued through the submucosal tissues with a cutting cautery. The incision is continued down to the bone of the premaxilla, and the tissues are elevated in the subperiosteal plane to identify the inferior portion of the piriform aperture (Fig. 3B).

The anterior nasal spine is identified and followed superiorly to the cartilaginous septum with a Joseph elevator or Cottle knife (Fig. 3B). The septal mucoperiosteal flaps are developed without additional nasal incisions. The caudal septum can be scratched with a Cottle knife or No. 15 blade to identify the plane between the mucoperichondrium and the cartilage (Fig. 3C). The mucoperichondrium can be developed on either the right or left side; if there is a pre-existing septal deviation, it is easier to develop it on the concave side.

Plate 50

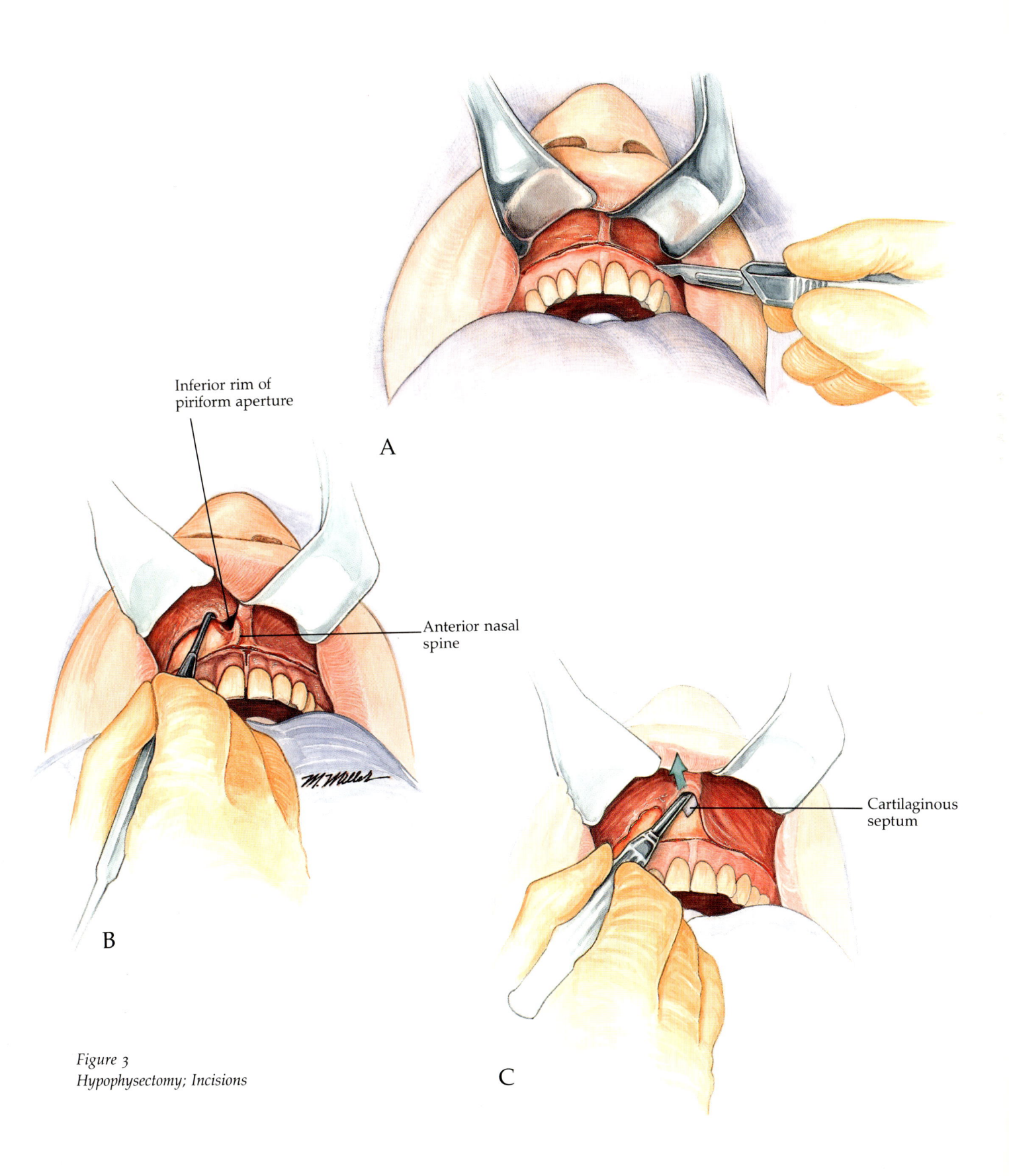

Inferior rim of
piriform aperture

Anterior nasal
spine

Cartilaginous
septum

A

B

C

Figure 3
Hypophysectomy; Incisions

Bilateral inferior nasal tunnels are elevated using a tunnel elevator with a curved tip (Fig. 3D). The tip of this instrument is kept in constant contact with the bone in order to avoid perforating the mucosa. The septal mucosa is widely elevated down to the vomer crest (Fig. 3E). It is important that the inferior tunnels extend above the attachment of the septal cartilage to the vomer on *both* sides (Fig. 3F). On one side this tunnel will connect with the septal mucosal elevation, and on the other side it must be high enough onto the septum to allow reflection of the septum without tearing the mucosa. The tight attachments at the mucosa at the bony cartilaginous junction must be divided carefully in order to avoid tearing the mucosa (Fig. 3F).

Plate 51

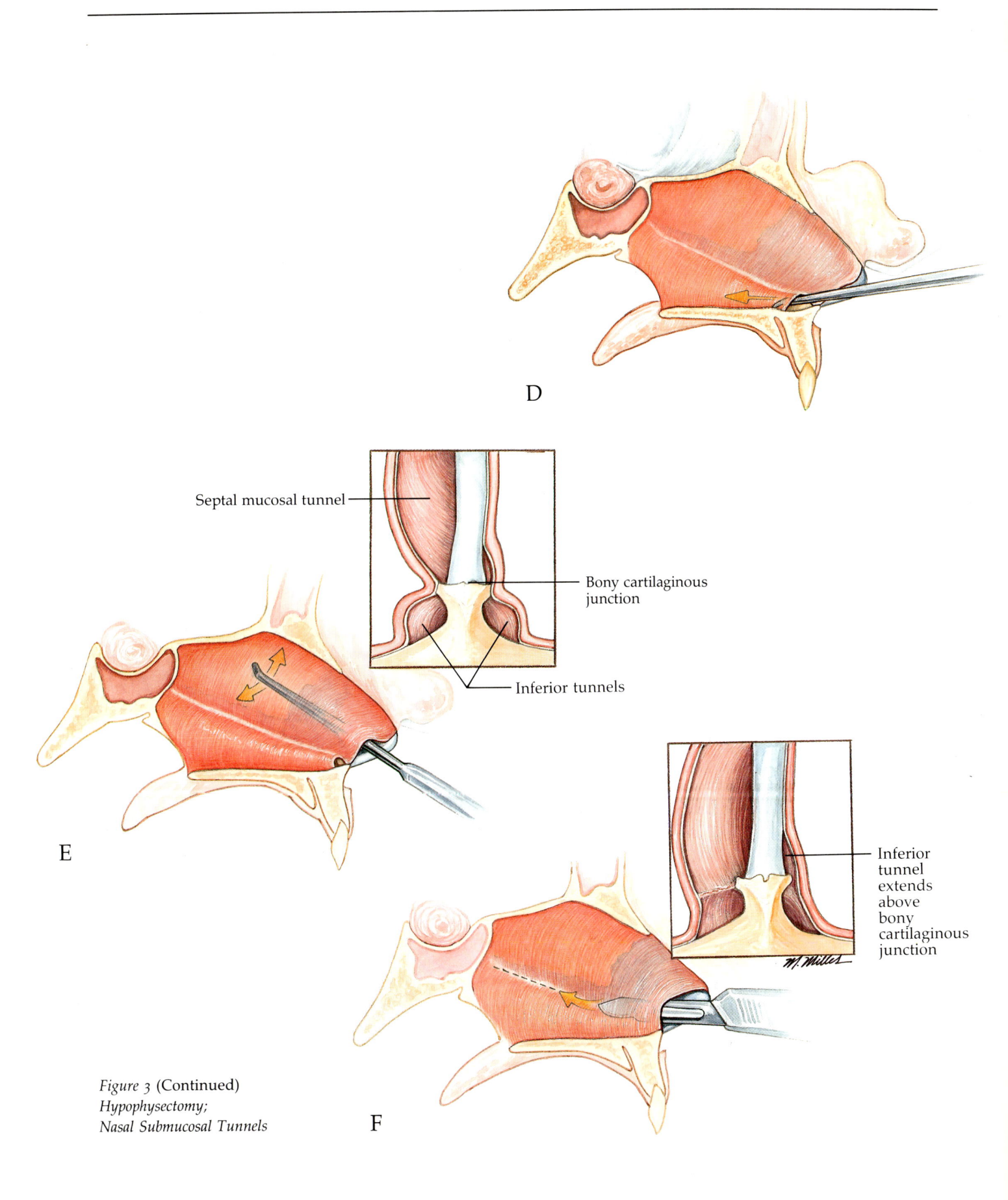

Septal mucosal tunnel

Bony cartilaginous junction

Inferior tunnels

Inferior tunnel extends above bony cartilaginous junction

D

E

F

Figure 3 (Continued)
Hypophysectomy;
Nasal Submucosal Tunnels

The septal mucoperichondrial elevation is continued back to the cartilaginous junction with the perpendicular plate of the ethmoid bone. When the bony cartilaginous junction is identified, the cartilage is separated from the maxillary crest inferiorly (Fig. 3G) and from the bone posteriorly (Fig. 3H). After the cartilage is fully mobilized, it will swing laterally toward the side on which the mucoperichondrium is undisturbed (Fig. 3I). The most superior attachment of the septal cartilage to the perpendicular plate of the ethmoid bone and its attachment to the upper lateral cartilages are not disturbed in order to prevent postoperative nasal collapse and a saddle nose deformity.

Once the cartilage is reflected to the side, the mucoperiosteal elevation is continued bilaterally from the vomer and the perpendicular plate of the ethmoid bone until the sphenoid rostrum is identified. The vomer and inferior portion of the perpendicular plate of the ethmoid are removed. If it is needed for additional exposure and room to manipulate the instruments, the premaxillary spine can be resected; however, this is not routinely required. Excessive removal of the premaxillary spine leads to some ptosis of the nasal tip and a more acute nasolabial angle.

The perpendicular plate of the ethmoid bone is cut with double-action or turbinate scissors (Fig. 3J) and is removed with forceps (Fig. 3K). It is important that the superior cut be performed first so that any twisting action as the bone is removed is not transmitted superiorly, where it could damage the cribriform plate. The perpendicular plate of the ethmoid should be removed in large pieces, which can be used later for reconstruction of the sella turcica and/or the anterior wall of the sphenoid sinus.

Plate 52

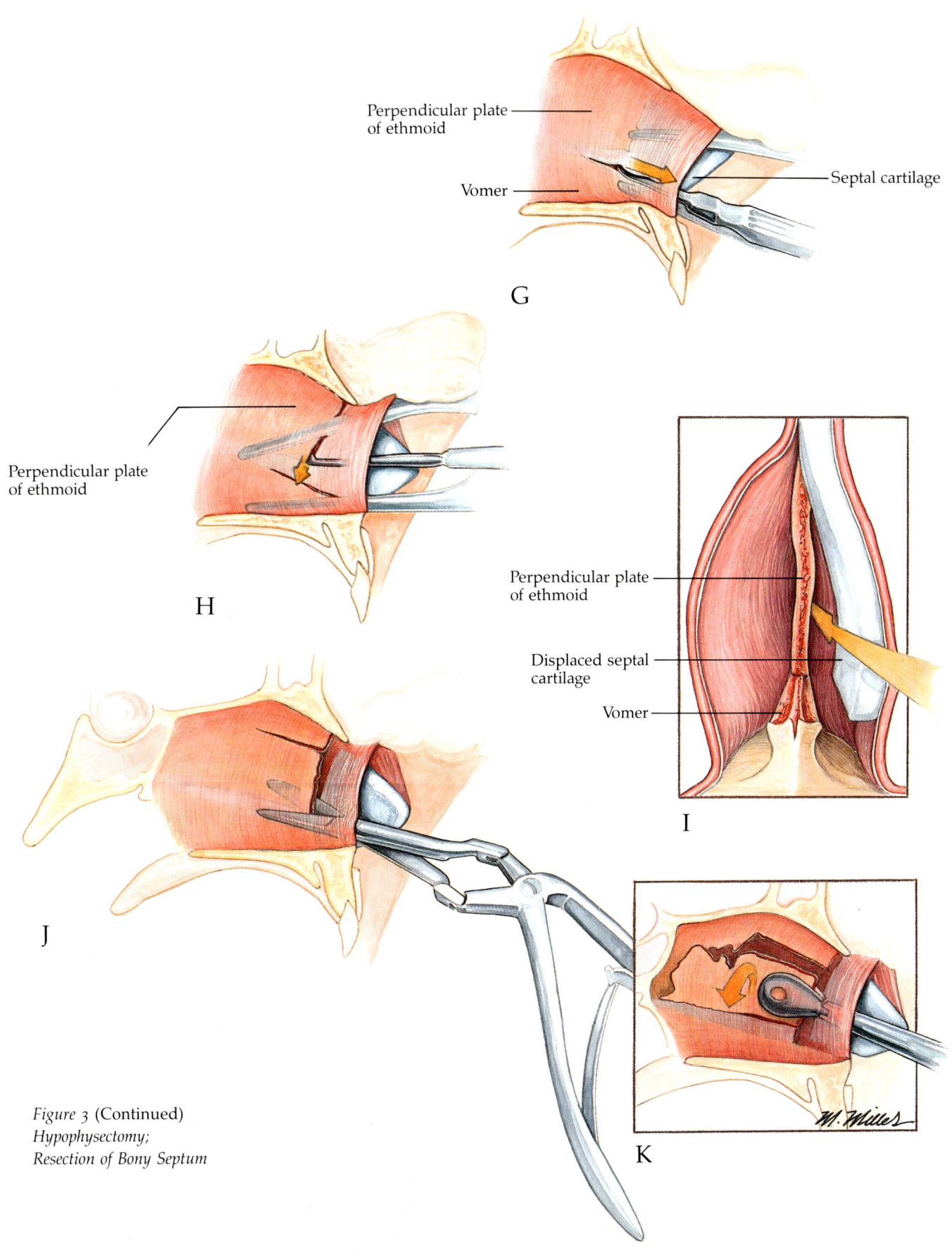

Perpendicular plate of ethmoid

Vomer

Septal cartilage

G

Perpendicular plate of ethmoid

H

Perpendicular plate of ethmoid

Displaced septal cartilage

Vomer

I

J

K

Figure 3 (Continued)
Hypophysectomy;
Resection of Bony Septum

The key to safe sphenoid surgery is identification of the sphenoid ostia before attempting to enter the sinus. As the perpendicular plate of the ethmoid is followed posteriorly, it develops a characteristic flaring as it fuses with the anterior face of the sphenoid bone. The sphenoid sinus ostia are identified on the superior medial aspect of the rostrum of the sphenoid. The mucosa is elevated laterally over the rostrum of the sphenoid bone until the ostia of the sphenoid sinus are identified (Fig. 3L). The ostia are frequently first seen as half-moon–shaped reflections of the mucosa within the sinus.

Once the sphenoid rostrum and the sinus ostia are identified, the Hardy retractor is inserted (Fig. 3M). Before inserting the retractor, a final check is made of the mucosal flaps, and any residual attachments along the vomer crest are lysed; otherwise, the retractor is likely to lacerate the mucosa. The Hardy retractor should be long enough to retract the mucosa off the face of the sphenoid, but an excessively long retractor only impedes passing the neurosurgical instruments into the sinus. The tension on the Hardy retractor should be adjusted to retract and compress the soft tissues of the nose and maintain exposure. Excessive tension cannot expand the bony walls of the nose or piriform aperture, and it risks complications of diastasis of the palate and fracture of the pterygoid plates or lesser wing of the sphenoid bone.

After the ostia are positively identified, the anterior wall of the sphenoid can be taken down by enlarging the ostia with a small sphenoid punch (Fig. 3N). Frequently the bone in the midline is thicker than the opening span of the punch or an intersinus septum prevents the punch from biting the bone. This midline bone can be quickly taken down with a 4-mm osteotome and mallet. As soon as the sphenoid sinus is open, the sella turcica should be apparent within it. If it is not, radiographic confirmation with a lateral view of the skull should be obtained. An instrument placed superiorly and inferiorly within the sinus defines the exposure in relation to the sella turcica. As much mucosa within the sinus as possible is removed; however, the lateral walls of the sinus are not scraped or otherwise manipulated because of the risk of dehiscence of the carotid artery or optic nerve.

Plate 53

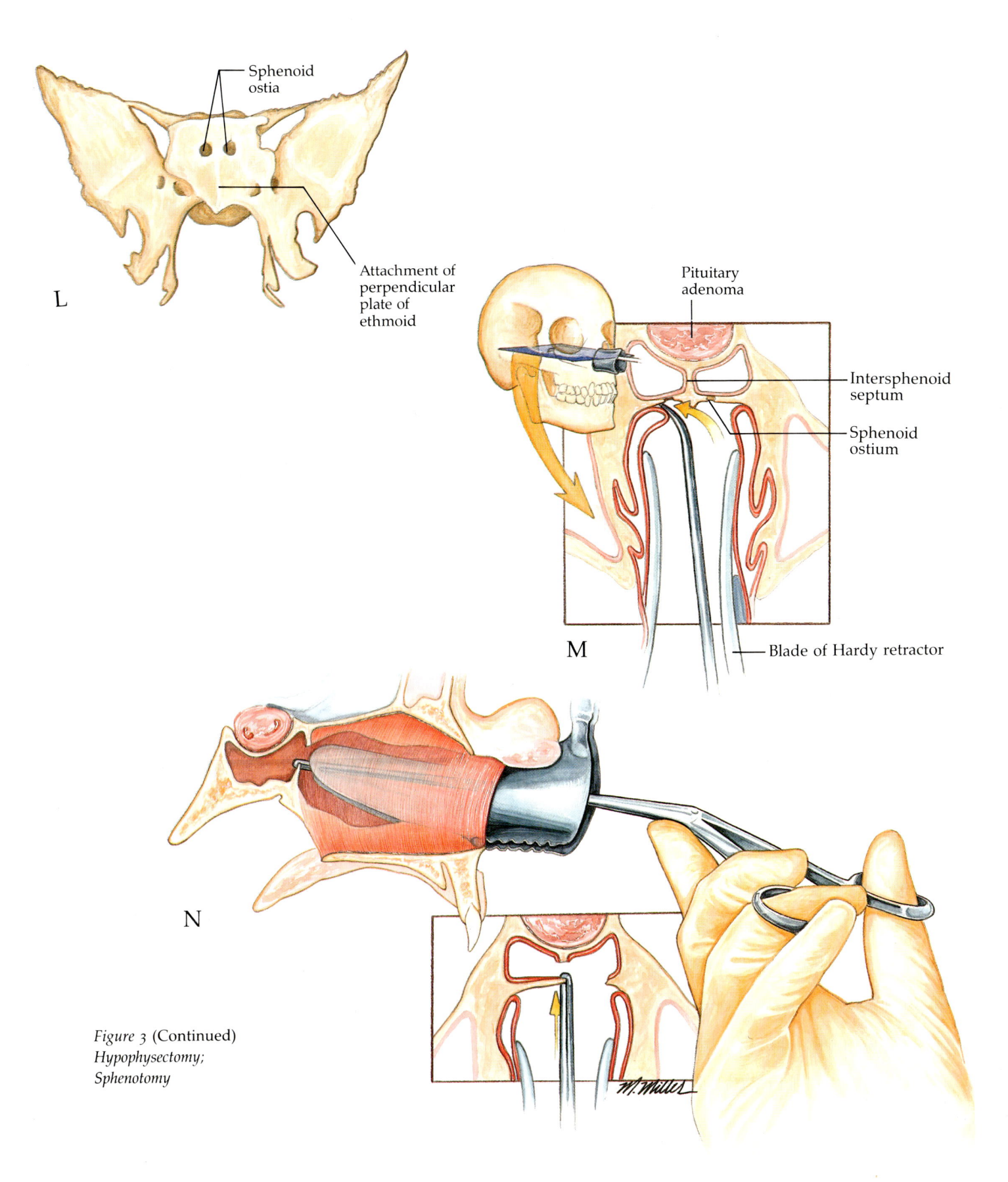

- Sphenoid ostia
- Attachment of perpendicular plate of ethmoid

L

- Pituitary adenoma
- Intersphenoid septum
- Sphenoid ostium
- Blade of Hardy retractor

M

N

Figure 3 (Continued)
Hypophysectomy;
Sphenotomy

The bone over the sella turcica is chipped with a 3-mm osteotome and mallet, care being taken not to lacerate the underlying dura mater. After a small opening is made in the bone, it is enlarged with a sphenoid punch. A cruciate incision is made in the dura to expose the tumor (Figs. 3O and 3P). The tumor is removed with ring curets and suction (Figs. 3Q and 3R). Particular care is taken with lateral dissection to avoid the cavernous sinus and optic nerve. A suprasellar extension will usually decompress into the sella turcica once the inferior portion of the tumor is removed. A gentle Valsalva maneuver by the anesthesiologist will help deliver the suprasellar portion of the tumor.

Plate 54

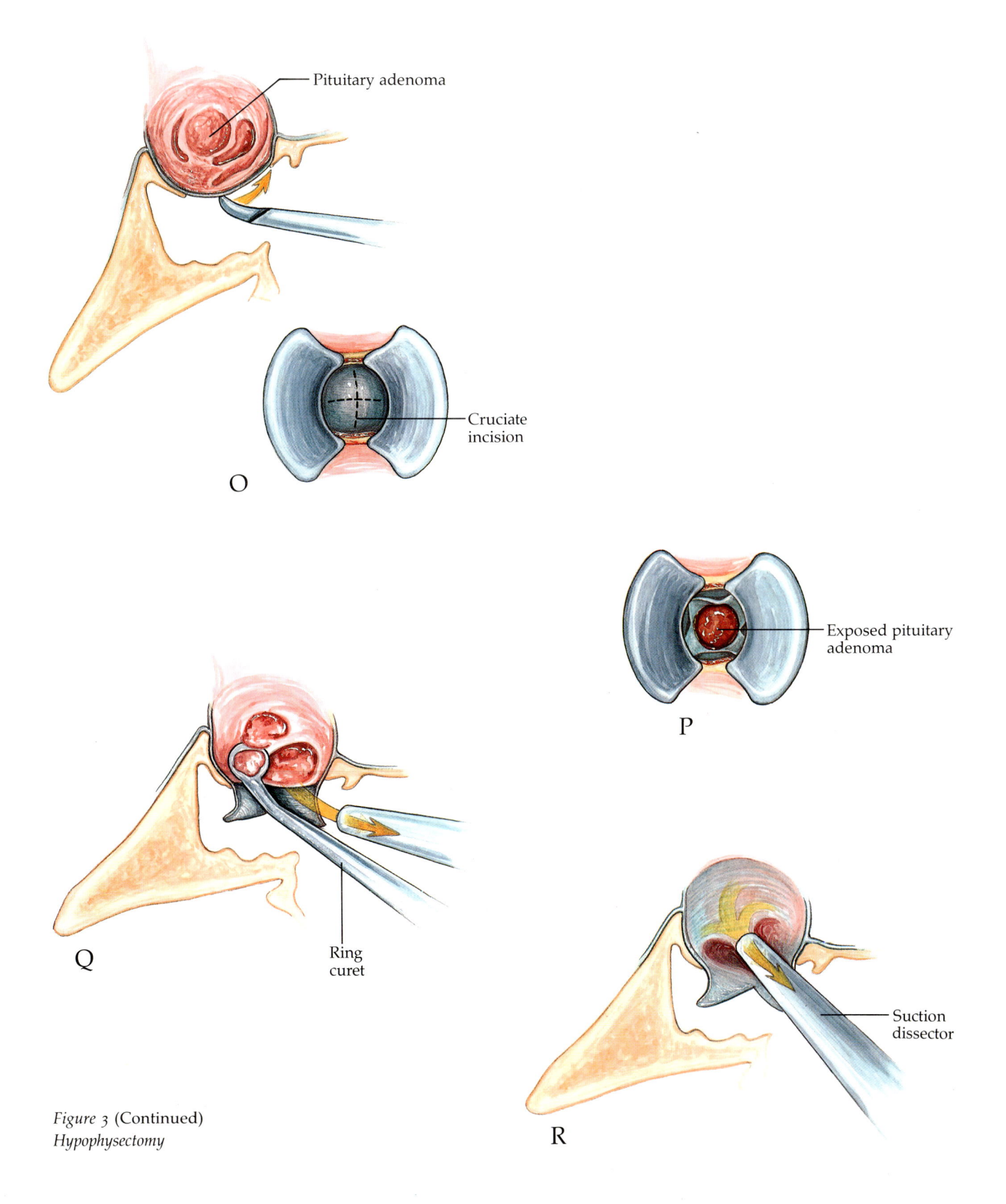

O — Pituitary adenoma / Cruciate incision

P — Exposed pituitary adenoma

Q — Ring curet

R — Suction dissector

Figure 3 (Continued)
Hypophysectomy

If no cerebrospinal fluid leak has occurred, the sella turcica is packed with abdominal fat and the posterior wall of the sinus is reconstructed with a piece of the perpendicular plate of the ethmoid bone (Fig. 3S). If a cerebrospinal fluid leak has occurred, both the sella turcica and the sphenoid sinus are packed, and the anterior wall of the sphenoid sinus is reconstructed with bone or cartilage.

Closure is started by permanently suturing the septal cartilage to the premaxillary spine in order to maintain its position in the midline. This is done with 3–0 nylon, which is drilled through the thin bone with a firm twisting action with a cutting needle in the needle holder (Fig. 3T). This maneuver is facilitated by pointing the needle forward parallel to the axis of the needle holder. The suture is passed through the cartilaginous septum and tied submucosally. The sublabial incision is closed with a running chromic suture (Fig. 3U). The nasal mucosa is quilted to the cartilaginous septum with transseptal 4–0 plain suture on a small straight needle. Septal splints can be added for additional septal stability (Fig. 3V). The nose is lightly packed, and the patient is extubated.

Postoperative Care

Patients may be kept in the neurosurgical intensive care unit overnight to monitor for cerebrospinal fluid leak, fluid and electrolyte imbalance (diabetes insipidus), and neurologic status. Visual field checks are made as soon as the patient is cooperative. Endocrine function is closely followed.

The nasal packing is removed the day after surgery if there is no significant postoperative oozing; otherwise it is removed at 48 hours. The internal splints are removed before the patient is discharged, usually between 6 and 8 days. The nasal and sublabial chromic sutures are left to dissolve unless they are bothering the patient.

Risks, Complications, and Sequelae

The infection rate with appropriate antibiotic coverage is negligible despite the fact that the procedure is done through a potentially contaminated oral and nasal cavity.

Nasal complications include loss of nasal tip projection from disarticulation of the upper portion of the septal cartilage from the perpendicular plate of the ethmoid bone or from excessive resection of the premaxillary spine. Posterior septal perforations can occur, but anterior perforations are uncommon because none of the septal cartilage is routinely resected.

Complications related to the Hardy retractor include diastasis of the palate and blindness from fracture of the lesser wing of the sphenoid bone through the optic canal. Diastasis of the palate is more likely to occur with patients with acromegaly and abnormally soft bone. Therefore, the retractor should be opened only until it meets firm resistance; excessive pressure should never be used.

Cerebrospinal fluid leak can occur, particularly in tumors with supradiaphragmatic extensions. Conservative management includes head elevation and repeated lumbar punctures or a lumbar drain. Most leaks seal spontaneously, but re-exploration and packing with additional fat usually repair persistent ones.

Plate 55

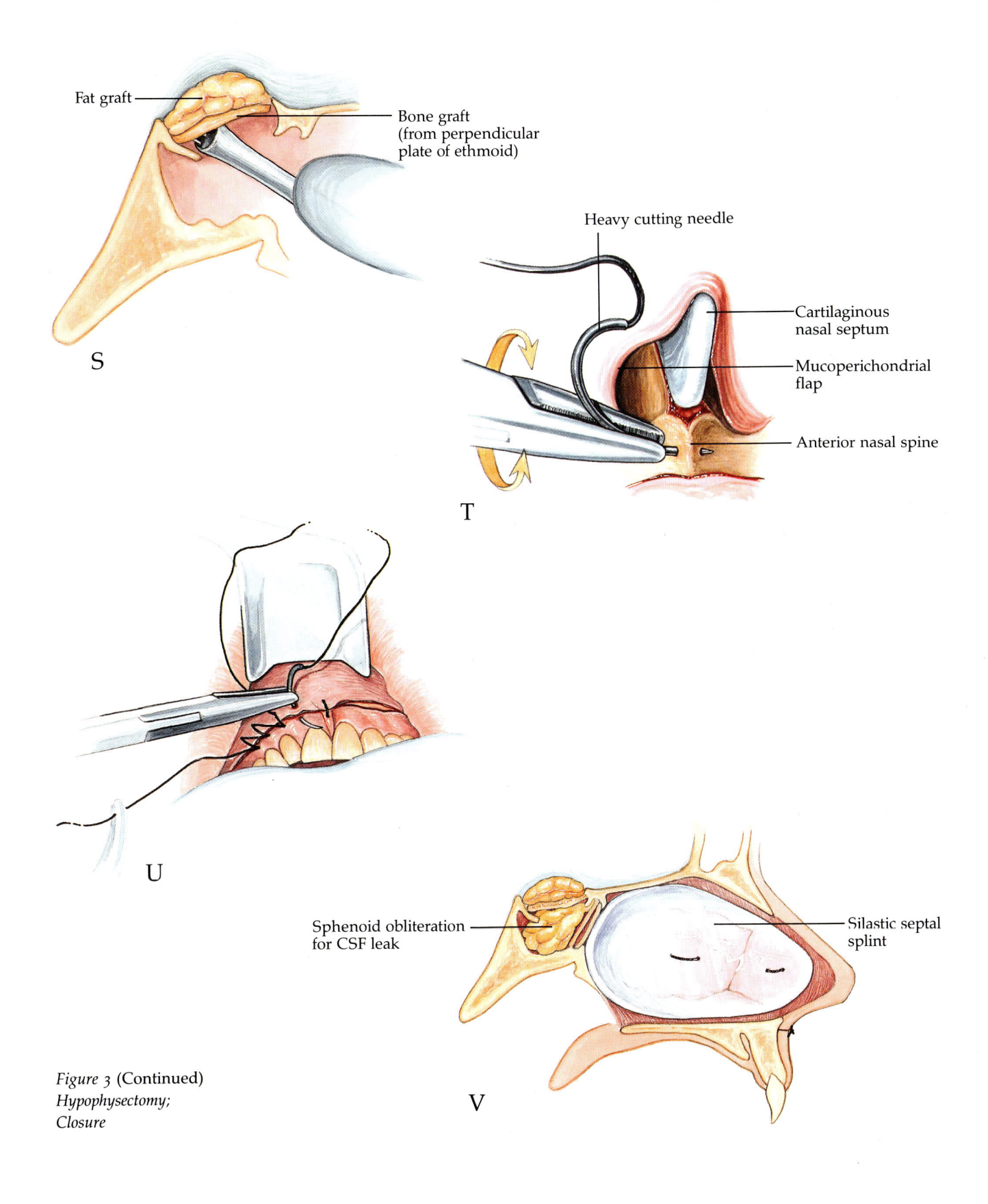

Fat graft

Bone graft (from perpendicular plate of ethmoid)

S

Heavy cutting needle

Cartilaginous nasal septum

Mucoperichondrial flap

Anterior nasal spine

T

U

Sphenoid obliteration for CSF leak

Silastic septal splint

V

Figure 3 (Continued)
Hypophysectomy;
Closure

133

Severe bleeding can occur from the cavernous sinus or internal carotid artery. The carotid artery can be damaged lateral to the sella turcica (and tumor), or it may be dehiscent within the sphenoid sinus. Visual loss can occur from damage to the optic nerve exposed within the sphenoid sinus or to the optic chiasm superior to the tumor.

Pearls and Pitfalls

Adequate vasoconstriction of the nasal mucosa is imperative for successful pituitary surgery. Adequate time should be allowed for the topical vasoconstrictor (cocaine) and the injected vasoconstrictor (lidocaine and epinephrine) to work before incisions are made. This is most conveniently done by applying the vasoconstrictive agents before the patient is prepared and draped. If there are cardiac contraindications to the use of lidocaine with epinephrine, phenylephrine (Neo-Synephrine) can be used; the optimal concentration is 0.05 mg per milliliter (1 to 20,000). This is conveniently prepared by adding 1 mg to 20 ml of local anesthetic.

The other key to adequate vasoconstriction is to infiltrate the floor of the nose thoroughly. This is most effectively done by bending a 1.5-inch 25-gauge needle so that the needle can be firmly inserted into the mucosa of the floor of the nose through the anterior naris.

In draping the patient, all towel clips should be kept in the midline and away from the side of the head in case an intraoperative radiograph is needed to confirm the operative position.

The initial mucosal incision should be kept just at the apex of the labial gingival sulcus. If the incision is lower than this, there will be insufficient tissue for closure of the wound. If the incision is higher, it will cause unnecessary trauma to the upper lip. A high incision will lead to complaints of stiffness of the upper lip and changes in the amount of teeth and gums that show when the patient smiles. These problems are usually treated with massage of the lip and waiting for the scar to soften.

A large septal branch of the sphenopalatine artery crosses the inferior portion of the rostrum of the sphenoid bone. The mucosa should be elevated only from the anterior and not the inferior surface of the sphenoid sinus to avoid injury to and hemorrhage of this vessel.

Suggested Reading

Kennedy DW, Cohn ES, Papel ID, Holliday MJ. Transsphenoidal approach to the sella: The Johns Hopkins Experience. Laryngoscope 1984; 94:1066–1073.

Kern EB, Pearson BW, McDonald TJ, Laws ER Jr. The transseptal approach to lesions of the pituitary and parasellar regions. Laryngoscope 1979; 89(Suppl 15):1–34.

Lee KJ. The sublabial transseptal transsphenoidal approach to the hypophysis. Laryngoscope 1978; 88(Suppl 10):1–65.

Ira D. Papel, M.D.

SEPTAL DERMOPLASTY

Hereditary hemorrhagic telangiectasia is an autosomal dominant disorder that affects the walls of small subepithelial blood vessels. Electron microscopy studies have shown that the affected vessels are dilated venules of capillary, postcapillary, and collecting vessels. There are defects in the endothelial lining as well as the smooth muscle walls of the vessels. These blood vessels are extremely fragile and thus are subject to bleeding with minimal trauma. The epithelial surfaces of the respiratory, gastrointestinal, and genitourinary tracts are affected. The most common symptom, however, is epistaxis from involvement of nasal septal mucosa. Transfusions for these patients may become common maintenance therapy.

In some patients pressure and local cautery application may suffice to control the epistaxis. At the opposite extreme are individuals who are constantly facing life-threatening complications due to hemorrhage. As a result of the serious potential of hereditary hemorrhagic telangiectasia, many surgical therapies have been proposed in the past. In 1960 Saunders described removal of the nasal mucosa and replacement with skin grafts. This procedure has been modified in this text but is essentially the same. In 1962 Heuston and Willis described excision of the anterior septum and lateral nasal mucosa. The CO_2 laser has been used to coagulate superficial telangiectasias in the nasal cavity. Argon and Nd:YAG lasers have also been used for therapy of hereditary hemorrhagic telangiectasia, with recommendations that repeat therapy may be necessary at 4- to 6-month intervals. More aggressive surgical therapy has been suggested, including labiobuccal flaps, amnion grafts, and facial flaps.

Indications

The major indication for septal dermoplasty is hereditary hemorrhagic telangiectasia. Other nasal disorders that cause diffuse nasal bleeding or cicatrix also may be considered for this procedure.

Preoperative Considerations

The diagnosis of hereditary hemorrhagic telangiectasia is clinical and is confirmed by family history. The clinical syndrome was well described by Osler in 1901. The disease is transmitted as an autosomal dominant disorder with variable penetrance. The recognizable features are multiple vascular lesions throughout the skin, mucosal surfaces, and viscera. The cutaneous lesions are typically macular or telangiectatic and blanch when pressure is applied. Macular vascular lesions are extremely common in Kiesselbach's area of the nasal septum, leading to the most common presentation of epistaxis. Visceral lesions such as arteriovenous malformations of the lungs may lead to hemoptysis. The hemostatic profile is normal.

Operative Steps

The patient is placed on the operating room table in the supine position with the head slightly elevated. General anesthesia is usually employed, but a local anesthetic is acceptable. The nasal mucosa is completely treated with topical 4 percent cocaine solution, and the membranous septum and submucosal tissues are infiltrated with 1 percent lidocaine with 1:100,000 epinephrine solution.

The nasal mucosa is then denuded with a ring curet as far back on the septum as possible. The mucosa is also removed from the floor of the nose and the lateral nasal wall (Fig. 4A). A rim of skin from the mucocutaneous junction is excised in order to provide an anchor site for the skin graft anteriorly (Fig. 4B). This incision is carried onto the floor of the nose just anterior to the inferior turbinate. Care should be taken to leave the perichondrium under the mucosa intact, as this layer will supply the skin graft with its new blood supply. There is usually steady bleeding from the bare perichondrial surfaces. The flow can be slowed or stopped by the application of thrombin spray solution to achieve hemostasis. The mucosa that lies in the inferior and middle meatuses is not removed in this procedure, as trauma to these areas is unlikely to occur in normal circumstances (Fig. 4C). A lateral alotomy can be considered to improve exposure (Fig. 4D). In an individual with small nostrils this may be a helpful maneuver, but in general it is not necessary.

Plate 56

A — Exposed septal perichondrium / Curet

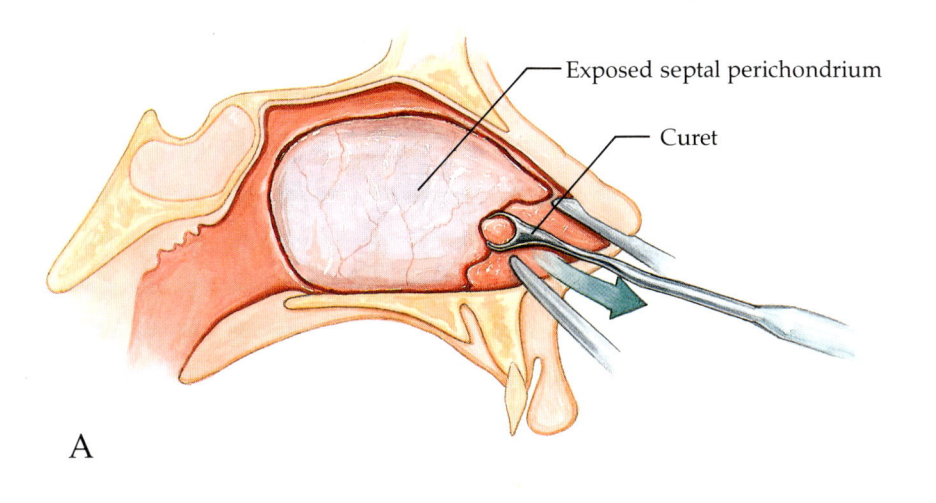

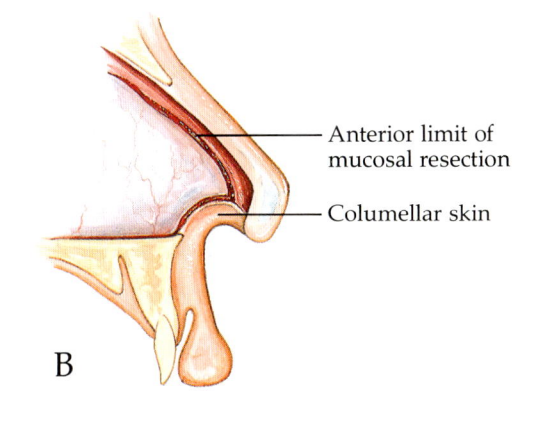

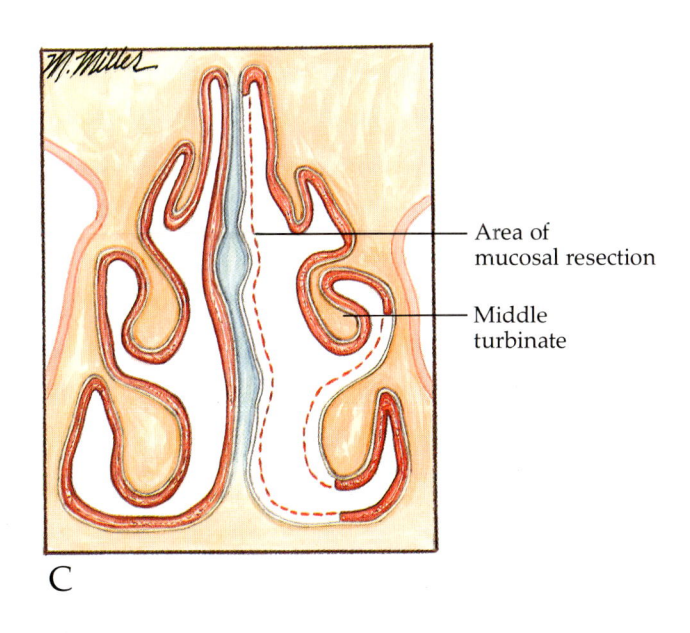

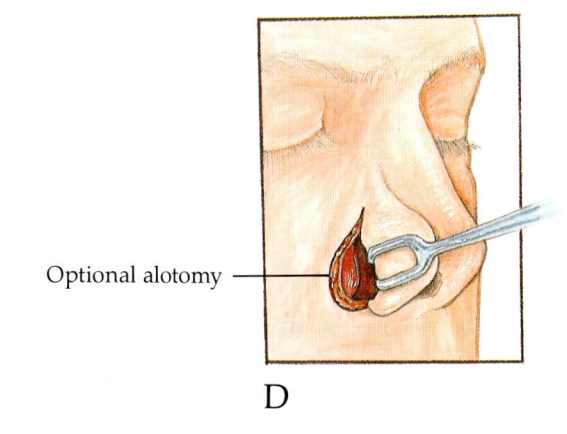

B — Anterior limit of mucosal resection / Columellar skin

C — Area of mucosal resection / Middle turbinate

D — Optional alotomy

Figure 4
Septal Dermoplasty; Mucosal Resection

A split-thickness skin graft with a thickness of 12 to 14 thousandths inch is then harvested from the lateral thigh with a dermatome. A graft of approximately 9 × 15 cm is usually adequate to provide coverage of both nasal passages. The donor site is then sprayed with thrombin solution and covered with an occlusive dressing. The graft is divided and carefully placed into the nasal cavity along the septum, around the floor of the nose, and onto the denuded areas of the lateral nasal wall (Figs. 4E and 4F). The anterior border of the graft is then sutured to the anterior skin at the membranous septum with 4–0 absorbable suture (Fig. 4E). A sheet of Silastic is then tubed and inserted into the nasal cavity after being coated with an antibiotic ointment. The placement of this sheeting must be meticulous so as not to displace the skin graft. The Silastic sheet is sutured to the nasal vestibule using 4–0 nylon mattress sutures. Packing can then be inserted into the interior of the Silastic sheet until moderate pressure is exerted around the entire nasal cavity (Fig. 4F). A drip pad is then applied, and the patient is transported to the recovery room. A mild oozing from the graft can be expected in the immediate postoperative period.

Postoperative Care

The packing is left inside the Silastic sleeve for 1 week. After its removal, the Silastic sheet is suctioned clean and left in place for 2 additional weeks. During this period the patient is encouraged to use a normal saline nasal spray several times a day to prevent crusting. After the Silastic sheet is removed, there will be areas of skin graft that have become necrotic if they were not overlying denuded areas. These can be trimmed at this time or left to undergo necrosis.

The patient will require instruction on how to maintain humidity in a nasal cavity stripped of most of its ciliated mucus-producing cells. The frequent use of saline or glycerine compound will help to keep the nasal cavity moist and free of crust and odors. This becomes a permanent task after septal dermoplasty. Occasional debridement of crust and debris by the physician may be necessary.

Since hereditary hemorrhagic telangiectasia is a systemic disease, a careful watch for recurrence of nasal lesions must be maintained for an indefinite period.

Risks, Complications, and Sequelae

The most likely complication intraoperatively is that excessive bleeding will prevent the surgeon from completing the procedure in a satisfactory manner. Because of the vascular nature of this disorder, the surgeon should always be prepared to deal with excessive blood loss in a timely and efficient manner. If the perichondrium over the nasal septum is damaged bilaterally, the cartilage will lose its blood supply and a septal perforation is likely to result. This can also lead to increased crusting and nasal obstruction later. Failure of the skin graft to survive may be secondary to inadequate removal of epithelial tissues. A hematoma or seroma under the graft may also jeopardize survival. Careless placement of the splints and packing may also compromise the final result. If the grafts are too thick, the patient may experience nasal obstruction. Care should

Septal Dermoplasty

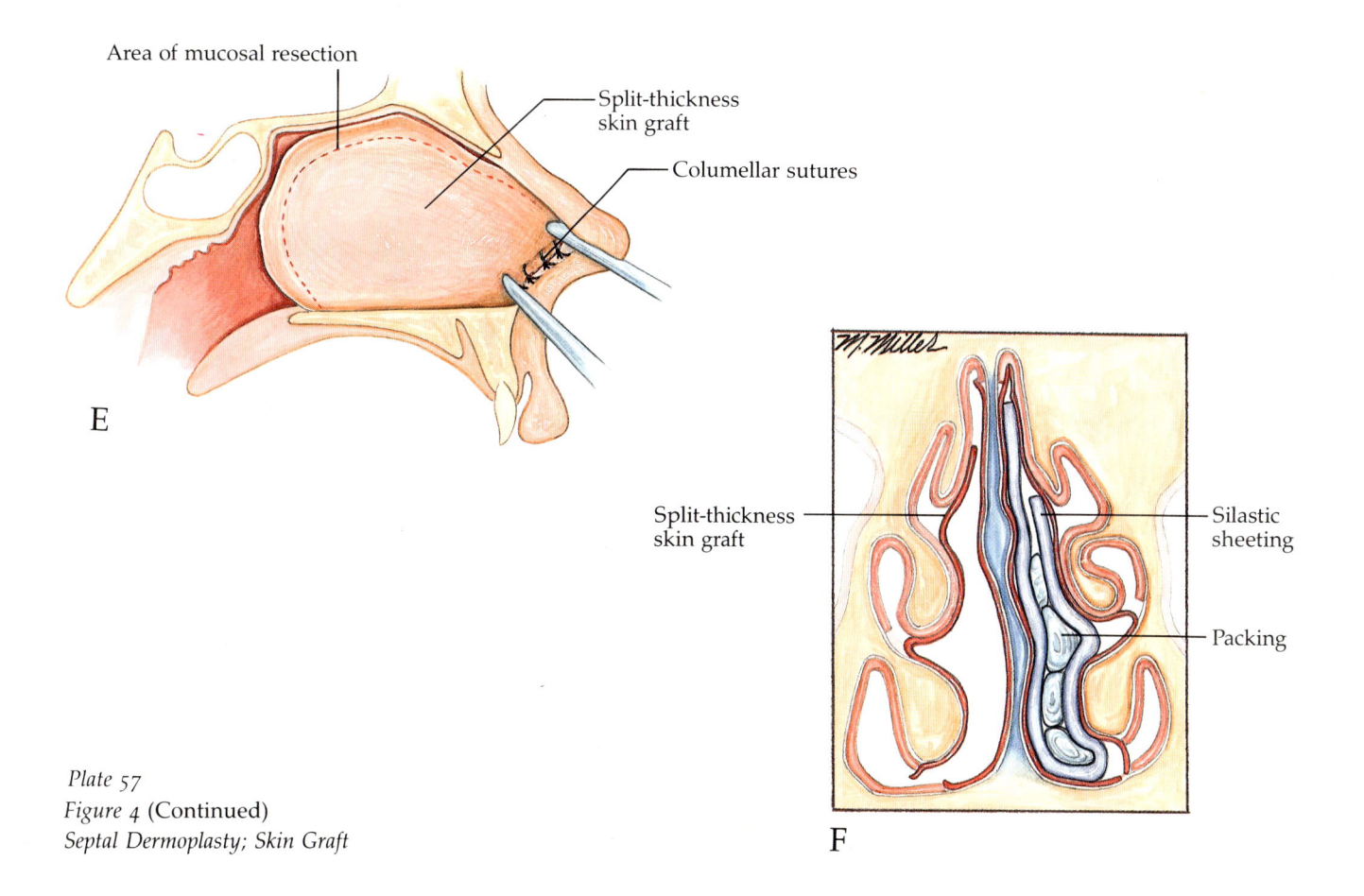

Plate 57
Figure 4 (Continued)
Septal Dermoplasty; Skin Graft

be taken to set the dermatome at the proper thickness prior to harvesting the skin grafts. As a result of the resection of respiratory epithelium, atrophic rhinitis and crusting may occur. The patient should be aware of the proper cleaning and maintenance techniques to keep these symptoms to a minimum. As with all procedures requiring the use of internal packing, an antibiotic with coverage of *Staphylococcus aureus* should be used in the perioperative period to avoid toxic shock syndrome or nasal infection.

Recurrence of telangiectatic lesions should always be expected. Telangiectasias have been seen to recur even in the skin graft material.

Pearls and Pitfalls

The treatment of hereditary hemorrhagic telangiectasia should be individualized. Whereas only gentle local therapy may be adequate for one patient, aggressive and invasive surgical procedures may be necessary for another. The severity of symptoms should determine if septal dermoplasty or other procedures will benefit the patient.

The best possible hemostasis should be maintained while performing the procedures. This allows for better exposure and greater accuracy in placing and fixing the skin grafts.

Use of thrombin topical spray has helped to reduce the bleeding from the perichondrium significantly. Silastic splints help reduce the trauma to the skin grafts while packing is placed, leading to better graft position and survival.

If trimming of the excess skin graft after packing removal is difficult, it is better to let the excess skin undergo necrosis rather than risk detaching the newly placed grafts.

Constant attention to and care of nasal toilet by the patient with help and advice from the physician are essential for comfort. The presence of septal perforations significantly complicates this cleansing activity.

Suggested Reading

Ben-Bassat M, Kaplan I, Levy R. Treatment of hereditary hemorrhagic telangiectasia of the nasal mucosa with the carbon dioxide laser. Br J Plast Surg 1978; 31:157–158.

Goldsmith MM, Fry TL. Tips on septal dermoplasty. Laryngoscope 1987; 97:994–995.

Heuston JT, Willis R. Excision of nasal lining and split-skin graft replacement in Osler's disease. Br J Plast Surg 1962; 15:314.

Hirshowitz B, Moscona R, Eliachar I. Closure of septal perforation in Osler-Weber-Rendu's disease by bilateral labial-buccal flaps. Plast Reconstr Surg 1978; 62:296–299.

Jahnke V. Ultrastructure of hereditary telangiectasia. Arch Otolaryngol 1970; 91:262–265.

Laurian N, Kalmanovitch M, Shimberg R. Amniotic graft in the management of severe epistaxis due to hereditary haemorrhagic telangiectasia. J Laryngol Otol 1979; 93:589–595.

McCabe WP, Kelly AP. Management of epistaxis in Osler-Weber Rendu disease: Recurrence of telangiectases within a nasal skin graft. Plast Reconstr Surg 1972; 50:114–118.

Meneffee MG, Flessa HC, Glueck HI, et al. Hereditary hemorrhagic telangiectasia (Osler-Weber-Rendu disease): An electron microscopic study of the vascular lesions before and after therapy with hormones. Arch Otolaryngol 1975; 101:246–251.

Osler W. On a family form of recurring epstaxis, associated with multiple telangiectases of the skin and mucous membranes. Bull Johns Hopkins Hosp 1901; 12:333–337.

Parkin JL, Dixon JA. Laser photocoagulation in hereditary hemorrhagic telangiectasia. Otolaryngol Head Neck Surg 1981; 89:204–208.

Zohar Y, Sadov R, Shvili Y, et al. Surgical management of hereditary hemorrhagic telangiectasia. Arch Otolaryngol Head Neck Surg 1987; 113: 754–757.

Saunders WH. Septal dermoplasty for control of nosebleeds caused by hereditary hemorrhagic telangiectasia or septal perforations. Trans Am Acad Ophthalmol Otolaryngol 1960; 64:500–506.

Manning Miles Goldsmith, M.D.

CLOSURE OF NASAL SEPTAL PERFORATIONS

Indications

Small, posterior septal perforations with well-healed edges often do not require any treatment. The symptomatic perforation is generally greater than 1 cm in diameter, located more anteriorly, and has thickened granulations at its edges. Temporary relief from intranasal crusting can be provided by frequent saline irrigations and petrolatum-based ointments. If these conservative measures fail to relieve the patient's symptoms, closure of the perforation is indicated.

A trial with a septal button is appropriate when the nature of the perforation (size and location) and the septal anatomy are suitable and when surgical closure is contraindicated. Generally, anterior septal perforations that are 2 cm or less in maximal diameter are appropriate for a button. Currently manufactured septal buttons (Xomed Inc, Jacksonville, Florida) are 3 cm in diameter and generally cover perforations up to 2 cm in size, allowing for 3 to 4 mm overlap of the margins. Septal deformities are relative contraindications to button placement, as the flange on the convex side of the deformity may increase nasal obstruction.

Contraindications to surgical closure include collagen vascular diseases (lupus erythematosus, Wegener's granulomatosis, polyarteritis nodosa, scleroderma), granulomatous diseases of the septum (sarcoidosis, tuberculosis), and patients who are poor operative risks. Placement of a septal button may also be appropriate for patients who are habitual drug abusers (persistent intranasal insufflation of cocaine) and for those perforations that are difficult to close surgically.

Preoperative Considerations

The etiology of the nasal septal perforation needs to be carefully evaluated prior to undertaking any corrective procedure. Common causes may be divided into four main categories: (1) trauma is the most common etiology and includes septal surgery, cautery for epistaxis, and persistent nose picking; (2) inflammation and infection, including septal abscess, collagen vascular diseases, granulomatous diseases, syphilis, and diphtheria; (3) inhalant irritants, which include cocaine, acidic fumes, and lime and cement dust; and (4) neoplasia, which includes carcinoma, leukemic infiltrates (chloroma), and polymorphic reticulosis. A biopsy of the margin of the perforation is indicated when the margin is clinically suspicious for neoplasia and when the etiology of the perforation is not clear from the history and/or physical examination.

Part I: Closure with Septal Buttons

The septal button offers an alternative means of septal perforation closure that is particularly useful in those patients who are poor candidates for surgical correction. In my experience, approximately 60 percent of selected patients are able to tolerate and continue to use a septal button on a long-term basis. The current septal buttons employed by the author are made of soft silicone material and come in the standard one-piece and the investigative two-piece models.

Operative Steps

INSERTION OF THE ONE-PIECE SEPTAL BUTTON

After adequate decongestion of the nose with cocaine, 1 percent lidocaine with 1:100,000 epinephrine is infiltrated around the margins of the septal perforation. The flanges of the button are trimmed to an approximate size that will permit 3 to 4 mm of overlap with respect to the margins of the perforation. The edges of one flange are then sewn together in a rosette fashion (Fig. 5A), and the suture is tied and left long. The sutured flange is directed into the nasal cavity, and the suture is passed through the perforation and retrieved from the contralateral side (Fig. 5B). Gentle traction is applied to the suture, and the rosette is pulled through the perforation while simultaneously a hemostat pushes it through from the contralateral side. The suture is then cut and the flange resumes its original configuration (Figs. 5C and 5D). Minor adjustments in the size of the flanges may be made. Care must be taken so that the flanges of the button do not abut the junction of the septum with the upper lateral cartilage, as this is a particularly annoying sensation for the patient.

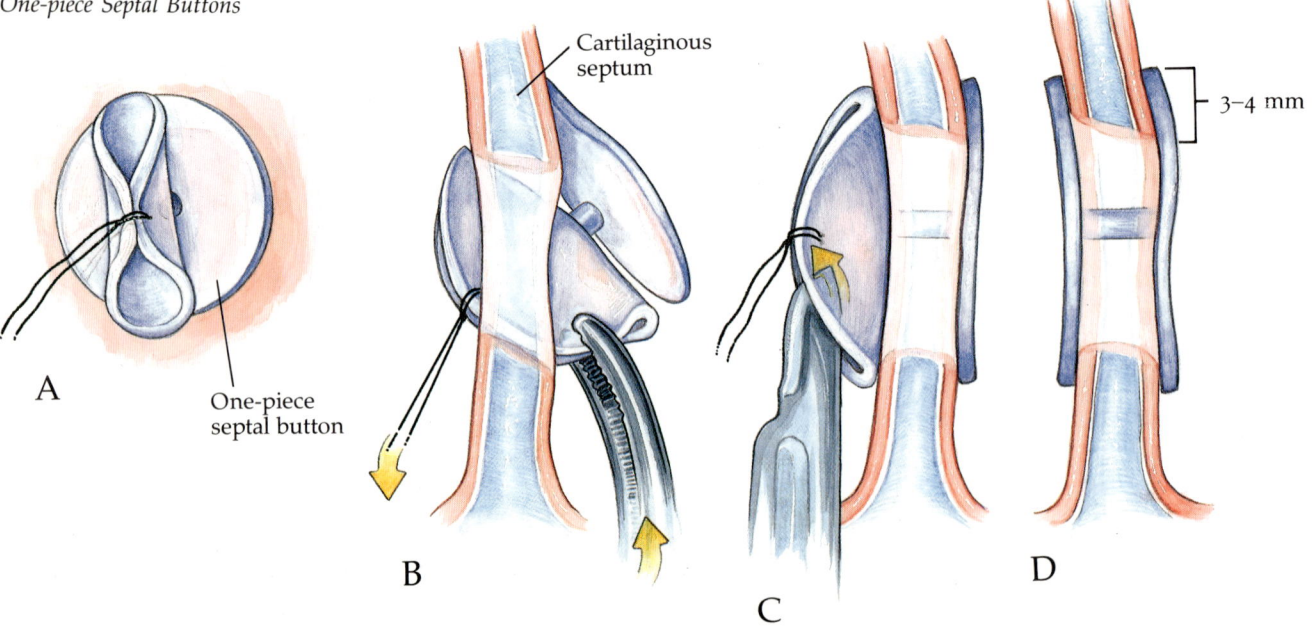

Plate 58
Figure 5
Closure of Nasal Septal Perforations;
Insertion Techniques for
One-piece Septal Buttons

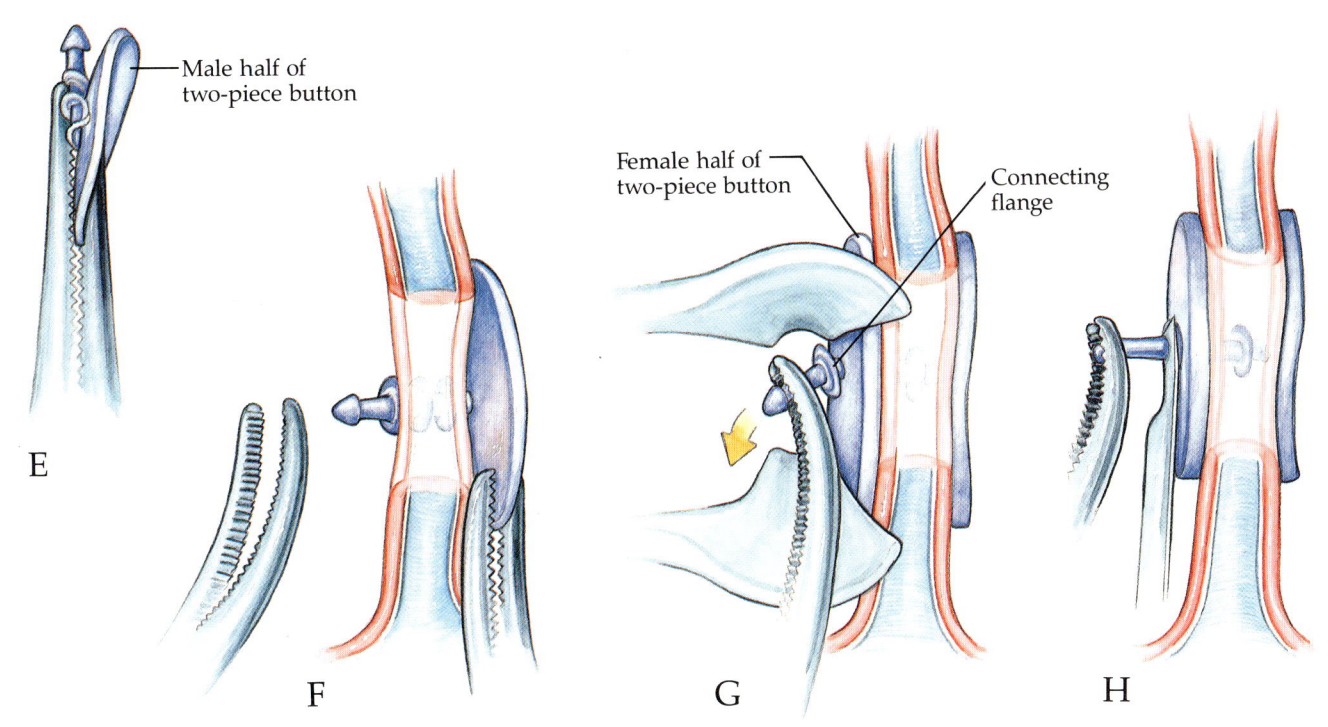

Plate 59
Figure 5 (Continued)
Closure of Nasal Septal Perforations;
Insertion Techniques for
Two-piece Septal Buttons

INSERTION OF THE TWO-PIECE SEPTAL BUTTON

The one-piece version of the septal button is rather difficult to insert as well as to remove. Furthermore, the width of the one-piece button is not adjustable, which may affect long-term patient tolerance, particularly if the button is too tight against the septum. An adjustable two-piece silicone septal button has been developed that obviates the disadvantages of the one-piece button.

After adequate decongestion of the nose by topical application of cocaine, 1 percent lidocaine with 1:100,000 epinephrine is infiltrated around the margins of the septal perforation. The pieces of the button are trimmed to an approximate size that will permit 3 to 4 mm of overlap with the margins of the perforation. The male connecting piece of the button is then grasped with a hemostat (Fig. 5E) and introduced through the perforation (Fig. 5F). The male piece is then introduced through the hole of the opposing female piece. A No. 1 nasal speculum is used to stabilize the female piece of the button as a hemostat pulls the male connecting piece through the female connector (Fig. 5G). The button is adjusted to the desired width by pulling the connecting flanges of the male piece sequentially through the hole in the female piece. The excess male connecting piece is then severed, leaving the most proximal connecting flange intact to secure the two pieces of the button (Fig. 5H). If removal is necessary, the connecting flange of the male piece is cut with a scalpel, and each piece of the button is delivered through a separate nostril.

Risks, Complications, and Sequelae

Immediate complications of septal button insertion are relatively minor and consist, for the most part, of epistaxis. Application of cocaine and infiltration with epinephrine prior to insertion help to prevent this complication, but on occasion the procedure will have to be aborted because of troublesome hemorrhage.

Crusting around the button is a variable problem that may limit long-term patient tolerance of the prosthesis. This can be somewhat alleviated by saline spray and petrolatum-based ointments. A tightly fitting button may conceivably cause enlargement of the perforation from pressure necrosis, although the author is not aware of any reports of this.

Pearls and Pitfalls

The etiology of the perforation must be established.

The septum should be relatively straight.

Be sure there is adequate topical application of cocaine and infiltration of the margins of the perforation with 1 percent lidocaine and 1:100,000 epinephrine prior to insertion of the prosthesis.

Trim the flanges so that there is 3 to 4 mm overlap with the margins of the perforation. If possible, the flanges of the button should not abut the junction of the septum with the upper lateral cartilage.

Part II: Surgical Closure of Septal Perforations

Operative Steps

After adequate nasal decongestion with cocaine, local anesthesia (1 percent lidocaine with epinephrine 1:200,000) is infiltrated in the usual manner. Relatively small (< 2 cm) and anterior perforations may be approached via a right hemitransfixion incision (Fig. 6A). Exposure is facilitated for larger and more posterior perforations by the external rhinoplasty approach. With either surgical approach, bilateral septal mucoperichondrial flaps are elevated as far back as the perforation (Fig. 6B). The anterior nasal spine of the maxilla is exposed, and the bilateral inferior subperiosteal tunnels are elevated (Fig. 6C). These inferior tunnels extend lat-

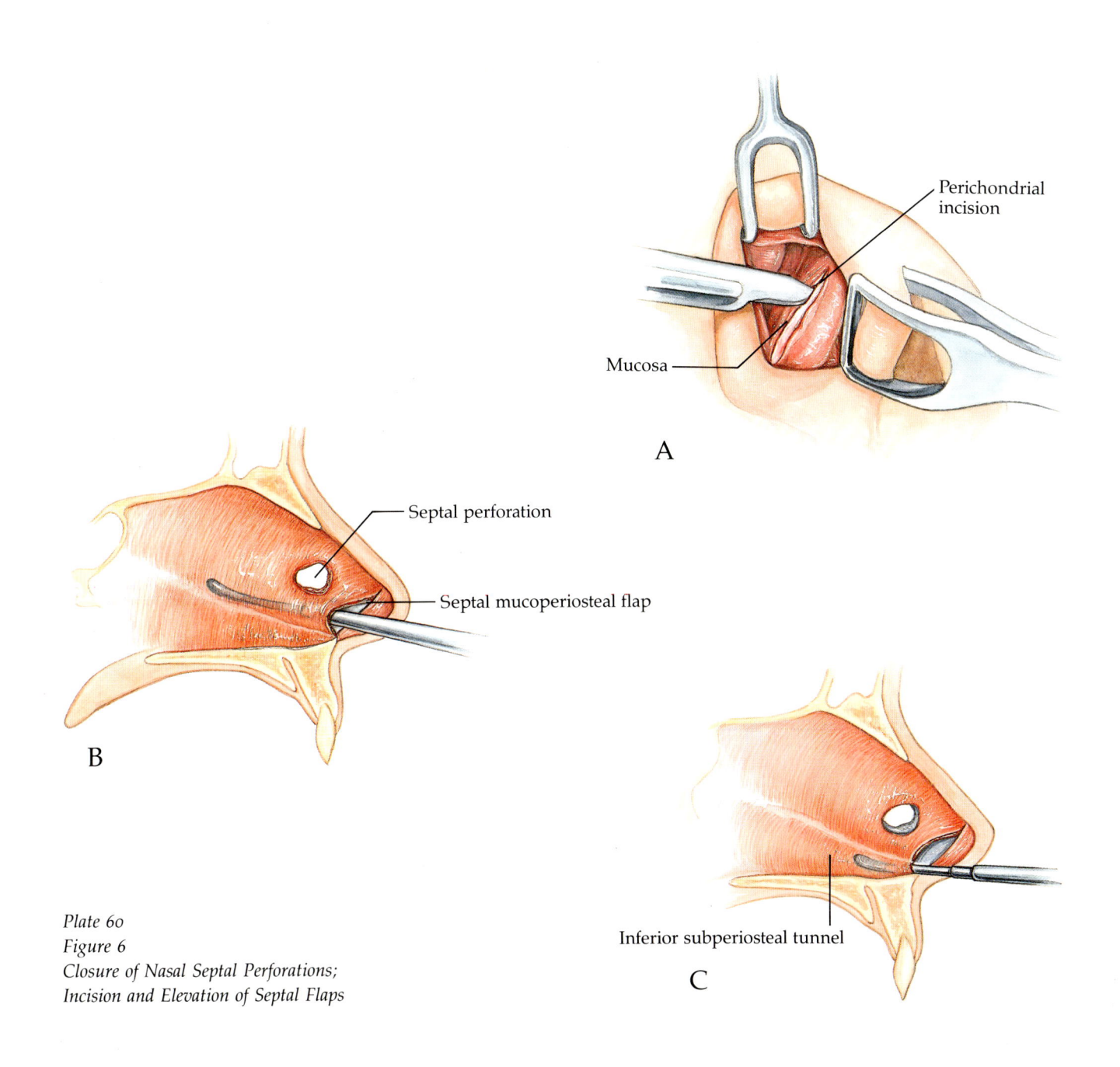

Plate 60
Figure 6
Closure of Nasal Septal Perforations;
Incision and Elevation of Septal Flaps

erally across the piriform aperture to include the periosteum of the inferior meatus and posteriorly for the length of the palate. The nasal septal and inferior septal pockets are connected. The septal mucoperichondrial flaps are then extended superiorly to the nasal dorsum and then posteriorly to the bony cartilaginous junction bilaterally. Bilateral submucoperiosteal elevation is then continued posteriorly to the sphenoid rostrum. Cartilaginous and bony septal deformities are corrected, which may afford extra mucosa for coverage. Relaxing incisions are now made laterally in the inferior meatus, high and just beneath the attachment of the inferior turbinate along its entire length. A second set of relaxing incisions is made superiorly at the junction of the septum and nasal dorsum or slightly lateral to this. At this point one has fashioned bilateral superior and inferior bipedicled flaps (Fig. 6D).

A composite graft designed to be slightly larger than the perforation is harvested from the conchal cartilage of the ear (Fig. 6E). Hydrodissection with a local anesthetic is first employed to lift the anterior perichondrium from the conchal cartilage. A postauricular incision is then made, and the composite graft is harvested with mastoid periosteum, intervening connective tissue, and the appropriately sized conchal cartilage with intact posterior perichondrium. The anterior perichondrium is left in place. A "sandwich" is then created by folding the mastoid periosteum over the bare cartilage and suturing this to the posterior perichondrium. Although we prefer the composite conchal graft, we have had success with temporalis fascia as well.

Plate 61

D — Superior relaxing incision

Superior relaxing incision

Relaxing incision (deep to inferior turbinate)

Conchal cartilage

Intact posterior perichondrium

Mastoid periosteum

E — Anterior conchal cartilage — Periosteum — "Sandwich" graft

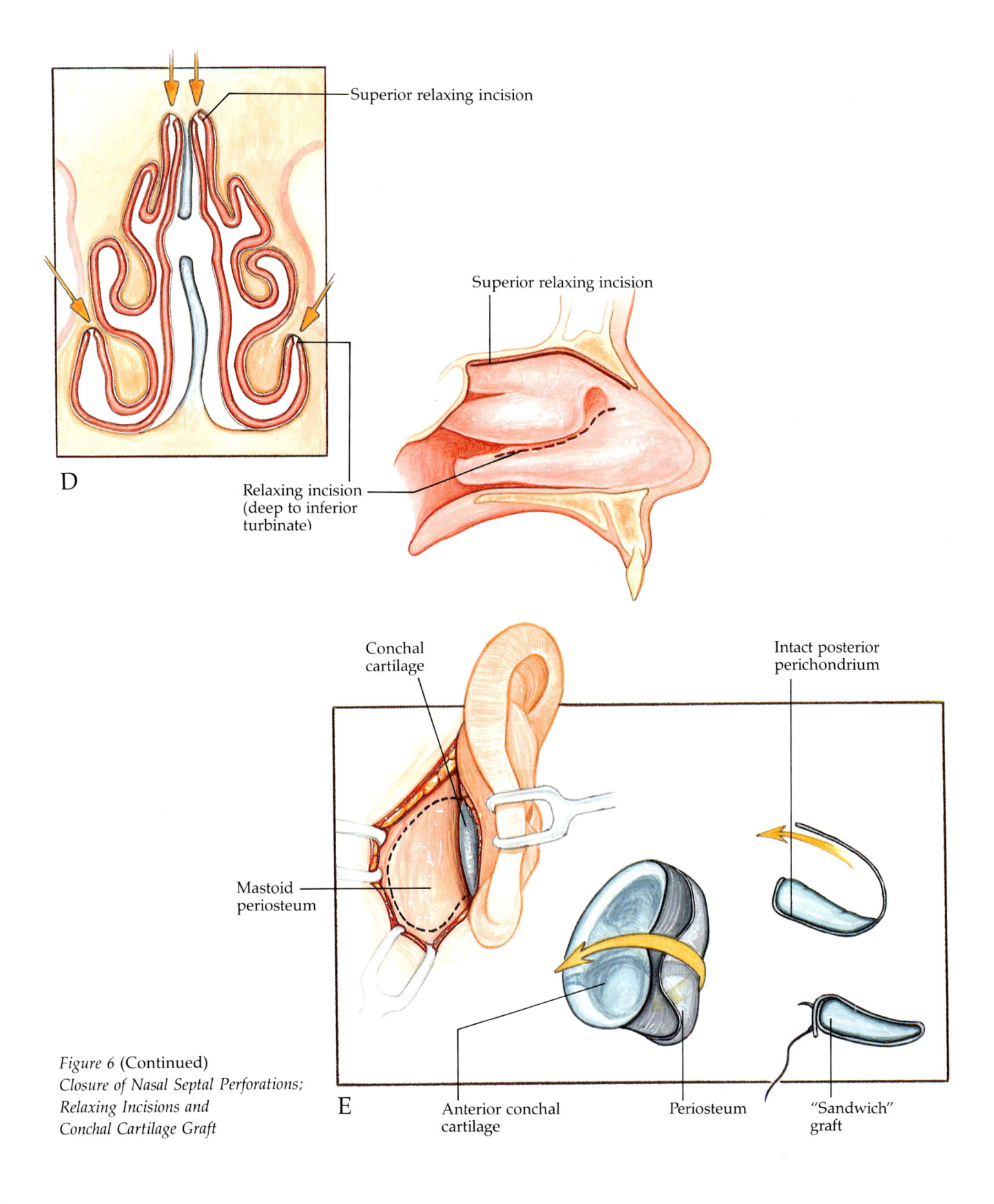

Figure 6 (Continued)
Closure of Nasal Septal Perforations; Relaxing Incisions and Conchal Cartilage Graft

147

Plate 62

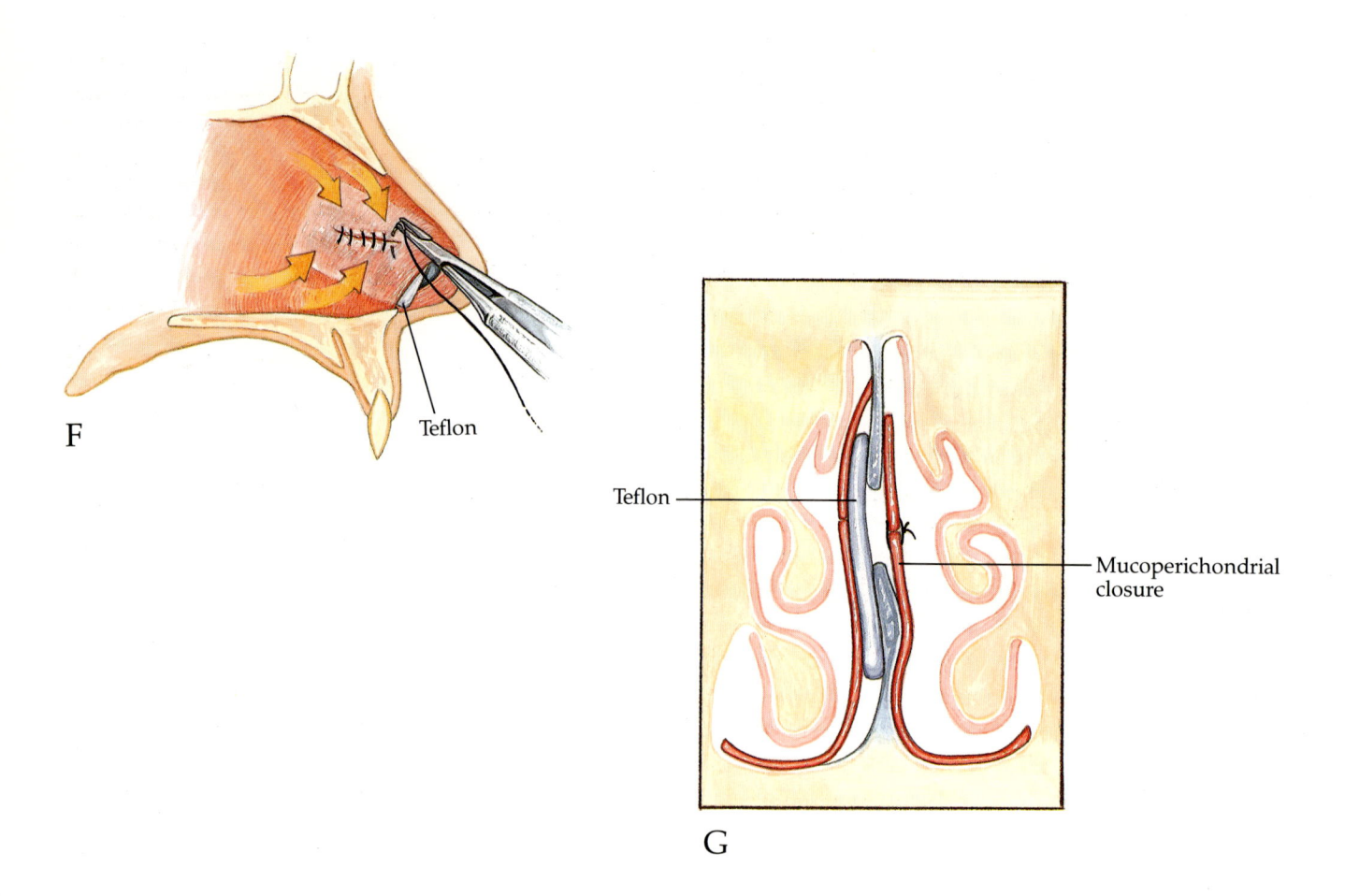

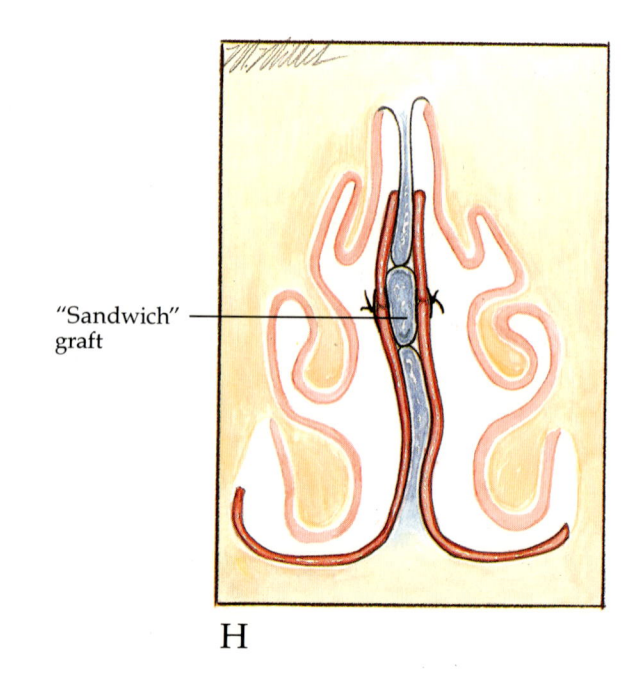

F — Teflon

G — Teflon, Mucoperichondrial closure

H — "Sandwich" graft

Figure 6 (Continued)
Closure of Nasal Septal Perforations; Closure

Polytef (Teflon) is temporarily placed within the septal pocket to facilitate suturing of the septal flaps (Figs. 6F and 6G). Permanent monofilament sutures (5–0 Prolene) are used to close the superior and inferior flaps on each side. Bilateral complete closure is usually possible for perforations less than 2 cm. For larger perforations, bilateral complete closure may not be possible, but at least one side must be completely closed. The Teflon is removed from the septal pocket and the sandwich graft is inserted (Fig. 6H). The hemitransfixion or external rhinoplasty incisions are closed in the usual fashion, and bilateral Teflon or soft Silastic splints are inserted and secured with a transseptal mattress suture. The septal splints stabilize the graft and septum as well as prevent graft desiccation and promote healing.

Postoperative Care

Patients are maintained on systemic antistaphylococcal antibiotics for 1 week postoperatively. Antibiotic-impregnated nasal packing is removed in 48 hours, but the septal splints are left in place for 2 to 10 weeks until healing is observed to be complete. The permanent monofilament sutures are then removed.

Risks, Complications, and Sequelae

Complications of this procedure are relatively minor, and include epistaxis and infection. Antibiotic-impregnated nasal packing for 48 hours postoperatively and a 1-week course of postoperative systemic antistaphylococcal antibiotics reduce the incidence of these complications. Poor healing is the other significant complication. With our technique, an 86 percent complete closure rate has been achieved.

Pearls and Pitfalls

There must be complete closure of the flaps on at least one side of the perforation.

Use of autogenous cartilage grafts with perichondrial and periosteal coverage appears to be ideal.

Leave the septal splints in place postoperatively until healing of the septal flap closure is observed. This may take 2 to 10 weeks.

Suggested Reading

Ward PH, Berman WE, eds. Plastic and reconstructive surgery of the head and neck. Proceedings of the Fourth International Symposium. Vol II. St. Louis: CV Mosby, 1984:542–546.

Rafael R. Portela, M.D.
Robert M. Naclerio, M.D.

CHOANAL ATRESIA

Choanal atresia is the most common congenital nasal anomaly but remains a rare clinical finding, with an incidence estimated to be about 1 in 8,000 births. It was first described by Johann Roederer in 1755 and ranges in presentation from a medical emergency to unilateral rhinorrhea appearing in childhood.

The differential diagnosis includes encephalocele, dermoid cyst, hamartoma, chordoma, teratoma, rhabdomyosarcoma, and traumatic septal displacement.

The embryologic basis for choanal atresia is not entirely clear, but the theories include (1) persistence of the buccopharyngeal membrane from the foregut, (2) persistence of the nasobuccal membrane of Hochstetter, (3) the abnormal persistence of mesoderm-forming adhesions in the choanal region, and (4) a misdirection of mesodermal flow secondary to local factors.

The disorder affects females more often than males and is more common on the right side when it occurs unilaterally. Unilateral atresia is more common than bilateral atrisia. A bony atretic plate is found 90 percent of the time, and a membranous plate is found in the remaining 10 percent. There is a 5 to 1 predominance of whites over blacks.

Patients with choanal atresia have a high incidence (50 percent) of other associated malformations, such as congenital heart deformities or other major organ malformations that must be recognized prior to surgical intervention. Associated abnormalities that significantly impact on survival may dictate prolonged conservative management.

Indications

Bilateral choanal atresia is a medical emergency. This diagnosis is suspected at birth by the characteristic cyclical apnea, cyanosis, and respiratory distress that is temporarily relieved by crying. The diagnosis is established when an attempt to pass a catheter (No. 6 French) into the nasopharynx is unsuccessful. Unilateral atresia may go unrecognized until later childhood, since associated respiratory distress is usually not encountered at birth. If the condition is unrecognized, patients present with unilateral rhinorrhea during early childhood. Unilateral choanal atresia is treated electively.

Preoperative Considerations

Numerous methods have been described to treat choanal atresia, including perforation and dilation of the atretic plate with an esophageal bougie, transnasal curettage, transantral repair, transseptal repair, and transpalatal repair with different modifications.

The transnasal procedures usually involve the use of a microscope or, more recently, an endoscope to improve visualization of the atretic plate. A choanal opening is then established using a variety of different instruments, including drills, lasers, and trocars. These transnasal procedures are usually performed in the neonate, in whom the bony atretic plate is soft, or in the adolescent, in whom a larger nasal airway allows for adequate exposure using microscopic surgical techniques.

For most children, we prefer the transpalatal approach, which offers the best exposure and the lowest incidence of re-stenosis. If the atretic plate is thick or if the posterior portion of the vomer is contributing to the deformity significantly, the transpalatal approach is preferred. In unilateral atresia, we initially use the transnasal route with a drill to remove the plate. If this fails, the transpalatal route is used.

If early surgical intervention is planned for a patient with bilateral choanal atresia, the "rules of 10" should be considered (10 lb, 10 weeks old, and 10 g of hemoglobin). This allows ample time for other organ anomalies to manifest themselves as well as for the infant to learn mouth breathing, which usually occurs at about 2 to 6 weeks of age. Some surgeons prefer to perform the needed repair as soon after birth as feasible.

Radiographic evaluation of the choanal atresia is best done using computed tomography (Fig. 7A). This method will delineate the degree of obstruction as well as the thickness and consistency of the atretic plate and show abnormalities of the vomer and medial displacement of the lateral nasal wall. Previous methods included the instillation of a radiopaque liquid into the nose, followed by a lateral radiograph taken with the patient lying on his or her back. This would identify the area of atresia provided retained nasal mucus was adequately removed. Linear tomography can also be used to demonstrate the atretic plate.

If the procedure is to be performed on a patient who has dentition, a palatal prosthesis can be made preoperatively using standard dental techniques. This prosthesis will help secure the palatal mucoperiosteal flap in the postoperative period.

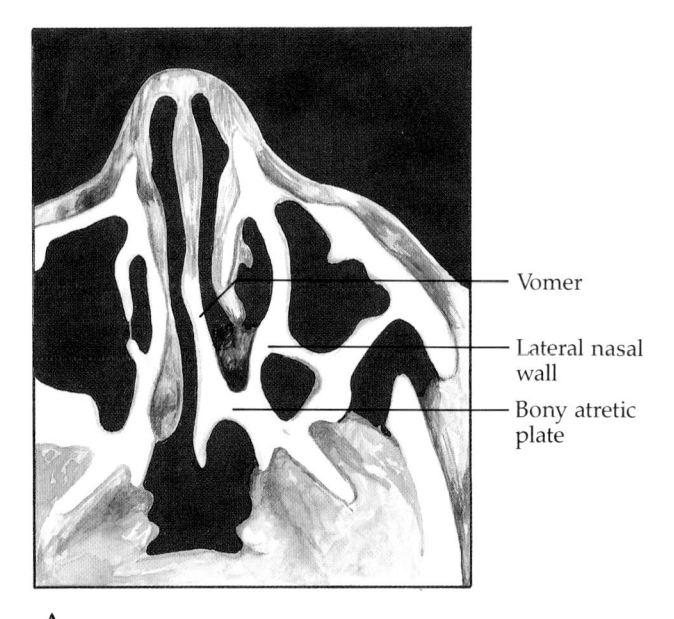

Plate 63
Figure 7
Repair of Choanal Atresia;
Radiographic Evaluation

Operative Steps

The procedure is performed under general endotracheal anesthesia. The patient's head is placed at the end of the table, in the Trendelenburg position (Fig. 7B). The face is prepared and the patient is draped allowing access to the nose and mouth. Nasal secretions are suctioned, and topical cocaine is used for decongestion. The oral cavity is exposed using a Dingman mouth gag (see Fig. 7E). The palate is infiltrated with 0.5 percent lidocaine with 1:200,000 epinephrine. Photographic documentation is made using the 0-degree and the 120-degree telescopes. The hypopharynx is packed with gauze to prevent aspiration. An operating microscope using a 300-mm lens is used to evaluate the atretic plate prior to making incisions.

A self-retaining nasal speculum is placed, and the inferior turbinates are outfractured. A laterally based mucoperiosteal flap is then elevated off the atretic plate using a Rosen knife and a No. 5 Frazier suction tube (Figs. 7C and 7D). Once this is completed, the nose is packed. Attention

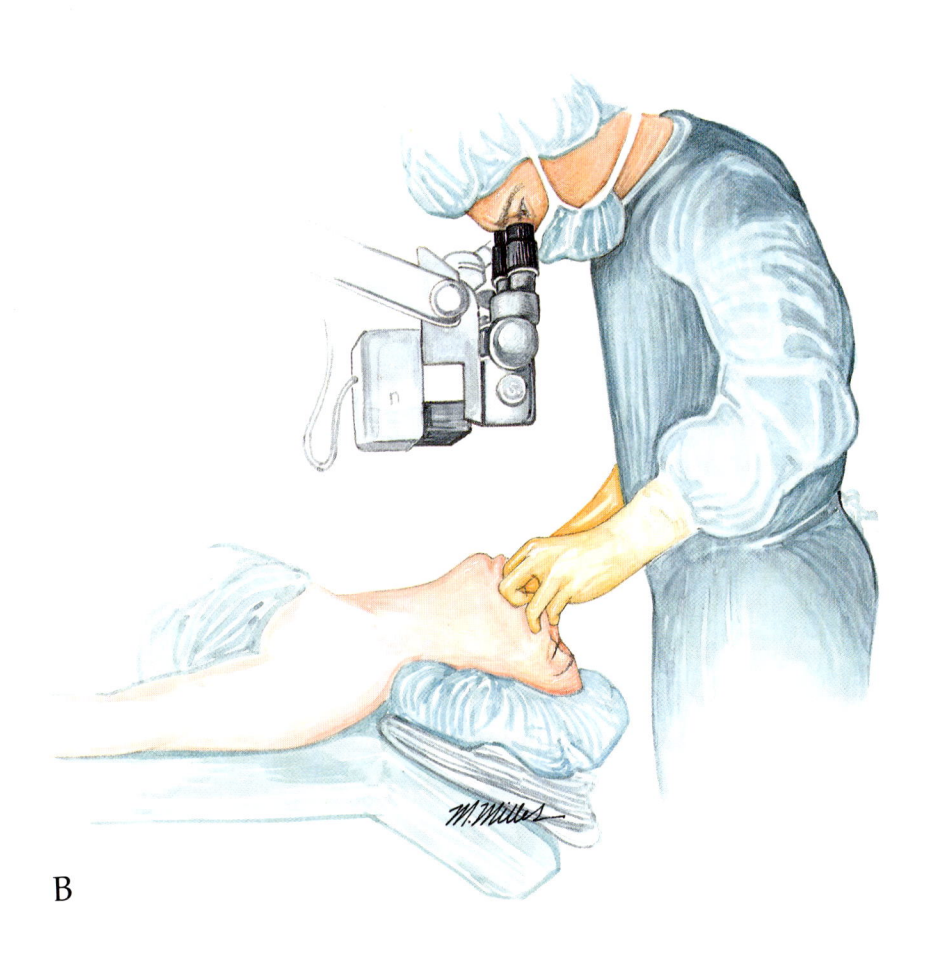

Plate 64

B

C

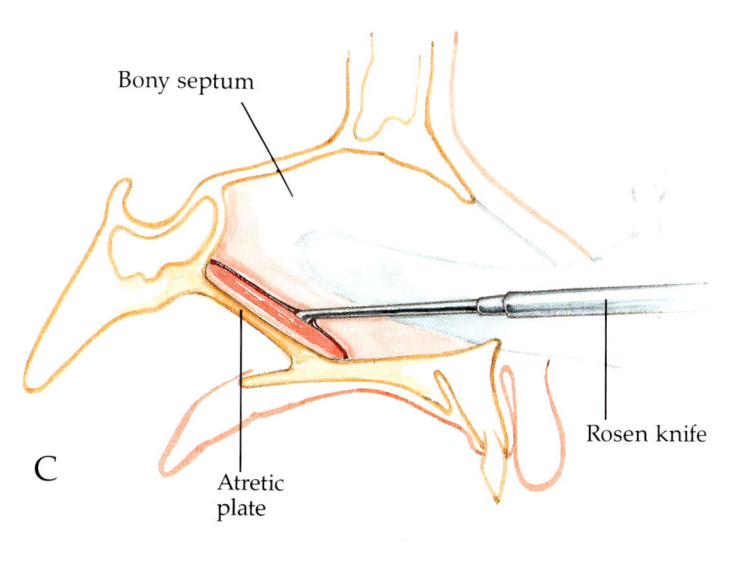

Bony septum

Rosen knife

Atretic plate

D

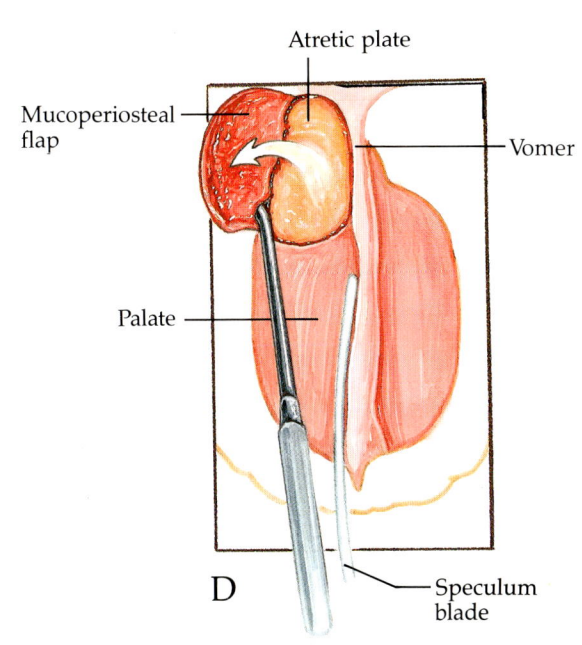

Atretic plate

Mucoperiosteal flap

Vomer

Palate

Speculum blade

Figure 7 (Continued)
Repair of Choanal Atresia;
Transnasal Exposure

Choanal Atresia

is directed to the intraoral procedure (Fig. 7E). A W-shaped palatal incision is made using a cleft palate blade, being careful to avoid the contents of the incisive foramen (Fig. 7F). The mucoperiosteal flap is elevated using a Freer or a Cottle elevator, to the greater palatine foramen (Fig. 7G). The greater palatine arteries are preserved. Utilizing the microscope and an elevator, the posterior end of the hard palate is identified and the muscular and mucosal attachments are elevated off the nasopharyngeal side of the atretic plates (Fig. 7H). The posterior edge of the hard palate, the atretic plate, and the posterior edge of the vomer are removed using cutting and diamond burs and continuous suction irrigation (Figs. 7I and 7J). The atretic plate is usually several millimeters anterior to the posterior bony choana. If necessary, the lateral nasal wall in the area of the atresia is thinned, being careful not to injure the sphenopalatine artery, the eustachian tube, or the sphenoid sinus. Using a sickle blade, an inferiorly based

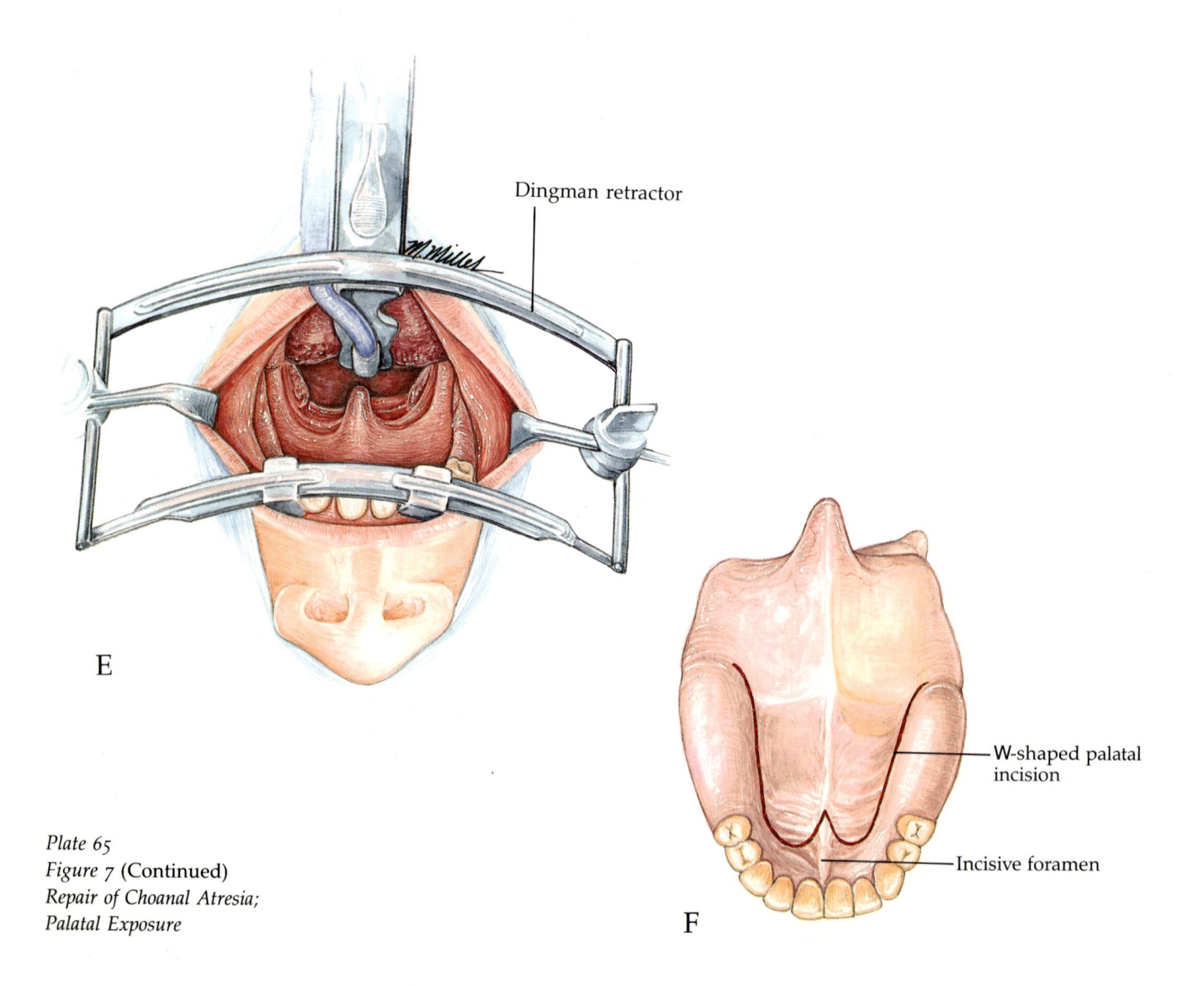

Plate 65
Figure 7 (Continued)
Repair of Choanal Atresia;
Palatal Exposure

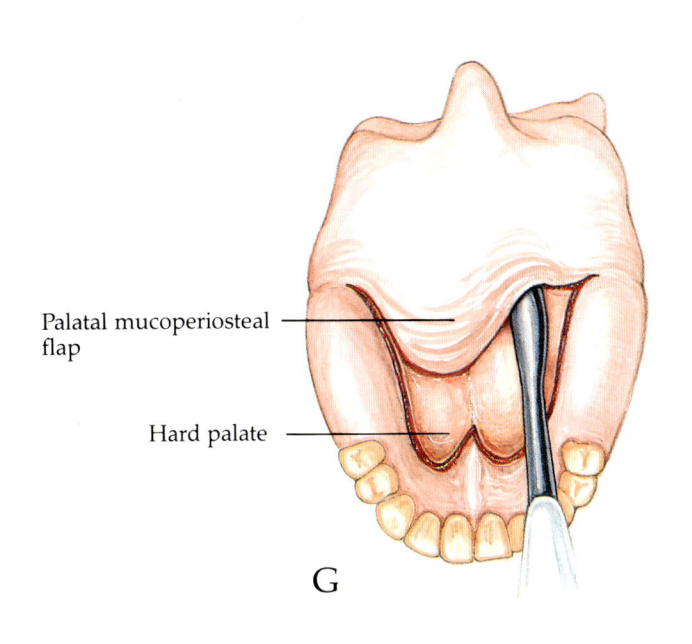

Plate 66

Palatal mucoperiosteal flap

Hard palate

G

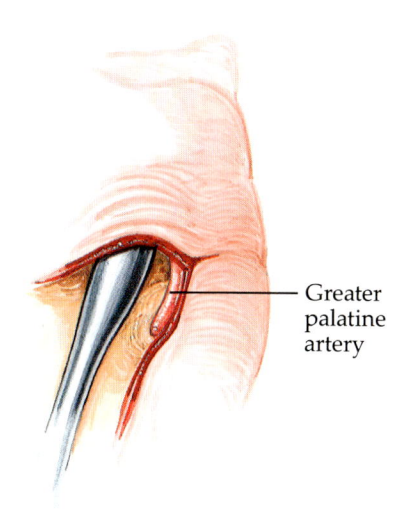

Greater palatine artery

H

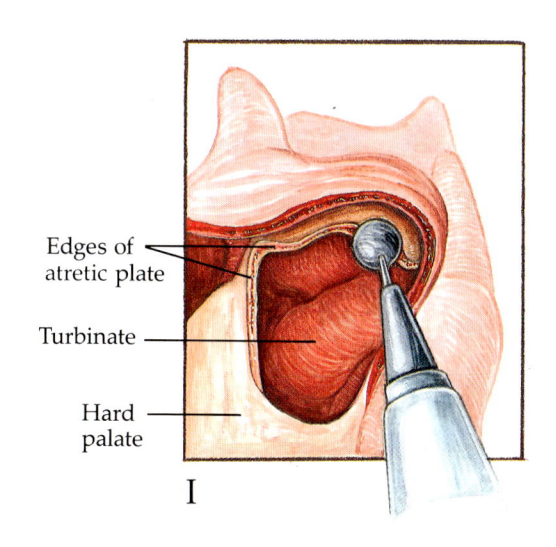

Edges of atretic plate

Turbinate

Hard palate

I

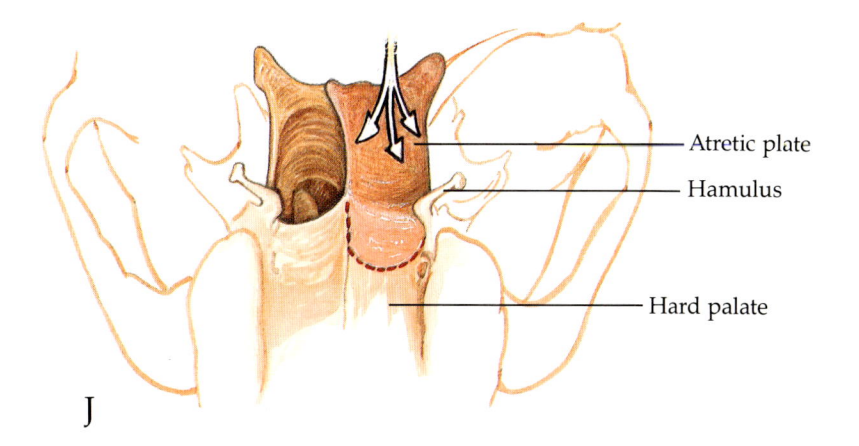

Atretic plate

Hamulus

Hard palate

J

Figure 7 (Continued)
Repair of Choanal Atresia;
Resection of Atretic Plate

155

flap is made on the nasopharyngeal portion of the mucoperiosteum to create an opening into the nasopharynx (Fig. 7K). Once an adequate opening has been established into the nasopharynx, two No. 10 French pediatric rubber catheters are passed through the nose and brought out through the mouth to use as guides for introducing the nasal stents. The largest Portex endotracheal tube that comfortably fits through the nose is used as a stent. The distance from the nasal ala to the posterior nasopharynx is measured and used as an estimate of stent length. A single stent partially transected in the midportion to create the posterior opening is used (Fig. 7L). Using the red rubber catheters, the stent is introduced into the nose from a posterior to an anterior direction (Fig. 7M). The posterior opening is visualized using the 120-degree telescope to assure proper stent placement. Catheters are now passed through the stents to ensure patency. The stents are secured anterior to the columella. The palatal incision is closed using interrupted 3–0 chromic catgut (Fig. 7N). The palatal prosthesis is secured to the teeth using 26-gauge wire or 2–0 Prolene suture. The hypopharyngeal pack is removed, and the patient brought out of anesthesia and extubated when fully awake.

Postoperative Care

The patient should be observed in the neonatal or pediatric intensive care unit for at least 24 hours if a bilateral repair has been performed or a transpalatal approach has been used, because of the potential for airway compromise caused by palatal edema. Meticulous suctioning of the catheters is required to assure patency. Local care using hydrogen peroxide is needed to control the crusting that develops at the nasal alae around the stents. Humidified oxygen will help alleviate oral mucosal dryness, and perioperative antibiotics decrease the potential for infection. The stent is removed in 2 weeks if an adequate choana has been established and healthy mucosal flaps are created. The stents are left in for 6 weeks if the choanal opening is small or there is poor mucosal coverage. The stents are removed under general anesthesia, and the choanae are visualized using the telescopes. Granulation tissue or redundant mucosa can be excised using the KTP laser with endoscopic guidance.

Risks, Complications, and Sequelae

Operative risks include bleeding from the greater palatine arteries, injury to the basiocciput during removal of the atretic plate, injury to the contents of the incisive foramen, or inadvertent extubation during manipulation of the mouth gag.

Early postoperative complications include airway obstruction secondary to edema of the soft palate or tongue, nasal infection, toxic shock syndrome, palatal mucosal necrosis, velopharyngeal incompetence from either muscular dysfunction or overly long stents, and pressure necrosis of the columella or the alar rim.

Late postoperative complications include re-stenosis of the choanae following stent removal (requiring dilations or revision surgery) and interference with palatal and midface growth (resulting in malocclusion).

Plate 67

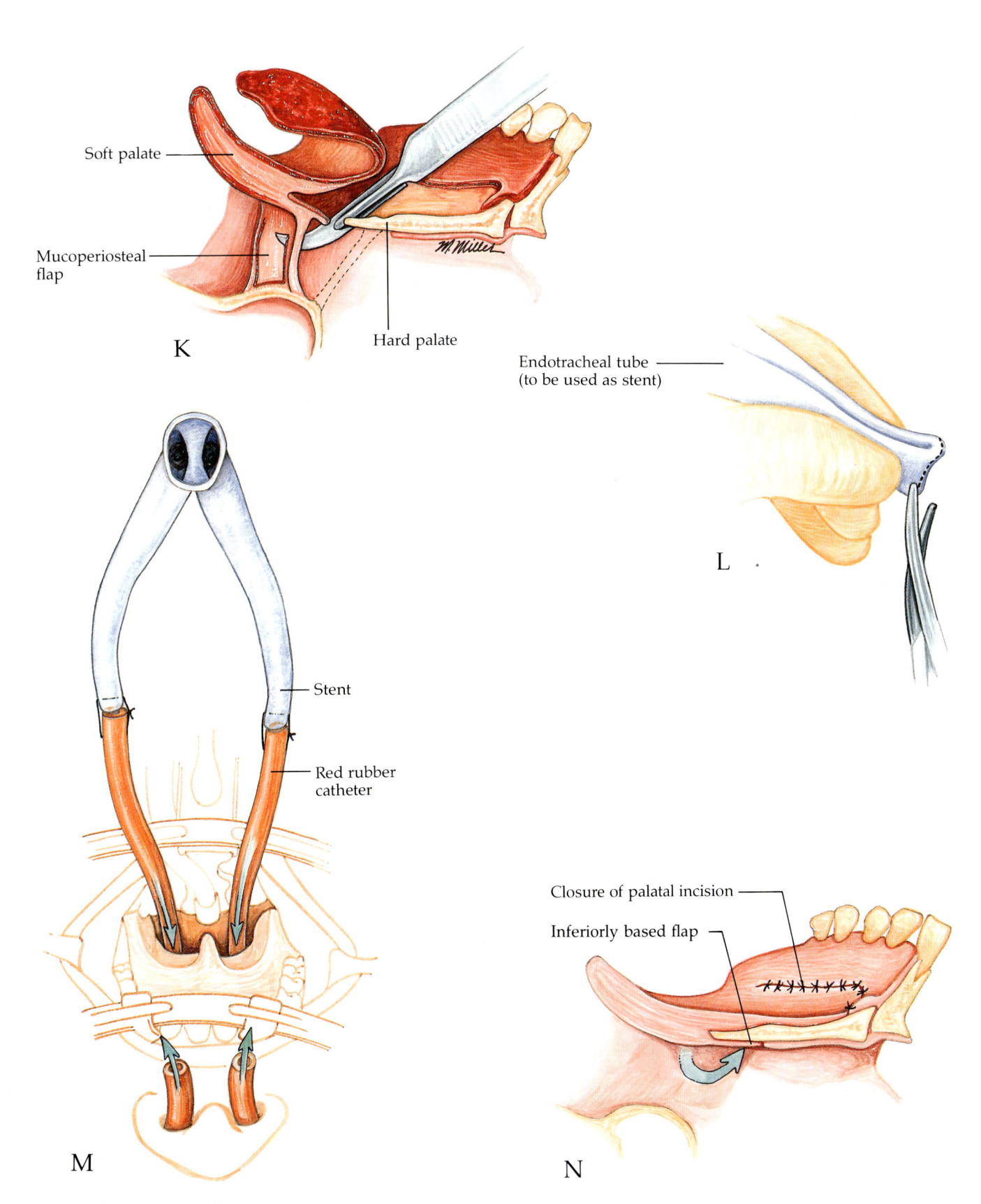

K — Soft palate, Mucoperiosteal flap, Hard palate

L — Endotracheal tube (to be used as stent)

M — Stent, Red rubber catheter

N — Closure of palatal incision, Inferiorly based flap

Figure 7 (Continued)
Repair of Choanal Atresia; Closure and Stent

Pearls and Pitfalls

The older the child, the higher the success rate and the better the intranasal exposure.

The microscope optimizes visualization of the deformities, and maximal nasal decongestion and palatal vasoconstriction help to provide the best exposure.

Incisions in the palate are best made using an angled cleft palate blade and the Dingman mouth gag for exposure.

Remember that the nasopharyngeal mucosal membrane is very thick and that this thickness as well as the deformity of the posteroinferior vomer must be resected.

The location of the stenosis relative to the posterior edge of the palate must be noted.

Major technical pitfalls include failure to remove the contributing portion of the vomer and the lateral nasal wall and improperly creating an adequate soft tissue aperture at the choana, particularly the nasopharyngeal mucosal membrane opening.

The stents pose problems if they are too long or if they apply pressure to the alar rims or the columella.

Associated major organ malformation may go unrecognized.

Suggested Reading

Alexopoulos KA. Choanal atresia. Lessons from five cases. Clin Pediatr 1967; 6:579–580.

Blegvad NR. Choanal atresia. Acta Otolaryngol 1959; 116(Suppl):46–49.

Carpenter RJ, Neel HB. Correction of choanal atresia in children and adults. Laryngoscope 1977; 87:1304–1311.

Flake CG, Ferguson CF. Congenital choanal atresia in infants and children. Ann Otol Rhinol Laryngol 1961; 70:1095–1110.

Grahne B, Kaltiokallio K. Congenital choanal atresia and its heredity. Acta Otolaryngol 1966; 62:193–200.

Hergerer AS, Strome M. Choanal atresia: A new embryologic theory and its influence on surgical management. Laryngoscope 1982; 92:913–921.

Hough IVD. The mechanism of asphyxia in bilateral choanal atresia: The technic of the surgical correction in the newborn. South Med J 1955; 48:588–594.

Johnsen S. Congenital choanal atresia. Acta Otolaryngol 1960; 51:533–540.

Kazanjian VH. The treatment of congenital atresia of the choanae. Ann Otol 1942; 51:704–711

McGovern FH, Fitzhugh GS. Surgical management of choanal atresia. Arch Otolaryngol 1961; 73:627–634.

Morrow RC. Bilateral congenital choanal atresia: Report of three cases corrected surgically in newborns. Ann Otol 1957; 66:135–138.

Owens H. Observations in treating 25 cases of choanal atresia by the transpalatine approach. Laryngoscope 1968; 78:1487–1499.

Ruddy LW. A transpalatine operation for congenital atresia of the choanae in the small child or the infant. Arch Otolaryngol 1945; 41:432–438.

Wright WK, Shambaugh GE, Green L. Congenital choanal atresia: A new surgical approach. Ann Otol Rhinol Laryngol 1947; 56:120–126.

Ira D. Papel, M.D.
John C. Price, M.D.

NASAL RECONSTRUCTION

Surgical procedures for nasal reconstruction can be dated as far back as 600 BC. The median forehead flap was used in India as a method of nasal reconstruction after amputation as a penalty for adultery. In the Middle Ages, the Brancas described the use of forehead flaps and delayed pedicle flaps from the upper arm. The arm flap method was described in detail by Gaspar Tagliocozzi in 1597, and this became commonly referred to as the Italian method. The work of Tagliocozzi and others during this period was suppressed and ridiculed because of religious restrictions in 16th-century Italy. The forehead flap was repopularized by Joseph Carpue of England in 1816; he described the use of median forehead flaps in two patients. Since that time a wide variety of forehead and scalping flaps have been described for total or near total reconstruction.

Indications

When planning reconstructive procedures of the nose, a surgeon must consider the status of three main components: the skin covering, the bone and cartilaginous skeleton, and the mucosal lining. The majority of procedures require repair of the skin only, but more serious injury or tumor eradication may result in full-thickness loss of part or all of the nose. The reconstructive surgeon must be able to formulate a plan for restoring the integrity of the nasal structure, form, and function.

Preoperative Considerations

In planning of the restoration of nasal skin, the nose should be considered as an esthetic unit on the face. At times it may be better to remove normal skin so as to create a unit that is of homogeneous color and integrity. Also of importance in planning surgery is the wide variation in skin characteristics on different parts of the nose and its surrounding structures. The cephalic nasal skin is thin and loose, with a paucity of sebaceous glands. The skin over the caudal nose is thick, poorly mobile, and filled with sebaceous glands. These characteristics influence the use of local flaps in repairing small to moderate nasal skin defects. Whenever possible, autogenous material should be used for providing skeletal support. Cartilage and bone are available from auricular, rib, cranial, and iliac sources in plentiful supply.

Operative Steps

PRIMARY CLOSURE
Smaller defects of the nasal skin can often be closed by primary closure. Regardless of whether the defect is caused by tumor ablation or trauma, wide undermining and incisions planned with respect to the relaxed skin

tension lines will enhance the results. Lesions on the lobular portion of the nose involve skin that is thick and inelastic. Scars in this area frequently heal with depressed characteristics that are easily noticed due to the shadows they create. Care in everting wound edges and postoperative splinting will minimize these defects, but some deformity usually exists even with the best technique. The skin of the upper nose is looser and more elastic. This allows for easier and more cosmetic closure of small defects.

SKIN GRAFTS. Skin grafts for the reconstruction of nasal defects are useful for coverage of any size defect. The color match of donor skin tends to be poor, and the thickness is usually insufficient to blend with the thick lobular skin. This mismatch usually results in a poor cosmetic result. When using full-thickness skin grafts to reconstruct partial nasal defects, the boundaries of esthetic units should be observed, resulting in a more natural appearance. Split-thickness skin grafts are also useful for temporary coverage after tumor excision, especially if total tumor control is not assured. An observation period before permanent skin coverage may be of benefit in some situations. Another limitation of skin grafts is that they cannot be used when the underlying soft tissue has been removed from the nasal skeleton. Only flaps with adjacent or distal blood supplies will survive. Shrinkage of the grafted site must also be considered in anticipation of the final result. This may cause retraction of the nasal ala in some situations, which will require later correction.

LOCAL FLAPS

Local skin flaps have the best chance of providing skin of similar color and thickness. This is more difficult to achieve in the tip area, for reasons outlined above. Careful planning of local flaps to take advantage of relaxed skin tension lines, areas of availability and elasticity, and esthetic units enhances the final result. Some flaps, especially the nasolabial flap, require secondary thinning or sculpturing at a later time. Whenever possible, the use of nasal skin to cover nasal defects will provide a better match of color and thickness than skin from the forehead or cheek. Most of these local flaps can be performed under local anesthesia with mild or no sedation. All require extensive subcutaneous undermining.

BILOBED FLAP. The bilobed flap is especially useful for transferring skin from the superior nose for reconstruction of more inferior defects (Figs. 8A and 8B). Midline defects can be reconstructed with lateral-based flaps. In general, it is important to preserve the nasofacial groove and the alar crease whenever possible. This will preserve the esthetic units in reconstruction. As shown in Figures 8C and 8D, this concept may need to be violated for certain defects just superior to the alar crease. The angle between adjacent flaps should range from 60 to 90 degrees (see Fig. 8C). This variance is necessary in order to tailor the flap to specific locations and esthetic units. Flaps with more than 90 degrees between segments risk poor blood supply and flap necrosis.

Plate 68

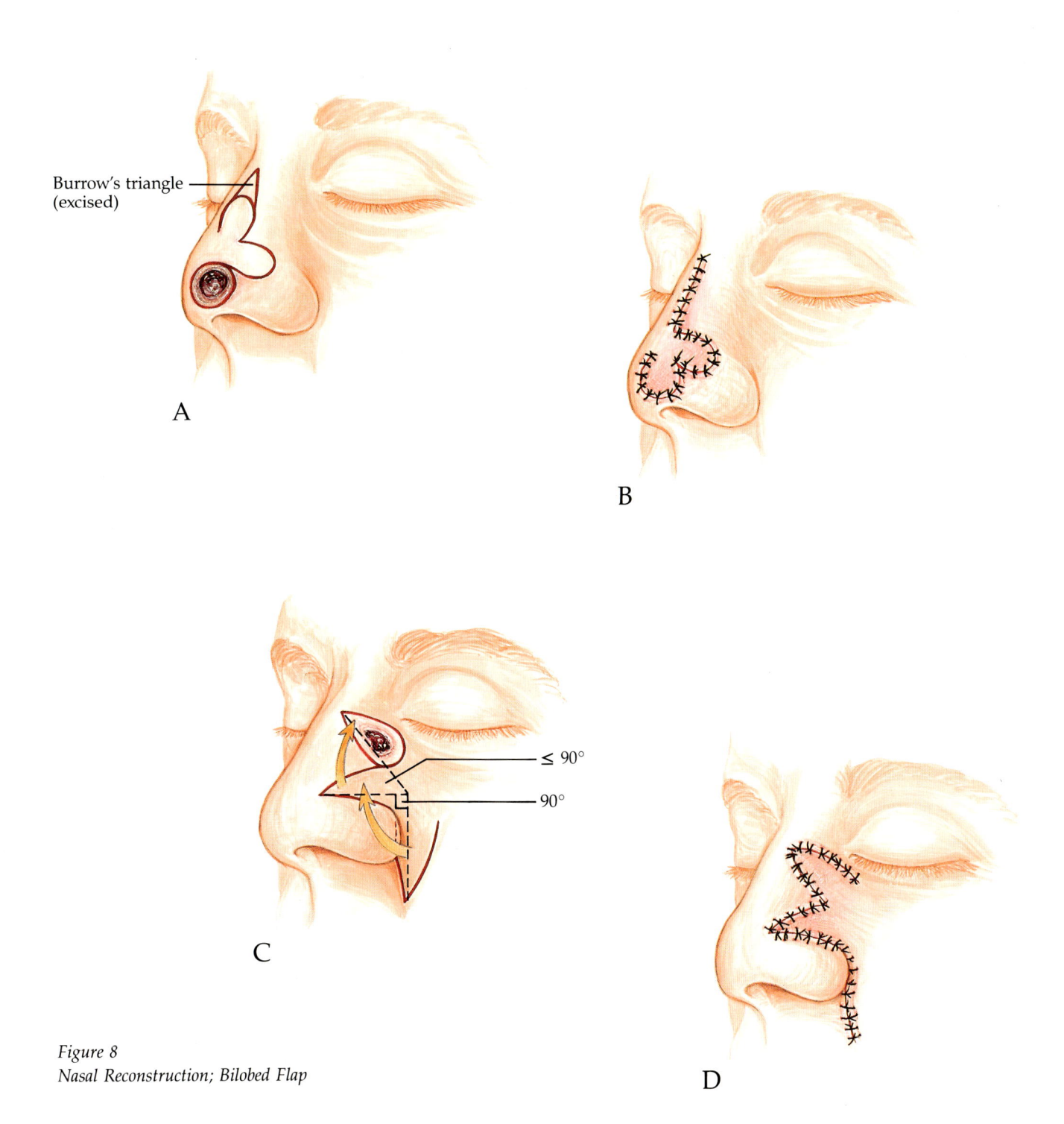

Burrow's triangle (excised)

A

B

C

≤ 90°
90°

D

Figure 8
Nasal Reconstruction; Bilobed Flap

RHOMBOID FLAP. For lesions of the cephalic nasal dorsum and lateral nasal areas, a rhomboid flap may provide a good color and thickness match (Fig. 9A). If the esthetic unit borders of the cheek and nose are left intact, the cosmetic result will usually be better. This flap will be successful only where there is enough skin elasticity to provide transposition and rotation (Fig. 9B). When designing the rhomboid flap, these esthetic borders should be respected. The classic design of a rhomboid flap dictates adjacent angles of 60 and 120 degrees, which provide equality of all sides and of the short axis. When planning individual flaps, careful measurement of angles and incision length will allow for an easier closure. This facilitates closure with minimal disruption of surrounding features (Fig. 9C).

Plate 69

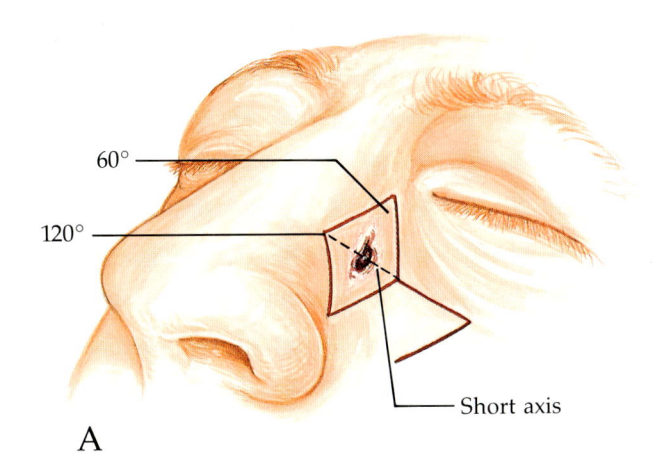

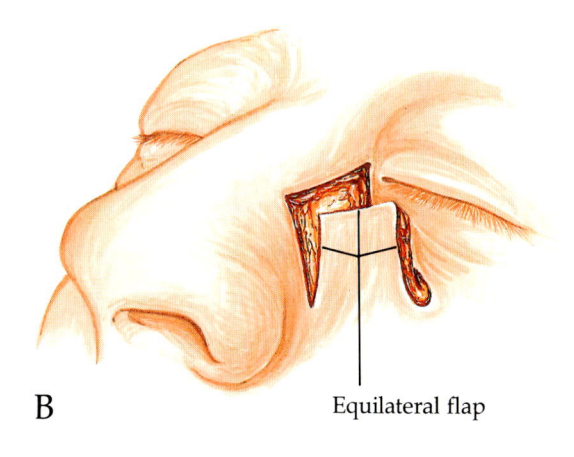

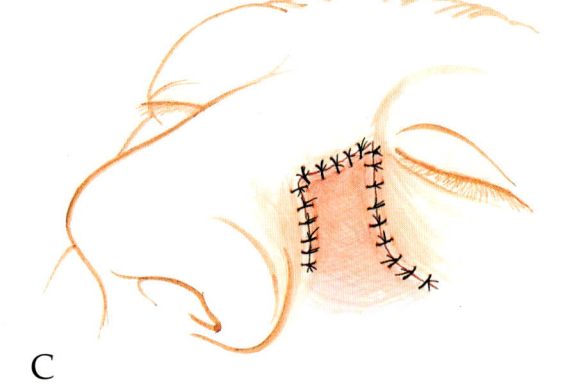

- 60°
- 120°
- Short axis

A

Equilateral flap

B

C

Figure 9
Nasal Reconstruction; Rhomboid Flap

GLABELLAR FLAP. This flap is useful for lesions that occur in the superior nasal dorsum and medial canthal areas (Fig. 10A). It provides skin of a good thickness and color for this region. The glabellar flap incorporates a V-Y advancement of the glabellar region with a rotation-transposition of the skin flap into the medial canthal or superior nasal defects (Fig. 10B). The flap should be designed so as to avoid the transposition of eyebrow hair into the medial canthus. A simultaneous Z-plasty of the donor area may avoid this problem and make the transposition easier, although it does create a longer total scar area.

MIDLINE TRANSPOSITION FLAP. This is a variation of the glabellar flap that provides skin that is slightly thinner and more workable in the medial canthal area. It is a transposition flap from the loose skin of the glabella to the medial canthal region. This skin is thin enough that it may be tailored to reconstruct the medial eyelids more easily than the classic glabellar flap.

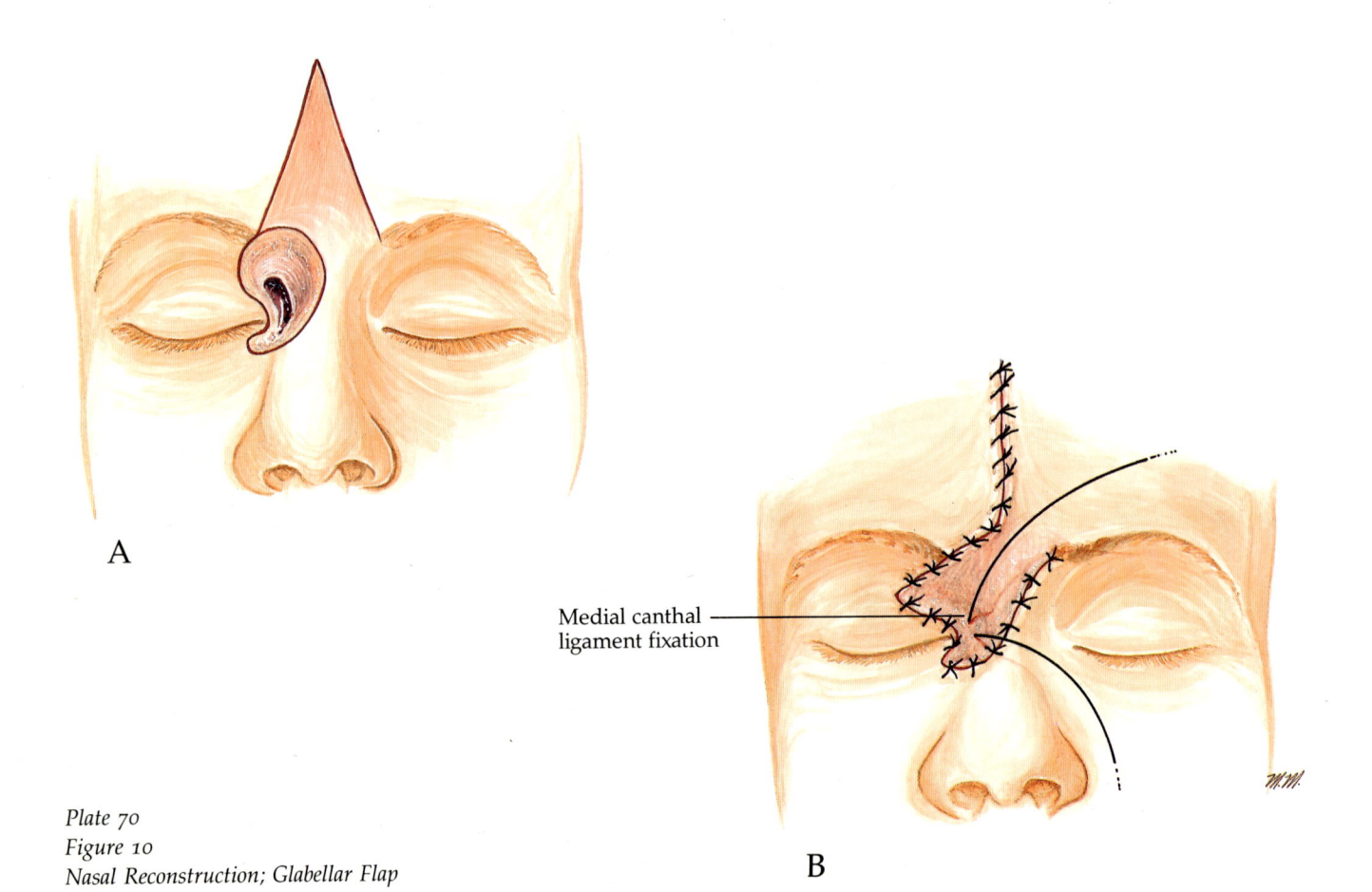

Plate 70
Figure 10
Nasal Reconstruction; Glabellar Flap

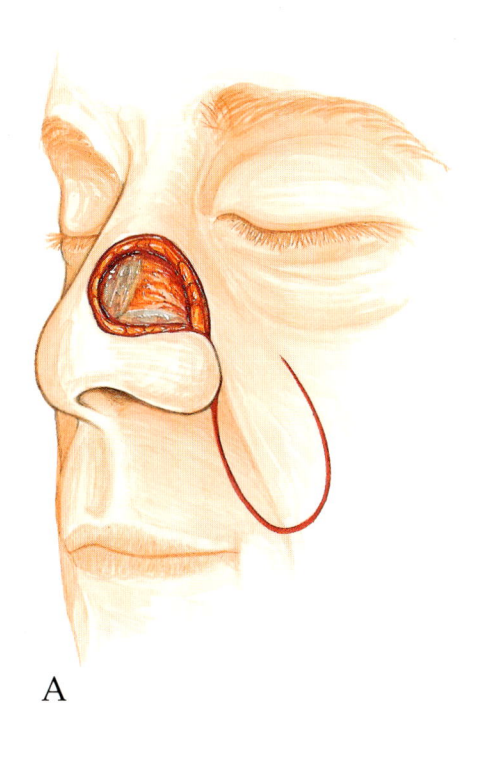

A

Wide undermining

Plate 71
Figure 11
Nasal Reconstruction; Nasolabial Flap

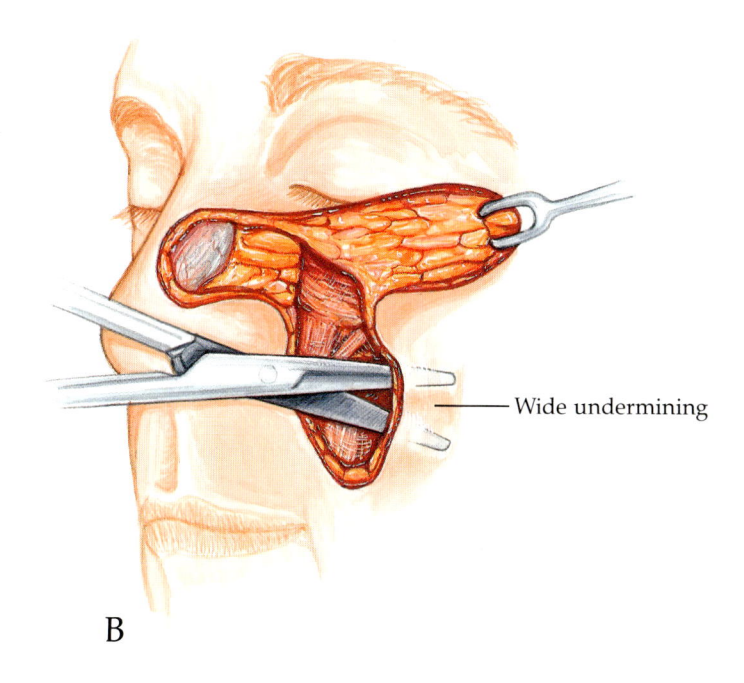

B

NASOLABIAL FLAP. The nasolabial flap is exceptionally useful and versatile in nasal reconstruction. The superiorly based flap is well suited to repair of lateral nasal skin defects and lateral nasal alar and full-thickness defects (Fig. 11A). The inferiorly based nasolabial flap is likewise well suited to repair of nasal floor, upper lip, and columellar defects. The nasolabial flap is generally developed as a random flap based on the subdermal vascular supply. A 2:1 length-to-width ratio should therefore be maintained. A greater length-to-width ratio may be attained by incorporating the facial vessels in the flap. These, however, lie deep to the facial sympathomimetic muscles, and this maneuver requires development of a significantly thicker pedicle. This is not usually necessary. Flaps should be designed to avoid resultant distortion of the lower lid, upper lip, oral commissure, nasal tip, or nasal ala by resultant tension. The final suture line should lie in the nasolabial crease. This may be achieved by widely undermining the skin of the cheek and advancing it forward (Fig. 11B). Removal of a Burrow's triangle at the inferior extremity of the in-

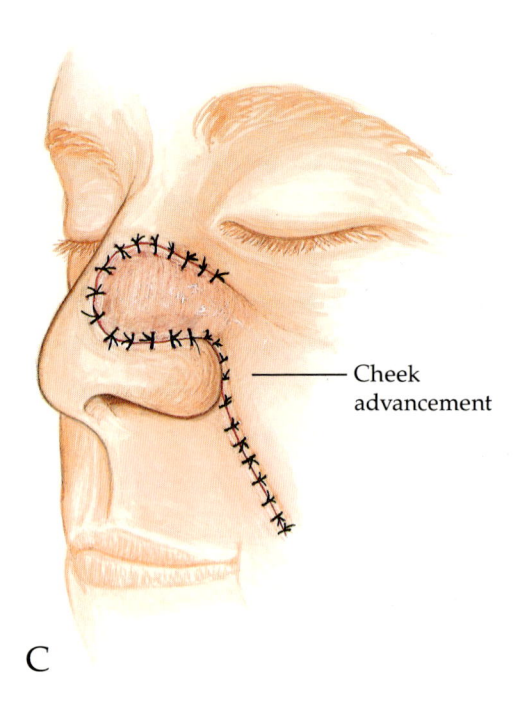

Plate 72
Figure 11 (Continued)
Nasal Reconstruction; Nasolabial Flap

C

Cheek advancement

cision may be necessary to avoid a "dog ear." A superiorly based flap of sufficient length may be turned in upon itself to repair alar margin and full-thickness defects. The tip of the flap should be sutured directly to the nasal mucosa. The alar margin is then positioned and the remainder of the skin closure accomplished (Fig. 11C).

CHEEK ADVANCEMENT FLAP. This technique is useful for closure of small to moderate defects in the nasolabial crease and lateral aspect of the nose. This is an advancement flap based on the subdermal blood supply. Lateral relaxing incisions are made superiorly along the inferior orbital margin and inferiorly along the nasolabial sulcus (see Figs. 14G and 14I). This allows for a very broad flap of excellent vascularity. The skin of the cheek may be undermined widely to achieve adequate relaxation and redraping of the flap. This flap has a tendency to form an undesirable "bow-string" effect at the nasal alar sulcus. Care must be taken to avoid undue tension at this point.

AURICULAR COMPOSITE GRAFT. Auricular composite grafts may be harvested from the helical rim or scapha to provide an excellent tissue match for the nasal ala (Figs. 12A, 12B, and 12C). The limitation of the composite graft is the size that can be successfully transferred without tissue necrosis. In general, a maximum width of 1.5 cm can be reliably transplanted. The recipient site must provide healthy vasculature in order to provide the graft with a chance for neovascularization (Fig. 12D). To achieve this state,

Plate 73

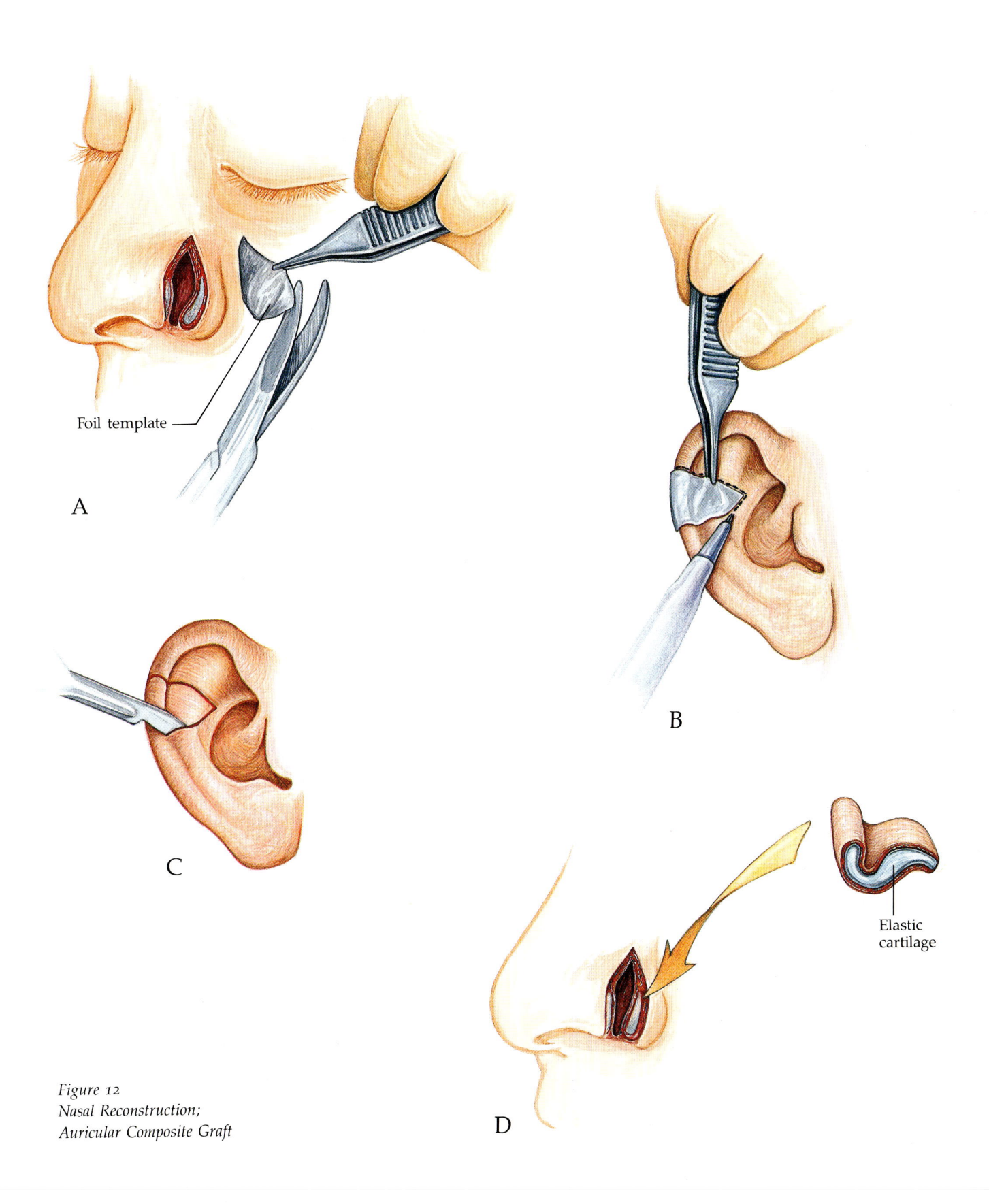

Foil template

A

B

C

Elastic cartilage

D

Figure 12
Nasal Reconstruction;
Auricular Composite Graft

169

both the graft and the recipient site must be treated with meticulous surgical technique to minimize tissue trauma (Figs. 12E, 12F, and 12G). Cautery and crushing forceps should not be used in this procedure. Local anesthetic is usually used for these reconstructions, but the use of epinephrine is discouraged.

The auricular composite graft with the least cosmetic defect is obtained from the crus of helix area. After simple incision extensions as shown (Fig. 12H), this defect can be closed primarily with minor changes in the auricular appearance (Fig. 12I). The graft can also be harvested from any area of the superior helical rim. In designing such a donor defect, the traditional simple wedge should not be used, as this will create a notching and distortion of the helical contour. All excisions in this area should be designed as advancement flaps, with staggering of the skin and cartilage incisions to avoid notching. These defects are usually closed by approximating the cartilage surfaces with fine Vicryl (5–0 or 6–0) sutures and the skin surfaces with either 6–0 nylon or fast absorbing gut 6–0 interrupted sutures.

Plate 74

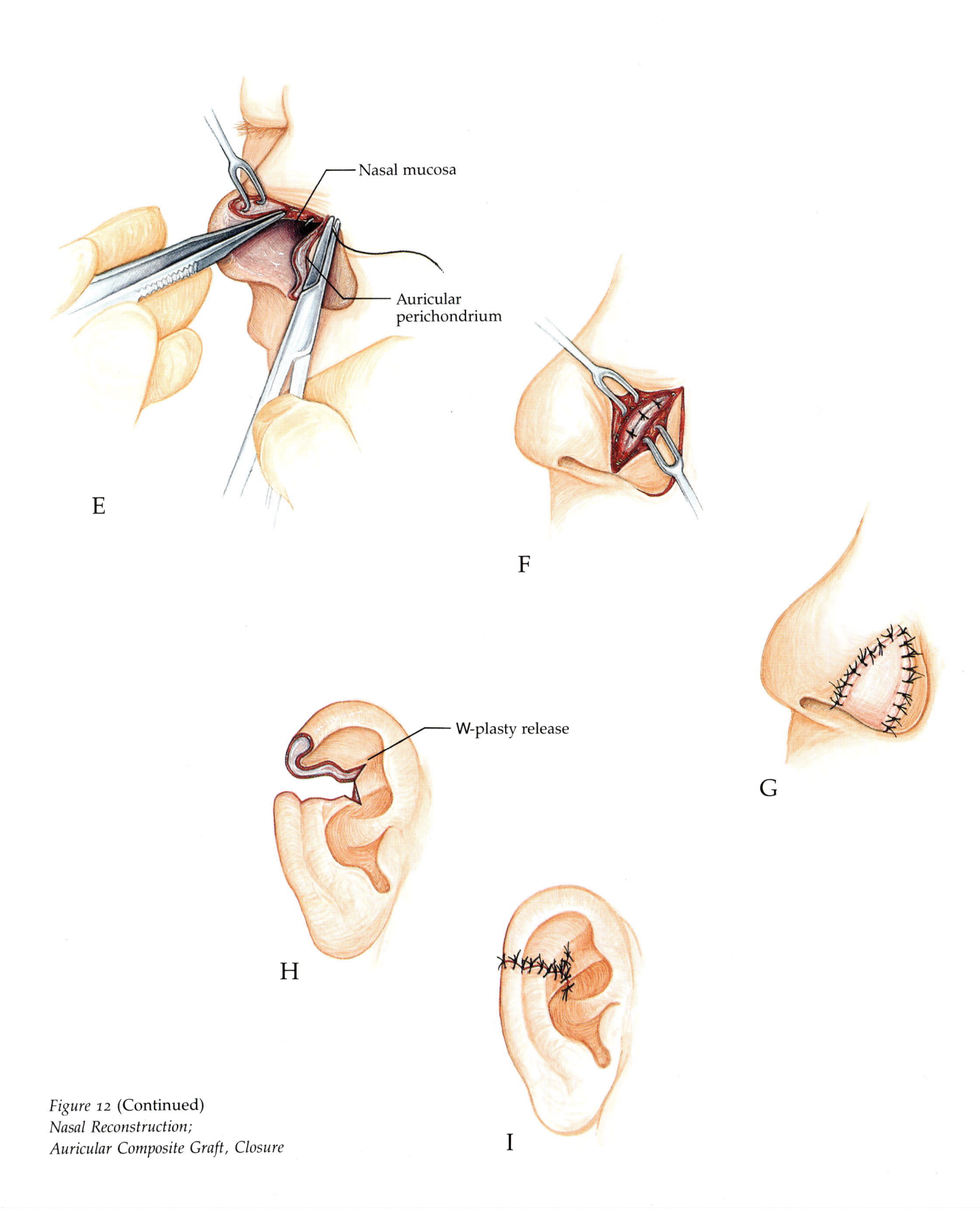

- Nasal mucosa
- Auricular perichondrium

E

F

W-plasty release

G

H

I

Figure 12 (Continued)
Nasal Reconstruction;
Auricular Composite Graft, Closure

171

REGIONAL FLAPS FOR LARGE NASAL DEFECTS

Subtotal or large nasal skin defects usually require more skin than can be obtained from local flaps. The regional skin of the forehead is the usual donor tissue. This provides a good color match, although it is thicker than existing nasal skin. Future thinning and contouring are usually necessary for optimal results.

MIDLINE ISLAND FLAP. This flap is uniquely applicable to repair of central nasal dorsal defects of intermediate and moderately large size. Blood supply is based on the frontal branch of the angular artery and the supratrochlear artery (Fig. 13A). Appropriate size and shape of the skin island are determined by a template, and the pedicle length is carefully measured from the base of the supratrochlear artery. Burrow's triangles are designed at either end of the skin island to permit either a vertical or a horizontal closure of the donor site defect. Skin only is incised initially, and wide undermining of the forehead and glabella down to the tumor defect is accomplished in the subcutaneous plane. The supratrochlear arteries may be located by intraoperative Doppler testing. One arterial pedicle is protected (Fig. 13A). Subcutaneous tissue and frontalis muscle are incised to the periosteum of the frontal bone around the opposite side of the skin island and parallel to the vascular supply so as to develop a subcutaneous pedicle for this island myocutaneous flap. The frontalis muscle is carefully elevated from the periosteal layer, and the skin island is delivered through the subcutaneous tunnel (Fig. 13B). Two-layer primary closure of both the skin island and the donor site is accomplished in a routine fashion (Fig. 13C).

Plate 75

- Burrow's triangle
- Skin island
- Supratrochlear vessels
- Subcutaneous pedicle

A

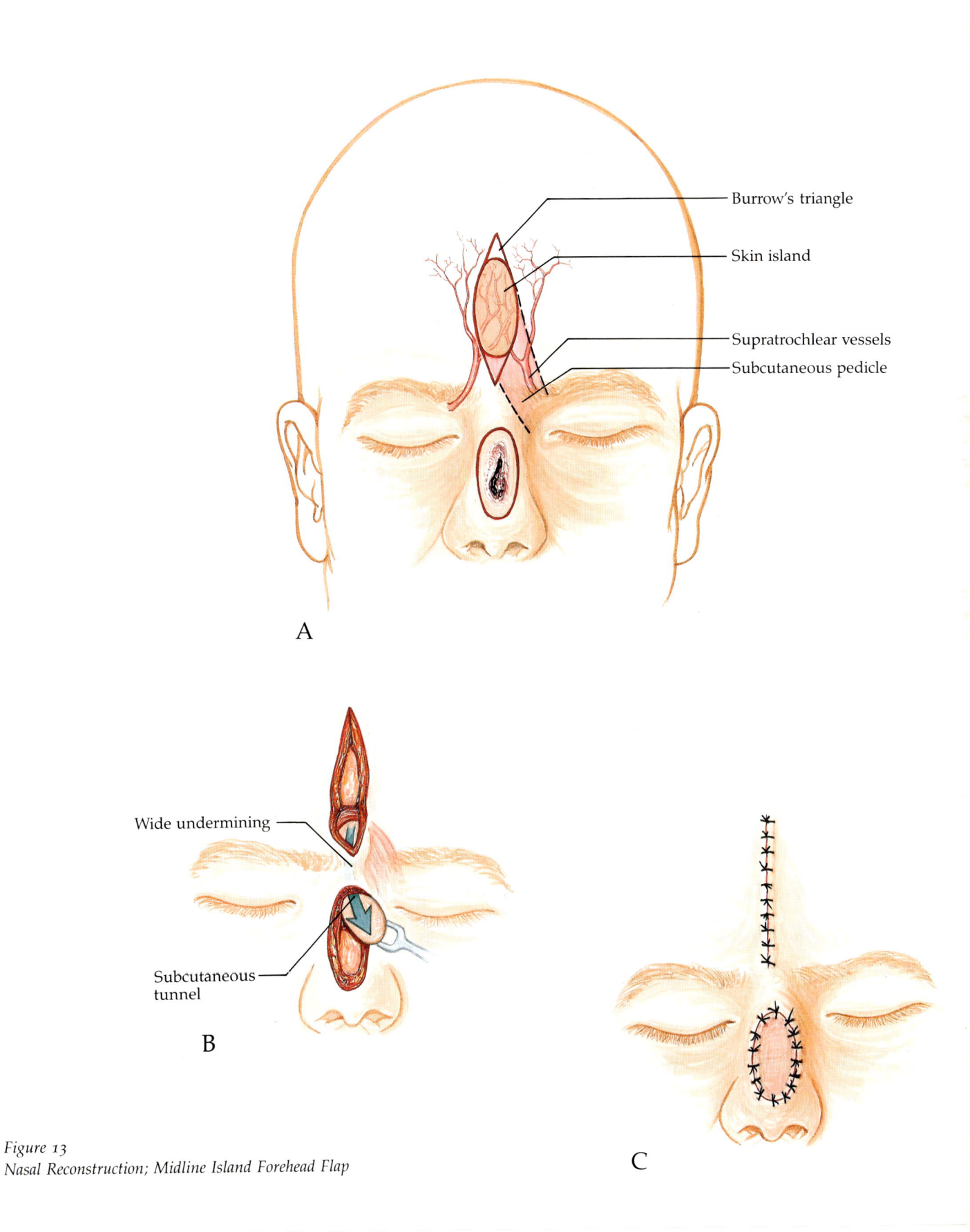

Wide undermining

Subcutaneous tunnel

B

C

Figure 13
Nasal Reconstruction; Midline Island Forehead Flap

MEDIAN FOREHEAD FLAP. The median forehead flap is useful for repair of more extensive cutaneous and full-thickness defects of the nose. It is based on the supratrochlear and supraorbital vessels from the internal carotid artery system and on the frontal branch of the angular (facial) vessels from the external carotid artery system (Fig. 14A). This is an axial flap that must incorporate the frontalis muscle as part of the pedicle and is therefore a myocutaneous flap. The flap should be 2 to 4 cm in width and may be 6 to 9 cm in length. This will bear a substantial skin island and may be pedicled from the ipsilateral, contralateral, or midline position. It may be employed to repair defects of the canthal and lid complex, median cheek skin, and nose. Design of the flap may vary according to length needed, hairline position, or balding pattern. An M-plasty may be necessary at the superior portion to avoid disrupting the hairline.

The flap is elevated deep to the frontalis muscle and above the frontal pericranium; it may therefore be of substantial thickness. The tip of the flap may be remodeled slightly by conservative beveling of the distal 5 to 6 mm to allow the cutaneous tip to be sutured along the distal defect without undue distortion (Fig. 14B). Developing the pedicle base to or into the brow may improve the length of flap available and facilitate rotation. This maneuver results in a malpositioning of the inner aspect of the brow, which must be corrected in a secondary procedure. The base of the pedicle may be primarily inset or it may require "tubing." The forehead defect can be closed primarily after extensively undermining the skin of the forehead and scalp (through its entire extent) (Fig. 14C). Three-layered closure should allow final approximation of the skin without undue tension.

Plate 76

- Supraorbital vessels
- Supratrochlear vessels
- Superficial defect
- Facial vessels

A

- Frontalis muscle
- Beveling of flap tip
- 5-6 mm

B

- Undermining of entire forehead

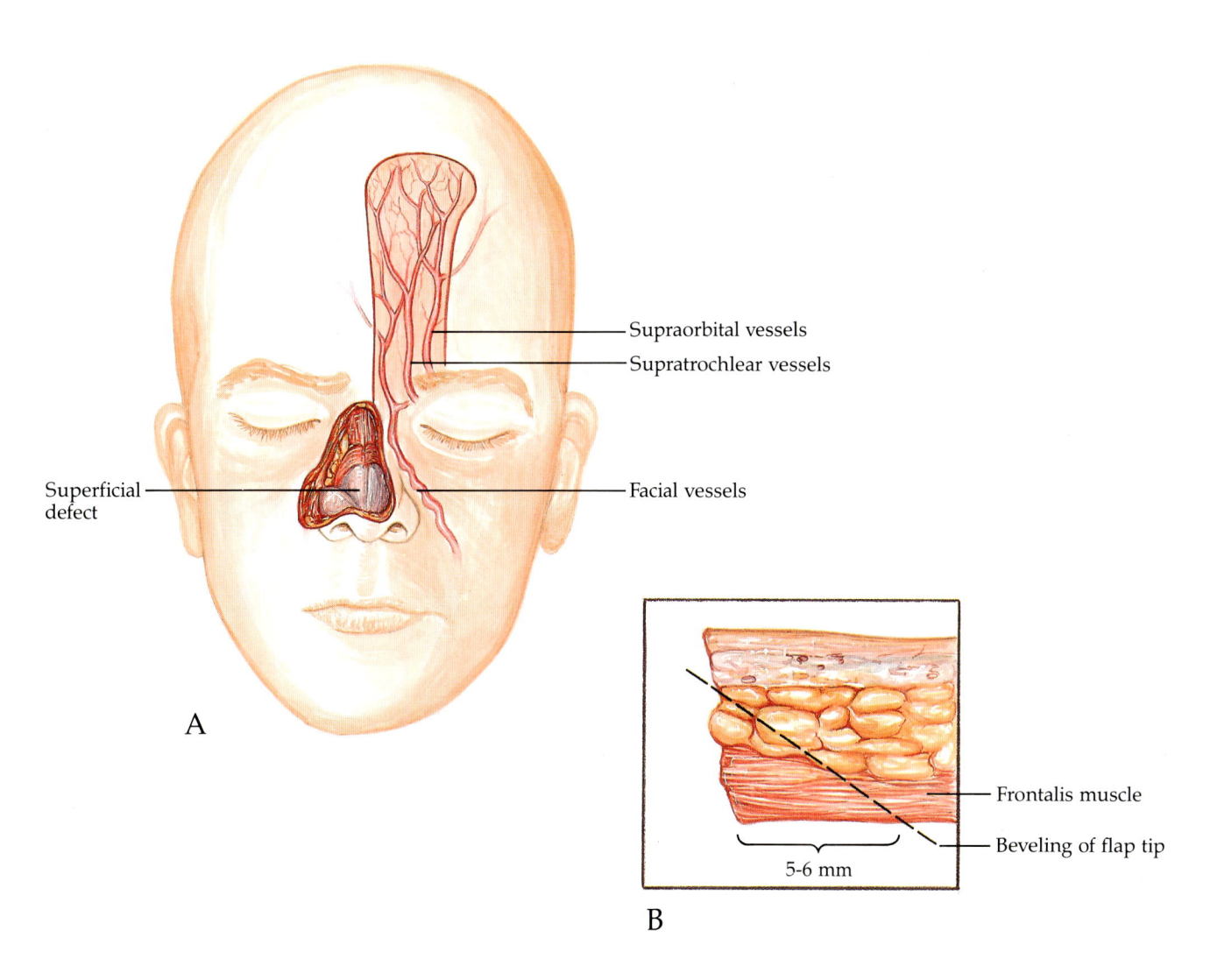

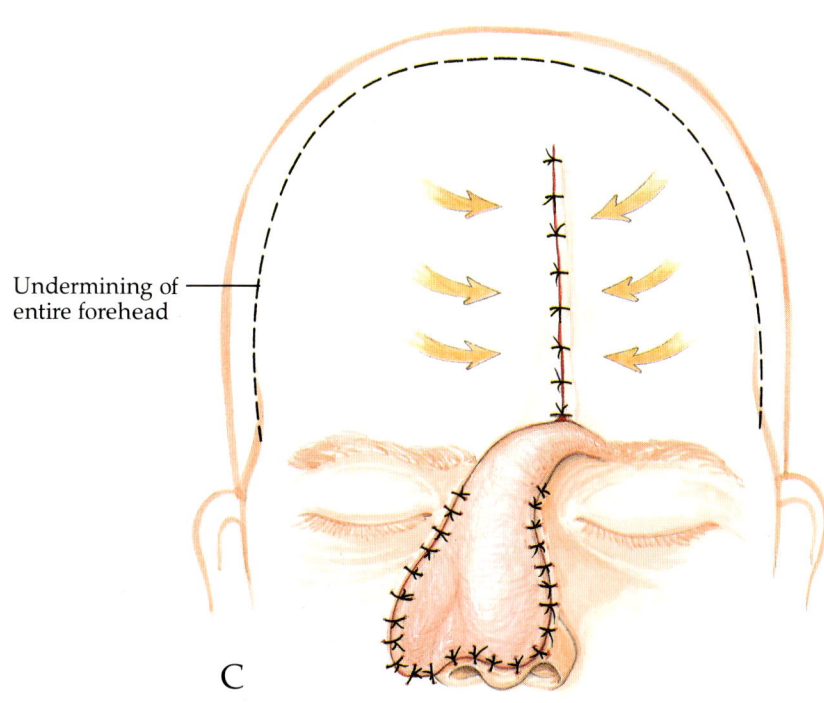

C

Figure 14
Nasal Reconstruction;
Median Forehead Flap, Superficial Defect

REPAIR OF DEFECTS OF THE NASAL LINING

Repair of full-thickness defects in the nose requires establishing an inner lining, structural integrity, and an external lining. The internal lining may be furnished by surfacing the back of a vascularized flap with split-thickness skin at primary reconstruction. It must be remembered, however, that split skin will retract substantially and may alter the external result or the patency of the internal nasal repair. Flaps from residual nasal mucosa are desirable (when adequate tissue exists), since they provide a moist surface with ciliary activity. An alternative method requires simple closure of the defect without reconstruction and then permits complete healing to occur. A minimum of 2 to 3 months should be allowed for development of vasculature across the excisional scar. The longer this interval, the better the ultimate results will be because of the improvement in vasculature and progressive maturation and contracture of the scar. The turn-in flaps are outlined around the perimeter of the nasal defect. These usually are no greater than 1 cm in width (Fig. 14D). The incision is carried down to the subdermal fat, and undermining is directed back toward the margin of the nasal defect. Caution is exercised to avoid transection of the base of the flap, which is the nasal mucosa (Fig. 14E). The flaps are then turned toward each other over the center of the defect and carefully approximated with interrupted 4–0 polyglycolic suture (Fig. 14F). External cutaneous closure is obtained by rotating a median forehead

Plate 77

Healed margin, full-thickness defect

Flap rotation

Undermining

Nasal dorsum

Nasal septum

Maxilla

D

E

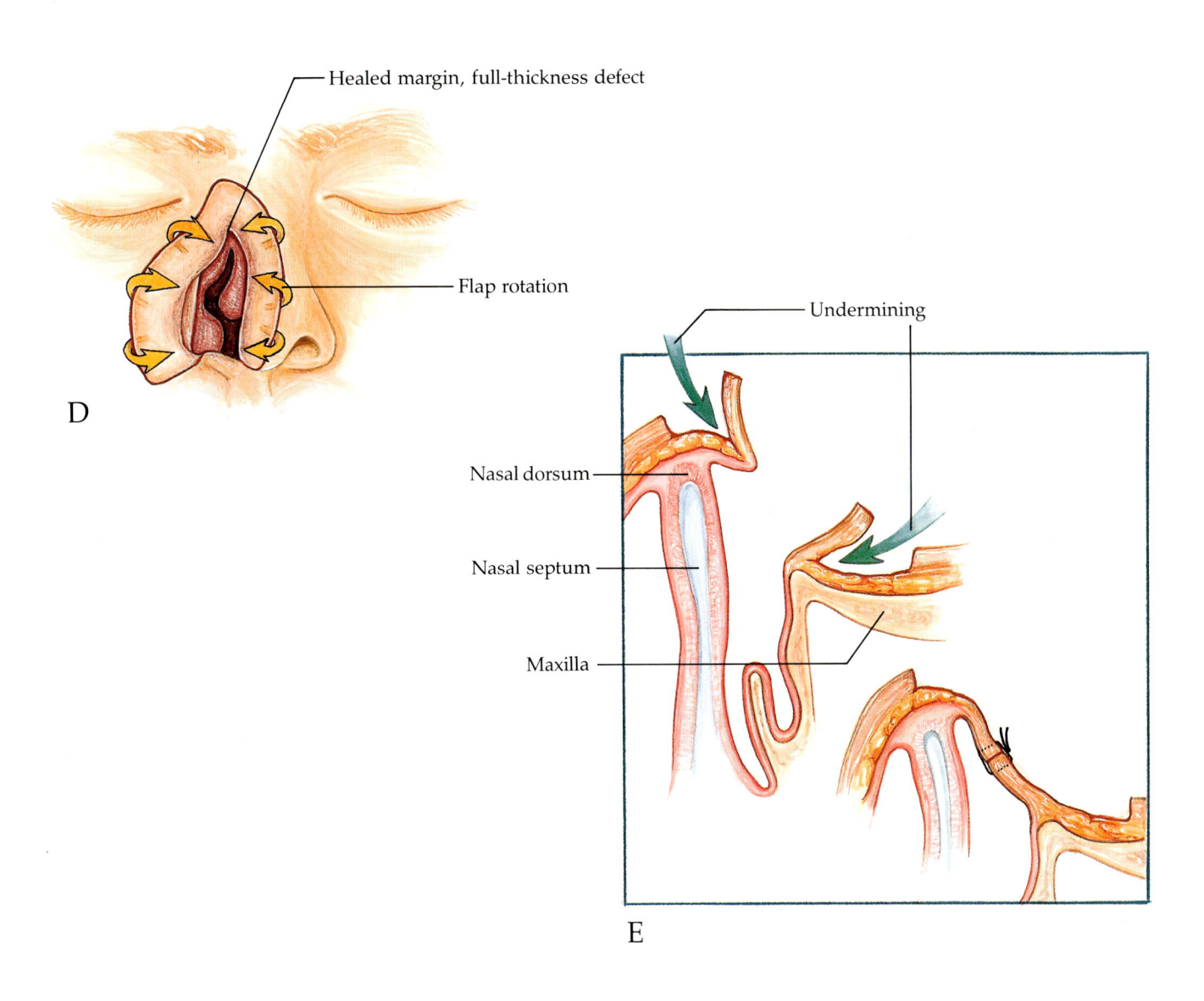

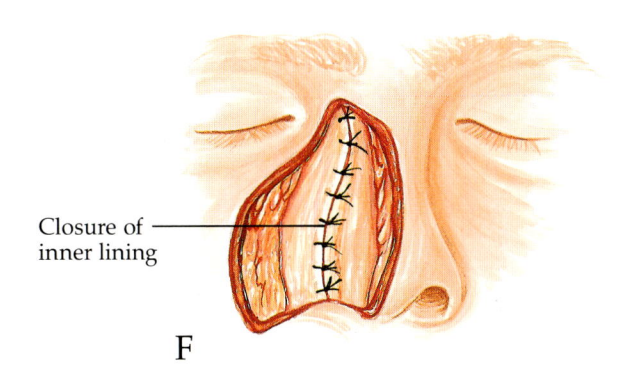

Closure of inner lining

F

Figure 14 (Continued)
Nasal Reconstruction;
Full-Thickness Defect, Inner Lining

flap into position (Fig. 14G). The alar margin is reconstructed by turning the flap tip inward upon itself and suturing it to the turn-in flaps and back of the median forehead flap (Fig. 14H). A cheek advancement flap then allows closure of the lateral aspect of the cutaneous defect with the best reconstitution of the esthetic units (Fig. 14I). When delayed reconstruction of full-thickness nasal defects is planned, a subcutaneous pocket may be developed near the anticipated flap tip and structural cartilage implanted or banked. This should be in the plane between the skin and the frontalis muscle, so that this pocket need not be disturbed at the time of deployment of the flap (Figs. 14J and 14K). Similarly, a split-thickness skin graft can be applied to the deep surface of the frontalis muscle to facilitate reconstruction of the inner lining of the nasal cavity (Fig. 14L).

Plate 78
Figure 14 (Continued)
Nasal Reconstruction;
Full-Thickness Defect, Outer Lining

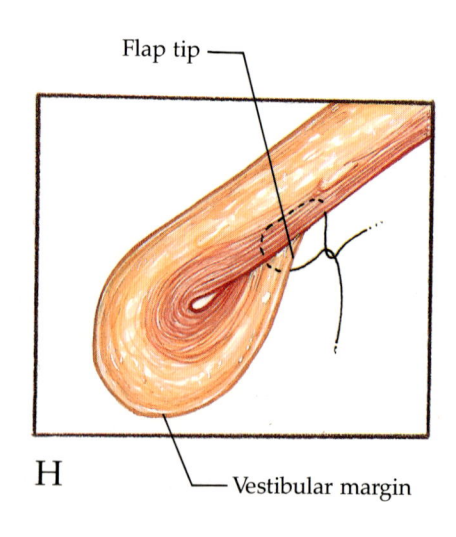

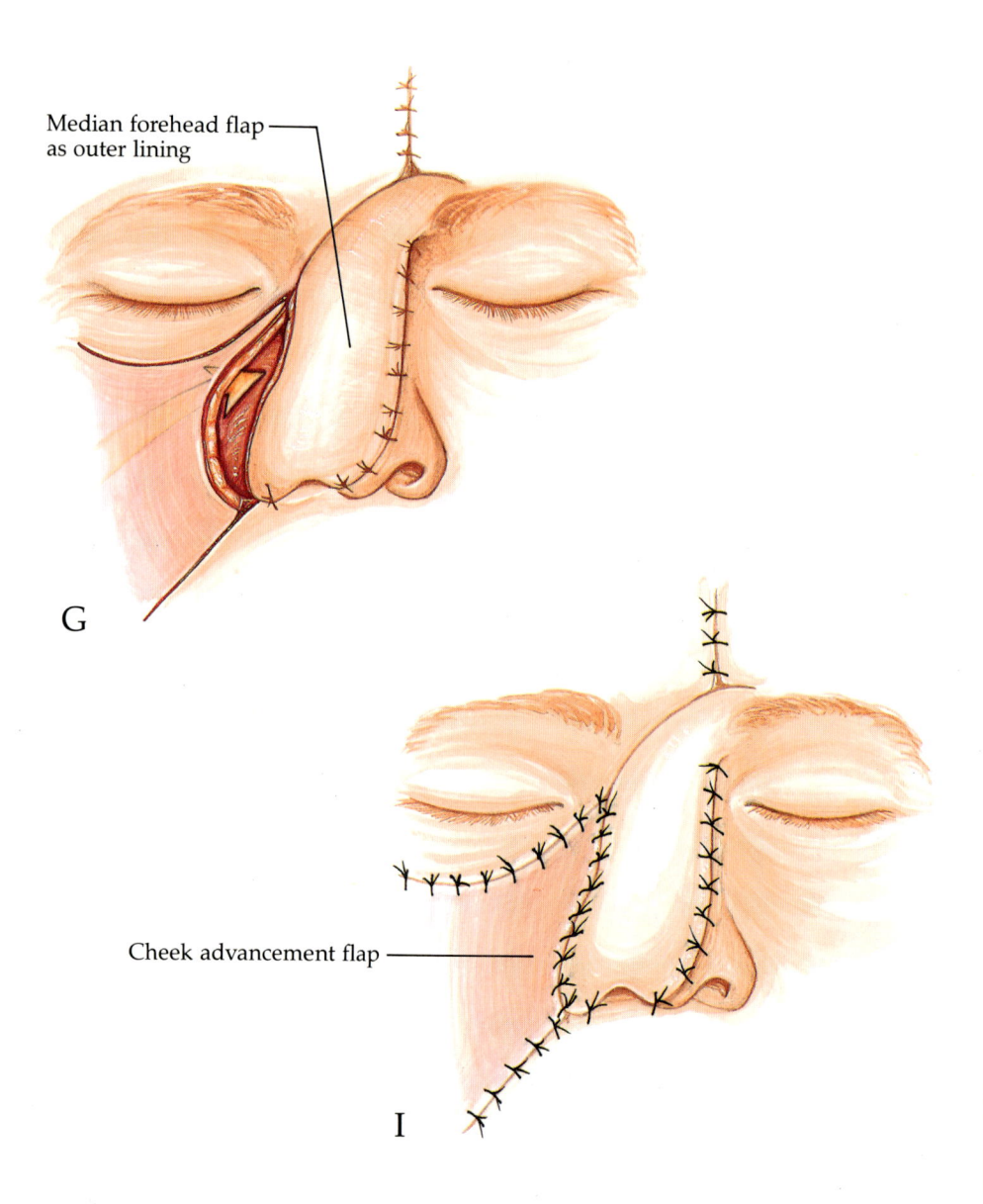

Plate 79

- Cartilage graft
- Subcutaneous pocket

J

- Banked cartilage

K

- Split-thickness skin graft

L

Figure 14 (Continued)
Nasal Reconstruction;
Full-Thickness Defect, Primary Closure

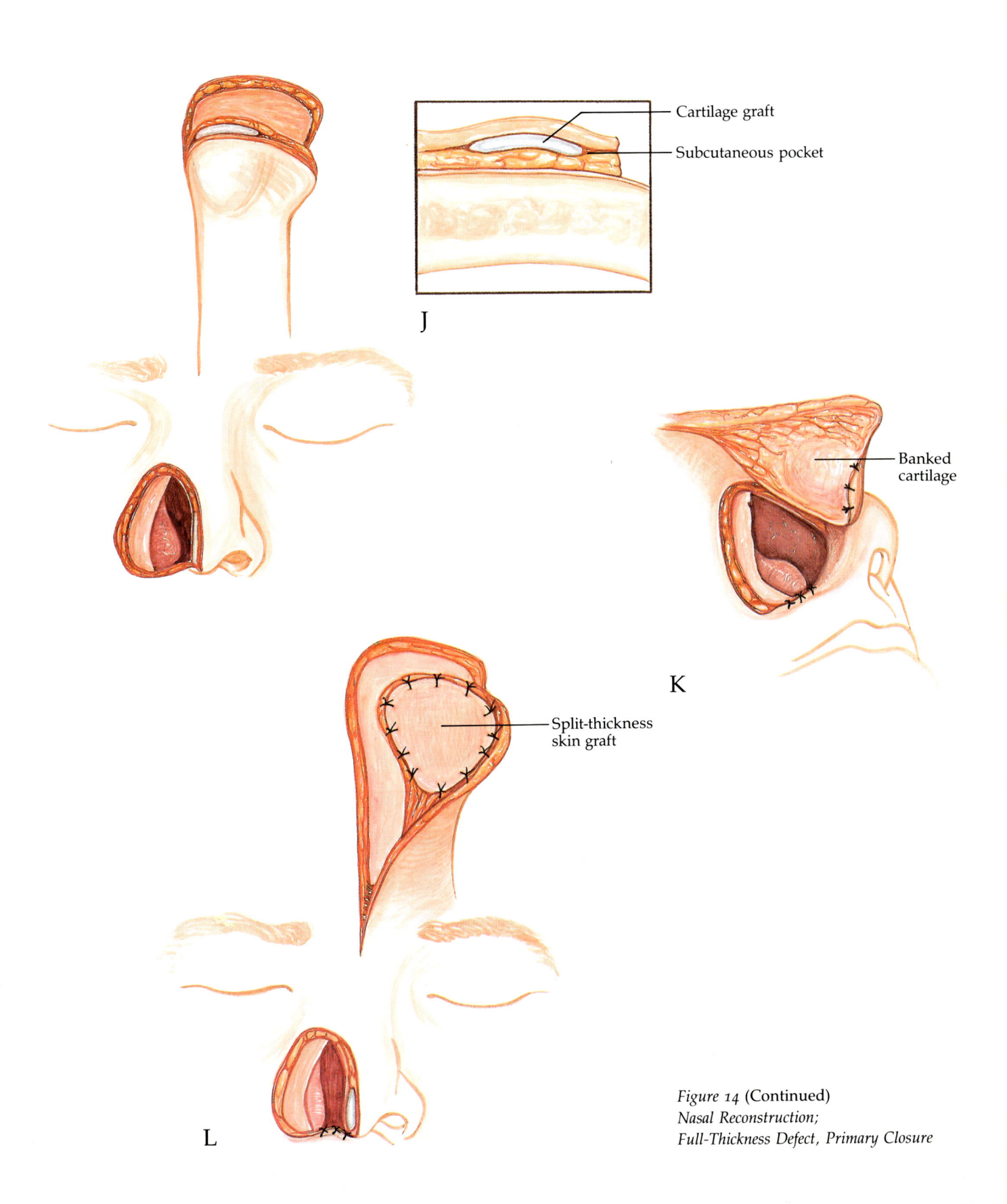

179

PEDICLE FLAP REVISIONS. The cosmetic disturbance of a flap pedicle in the central face is considerable. Visual compromise may also result from a pedicle overhanging a portion of the eye. It is desirable to amputate the pedicle as soon as physiologically feasible. Testing of the adequacy of distal vascular ingrowth is begun 2 weeks postoperatively. A thin, rubber surgical drain or wide rubberband is passed around the pedicle, tension-placed, and fastened into position with a hemostat. When no blanching of the distal flap occurs, the pedicle may be amputated. This usually takes place between 2 and 4 weeks following the primary surgery. If radiation has been delivered to the operative field, or if there is underlying small vessel disease, this interval may be considerably longer. The revisions can be done under local anesthesia. The flap is simply amputated distally, taking care to leave ample tissue on the recipient side for appropriate remodeling and wound closure. The same principles are applied at the base of the flap, taking care to preserve the inner aspect of the eyebrow (Fig. 14M). The subcutaneous fat is carefully trimmed from the skin margins (Fig. 14N). The inner aspect of the brow is carefully repositioned by opening the inferior limb of the forehead incision and back cutting just above the brow margin as necessary (Fig. 14O). Subcutaneous tissue is approximated with interrupted 4–0 polyglycolic acid suture, and the skin is closed with interrupted 6–0 monofilament nylon sutures.

FLAP REVISIONS. Many regional flaps are thicker than the pre-existing nasal skin. This may create a contour irregularity that is distressing to the patient. Depressed scars, especially on the nasal tip, are extremely common after reconstruction. The surgeon should wait at least 6 months following pedicle division to allow the flap edema to subside. Defatting of the flap is then undertaken if it is still too thick (Fig. 14P). This maneuver can be combined with W-plasties, Z-plasties, and geometric closure where appropriate to refine the scars further. Care should be taken not to devitalize grafted tissue in an effort to accomplish too much at one sitting.

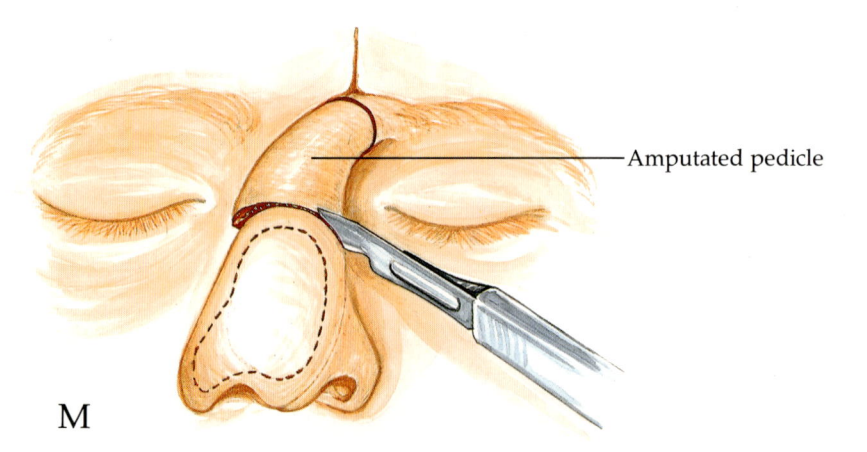

Plate 80
Figure 14 (Continued)
Nasal Reconstruction;
Median Forehead Flap, Revision

Plate 81

N

O

P

Subcutaneous fat

Repositioned brow

Subcutaneous fat

Figure 14 (Continued)
Nasal Reconstruction;
Median Forehead Flap,
Revision, and Flap Debulking

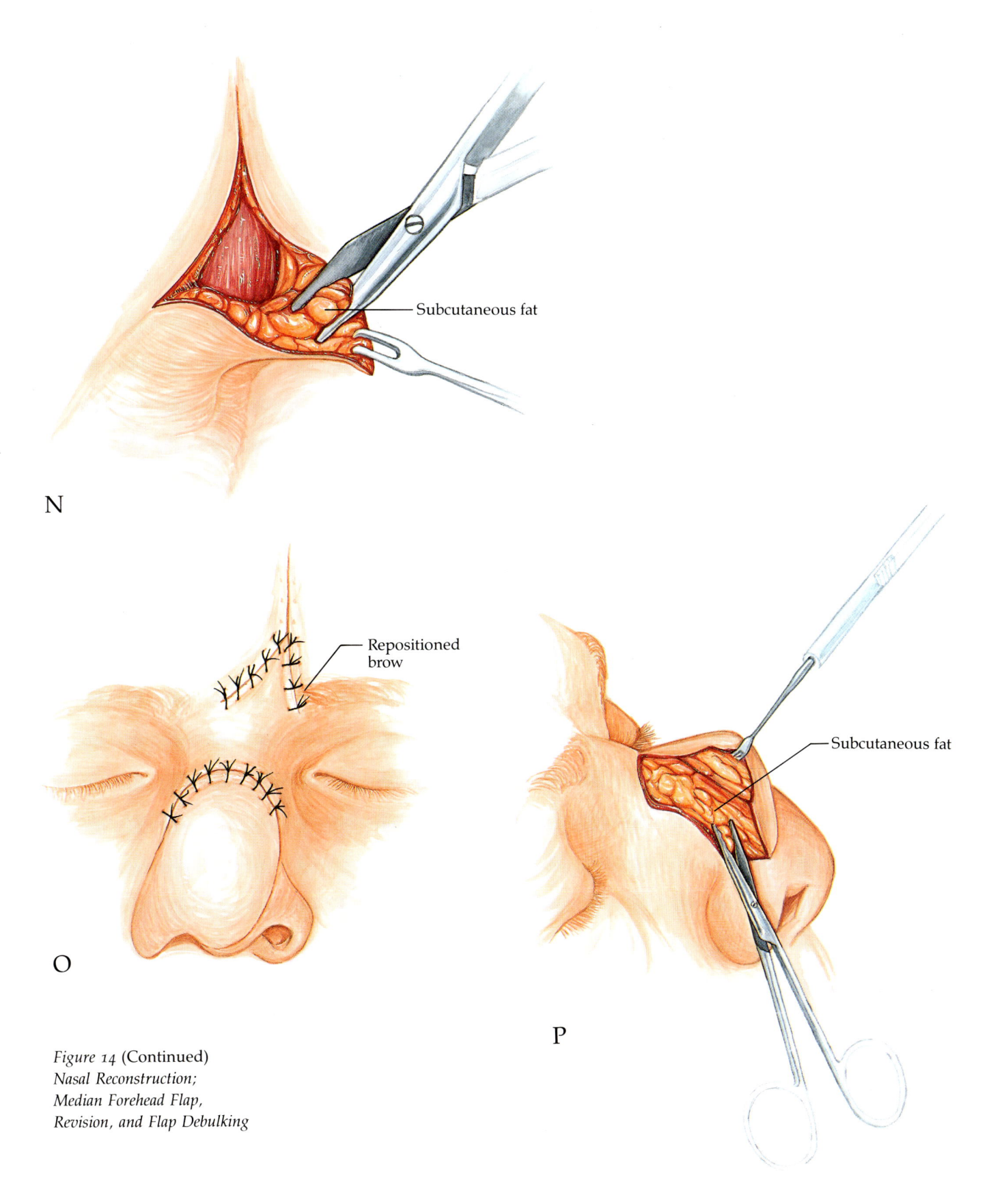

CONVERSE SCALPING FLAP. The Converse scalping flap is our preferred method for reconstruction of the total nasal defect. The rich blood supply of this flap is provided by the superficial temporal, supraorbital, supratrochlear, and facial arteries (Fig. 15A). This provides a significant advantage over flaps that rely on only one set of vessels, such as the oblique forehead flap, the lateral forehead flap, the sickle flap, and the up and down flap. The forehead skin provides an excellent color, thickness, and texture match to the skin of the middle third of the face. The actual donor site itself may be varied in thickness by either incorporating or eliminating the frontalis muscle (Fig. 15B). The flap tip may be delayed to increase the reliability of tissue transfer, and cartilage strips for dorsal nasal and columellar support may be implanted before or after pedicle transfer, as may a split-thickness skin graft for internal lining.

The central back cut in the skin of the forehead is essential for adequate development of pedicle length (Fig. 15B). This poses a critical danger to the flap's vasculature, however, and the path of the main branch of the superficial temporal artery should be mapped out with Doppler testing prior to making this or the coronal incisions. The flap pedicle is rolled on itself as much as possible during development, and the nasal tip and columella are fashioned and sutured into position (Fig. 15C). The actual skin donor site is covered with split-thickness skin graft with a few "piecrust" incisions, and the remainder of the flap donor site is covered with meshed split-thickness skin graft (Fig. 15C). The pedicle is retrieved in 3 to 4 weeks when it passes the tourniquet test. The meshed skin graft is stripped away from the pericranium, and the hair-bearing skin is returned to the scalp and the hairline re-established. The skin of the forehead on the side of the pedicle redrapes to its natural position.

Plate 82

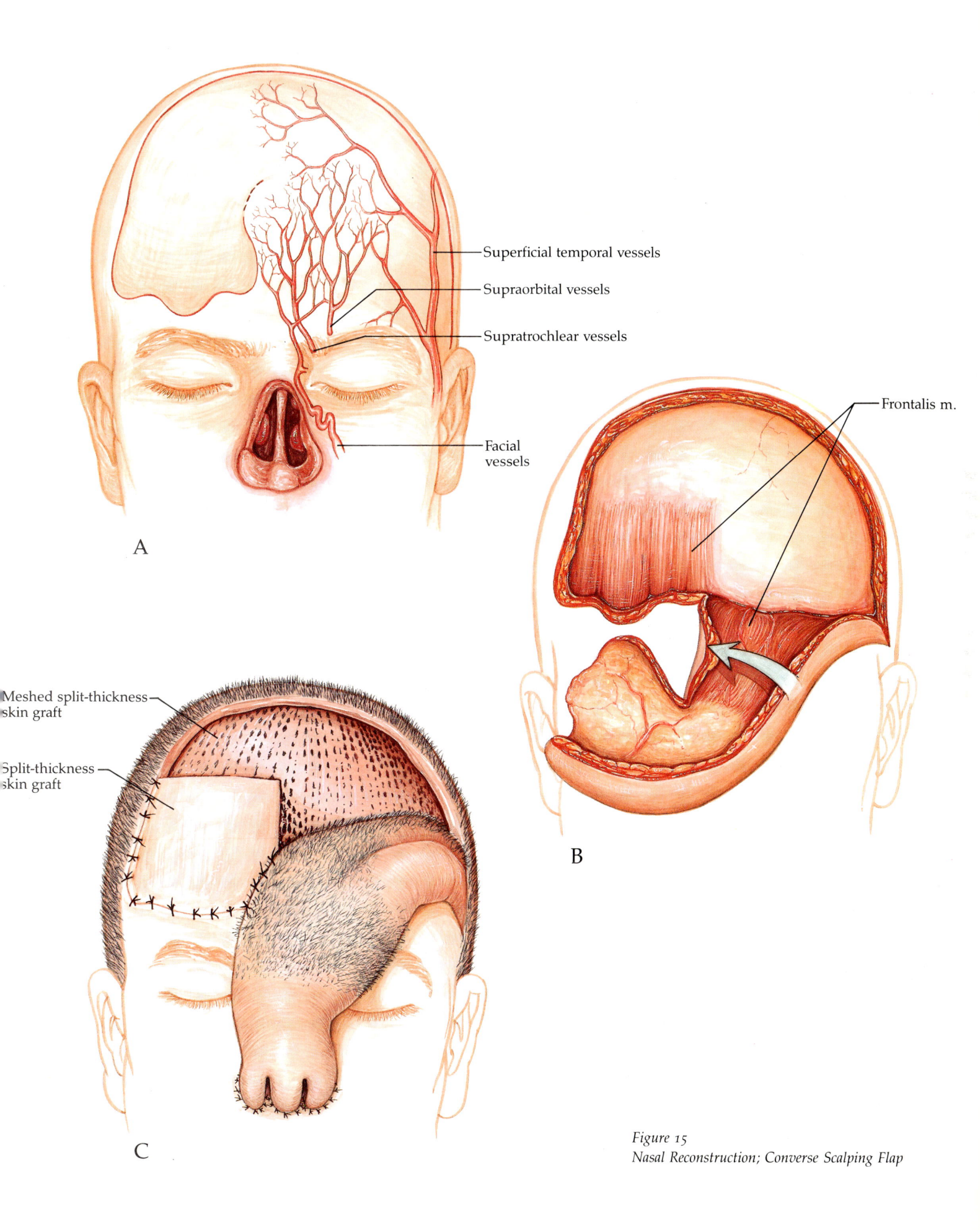

- Superficial temporal vessels
- Supraorbital vessels
- Supratrochlear vessels
- Facial vessels

A

Frontalis m.

B

Meshed split-thickness skin graft
Split-thickness skin graft

C

Figure 15
Nasal Reconstruction; Converse Scalping Flap

FASHIONING THE NASAL TIP. Fashioning the nasal columella and tip in total and subtotal nasal reconstructions is perhaps the most difficult area in which to achieve adequate esthetic restoration. This must begin by providing a flap of adequate length and width. The flap is turned downward, with the epithelial surface against the face. This flap tip is folded on itself with the skin facing outward, and the corners of the cut margins are sutured together with absorbable material (Fig. 16A). This same anchor point is turned back toward the raw surface of the flap (Fig. 16B) and sutured to the center of the flap at its point of contact (Fig. 16C). Anchoring sutures are placed in what will be the dome area. The flap is rotated 180 degrees (Fig. 16D), and the lateral margins are folded downward to where they are sewn into their positions at the lateral nasal border (Fig. 16E).

REPAIR OF SUPPORT STRUCTURES
The skeletal support of the nose is composed of the cartilaginous lobule and the bony pyramid. The cartilage structures include the paired lower and upper lateral cartilages, which interact with a hinge mechanism and form the internal nasal valve. The quadrangular cartilage of the septum and the lateral sesamoid cartilages complete the set. These cartilages as a whole not only provide skeletal support but also play an important role in nasal physiology. The nasal bones are attached to the frontal process above and the maxilla laterally and posteriorly. At their caudal end, the nasal bones join with the upper lateral cartilages, with the cartilages resting interior. The bony septum consists of the perpendicular plate of the ethmoid bone and the vomer and plays little role in external nasal support if the nasal bones are intact.

When part of the nasal ala is deficient, a composite graft of auricular origin may be utilized. Up to 1.5 cm of area may be reconstructed with a good expectation of graft survival. The thickness of the skin and cartilage of the auricle is quite similar to that of the nasal ala. A superiorly based nasolabial flap folded into the defect may also be used for alar reconstruction, but it will need thinning later.

When the skin is intact and the cartilaginous framework is deficient, free autogenous grafts of auricular, septal, or costal cartilage may be utilized. These may be shaped and inserted into soft tissue pockets as needed to provide support or contour or both.

Struts of cartilage can be used to augment and support nasal skeletal deficiencies as necessary. This may take the form of columellar struts to improve nasal projection or dorsal struts to provide support. These dorsal grafts can be anchored to the frontal bones or the columellar structures or both.

Figure 16
Nasal Reconstruction; Nasal Tip Fashioning

Plate 83

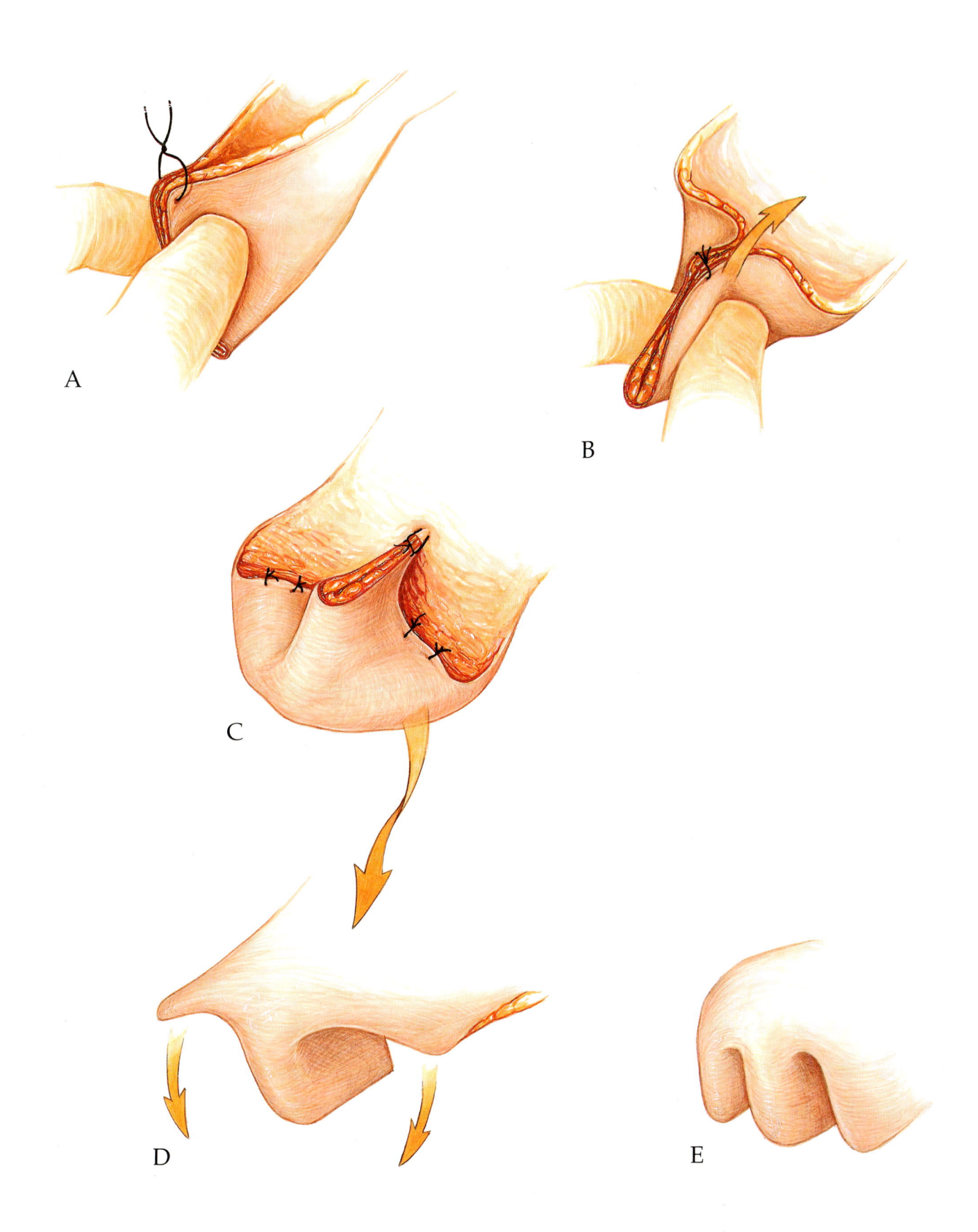

A

B

C

D

E

Butterfly grafts of auricular cartilage may be used to lengthen the lobule and provide support for the nasal valve.

When planning nasal reconstruction that will require both skin and skeletal tissues, the procedures may be staged to add the support either primarily or secondarily. Cartilage may be banked under a delayed flap so that when the flap is transferred, the support is already vascularized and stable. Autogenous bone of the cranial iliac crest or rib origin may also be used for support. The bone grafts can be wired to the frontal process as a cantilever.

Suggested Reading

Carpue J. An account of two successful operations for restoring a lost nose from the integuments of the forehead. London: Longman, Hurst, Rees, Orme, and Brown, 1816.

Converse JM. Reconstruction of the nose by the scalping flap technique. Surg Clin North Am 1959; 49:2.

Denecke HJ, Meyer R. Plastic surgery of the head and neck, corrective and reconstructive rhinoplasty. Berlin: Springer, 1967.

Tagliocozzi G. De curtorum chirurgia per insitionem. Venice: Bindoni, 1597.

John C. Price, M.D.

RHINECTOMY

Indications

Total rhinectomy is indicated for removal of malignant lesions of the nasal skin that have penetrated the skeletal framework of the nose, for anterior intranasal malignancies of intermediate and larger size, and for sarcomas involving the external nose. Rhinectomy may be required in conjunction with maxillectomy or craniofacial surgery.

Preoperative Considerations

Cutaneous margins vary with the origin and histopathology of the malignancy. As a general rule, the larger the lesion, the larger the margin required. The morphea variety of basal cell carcinoma requires more extensive margins than other types. The size and depth of penetration of cutaneous melanoma should be considered when planning skin margins. Infiltration of skin by tumor arising within the nasal cavity should be considered a serious sign, carrying with it an increased risk of spread of tumor along the subdermal lymphatics. Two-centimeter skin margins should be considered minimal in this circumstance. Larger margins would be indicated if there is any sign of cutaneous edema or erythema beyond the tumor margin. Bone margins should be generous but not needlessly excessive. High-resolution computed tomographic scanning of the nasal and facial bones is an invaluable adjunct to operative planning.

The area is highly vascular, and brisk bleeding may be anticipated. Infiltration of the incision lines (only) with local anesthetic and epinephrine should be considered. The patient's blood is routinely typed and cross-matched for 4 U of packed red blood cells.

Administration of perioperative antibiotics is indicated, as nasal packing is maintained for a variable period during the postoperative course. The potential for development of toxic shock syndrome exists; therefore the patient should be covered for *Staphylococcus aureus* and other potential skin pathogens. Coverage of gram-negative and anaerobic organisms is not essential in this case.

Operative Steps

General anesthesia is induced by peroral placement of an endotracheal tube of either the RAE or armored variety. The tube is then fixed anteriorly in the middle to the chin with tape or anchored to a mandibular incisor tooth with a 0 silk suture. Cutaneous margins are marked and infiltrated with local anesthetic and epinephrine solution. Suture tarsorrhaphies are placed bilaterally. The face is prepared in the usual fashion and the head drape positioned. Sterile towels are applied so as to exclude the endotracheal tube from the operative field while allowing adequate exposure of the midportion of the face. Placement of a split sheet completes the draping procedure.

The skin incision is carried down through bone with a single motion (Fig. 17A). Any bleeding at this point will be high pressure arterial or from intermediate to large veins. Finger pressure along the skin assists in controlling this while hemostats are applied. An electrocautery or an argon beam coagulator is quite helpful in obtaining hemostasis. The periosteum of the nasal and maxillary bones is then elevated away from the tumor so as to improve exposure and facilitate the bone cuts (Fig. 17B). Sectioning of the bone is accomplished with either sharp osteotomes or with a sagittal saw (Fig. 17C). These cuts transect the nasal bone, the frontal process of the maxilla, and the anterior nasal spine. They are planned so that any extension of tumor along the nasal septum is removed with adequate margin. The cartilaginous septum may be transected with

Plate 84

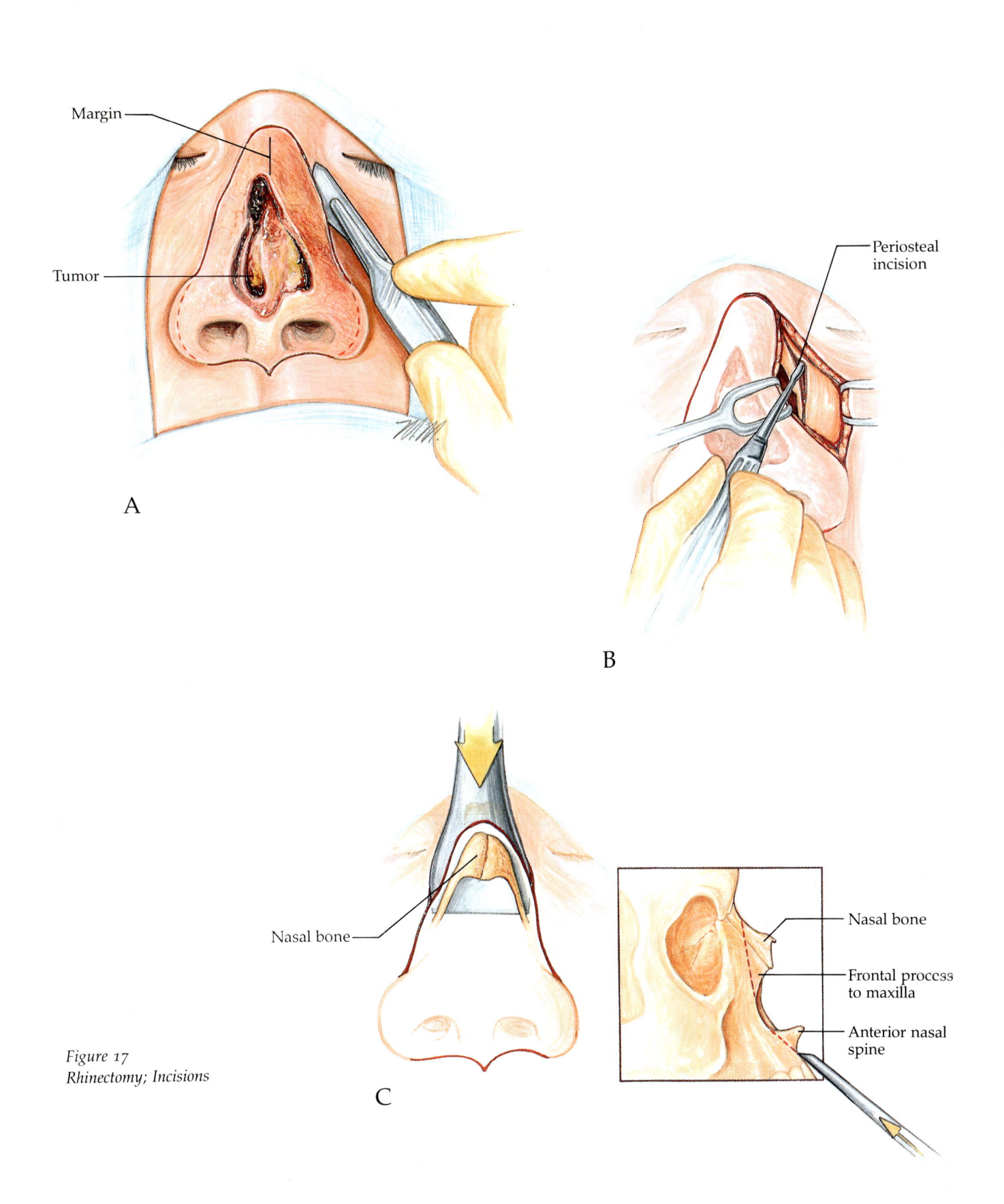

A

B

C

Figure 17
Rhinectomy; Incisions

Labels: Margin, Tumor, Periosteal incision, Nasal bone, Nasal bone, Frontal process to maxilla, Anterior nasal spine

189

heavy surgical scissors (the Mayo scissors is preferable) (Fig. 17D). This should complete the removal of the specimen, which is forwarded to the pathologist (or Moh's dermatologist) for frozen section inspection of the margins to confirm adequate tumor removal. A laparotomy sponge is placed in the resection cavity, and firm pressure is applied. The margins of resection are carefully examined in a systematic clockwise fashion, and complete hemostasis is obtained. The cutaneous and nasal mucosal edges are undermined with a periosteal elevator around the circumference of the defect (Fig. 17E). Bone and cartilaginous edges are further reduced with the rongeur. Residual septal mucosa is approximated to the mucosa of the opposite side, thereby covering the transected margin of septum. The facial skin and nasal mucosa are approximated in a similar fashion, thereby achieving a final closure with no exposed bone or cartilage (Fig. 17F). Absorbable suture (4–0) is preferred for this closure. If direct closure produces excessive tension on facial structures (e.g., retraction of the upper lip into the nasal cavity), a split-thickness skin graft should be interposed between the facial skin and nasal mucosa.

Postoperative Care

Application of antibiotic-saturated Vaseline gauze packing allows for additional hemostasis and helps to prevent seroma and hematoma formation. It is desirable to mold an additional quantity of this packing into a rough nasal shape prior to the application of an external bandage. This may relieve some of the immediate postoperative anxiety of the patient and his or her family. This camouflage may be continued through the postoperative course until the resection cavity has matured enough for surgical or prosthetic reconstruction. Final pathologic confirmation of the adequacy of the margins is essential.

Risks, Complications, and Sequelae

Significant bleeding occurs from this operation, and transfusion may be required. Substantial cosmetic defect also occurs, and the patient must be cognizant of this through informed consent. Risk of injury to or infection of the eyes or central nervous system exists but is less likely to occur than with other forms of internasal and paranasal sinus surgery. The surgeon and the patient alike must be aware that the worst complication is failure to attain adequate margins to control malignant disease. Firm understanding must exist regarding the indications and necessity for extending surgery to the orbit, face, palate, or other adjacent structures.

Plate 85

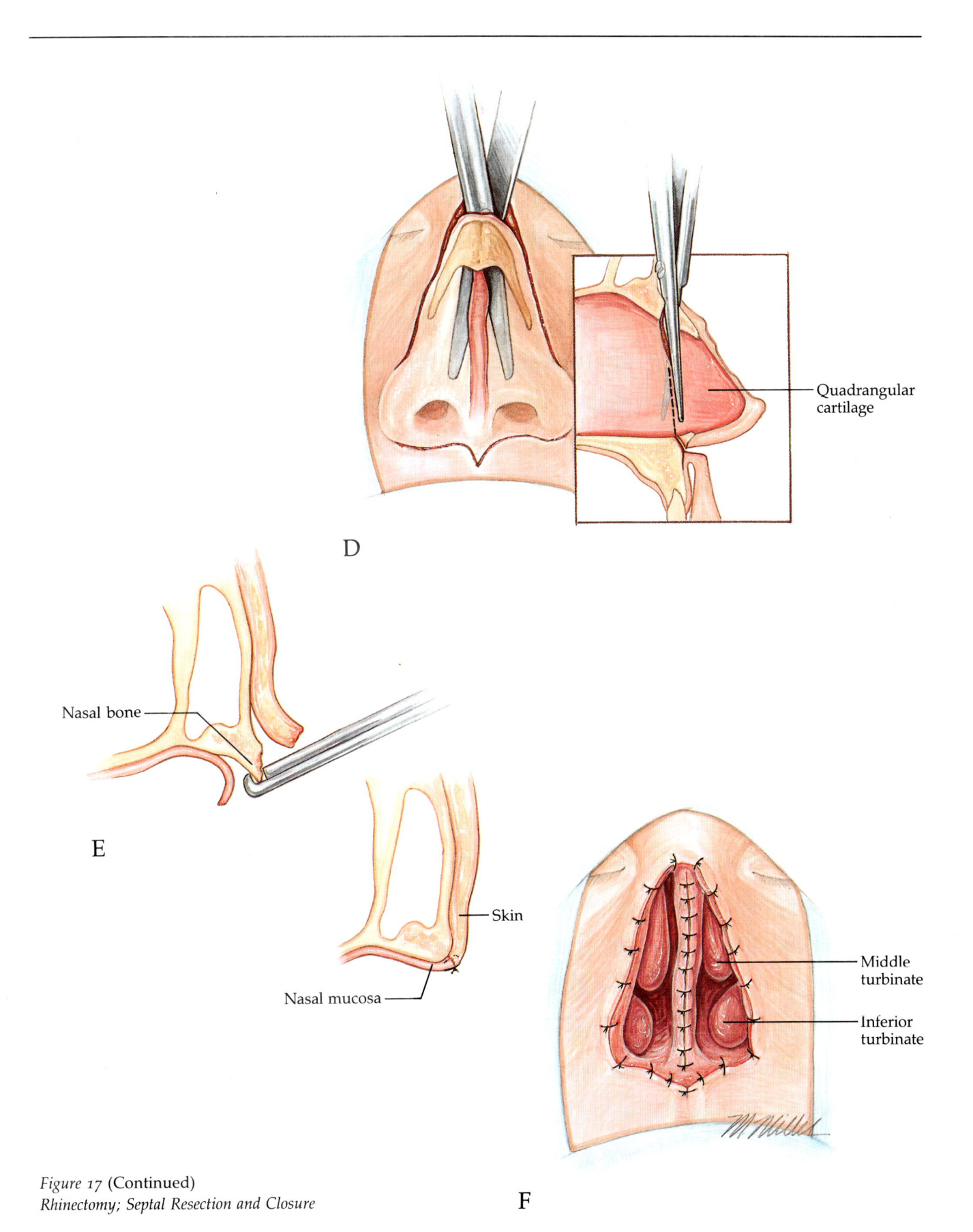

D

Quadrangular cartilage

Nasal bone

E

Skin

Nasal mucosa

F

Middle turbinate

Inferior turbinate

Figure 17 (Continued)
Rhinectomy; Septal Resection and Closure

Pearls and Pitfalls

Inadequate disease control is the greatest peril of this operation. Careful preoperative planning is essential and meticulous pathologic examination of margins is critical.

Since operative hemorrhaging is brisk, the operation must be well planned and quickly executed.

Hemostasis is facilitated by using vasoconstrictive agents with the local anesthetic, the electrocautery, the argon beam coagulator, and firm finger pressure around the cutaneous incisions.

Surgical reconstruction should not be attempted until final pathologic margin clearance has been obtained. Frozen section analysis is frequently deceptive.

Prosthetic reconstruction of the nose should be delayed until adequate wound and scar maturation has occurred, usually between 3 and 6 months postoperatively.

Mark M. Miller, M.A.

FABRICATION OF A NASAL PROSTHESIS

The history of facial prosthetics is a long but poorly documented one. Nevertheless, according to Chalian, Egyptian mummies have been discovered with prosthetic ears, eyes, and noses, thus dating these devices back to antiquity. It is also known that the prosthetic material of choice reflected the technology of the day. Tycho Brache, a 16th-century Danish astronomer, lost his nose during a duel and subsequently replaced it with an artificial nose made of silver and gold. The Chinese are known to have made facial prostheses from waxes and resins. Additionally, the story is told of one Anna Coleman Ladd, an American sculptress and socialite, who in the aftermath of World War I created beautiful metallic masks for the facially disfigured. These masks were galvanized in silvered copper, then painted realistically in oils to "reproduce, as faithfully as possible, the former appearance of the mutile." However, it was not until the advent of 20th-century technology that flexible materials came into considerable use for the creation of facial prostheses. With the discovery of vulcanized natural rubber by Charles Goodyear in 1834 and continuing on to the current use of synthetic organic polymers, especially silicone, the progress of facial prosthetics can be characterized by the continual search for the best available material.

Indications

The patient who has been or will be heavily irradiated or who is a poor risk for additional surgery because of advanced age or ill health is a good candidate for prosthetic nasal reconstruction. The use of a nasal prosthesis may also be advantageous in cases in which disease recurrence is a possibility. In addition to the cosmetic restoration of the patient, the nasal prosthesis serves to help restore the natural humidity of the nasal sinus and to improve voice resonance, while offering protection to the nasal wound. Nasal prosthesis candidates should be at least 6 weeks postoperative and have no residual edema. The wound should be free of crusting.

Fabrication Steps

All successful facial prostheses begin with good impression-taking techniques. The patient is placed in an upright sitting position with the head slightly tilted back. All exposed facial hair is coated lightly with petroleum jelly. The hair is covered with a nurse's bouffant, and the clothing is shielded with a protective drape. The nasal wound is thoroughly cleaned of mucus and packed with sterile lubricated gauze to occlude the choanae. Steps must be taken to ensure that no impression material flows into the throat. Normal set irreversible hydrocolloid impression material is mixed with room temperature water to a relatively thin consistency. The mix is spatulated against the sides of the mixing bowl to ensure freedom from lumps. The material is applied to the skin above the wound and allowed to flow freely over the skin margins into and filling the wound (Fig. 18A). Pouring the material directly into the wound increases the likelihood of trapping air and thus compromising the exactness of the impression. it is important to reassure the patient by maintaining verbal and tactile communication with him or her during the molding process. Before the first coat of material has solidified, a heavier layer of alginate is applied, with a thin layer of gauze being utilized between the two coats as a binder. Once the material is set, fast-set plaster bandages are layered upon the external surface of the impression for support (Fig. 18B). The patient is assisted to a fully upright position, and the impression is carefully removed, paying specific attention to any undercuts that may tear it.

Dental stone is mixed to a heavy consistency and slowly vibrated into the mold, allowing all air to escape from the lowest recesses and undercuts. The plaster is poured up to but not over the highest point of the upturned mold. This creates a channel in the cast through which access is gained to the back of the sculpted prosthesis (Fig. 18C). The cast is allowed to set, and all outside edges and flashing are trimmed with a model trimmer or dental bur.

Sculpting of the nasal prosthesis is preceded by applying a thin coat of petroleum jelly to the stone cast over the area to be covered with the sculpted prosthesis. To this, a layer of aluminum foil is burnished down, using the blunt face of a dental elevator. This foil layer aids in the removal of the sculpted prosthesis from the stone cast during subsequent trial fittings. Sulfur-free modeling clay is used as a sculpting medium. Preoperative photographs of the patient as well as any preoperative casts are used as references. (If possible, the patient should see the prosthetist prior to ablative surgery, at which time a preoperative cast is made as a sculpting reference.) Sculpting should proceed with careful attention to facial proportions and bone structure. The sculpture is rotated in space as sculpting progresses, so that frontal, lateral, superior, and inferior views are examined and adjusted accordingly. Where possible, edges are made to lie in natural skin creases for a less noticeable transition between skin and prosthesis. Occasionally the sculpture is refrigerated to harden the clay for enhanced sculpting of finer details. Final sculpting and smoothing are done with a No. 1 or 2 flat sable brush dipped in xylene. Skin texture is created with a bristle brush or by pressing small silicone impressions of actual skin into the clay surface.

During a second visit, the sculpted prosthesis is removed from the stone face cast and placed directly on the patient's face to check the fit,

Plate 86

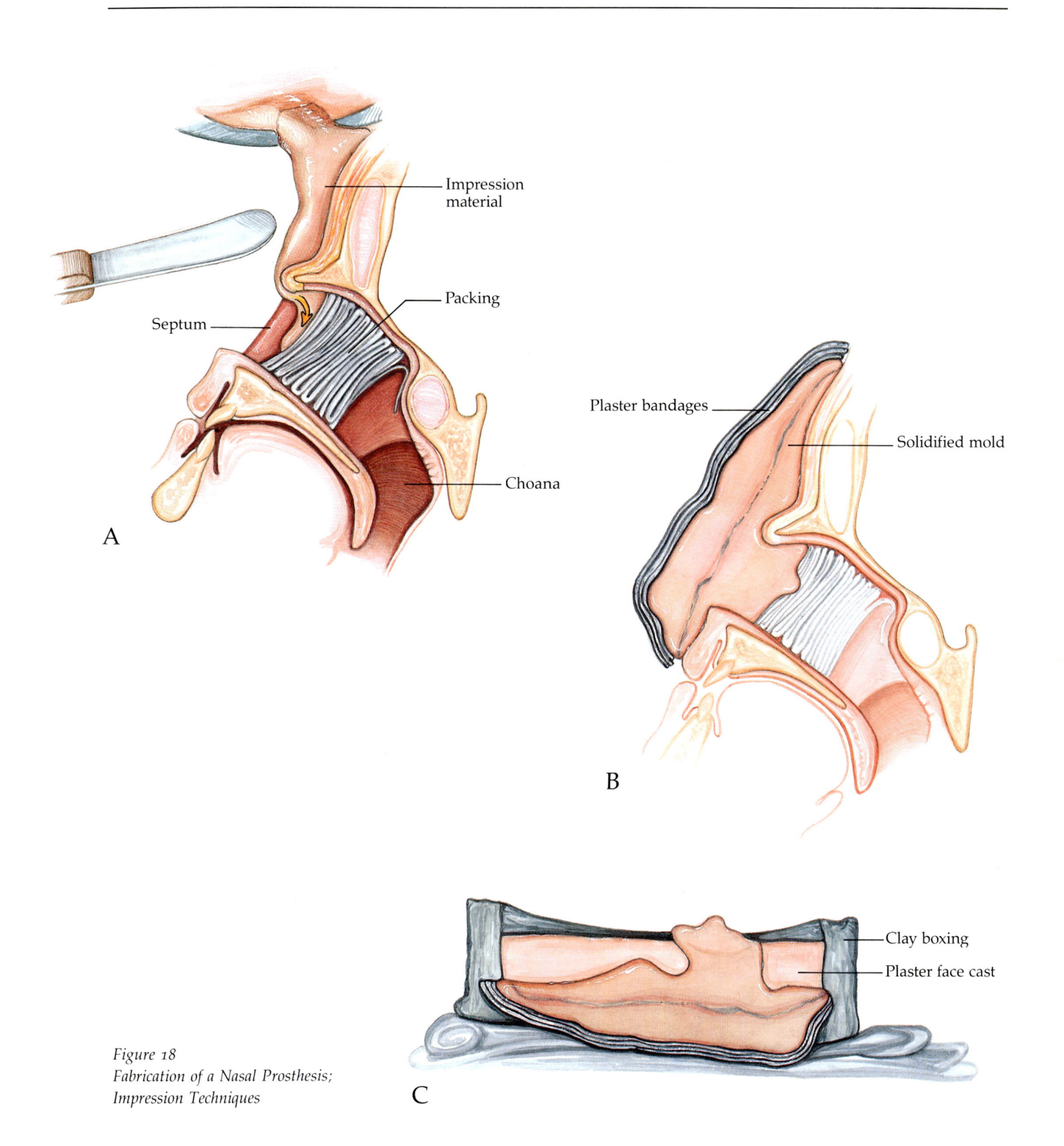

- Impression material
- Septum
- Packing
- Choana

A

- Plaster bandages
- Solidified mold

B

- Clay boxing
- Plaster face cast

C

Figure 18
Fabrication of a Nasal Prosthesis;
Impression Techniques

195

shape, and alignment. All final adjustments are made, and the sculpture is returned to the cast. Also during this second visit, an intrinsic skin color sample is created by mixing the appropriate pigments with silicone until the desired hue is achieved, namely, the lightest overall color value adjacent to the prosthesis area. This should be done under natural light. The final color formula is recorded in a log and later referred to when the base silicone is intrinsically colored prior to packing in the mold.

To initiate the molding process, the sculpted prosthesis is boxed with modeling clay or dental boxing wax. A generous coat of liquid separator is painted on the frontal surface of the stone cast and allowed to dry. Separator applied to the clay prosthesis is unnecessary, since this only masks the delicate skin texture already achieved. If the clay prosthesis has been refrigerated, it is allowed to warm to room temperature until all condensation has evaporated.

Dental stone is again mixed to a heavy consistency and gently vibrated over the sculpted prosthesis until coverage of at least 2 cm is obtained. Care must be taken to avoid trapping air in the nares. The anterior mold is allowed to solidify and cool.

Through the back opening in the cast, two "nasal passages" are sculpted from the bulk clay, leaving a midline "septum" for structural support (Fig. 18D). These nasal passages are continuous with the nares previously sculpted on the frontal side (Fig. 18E). The depth of the prosthesis skin represented in clay should be 2- to 3-mm, with the nasal tip somewhat thicker. The posterior mold is now poured in the same manner as the anterior one; however, in this case, no separator is used, since the posterior mold should remain permanently attached to the back of the patient's cast. The posterior mold is allowed to solidify and cool.

The anterior mold is removed, the clay prosthesis is discarded, and both molds are thoroughly cleaned of all clay residue using a mild detergent and hot water. With a dental bur, a 1-cm wide trough is made in the face of the anterior mold, circumferentially around the site of the prosthesis. This trough is connected with the perimeter by burring outward several connecting troughs. These channels allow for the escape of excess casting material. Again the mold halves are washed of all plaster dust, then dried and lightly sprayed with a separator (Fig. 18F).

Silicone base is mixed with pigment to the predetermined intrinsic color proportion. The mold halves are packed with this mix, then reapproximated. Excess silicone is extruded with hand pressure until the mold halves are firmly seated against each other. The mold halves are then clamped, and the silicone is allowed to cure.

Plate 87

Sculpted nasal prosthesis within anterior mold

Nasal passage

Face cast

D — Dental elevator

"Septum"

E — Air flow through nasal passage

Face cast

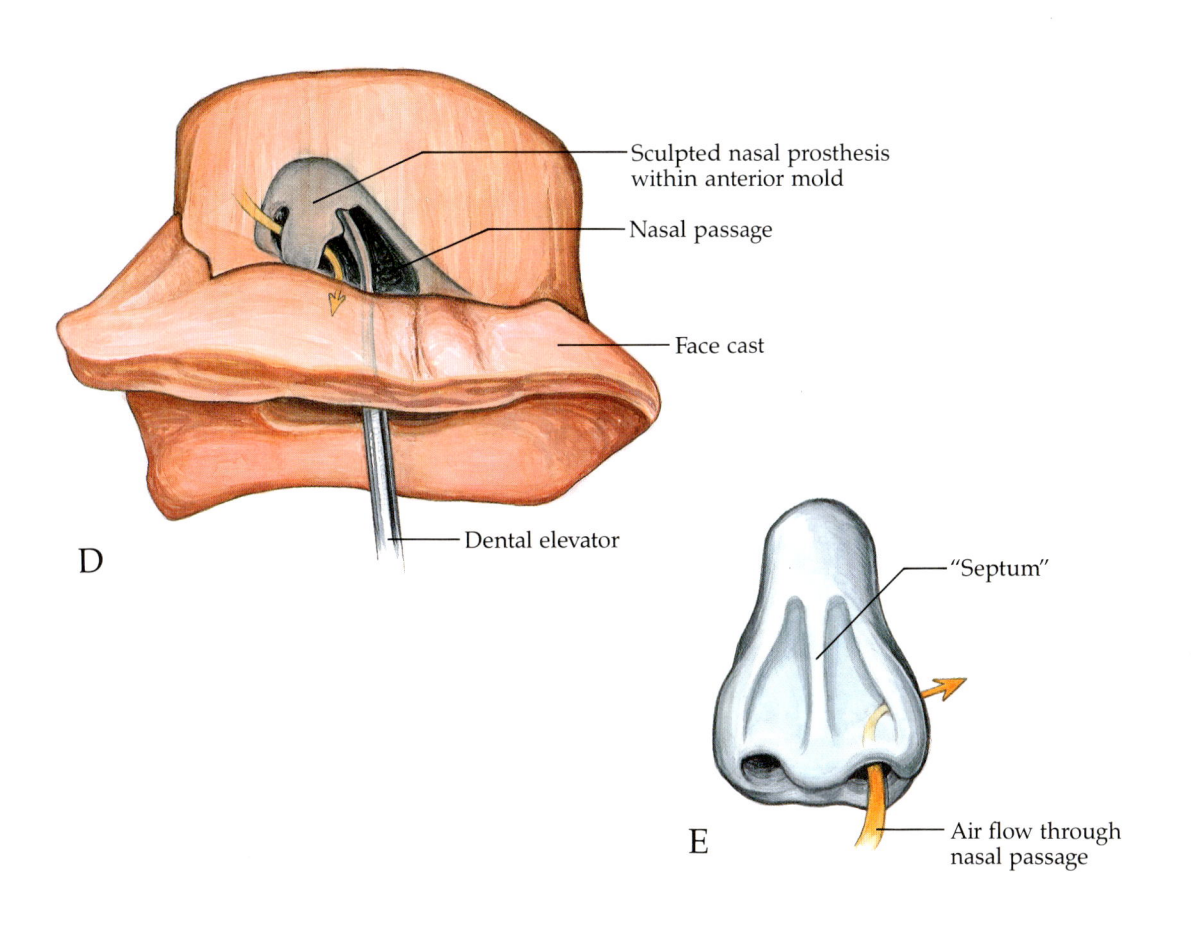

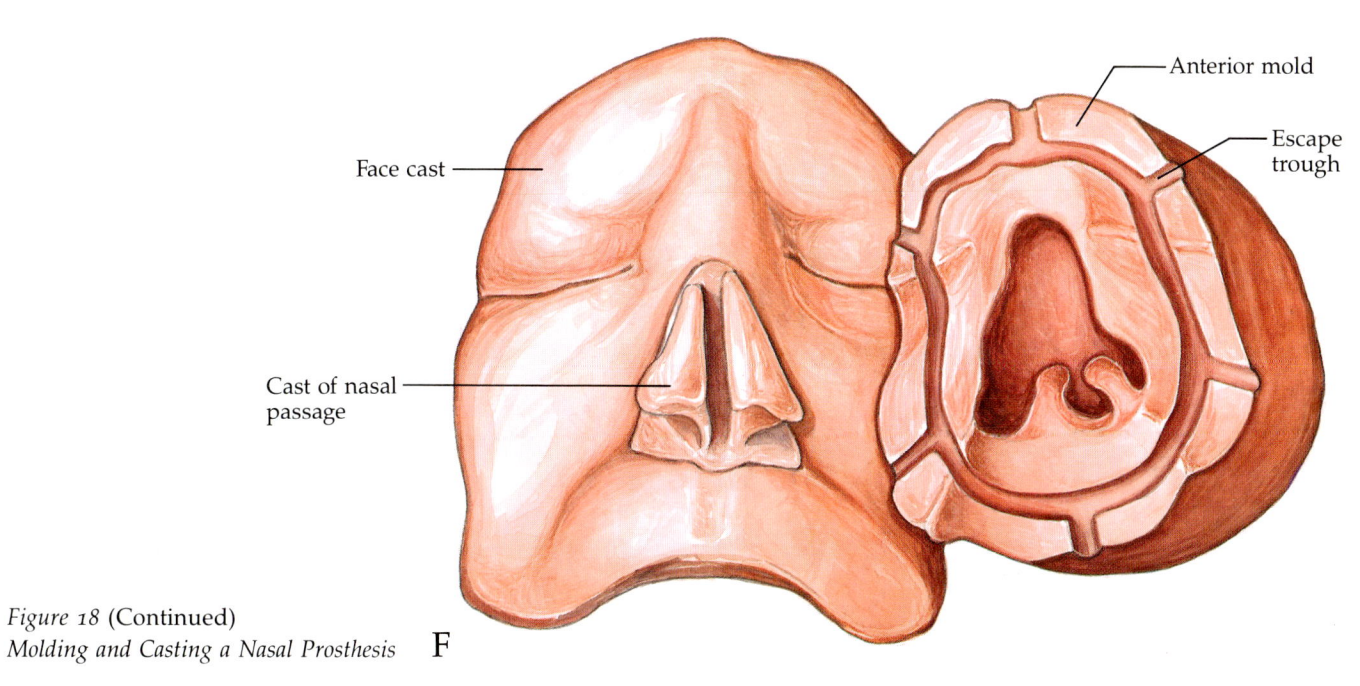

Cast of nasal passage

Anterior mold

Escape trough

Figure 18 (Continued)
Molding and Casting a Nasal Prosthesis F

Fabrication of a Nasal Prosthesis

Once cured, the prosthesis is removed and an excess flashing is trimmed. With the patient present, external coloration is applied to the prosthesis with a mixture of pigment, silicone base, and xylene as a thinning agent. This mixture is applied with a number one or two sable watercolor brush utilizing a stipple technique. The perimeter is painted with the prosthesis in place on the patient to ensure an exact color match by direct comparison of prosthesis to skin (Fig. 18G). Again, all coloration is done under natural light. The painted prosthesis is placed under a heat lamp or hot air gun to accelerate drying. When the external coloration has dried to the touch, the entire prosthesis is sealed with a light coat of Dow Corning Adhesive A (Dow Corning Corp., Midland, Michigan) thinned with xylene. Before this sealing layer has dried, the surface is dabbed with a damp gauze sponge to eliminate sheen.

With the prosthesis now complete, the patient's wound margins are cleaned with an alcohol sponge and the prosthesis is applied with an appropriate adhesive. Although adhesives are the most frequently used mode of prosthesis retention, osseointegrated titanium implants and magnets are also currently being utilized for the retention of facial prostheses. Spectacles may be suggested for improved retention and cosmesis. Upon completion, the patient is thoroughly instructed as to the proper care and maintenance of the prosthesis.

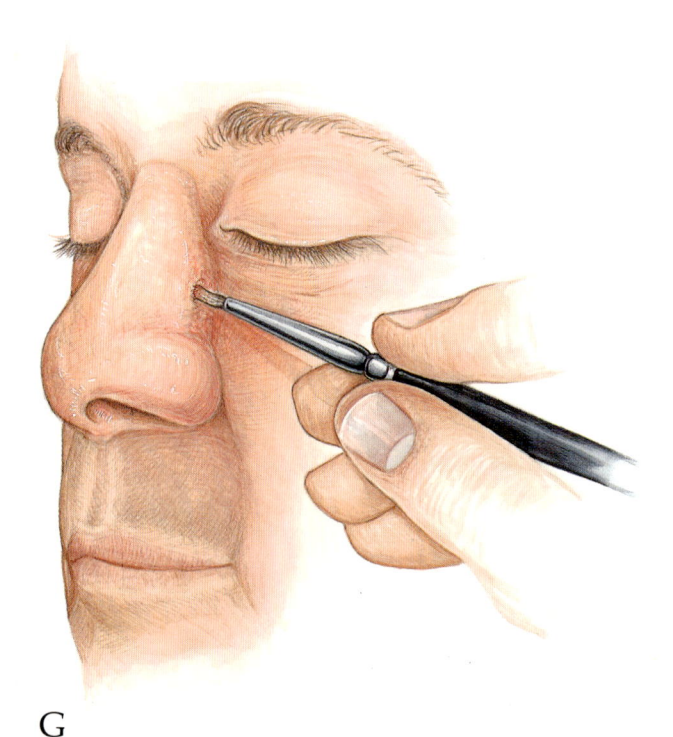

Plate 88
Figure 18 (Continued)
Extrinsic Coloration
of a Nasal Prosthesis

G

Pearls and Pitfalls

Prosthetic rehabilitation is much less debilitating for the already surgically traumatized patient. Many infirm and elderly patients are poor candidates for the rigors of lengthy reconstructive surgery.

Prosthetic rehabilitation is noninvasive and can be accomplished on an outpatient basis.

In patients with cancer, prosthetic rehabilitation allows for the continual inspection of the surgical wound for disease recurrence.

Prosthetic rehabilitation can be accomplished in 2 to 3 weeks once the tissues have stabilized.

A prosthesis is much less expensive than the combined costs of hospitalization and the professional fees involved in one or many reconstructive procedures.

Moreover, a prosthesis often results in a more esthetic and natural appearance.

Prosthetic rehabilitation allows the patient the opportunity to choose reconstructive surgery at any time.

A prosthesis is subject to deterioration by physical wear and tear and therefore must be periodically replaced. Obviously it is not self-replicating, as is skin.

Current technology has not provided a material that can match skin in its remarkable elasticity, tensile strength, and durability.

A prosthesis must be reattached to the face daily and is maintenance-intensive.

Most retention methods are far from foolproof, and therefore the patient often lives with the fear that the prosthesis may dislodge in public.

Some patients, no matter how successful the prosthesis, simply will not accept a device that is artificial and not of themselves. Chen, Udagama, and Drane have indicated that 12 percent of patients with facial prostheses never wear them because of this lack of acceptance or other dissatisfactions.

Suggested Reading

Albrektsson T, Brånemark P-I, Jacobsson M, Tjellström A. Present clinical applications of osseointegrated percutaneous implants. Plast Reconstr Sur 1987; 79:721.

Birnbach S, Herman GL. Coordinated intraoral and extraoral prostheses in the rehabilitation of the orofacial cancer patient. J Prosthet Dent 1987; 58:347.

Chalian VA, Drane JB, Standish SM. Maxillofacial prosthetics: Multidisciplinary practice. Baltimore: Williams & Wilkins, 1971:1.

Chen M, Udagama A, Drane J. Evaluation of facial prostheses in head and neck cancer patients. J Prosthet Dent 1981; 46:538.

Eaton LD. Functional anatomical reconstruction in an oculofacial prosthesis. Ophthalmology 1984; 91:985.

Romm S, Zacher J. Anna Coleman Ladd: Maker of masks for the facially mutilated. Plast Reconstr Surg 1982; 70:106.

Schaaf NG. Maxillofacial prosthetics and the head and neck cancer patient. Cancer 1984; 54(Suppl):2690.

Swartz B, Udagama A. Magnetic prostheses: An alternative fixation and orientation method. Plast Reconstr Surg 1982; 69:755.

Chapter IV
PARANASAL SINUSES

Douglas E. Mattox, M.D.

CALDWELL-LUC WITH TRANSANTRAL ETHMOIDECTOMY

Indications

The Caldwell-Luc (sublabial maxillary antrotomy) procedure has been the mainstay in the management of maxillary sinus disease for six decades. Although its role in the treatment of inflammatory sinus disease has decreased since the advent of endoscopic techniques, it remains the basis for many other procedures, including the facial degloving technique, medial maxillectomy, and transantral internal maxillary artery ligation.

Preoperative Considerations

The preoperative evaluation should include radiographic documentation of maxillary sinus disease. The right-handed surgeon is usually most comfortable standing on the patient's right side, regardless of which sinus is being operated on.

Operative Steps

CALDWELL-LUC PROCEDURE

Although it is possible to perform the procedure under local anesthesia, general anesthesia with orotracheal intubation is preferred. A pharyngeal pack can be used to prevent swallowing or aspiration of blood. The sublabial sulcus and the face of the maxilla are infiltrated with local anesthetic and vasoconstrictor. An attempt should be made to infiltrate beneath the periosteum, or at least as close to it as possible. During the injection, the orbital rim and infraorbital foramen should be palpated with the opposite hand to prevent injury of the infraorbital nerve and orbital contents by the needle.

A sublabial incision is made from the medial incisor to the second bicuspid (Fig. 1A). The incision should be well above the gingiva so that an adequate cuff of mucosa remains below the incision for a secure closure. The incision is made directly down onto the underlying bone; hemostasis is obtained with electrocoagulation. The periosteum is elevated off the face of the maxilla with a soft tissue elevator or sponge (Fig. 1B), and the tissues are retracted with an Army-Navy or similar retractor. The elevation is continued until the infraorbital nerve is identified.

Plate 89

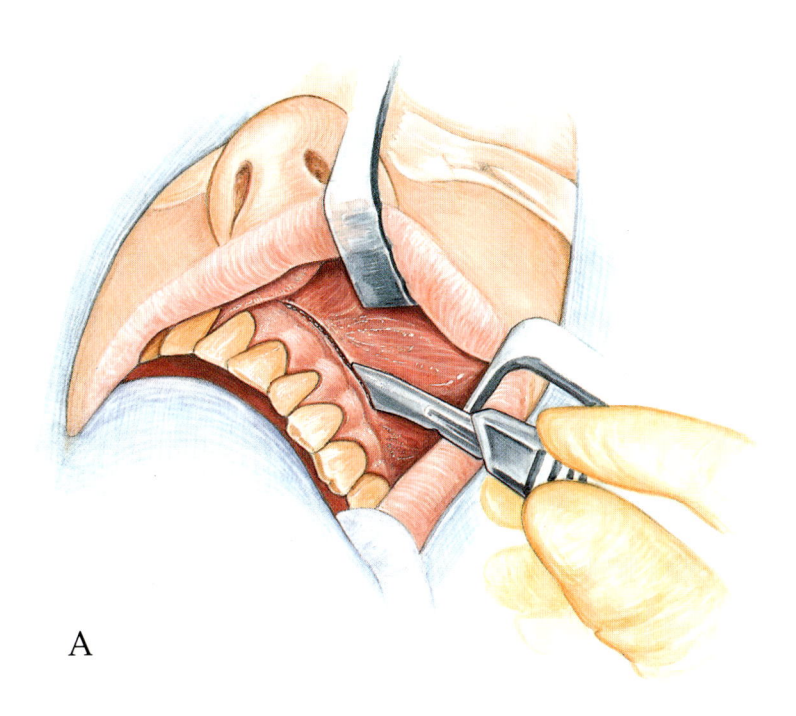

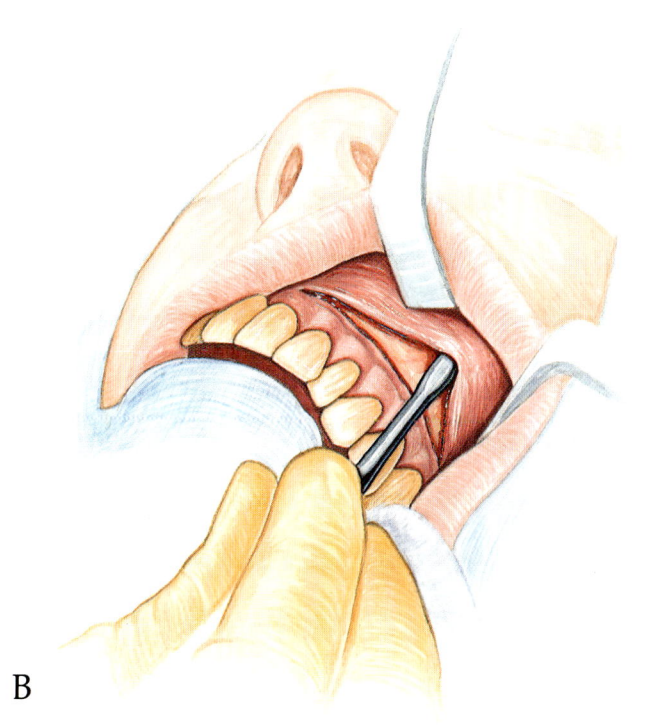

A

B

Figure 1
Caldwell-Luc; Incision

The antrotomy is performed in the face of the maxilla above and lateral to the root of the canine tooth with a small osteotome (Fig. 1C), and the opening is enlarged with a Kerrison punch or a high-speed drill (Fig. 1D). The size of the opening should match the task at hand. No cosmetic deficit or loss of structural strength will result from removing the anterior wall as long as the medial buttress (maxillary process) and the lateral buttress are preserved.

Once the antrotomy is completed, the operation is continued according to the pathology found. Inflammatory disease of the maxillary sinus is managed by removing the inspissated secretions and all the irreversibly hypertrophic mucosa (Fig. 1E). Mucosa that is normal or min-

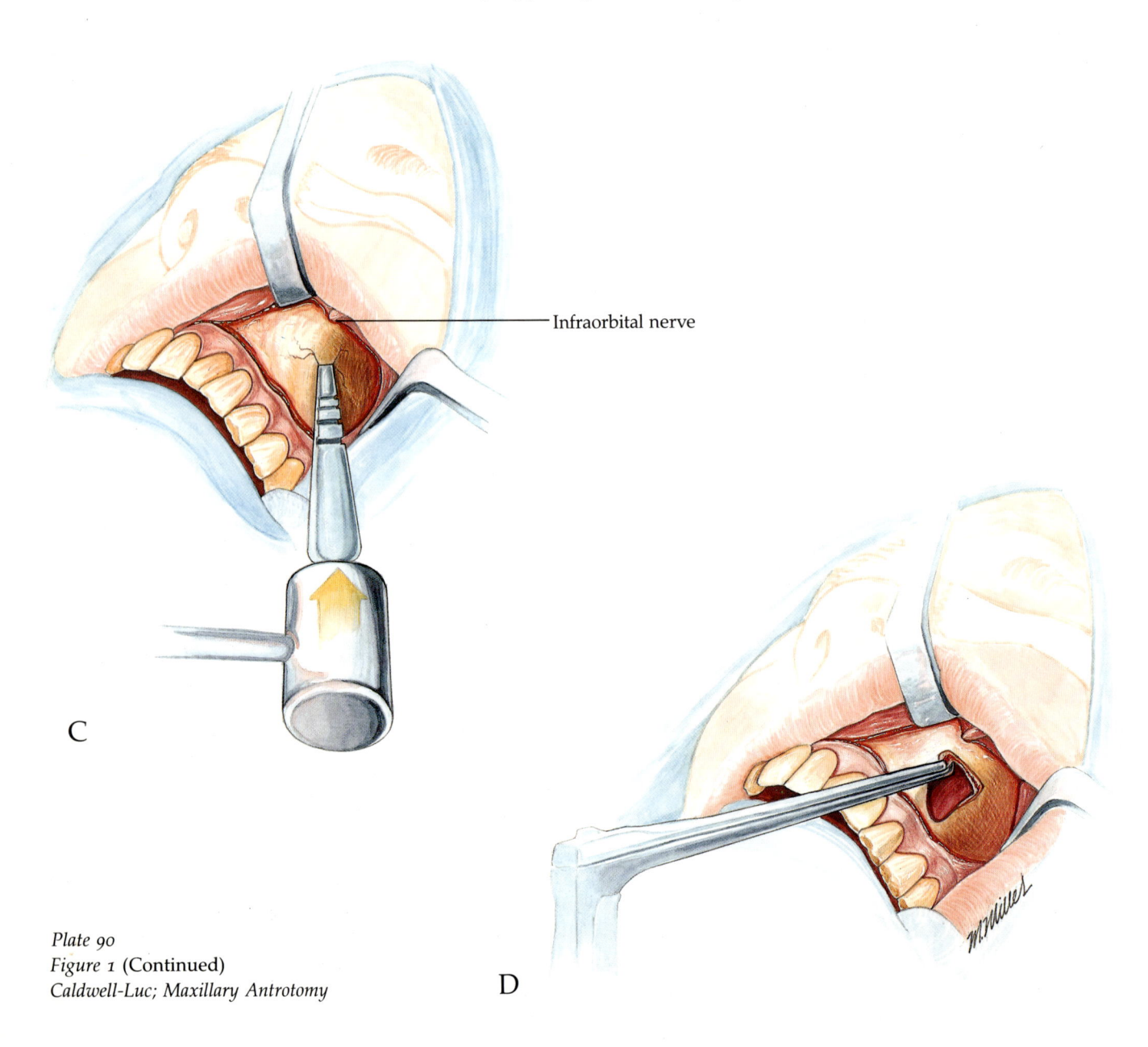

Plate 90
Figure 1 (Continued)
Caldwell-Luc; Maxillary Antrotomy

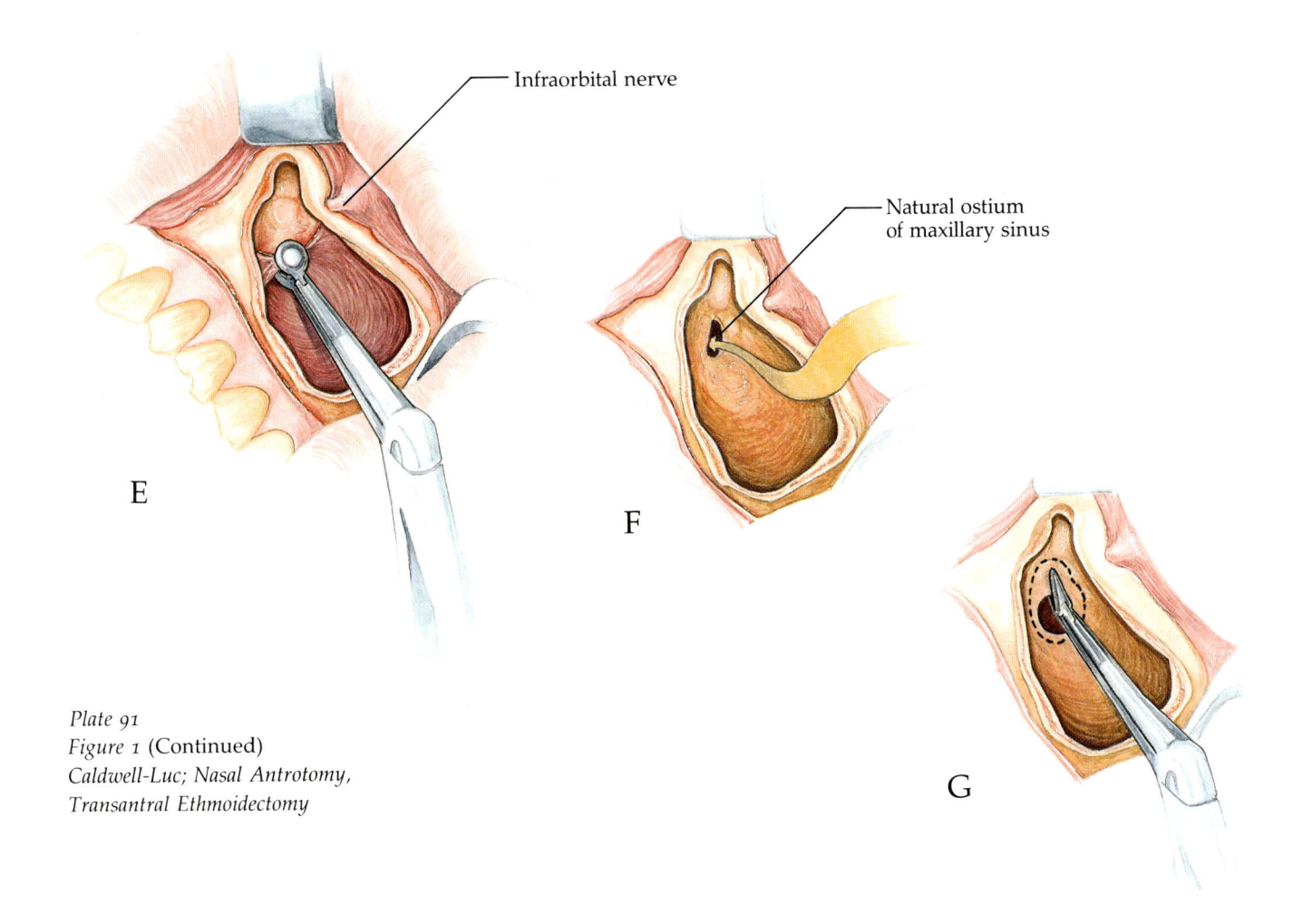

Plate 91
Figure 1 (Continued)
*Caldwell-Luc; Nasal Antrotomy,
Transantral Ethmoidectomy*

imally thickened should be preserved to allow a source for remucosalization of the sinus. If the procedure is performed for access to deeper structures (e.g., the pterygomaxillary fossa), the mucosa of the sinus should be preserved.

Adequate drainage of the sinus should also be ensured regardless of its preoperative condition. Although traditionally this has been done through an inferior meatal nasal-antral window, a middle meatal nasal antrostomy is probably physiologically more natural. The natural ostium can be identified in the medial wall of the sinus (Fig. 1F) and is easily enlarged with Kerrison's punches or upbiting forceps (Fig. 1G). If an inferior meatal antrotomy is made, care should be taken to avoid trauma to the adjacent inferior turbinate because adhesions from the turbinate to the lateral wall of the nose can obstruct the antrostomy. It should be remembered that inflammatory disease of the maxillary sinus rarely occurs in isolation, and careful evaluation and management of the adjacent ethmoid sinus should be performed before contemplating maxillary sinus surgery.

The sinus is packed with gauze soaked in antibiotic ointment or a long (3-foot) Penrose drain. The packing is brought through the maxillary antrotomy into the nose and out the nostril.

TRANSANTRAL ETHMOIDECTOMY

The inferior portion of the ethmoid sinus abuts against the superior medial border of the maxillary sinus, allowing easy access to the middle and posterior ethmoid cells and sphenoid sinus through the maxillary sinus. The most anterior cells cannot be reached through the maxillary sinus. Therefore for complete exenteration, the transantral approach must be combined with an external or intranasal ethmoidectomy. The party wall between the maxillary and the ethmoid sinus is removed with Takahashi forceps and the ethmoid sinus entered under direct vision (Fig. 1H). An advantage of this technique is that the position of the medial wall of the orbit is known from the outset, reducing the risk of damaging the intraorbital contents. The dissection can easily be extended through the posterior ethmoid cells into the sphenoid sinus.

Postoperative Care

The packing is removed 24 to 48 hours after surgery. The nose should be regularly inspected during the postoperative healing period to ensure that the antral window does not close and that adhesions from the middle or inferior turbinate do not obstruct drainage from the maxillary sinus.

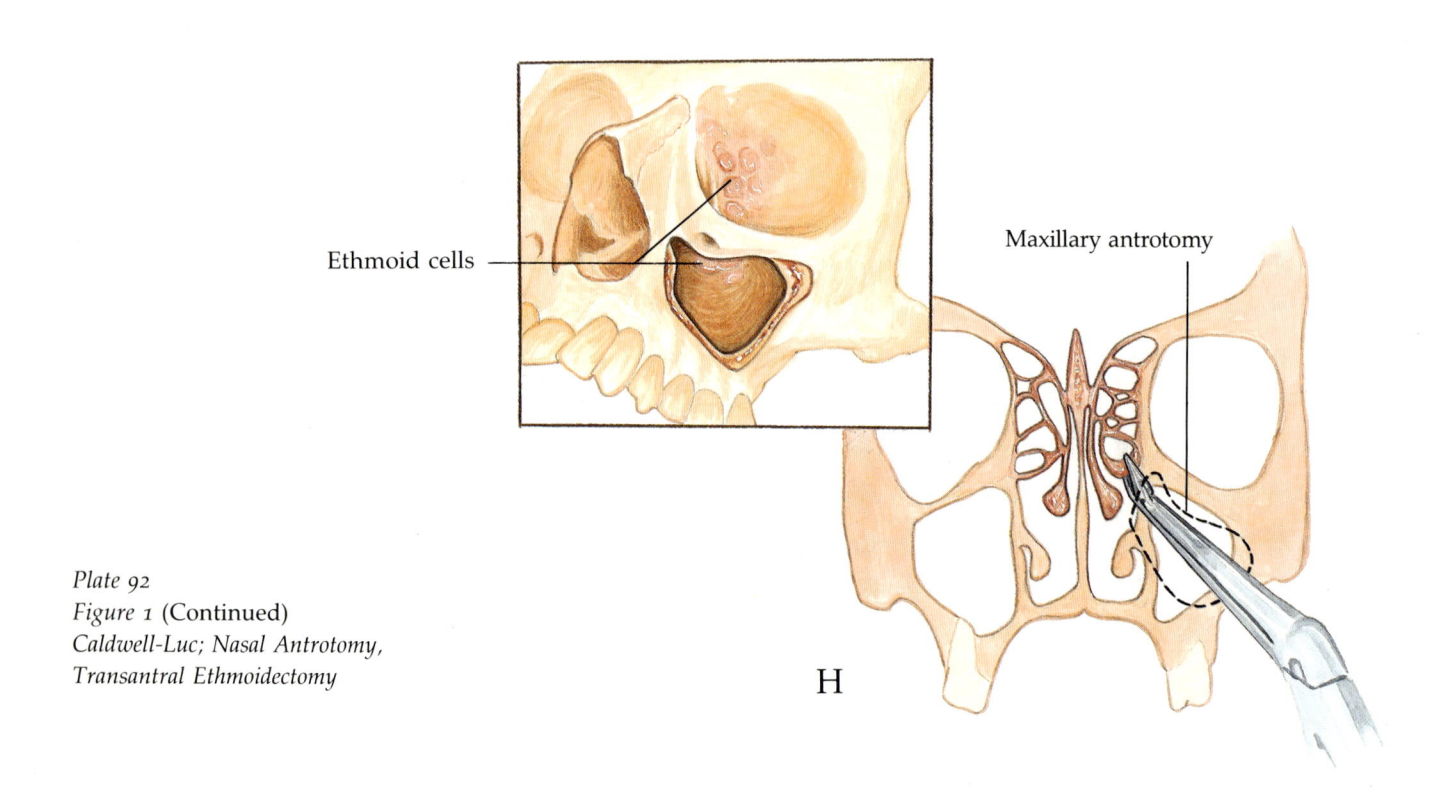

Plate 92
Figure 1 (Continued)
Caldwell-Luc; Nasal Antrotomy, Transantral Ethmoidectomy

Risks, Complications, and Sequelae

Postoperative antral infection is preventable by providing adequate drainage of the sinus into the nose through the inferior meatus or preferably through the middle meatus. The antrostomy can also close or stenose. This can be prevented by creating an adequately large antrostomy in the first place and by following the patient carefully and lysing any adhesions forming around the antrostomy. Particular care must be taken with inferior meatal antrostomies because if the inferior turbinate is abraded, it can scar to the lateral wall of the nose, occluding the opening.

Oral antral fistulas are exceedingly rare. This complication should not occur if the mucosal edges are properly everted and the sinus is adequately drained into the nose to prevent postoperative antritis.

Hypoesthesia or anesthesia of the cheek and lip is caused by damage or stretching of the infraorbital nerve. The patient should always be warned of this possibility because the amount of hypoesthesia does not always correlate with the surgeon's perception of the amount of traction put on the nerve. This hypoesthesia should disappear over a few months if the infraorbital nerve is not transected. Hypoesthesia of the teeth and gingiva frequently occurs because small branches of the superior alveolar nerve pass through the face of the maxilla above the teeth.

Pearls and Pitfalls

Appropriate placement of the sublabial incision is important. If it is made too low, there will not be a sufficient cuff for resuturing of the incision. Conversely, if it is too high, it may lead to unnecessary scarring and stiffness of the upper lip. An incision that is carried too far superiorly and laterally may enter the buccal fat pad. If this occurs, the tissue should be resutured because the fat will continue to ooze into the wound and constantly become trapped in the suction.

Anesthesia of the infraorbital nerve is the most common complication of Caldwell-Luc surgery. The nerve should be positively identified to protect it, and no instrument should be allowed to slip into the foramen, which would severely damage the nerve. Some anesthesia of the gums and teeth may be unavoidable. Although the superior alveolar nerve is supposed to travel just above the tips of the maxillary teeth, some branches appear to travel higher and can be damaged when the maxillary osteotomy is performed.

Severely infected and hypertrophic mucosa should be removed from the antrum, but normal-appearing mucosa should be retained. Routine stripping out of all the mucosa from the sinus only leads to problems with delayed healing, inspissation of secretions within the sinus, and postoperative discomfort.

The Caldwell-Luc procedure is contraindicated in children with primary dentition because of the high probability of damaging the roots of the unerupted permanent teeth.

As in any ethmoidectomy procedure, the most important landmark is the middle turbinate. The root of the middle turbinate should always be preserved in order to avoid damage to the cribriform plate. If the entire turbinate is preserved, its lateral surface should not be scraped or abraded in order to prevent adhesions between the turbinate and the lateral wall of the nose, which, in turn, would lead to recurrent sinusitis.

Extensive removal of both the medial orbital wall and the roof of the maxillary sinus can lead to enophthalmos because of herniation of the orbital fat into the ethmoid and maxillary sinuses. This, of course, is the procedure of choice for decompression in Graves' disease.

As in any ethmoid procedure, one should proceed carefully and remove bony septa slowly with small biting forceps, checking landmarks at each stage.

Douglas E. Mattox, M.D.

TRANSANTRAL MAXILLARY ARTERY LIGATION

The majority of uncontrollable posterior nose bleeds arise from the sphenopalatine branch of the internal maxillary artery. Usually the bleeding arises from the posterior lateral nasal wall in the vicinity of the posterior end of the middle turbinate, but it may come from the rostrum of the sphenoid or the posterior nasal septum. The bleeding in this area can be brisk, and the patient is at risk not only for hypovolemia from blood loss but also for pulmonary complications secondary to aspiration of blood. Most posterior nose bleeds can be managed with posterior nasal packing or tamponaded with an inflatable nasal balloon or Foley catheter. Patients with persistent bleeding despite adequate packing are candidates for arterial ligation. Before surgical intervention is seriously considered, the site of the bleeding must be determined, particularly whether it is low and posterior from the internal maxillary artery or high and anterior from the anterior or posterior ethmoidal arteries.

Surgical Anatomy

The pterygomaxillary space is a shallow cleft between the back wall of the maxillary antrum and the pterygoid plates. It contains the terminal branches of the internal maxillary artery, the infraorbital nerve, and the pterygopalatine ganglion (Figs. 2A and 2B). The important branches of the internal maxillary artery are the infraorbital, vidian, sphenopalatine, descending palatine, and superior alveolar. The infraorbital nerve exits from the foramen rotundum; the vidian canal and nerve are slightly medial and inferior to the infraorbital nerve. Fortunately, the arteries are superficial to the nerves as the fossa is approached from anteriorly.

Indications

Arterial ligation (internal maxillary artery and/or ethmoidal arteries) is indicated by epistaxis that continues despite adequate attempts at local control with anterior and posterior nasal packing and use of a cautery locally.

Evidence of acute or chronic infection of the maxillary antrum contraindicates this approach. After an acute episode of epistaxis, particularly if the patient has had his or her nose packed, opacification or an air-fluid level within the maxillary sinus is a common radiographic finding. This should not be overinterpreted as indicative of acute infection.

Preoperative Considerations

The patient should be intubated with a right-angled endotracheal (RAE) tube so that the endotracheal tube is not in the surgeon's way. The patient is placed on the table in a semisitting position such that the operating microscope can easily be directed into the sinus. A 300-mm lens should be used on the microscope because of the depth of the operative cavity.

Operative Steps

The maxillary antrum is approached as for a Caldwell-Luc procedure. Local anesthetic with epinephrine is infiltrated in the soft tissues over the canine fossa. The sublabial incision is made, leaving sufficient gingival tissue for easy closure. The maxillary antrum is entered, and bone is widely removed from the entire face of the antrum. A small rim of bone is left around the infraorbital nerve, but the bone removal should extend up to the thick bone of the infraorbital rim on each side of the nerve. The mucosa on the back side of the sinus is incised to develop an inferiorly based flap.

The bone of the back wall of the sinus is cracked with a chisel and removed with Kerrison punches (Fig. 2C). Medially, the dissection is limited by the thick orbital process of the palatine bone. Care must be taken in removing the posterior wall of the antrum not to penetrate the periosteum of the pterygopalatine fossa and lacerate the artery.

Plate 93

- Pterygomaxillary fossa
- Internal maxillary artery

A

- Sphenopalatine ganglion
- V$_2$
- Vidian artery and nerve
- Sphenopalatine artery
- Descending palatine artery and nerve
- Infraorbital artery and nerve
- Internal maxillary artery
- Superior alveolar artery

B

- Orbital process of palatine bone
- Infraorbital nerve
- Posterior ostectomy
- Maxillary mucosal flap

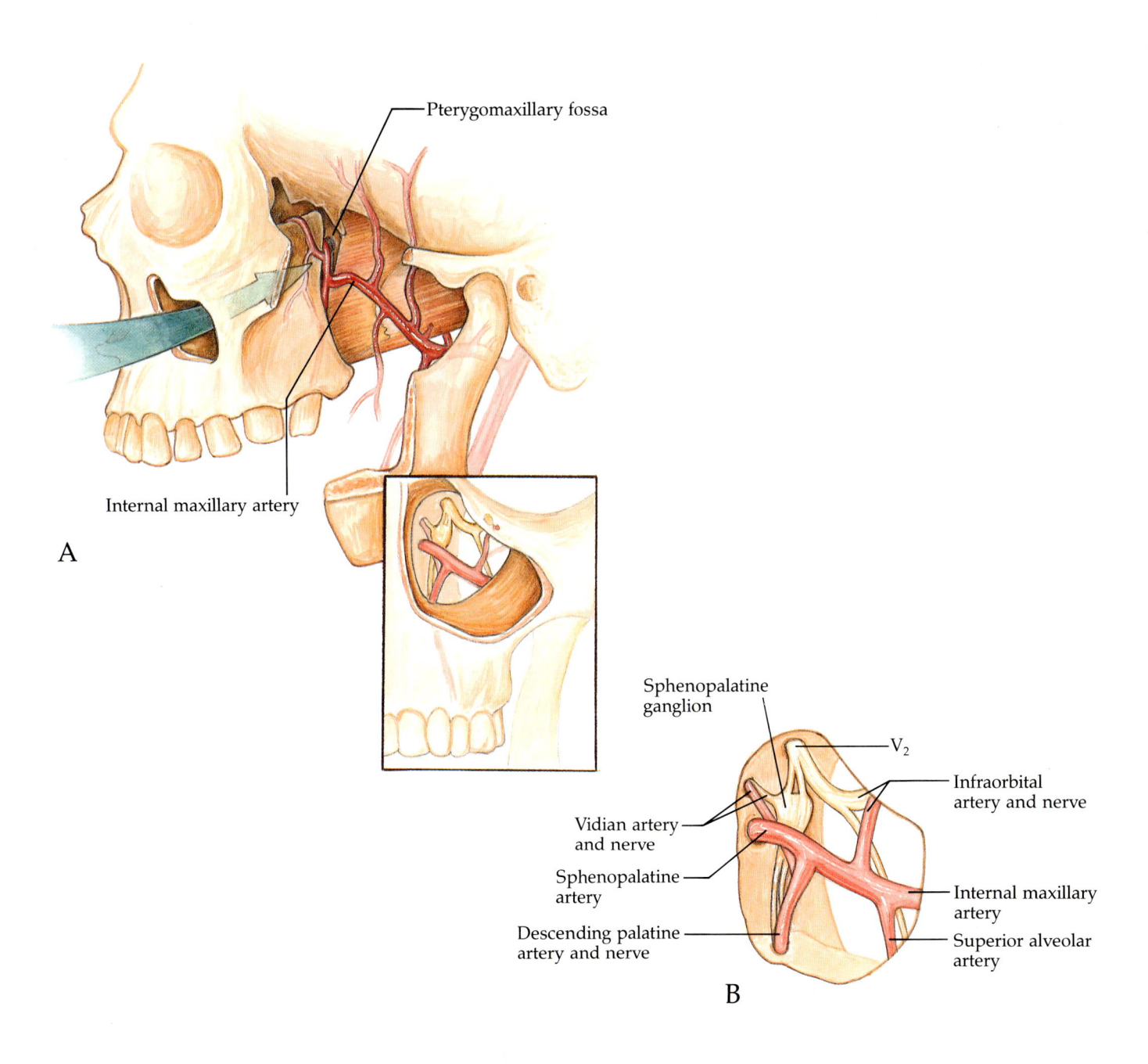

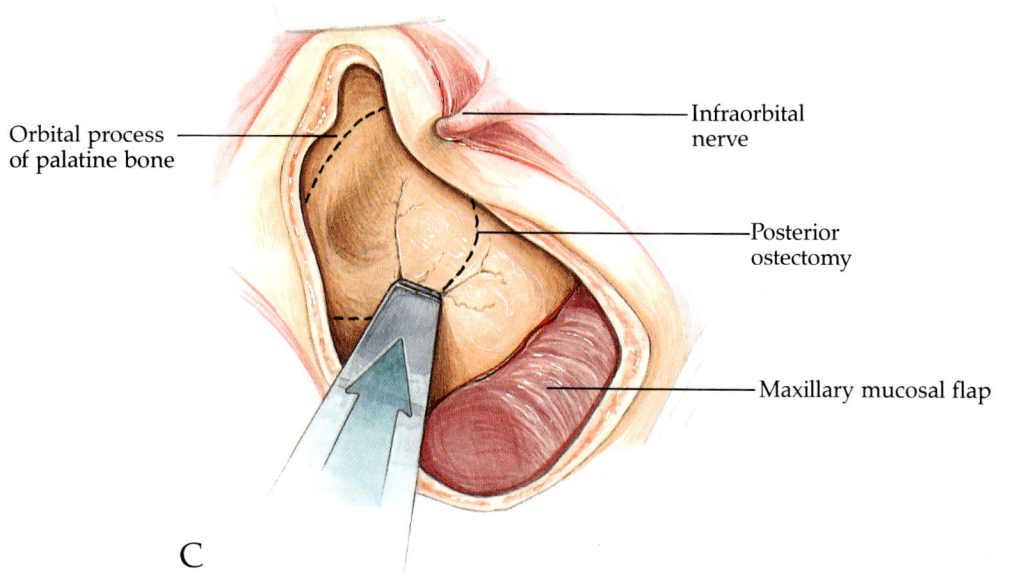

C

Figure 2
Transmaxillary Ligation;
Anatomy and Approach to
Pterygomaxillary Fossa

After the posterior bone is fully removed, a cruciate incision is made in the periosteum (Fig. 2D). Frequently there are small venous branches in the periosteum that should be cauterized with bipolar forceps before it is incised. After the periosteum is open, a nerve hook is used to dissect through the fibrous and fatty tissue and to identify the internal maxillary artery and its branches (Fig. 2E). The internal maxillary artery enters the lateral portion of the fossa, and as many branches as possible should be identified, including the infraorbital, descending palatine, and sphenopalatine. In addition to these branches, the internal maxillary artery may have a tortuous and folded path within the fossa. The artery is always found superficial to branches on the infraorbital nerve. It is generally found that dissecting the fibrofatty tissue of the fossa is easier in females than in males. Standard ear instruments are particularly useful for the dissection, including a slightly blunt round knife and a ball-tip mastoid seeker.

After the artery is skeletonized (Fig. 2F), the main trunk of the artery and the sphenopalatine branch are clipped with hemoclips (Fig. 2G). There can be nasal branches from the descending palatine artery; therefore, it should also be clipped. Two clips are placed on each artery; the artery is *not* divided. Care should always be taken not to lacerate the artery because it would be extremely difficult to obtain control of a hemorrhaging artery.

The sinus mucosal flap is reflected back over the pterygomaxillary fossa. Secondary drainage of the maxillary antrum should always be provided through a middle or inferior meatal window. The antrum can be lightly packed with gauze, or a Penrose drain can be brought out through the nose. The sublabial incision is closed with a running chromic suture.

Postoperative Care

The nasal packing should be removed in the operating room and the nose carefully examined for bleeding. The patient can usually be discharged in 24 to 48 hours postoperatively.

Risks, Complications, and Sequelae

Bleeding can occur if the site of bleeding has not been accurately identified and the incorrect artery has been ligated. Since on occasion arterial pressure can open hemoclips, it is important to inspect the hemoclips carefully for complete closure before the wound is closed. The artery is never cut between the clips.

Hypoesthesia of the infraorbital nerve can occur from retraction or direct damage during the antrotomy or damage of the nerve within the pterygomaxillary space.

Acute infection of the maxillary antrum risks spread of infection to the pterygoid palatine space.

Pearls and Pitfalls

There is no question that transantral maxillary ligation, combined with ethmoidal artery ligation, is an effective method of managing nasal epistaxis. However, the proper timing of the procedure is widely debated. Advocates of arterial ligation point out that hospitalization and total pa-

Plate 94

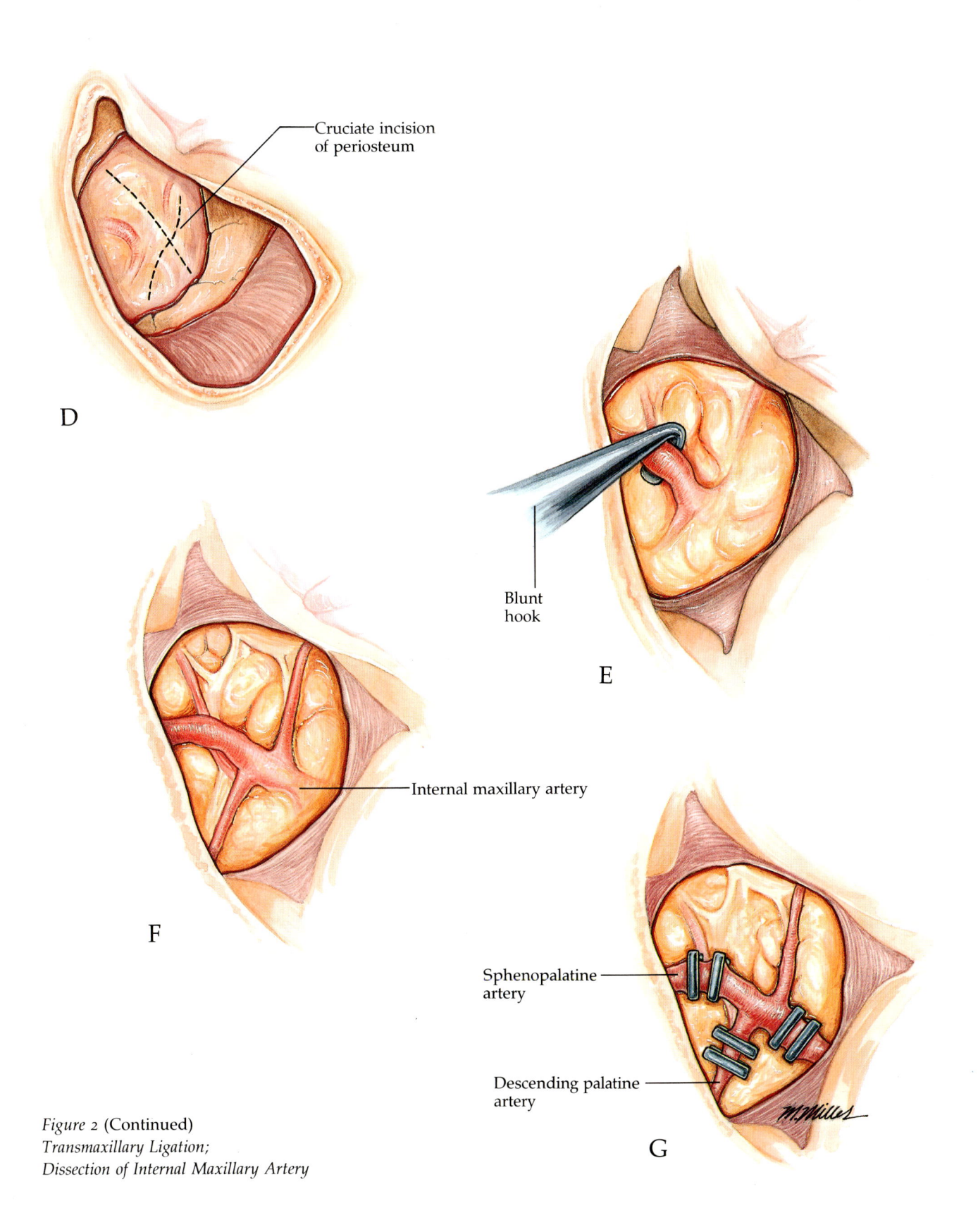

D — Cruciate incision of periosteum

E — Blunt hook

F — Internal maxillary artery

G — Sphenopalatine artery; Descending palatine artery

Figure 2 (Continued)
*Transmaxillary Ligation;
Dissection of Internal Maxillary Artery*

213

tient cost can be reduced by early surgical intervention, whereas the procedure's detractors point out the potential risks and morbidity resulting from the surgery.

My own algorithm is to administer anterior and posterior nasal packing to every patient with posterior epistaxis. If the patient continues to bleed despite the packing or rebleeds promptly after its removal, surgical ligation is employed. I have discussed surgery versus packing with many patients postoperatively. They relate that packing the nose is uncomfortable, and that a repeat packing after the nasal mucous membranes have been traumatized is very painful. Topical anesthetics and vasoconstrictors are of little value in the face of active bleeding that washes them away before they have an effect. Among the patients to whom I have spoken, all would have chosen immediate surgery over nasal packing.

The operation is much easier to perform in women than in men. The pterygopalatine space is filled with a soft fatty tissue in women, whereas in men the surrounding tissue is much more fibrous and adherent to the artery, making the dissection more difficult.

Never transect the artery. The clips can be loosened by the pulsatile action of the artery, and if they should slip off a transected artery, it would be very difficult to recontrol the bleeding within the pterygomaxillary space.

It is important to clip all arterial branches to the nose. Although the sphenopalatine is the main arterial branch to the nose, branches from the descending palatine artery can cause persistent bleeding despite successful ligation of the sphenopalatine branch.

The most difficult question is the management of the patient with persistent bleeding despite adequate ligation of the internal maxillary and ethmoidal arteries. The nose should be re-examined to ensure that the proper site of the bleeding has been identified. Arteriography may be of value to determine if a branch of the internal maxillary artery has been missed. If the site of bleeding can be identified with arteriography, embolization is an alternative if the arteriographer is experienced in selective embolization in the head and neck. Patients with persistent bleeding should also be re-examined for occult bleeding diatheses such as von Willebrand's disease or Osler-Weber-Rendu syndrome. External carotid ligation can also be considered if the distal point of hemorrhage cannot be otherwise identified.

Suggested Reading

Chandler JR, Serrins AJ. Transantral ligation of the internal maxillary artery for epistaxis. Laryngoscope 1965; 75:1151–1159.

Montgomery WW, Reardon EJ. Early vessel ligation for control of severe epistaxis. In: Snow JB, ed. Controversy in otolaryngology. Philadelphia: WB Saunders, 1980:315–319.

Ward PH. Routine ligation of the maxillary artery is unwarranted. In: Snow JB, ed. Controversy in otolaryngology. Philadelphia: WB Saunders, 1980:320–326.

Douglas E. Mattox, M.D.

LIGATION OF ETHMOIDAL ARTERIES

Indications

The ethmoidal arteries are a less common source of severe nasal epistaxis than the sphenopalatine artery. However, if preoperative evaluation indicates the bleeding is coming from high within the nose, ethmoidal artery ligation should be included with sphenopalatine artery ligation. Ethmoidal artery hemorrhage can also occur after acute injuries of the frontal ethmoid area from blunt instruments or moving vehicle accidents.

Preoperative Considerations

The nose should be carefully examined with a headlamp to identify the exact source or at least the region where the hemorrhage is coming from. A tarsorrhaphy will protect the cornea during the procedure. The preoperative note should include an evaluation of visual acuity.

Operative Steps

A medial canthal incision, elevation of the lacrimal sac, and elevation of the orbital periosteum are carried out as for external ethmoidectomy (see Chapter 5). The periorbita is gently elevated taking care not to interrupt its surface. The frontoethmoidal suture line is identified starting with the upper portion of the lacrimal fossa and traced posteriorly. The anterior ethmoidal artery is found approximately 24 mm posterior to the anterior crest of the lacrimal fossa.

Once the artery is identified, it is gently exposed by dissection above and below with a Freer or Cottle elevator. Small arteries can easily be coagulated with a bipolar cautery (Fig. 3). A large artery can be tied with a 4–0 silk suture. The sutures are passed behind the artery with a small curved clamp. The ties should be placed against the periorbita and the artery divided close to the bone. Additional dissection for approximately another 12 mm will reveal the posterior artery, which can also be coagulated. Unipolar coagulation should not be used for the posterior artery because of its close proximity to the optic nerve.

The wound is closed in layers with a cosmetic skin closure. No special wiring or suturing of the medial canthal tendon is needed as long as it has been elevated subperiosteally and the ligament itself has not been disrupted.

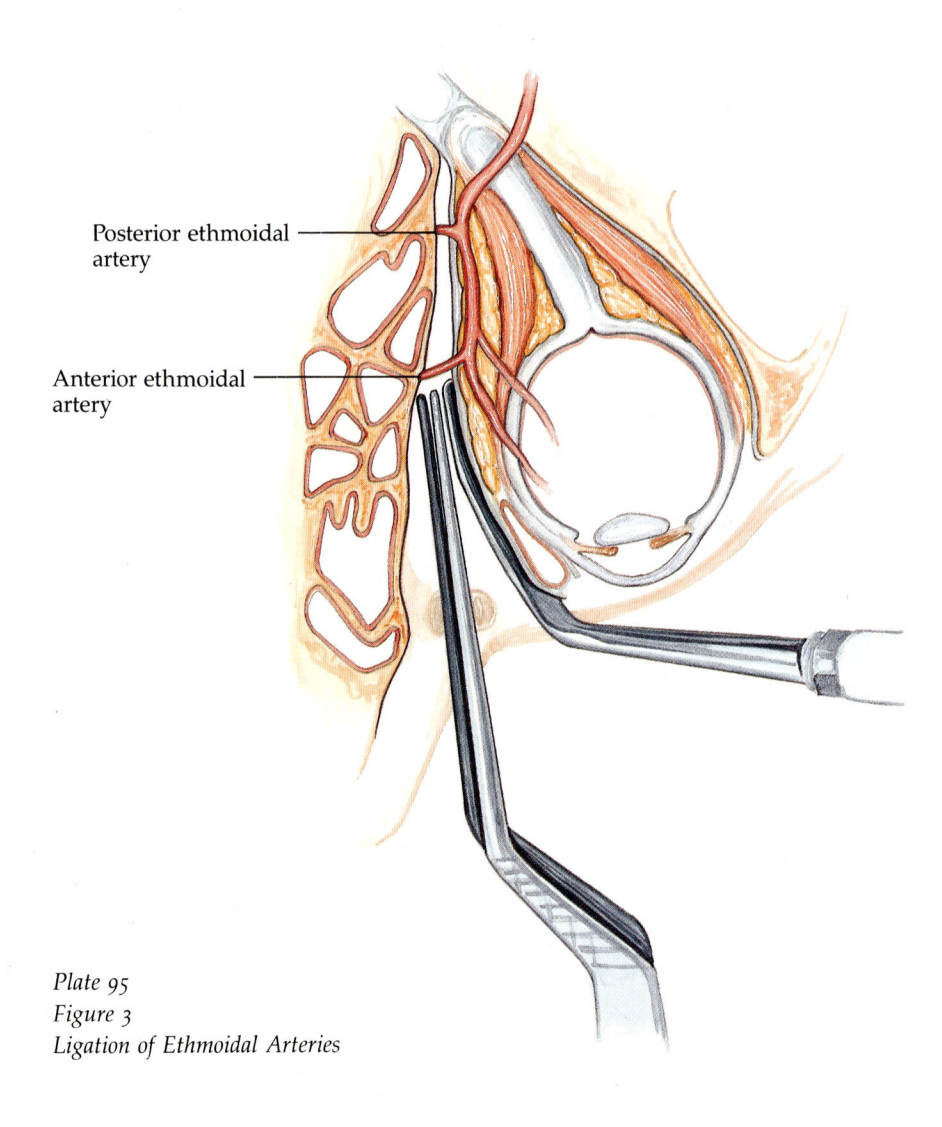

Plate 95
Figure 3
Ligation of Ethmoidal Arteries

Postoperative Care

The nasal packing should be removed in the operating room and the nose carefully examined for bleeding. The patient can usually be discharged in 24 to 48 hours postoperatively.

Risks, Complications, and Sequelae

Recurrent bleeding can occur if the artery is avulsed without control. Recurrent epistaxis is indicative of a misdiagnosis of the origin of hemorrhage.

The medial canthus can be blunted and the telecanthus developed if the medial tendon is damaged during the elevation. Blindness can occur with any ethmoidal procedure if the optic nerve is damaged.

Pearls and Pitfalls

General guidelines for the location of the interior and posterior ethmoidal arteries relative to the lacrimal crest and optic nerve have been given, but it should be remembered that this anatomy is extremely variable and one or another of the arteries may be absent.

Ethmoidal artery hemorrhage severe enough to require surgery is unusual, and ethmoidal ligation is rarely indicated alone. The procedure should usually be combined with transantral ligation of the internal maxillary artery. An exception to this rule is in patients with acute nasofrontal trauma who may have severe bleeding from the ethmoidal arteries.

As in any ethmoidal surgery, the patient's visual acuity and extraocular mobility should always be checked in the immediate postoperative period. An intraorbital hematoma will manifest as unilateral proptosis. This complication should be treated immediately with a lateral canthotomy for decompression of the orbit, and an ophthalmologic consultation should be obtained.

Suggested Reading

Kirchner JA, Yanagisawa E, Crelin FS Jr. Surgical anatomy of the ethmoidal arteries: A laboratory study of 150 orbits. Arch Otolaryngol 1961; 74:382–386.

Montgomery WW, Reardon EJ. Early vessel ligation for control of severe epistaxis. In: Snow JB, ed. Controversy in otolaryngology. Philadelphia: WB Saunders, 1980:315–319.

Douglas E. Mattox, M.D.

EXTERNAL ETHMOIDECTOMY

Indications

External ethmoidectomy, despite its mild cosmetic disadvantages, is the safest and most complete access to the ethmoid sinus. It is the technique that every resident should learn first because of its safety and clearly identifiable landmarks. If the surgeon should become disoriented during an intranasal procedure, or fear operative complications because of abnormal patient anatomy, or need to manage a complication, the external approach is the procedure of choice. A paranasal skin incision is a small price to pay for the additional exposure and preservation of the dura mater or optic nerve.

Anatomic Relationships

Anatomic relationships of the ethmoid sinus to the medial orbital wall and anterior cranial fossa are shown in Figure 4A. The level of the cribriform plate is marked by the foramina of the anterior and posterior ethmoidal arteries. The cribriform plate may be several millimeters lower than the level of the fovea ethmoidalis (roof of the ethmoid sinus); therefore dissecting directly medially at the level of the fovea almost assures penetration of the dura mater adjacent to the cribriform plate.

The anterior and posterior ethmoidal arteries are also roughly in line with the optic canal. A mnemonic for the locations of the foramina of the medial orbital wall is the number series 24-12-6, which are, respectively, the average distances in millimeters from the anterior lacrimal crest to the anterior ethmoid foramen, from the anterior to the posterior ethmoid foramina, and from the posterior foramen to the optic canal (see Fig. 4F farther on). The ranges in these measurements, however, are highly variable and there is no substitute for careful surgery. Harrison noted that the anterior ethmoid foramen was absent in 16 percent of orbits and that over 30 percent had multiple foramina for the posterior artery.

The area of bone removal is shown in Figure 4A and includes the anterior and posterior lacrimal crest and lamina papyracea far back on the anterior ethmoid foramen. Beyond this landmark, the dissection is continued on the medial side of the lamina papyracea within the sinus to reduce the herniation of the orbital fat into the sinus and prevent enophthalmos.

Operative Steps

Temporary tarsorrhaphy sutures protect the cornea during the procedures. The medial canthal area of the nose is infiltrated with 1 percent lidocaine with epinephrine 1:100,000. A curved incision is made from the medial end of the eyebrow to the level of the inferior portion of the lacrimal crest. A small M-plasty in the center of the wound will decrease postoperative bow stringing of the scar (Fig. 4B).

The incision is extended through the subcutaneous tissues directly to the lateral nasal bone (Fig. 4C). The angular vein and artery are encountered and ligated. The periosteum is elevated from the nasal bone toward the medial canthal tendon (Fig. 4D). The tendon should be carefully elevated in the subperiosteal plane. No telecanthus will occur if the tendon itself is not damaged. The elevation is continued posteriorly to identify the anterior and posterior ethmoid foramina. The anterior ethmoidal artery can be ligated, clipped, or coagulated with a bipolar cautery.

Plate 96

- Anterior ethmoid foramen
- Posterior ethmoid foramen
- Optic canal
- Superior orbital fissure
- Anterior lacrimal crest
- Posterior lacrimal crest
- Area of bone removal

A

- M-plasty incision
- Suture tarsorrhaphy

B

- Periosteum

C

- Medial canthal tendon

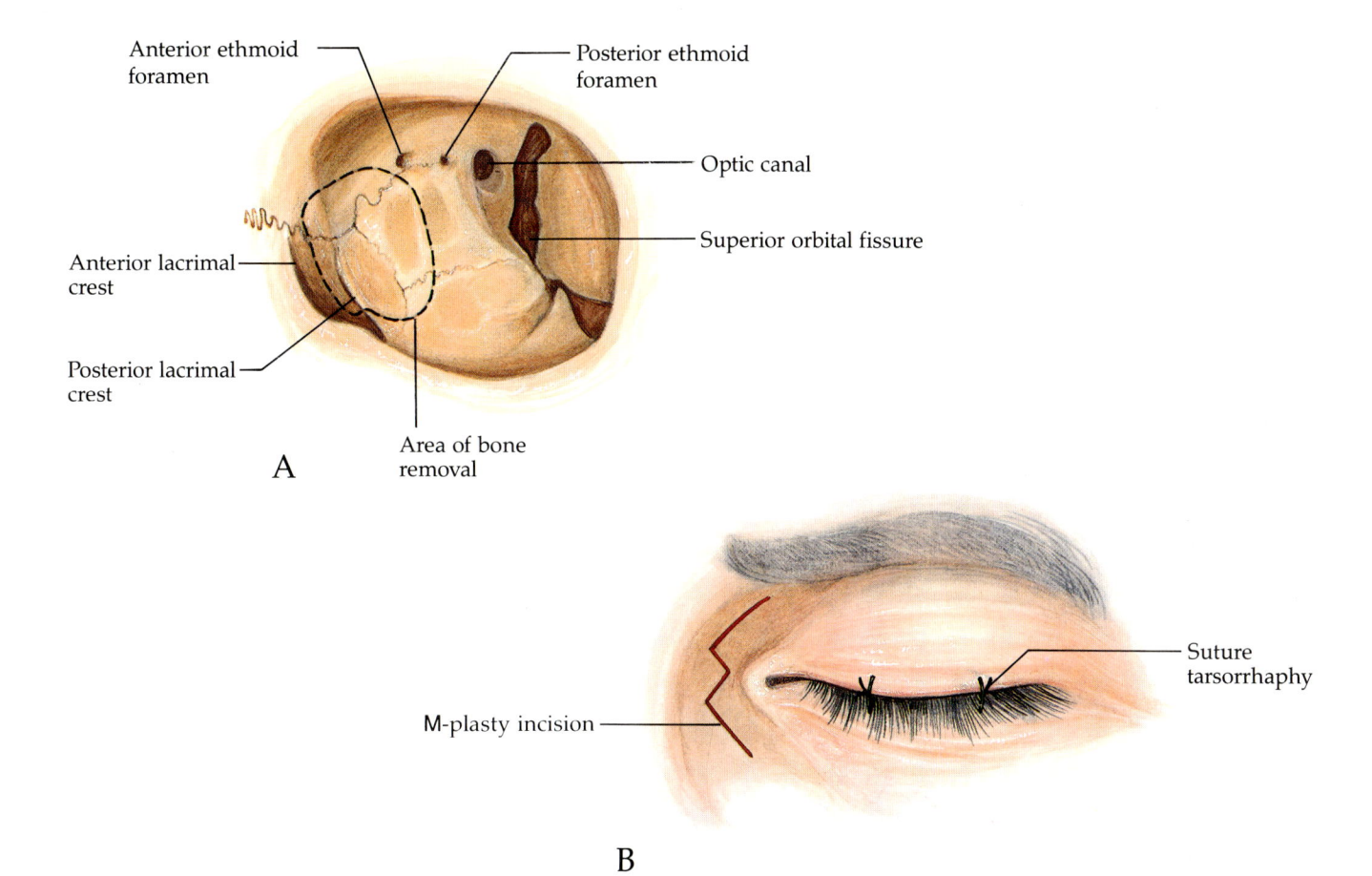

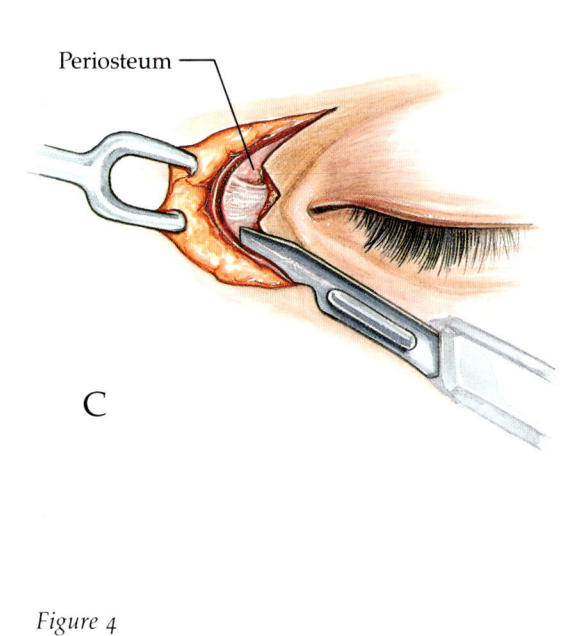

D

Figure 4
External Ethmoidectomy;
Anatomy and Incision

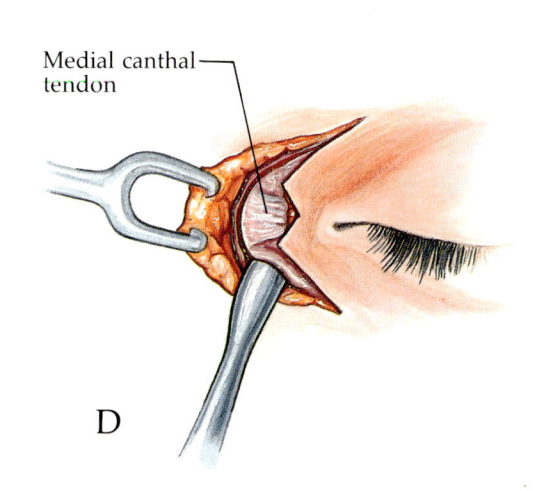

The lacrimal sac is gently elevated from the lacrimal fossa. The bone of the medial wall of the orbit is removed, as indicated in Figure 4A. Initially a small osteotome is used to crack the bone of the posterior lacrimal crest. The more posterior bone of the lamina papyracea is easily removed with small biting forceps (Fig. 4E). Posterior to the level of the anterior ethmoidal artery, the dissection is continued within the sinus and further elevation of the periorbita is not necessary. It is important to keep the periorbita intact in order to prevent the orbital fat and the medial rectus muscle from herniating into the sinus. Retraction of the globe and periorbita is best obtained with Sewall orbital retractors. The globe will tolerate reasonable retraction sufficient to give exposure into the ethmoid sinus; however, excessive retraction should be avoided.

Once the ethmoid sinus is entered, the mucosa of each ethmoid cell is removed, which will reveal the bony partitions for the next ethmoid cell (Fig. 4F). The dissection can easily be carried posteriorly into the sphenoid sinus. The middle turbinate is visualized and preserved in order to protect the cribriform plate lying medial to the superior attachment of the middle turbinate.

The most anterior ethmoid cells and agger nasi cells are not well visualized with the external approach. The external approach can be combined with an intranasal approach, as shown in Figure 4G, for the combined removal of the anterior and posterior cells.

Postoperative Care

The nose is packed with gauze soaked in antibiotic ointment or with gauze inside a finger cot. The packing may be removed the next day or left in for an additional 24 hours if the area is still oozing. Intermittent cleaning of the nose during the postoperative period promotes healing and prevention of adhesion formation. The nose should also be inspected for recurrent polyps, and these should be removed before they obstruct drainage of the ethmoidectomy cavity.

Risks, Complications, and Sequelae

External ethmoidectomy is generally reserved for cases of severe infection, fungal sinusitis, and nasal polyposis. During the procedure, blood loss is often substantial. Control of the bleeding can be obtained by temporary packing of the nose with gauze packing soaked in local anesthetic with epinephrine.

Blindness can also occur with any ethmoid surgery. The most common place for the optic nerve to be injured is within the sphenoid sinus, but occasionally the nerve is dehiscent within the posterior ethmoid sinus. There is some risk to the globe from overly vigorous retraction during the procedure. Telecanthus can occur if the medial canthal tendon is traumatized; this can be prevented by subperiosteal elevation of the tendon over the lacrimal bone.

Bleeding can also occur as a result of damage of the internal carotid artery within the sphenoid sinus. Management is by immediate packing of the sinus and arteriographic occlusion of the artery.

Cerebrospinal fluid leak can occur from penetration of the dura mater, either in the fovea ethmoidalis or the cribriform plate. The danger of such

Plate 97

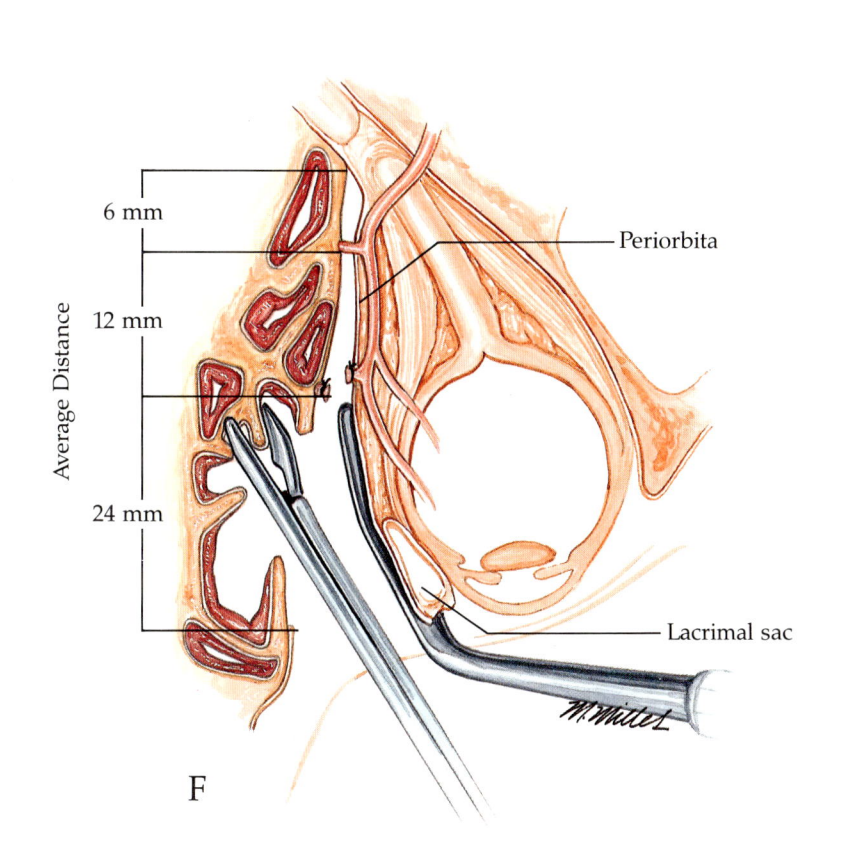

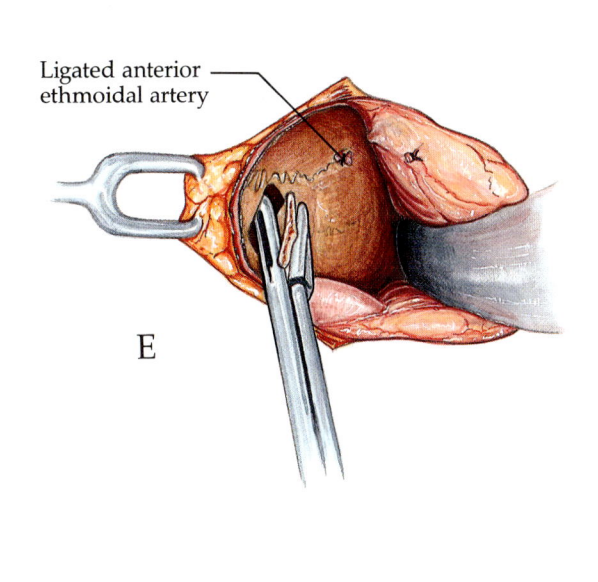

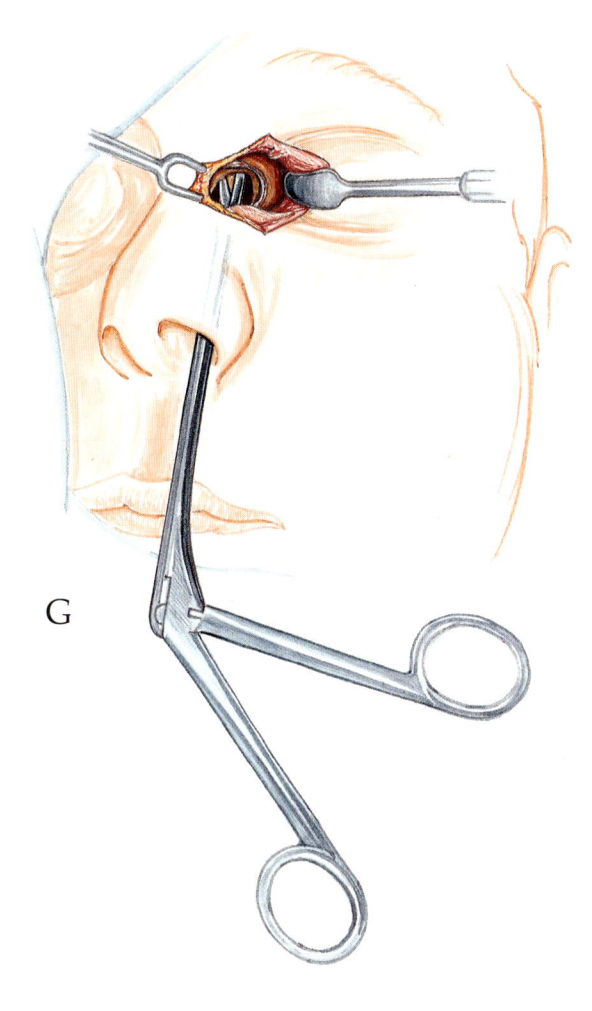

Figure 4 (Continued)
External Ethmoidectomy; Ethmoidectomy

221

leaks is minimal during external ethmoidectomy because these structures are easily visualized and protected during the dissection. External ethmoidectomy is the approach of choice for repair of traumatic or iatrogenic cerebrospinal fluid leaks of the ethmoid.

Pearls and Pitfalls

As with any ethmoidectomy procedure, the most important landmark is the middle turbinate, and the root of the middle turbinate should always be preserved in order to avoid damage to the cribriform plate. If the turbinate is preserved, its lateral surface should not be scraped or abraded to prevent adhesions between the turbinate and the lateral wall of the nose, which, in turn, would lead to recurrent sinusitis.

Lessons learned from endoscopic surgery of the ethmoid sinus are applicable to standard surgical therapy. The patient should be checked carefully in the postoperative period for adhesions between the middle turbinate and the lateral wall. If these occur, they should be divided to promote drainage of the sinus. Areas of granulation tissue within the ethmoid cavity may indicate osteitic bone underlying this area. If this bone can be removed, healing will be promoted. Recurrent polyps, especially in the area of the frontal or the maxillary sinus ostia, should be removed as they appear in order to prevent obstruction of the sinus.

If cerebrospinal fluid leak is recognized intraoperatively, it should be repaired immediately. This is done by first carefully cleaning the mucosa from the bone and surrounding the area of dural injury and covering the area with a free or pedicled mucosal graft from the turbinate or nasal septum. If there is a gross defect in the dura mater and bony plate of the fovea ethmoidalis, a musculofacial graft from the temporalis muscle can be gently inserted through the defect and then covered with a mucosal graft. The graft should be covered with Gelfoam soaked in Terramycin ointment and the nose packed firmly with gauze. The Gelfoam will prevent the graft from being dislodged when the packing is removed. If the patient remains afebrile, the packing should be left in for 4 to 5 days until it has been thoroughly soaked with secretions and slips from the nose without sticking. Persistent cerebrospinal fluid drainage while the nose is packed can be treated with repeated lumbar punctures or subarachnoid lumbar drain to reduce the pressure on the repair.

Cerebrospinal fluid leaks with significant bleeding may indicate injury of an intracranial vessel and should be evaluated immediately with computed tomography, magnetic resonance imaging, and arteriography. Injuries of this magnitude are best repaired through a frontal craniotomy.

Suggested Reading

Harrison DFN. Surgical approach to the medial orbital wall. Ann Otol Rhinol Laryngol 1981; 90:415–419.

Neal GD. External ethmoidectomy. Otolaryngol Clin North Am 1985; 18:55–60.

Loring W. Pratt, M.D.

FRONTAL SINUS TREPHINATION

Indications

Historically, purulent frontal sinusitis has been one of the most serious and one of the most lethal forms of sinusitis. In the course of finding methods to manage this disease, which often developed into osteomyelitis, meningitis, and brain abscess, many surgical procedures have been utilized. In the past, before the use of antibiotics, surgical exploration and drainage of the infected region was the only possible salvation for the patient. Morbidity was extremely high, and both continuing morbidity and recurrence were common in those who survived the initial attack. Mortality from intracranial spread of infection was frequent.

With the advent of antibiotics, mortality figures were improved, but morbidity and recurrence rates were still unsatisfactory. The accepted procedure during those years was simple trephination of the frontal sinus for acute infections, and a variety of surgical approaches to the frontal sinus and the nasofrontal duct were devised to improve the drainage of the nasofrontal duct and better ventilate the frontal sinus. Some procedures were planned to eliminate or minimize the cosmetic defect that often accompanied radical frontal sinus collapse surgery. Attempts to reconstruct the nasofrontal duct and maintain its patency were made with gold foil tubes and included the Dench, Denker, and collapse procedures. It was necessary to cut away with a rongeur any necrotic or osteomyelitic bone located in sites distant to and/or discontinuous with the sinus.

Preoperative Considerations

Accuracy of diagnosis is the most important preoperative consideration. It is essential that patients undergo trephination of the frontal sinus only for acute purulent frontal sinusitis. The diagnosis is made from the patient's history and physical and laboratory findings.

The history reveals a recent and usually sudden onset of excruciating pain in the region of the frontal sinus. This is most commonly associated with a history of recent acute upper respiratory infection. Percussion over the frontal sinus reveals exquisite tenderness, and jarring or walking produces severe pain. If the patient is asked to jump and land flat-footed, the jarring produces excruciating pain. X-ray study of the sinus shows clouding and often a fluid level. It must be remembered that complete clouding of a frontal sinus may mean that the sinus is full of pus, absent, or very shallow and that clouding alone is not diagnostic of acute purulent sinusitis. A complete blood count shows elevation of the leukocyte count with a shift to the left.

Using the usual skin preparation, and without shaving the eyebrow, an incision is made transversely in the skin at the medial end of and just below the eyebrow, following the contour of the lower margin of the eyebrow, deep enough to pass through only the skin (Fig. 5A). Approximately 1.5 cm is sufficient length to allow trephination of the sinus. After hemostasis has been secured with a cautery or ties and the wound edges have been retracted, a vertical incision is made in the subcutaneous tissues down to the frontal bone (Fig. 5B). A vertical incision is chosen because it lessens the chance of injury to the trochlear and supraorbital nerves. The periosteum is elevated laterally and medially with a septal elevator, and small retractors are used to expose the bone (Fig. 5C). Care is taken to ensure that the elevation and retraction are done in the subperiosteal plane and that no dissection is carried out in more superficial layers, thus reducing the hazard of trauma to the nerves. When an adequate area of bone has been exposed, as large a dental bur as possible is used to open the frontal sinus (Fig. 5D). The diamond bur works especially well for this purpose. The large bur is used to reduce the possibility of inadvertent penetration of both anterior and posterior walls of the sinus. It is moved gently around the surface, thinning the bone and making an opening of

Plate 98

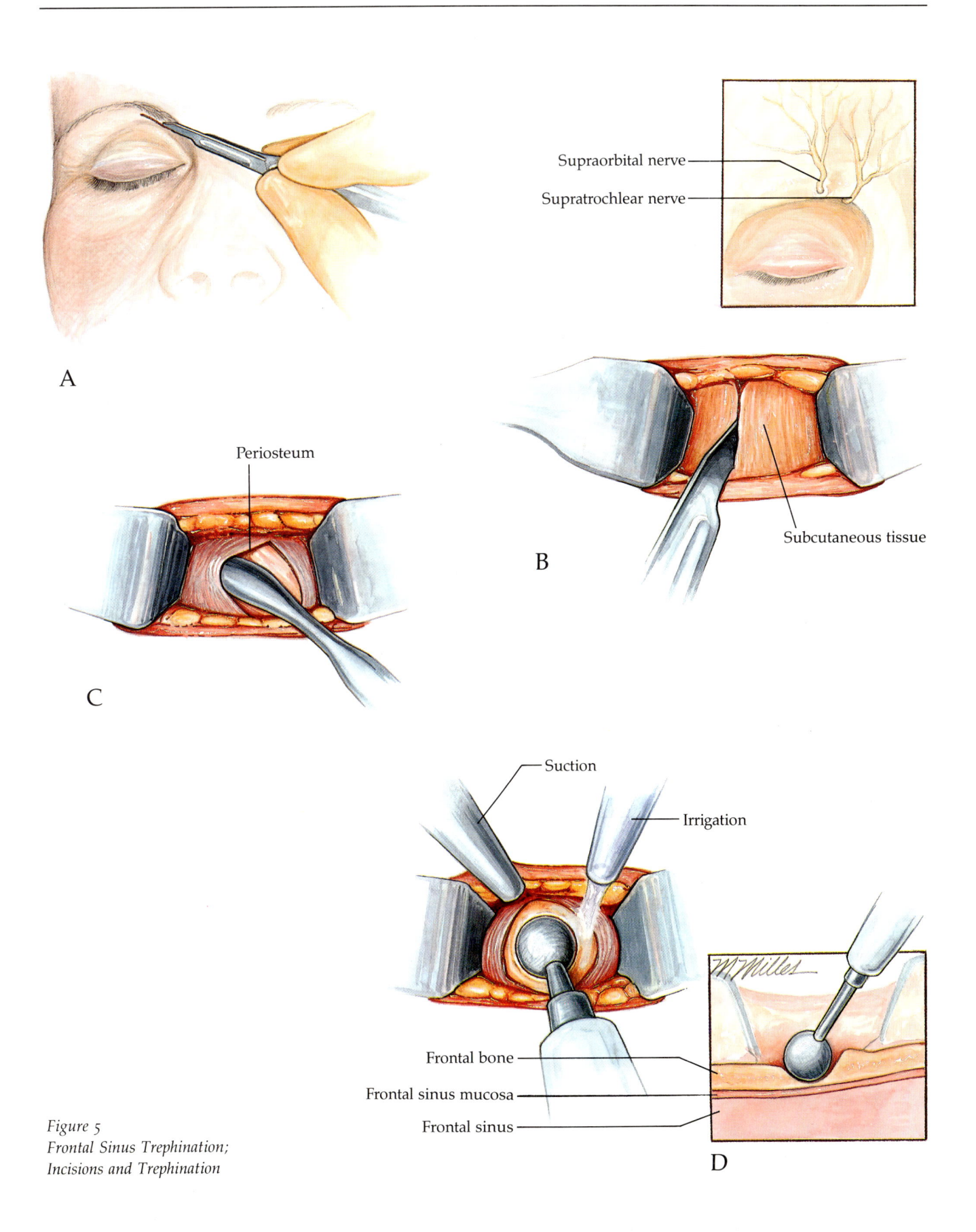

A

B
Supraorbital nerve
Supratrochlear nerve
Subcutaneous tissue

C
Periosteum

D
Suction
Irrigation
Frontal bone
Frontal sinus mucosa
Frontal sinus

Figure 5
Frontal Sinus Trephination;
Incisions and Trephination

5 to 6 mm without opening the mucosa of the sinus. A small curet, such as is used to remove the annulus of the tympanic bone in middle ear surgery, is used to remove the remaining eggshell-thin bone at the periphery of this dissection (Fig. 5E). Often as the bone is removed the mucosa bulges through the bony incision and may be incised to expose the lumen of the sinus. Sometimes pus runs from the sinus or gas escapes, but on occasion pus lies on the posterior wall of the sinus and must be removed by irrigation. A small piece of red rubber catheter, No. 8 French, attached to a syringe is used to direct a stream of saline into the sinus, washing the pus out of the sinus (Fig. 5F). Sometimes the tip of the catheter must be introduced into the sinus in order to accomplish this. Culture samples should be taken and studied for both aerobic and anaerobic organisms. The region of the nasofrontal duct must not be explored, dilated, or manipulated in any way. Mosher's dictum, "preserve the virginity of the nasofrontal duct," should be strictly followed. The tip of the catheter is left in the sinus, and the catheter is sutured to the skin with a 16-gauge catheter lying beside it; it is left protruding from the sinus as a drain. A dry dressing is applied both under and over the free end of the catheter to absorb any drainage (Fig. 5G). A turban type of bandage using elastic gauze (Kerlix) stays in place best.

Postoperative Care

The patient should be kept on high doses of the appropriate antibiotic postoperatively. As a rule, these infections are streptococcal, pneumococcal, or caused by *Haemophilus* organisms, and the antibiotic chosen should cover this group of pathogens until the results of the culture can be obtained.

Care of the wound is specific. The catheter drain should be removed in 24 hours and the sinus irrigated by way of the indwelling 16-gauge catheter. The wound edges should be separated with a mosquito clamp, so that there is free access to the sinus cavity. Irrigation with normal saline is accomplished *without using any pressure,* which might spread infection or irrigant into the intracranial space. The patient is asked to report if he or she tastes salt or feels water running down into the nose while the irrigation is in progress. Irrigations should be performed on a daily basis. If the 16-gauge catheter slips out another may be inserted, or a blunt needle may be used, but spreading the wound to allow for easy egress of the irrigating fluid is essential prior to the irrigation. Usually fluid runs through the nasofrontal duct after two or three irrigations, and after two consecutive irrigations that cause fluid to run into the back of the throat, they may be discontinued.

Risks, Complications, and Sequelae

Infections are often seen with this procedure. Most common are those in the region of the incision, involving the brow, which may vary from cellulitis and subperiosteal abscess to more serious problems involving the orbit, which also vary from cellulitis to abscess. Involvement of bone with infection may produce either local or distant osteomyelitis. Occasionally intracranial infections are seen, which involve direct spread from the original site, by direct extension, producing epidural abscess, meningitis, arachnoiditis, subdural abscess, and brain abscess.

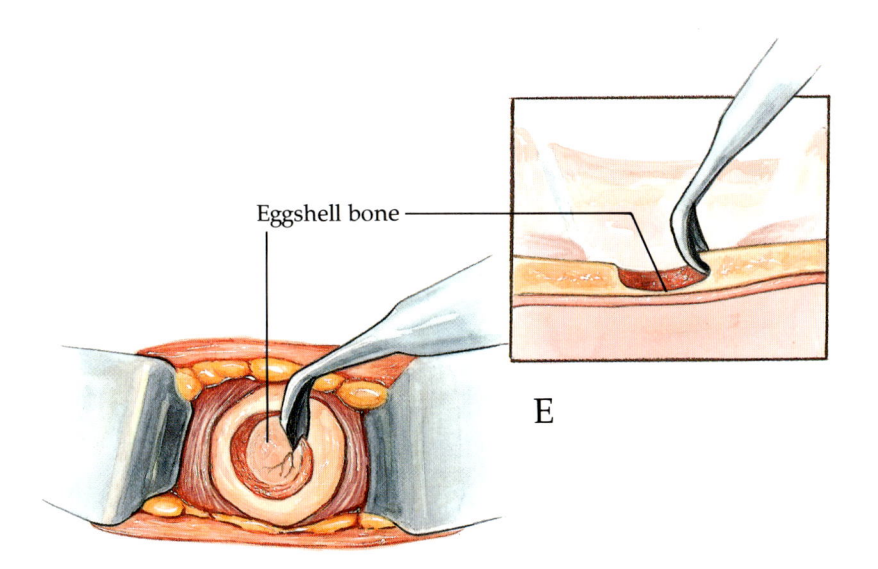

Plate 99

Eggshell bone

E

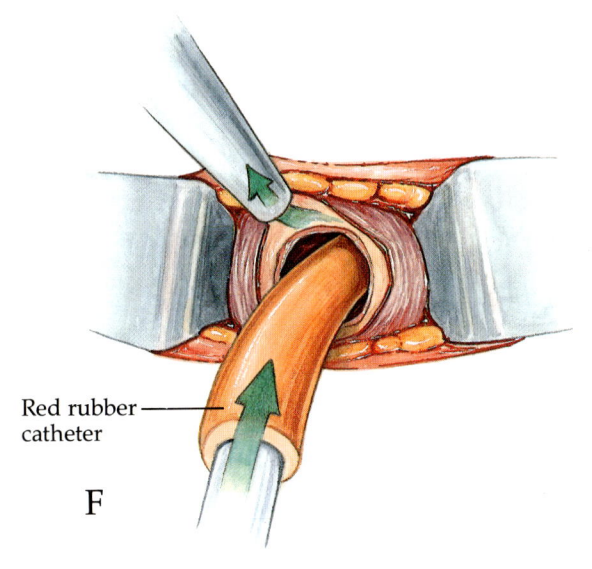

Red rubber catheter

F

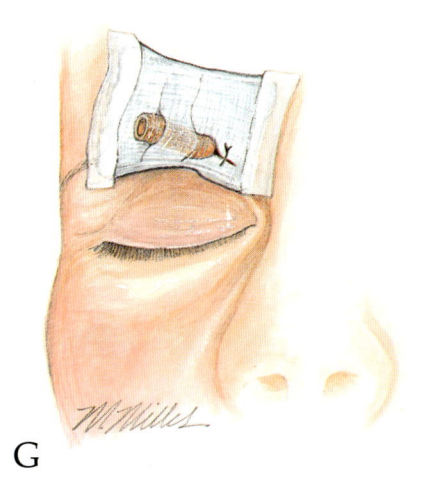

G

Figure 5 (Continued)
Frontal Sinus Trephination;
Sinus Irrigation and Drainage

227

Hematogenous spread of infection produces septicemia, subdural abscess, and epidural abscess. The diploic veins of Breschet may be the corridor through which infection is spread to distant parts of the skull. Retrograde venous spread also leads to cavernous sinus and sagittal sinus thrombosis.

The most common neurologic sequelae are areas of anesthesia and paresthesia of the brow. The trauma of surgery may cause spread of infection, producing epidural abscess, meningitis, subdural abscess, and brain abscess of the frontal lobe.

Complications of the orbital area include hair loss (from shaving), edema, cellulitis, and abscess of the upper lid, and orbital cellulitis and orbital abscess, which may lead to ophthalmoplegia and/or to proptosis.

Complications from postoperative care are unusual. Bacterial meningitis may result from the introduction of bacteria into the meningeal space by postoperative irrigations, and chemical meningitis from the extravasation of irrigating fluid into the meningeal spaces. Infection may lead to brain abscess from erosion of the posterior table of the skull from the necrotizing pressure of the indwelling drain. Hematoma, orbital cellulitis, and orbital abscess are occasional complications.

Pearls and Pitfalls

A careful preoperative examination for neurologic abnormalities must be performed.

Preoperative x-ray films and/or computed tomograms of the sinus should be obtained.

Following Mosher's dictum, be especially careful to preserve the virginity of the nasofrontal duct.

Do not use pressure to irrigate the wound.

Never use an irrigant that is not well tolerated intrathecally; use normal saline.

Pressure dressings should be firm but not too tight, and especially not tight over the orbit.

When discussing the informed consent form, tell the patient that he or she may have numbness of the forehead following the procedure and warn of possible intracranial and optic complications in addition to the possibility of recurring infection.

W. J. Richtsmeier, M.D., Ph.D.

FRONTOETHMOIDECTOMY

The reversal of chronic frontal sinusitis incorporates the concept of drainage of the frontal sinus through the frontal sinus recess into the ethmoid sinus. The path through the ethmoid sinus must be cleared if there is to be restoration of the normal mucociliary transport of the frontal sinus. There is no simple structure identified in most patients that can be labeled as a "nasofrontal duct." In that regard, decisions concerning the obliteration of the frontal sinus for irreversible mucosal or ostial disease are based on the inability to perform a functional procedure because the sinus cannot be drained into the nose.

Because mucociliary transport is an important clearance mechanism of the frontal sinus, performing a septectomy in an effort to ventilate one sinus with the other is usually not indicated. Since mucociliary transport usually brings mucus up the medial wall of the frontal sinus, a septectomy may improve unilateral disease by allowing mucociliary transport to move material from the diseased to the healthy side of the sinus, which can drain into the nose. Simple ventilation of the sinus rarely provides complete improvement, and, therefore, if there is no mucociliary transport on the diseased side, because of extensive polypoid disease, septectomy will not improve the involved side. It is also important to realize that surgery does not reverse the medical-mucosal problems of allergy or hyper-reactivity. The reversibility of otherwise hyperplastic mucosa is remarkable. Underlying osteitis or osteomyelitis can defeat the best surgical decompression efforts, and bone cultures obtained at the time of surgery may be invaluable.

Indications

Frontal ethmoidectomy is a procedure for which there are relatively few indications in contrast to other approaches to the ethmoid and frontal sinuses. A relative indication is that of chronic mucosal disease in a small frontal sinus. It is best to limit the extent of the facial incision as much as is feasible. Neither the endoscopic approach to the frontal sinus nor the bicoronal-osteoplastic flap (in patients who are not bald) leaves visible scars, and these approaches should be considered first in surgery of benign disease. A patient with male pattern baldness may not be a suitable candidate for a bicoronal flap, nor would an individual with significant scalp or cranial diseases. Trauma may provide access through lacerations and offers direct exposure of potential posterior traumatic defect. Individuals who have significant (or predominant) ethmoid disease would benefit more from the ethmoidectomy extension than from a primary bicoronal frontal sinus approach. In addition, those with disease that has penetrated into the orbit, such as an infected mucopyocele, may also be candidates for this approach. Patients who are not suitable for an endoscopic approach but require a local anesthetic because of medical problems are more easily treated through the frontal ethmoidectomy approach.

Relative contraindications to this approach include extensive bilateral disease, a need to preserve the forehead blood supply for possible flaps in other areas (such as in a patient with multiple basal cell carcinomas of the nose), and situations in which malignancy is suspected (biopsies are better obtained through the transnasal approach, when possible, avoiding contamination of a cutaneous incision).

Preoperative Considerations

A radiologic study of the frontal sinus and frontal sinus-ethmoid complex in order to identify the frontal sinus recess is required; it also clarifies the various anatomic relationships. This is best performed using coronal views; however, axial, sagittal, and three-dimensional reconstruction can provide valuable conceptual information for the surgeon. Computed tomographic scanning is recommended over magnetic resonance imaging, since bone is not detailed well with the latter. Information regarding the presence or absence of tumors, soft tissue invasion, and inflammatory changes may be better distinguished on magnetic resonance imaging. The 6-foot Caldwell view of the frontal sinus is important so that a template can be made of the frontal sinus.

The patient is informed about the anatomic relationship of the operative site to the skull base and orbit and the risks of injury to these structures. The patient needs to be counseled about possible recurrence and the potential need for a combined intranasal or an extended external incision or for obliteration of the sinus (using an abdominal fat graft). The likelihood of visible scars and persistent forehead anesthesia should be explained. Decisions regarding local or general anesthesia are made on medical grounds, although this procedure is usually performed under general anesthesia. Standard instruments used for sinus procedures are employed. Sewall retractors are recommended for the orbit.

The anesthesia service should be requested to provide the patient with an orotracheal tube in the midline, usually extending directly inferior such as that provided by a RAE tube. After placing ophthalmic ointment in the eyes, the eyelids are sutured closed with a tarsorrhaphy suture at the lateral limbus to reduce the likelihood of ocular injury. Once the patient is anesthetized, he or she is prepared in the standard fashion. Strict aseptic technique is not critical; however, contamination of the wound from the skin into the sinus may confuse cultures taken intraoperatively and thus should be minimized.

Once the patient is anesthetized, an oropharyngeal pack should be placed so that drainage from the sinus is not swallowed or aspirated. A head drape is sewn or stapled to the hairline, and the abdomen is prepared for possible fat graft harvesting.

Operative Steps

One should consider both the supratrochlear and supraorbital arteries in determining placement of the incision. The incision follows the approach described by Lynch (Fig. 6A). A notch at the level of the medial canthus helps in the postoperative reapproximation of the incision and breaks up the vertical suture line.

When the incision is extended superiorly, consideration must be given to its placement within or outside the brow. If the incision is placed inside the brow, the knife needs to be beveled in order to follow the plane of the hair roots, which angle more superiorly. Hair roots transected by a knife held perpendicular to the skin edge do not regenerate. This leaves an undesirably wide non–hair-bearing scar inside the brow. Bilateral disease requires extension of the incision inferiorly onto the nasion, inferior to the glabella, where the horizontal midline connection is placed. Placing the horizontal portion lower and in a skin crease minimizes the visibility

Frontoethmoidectomy

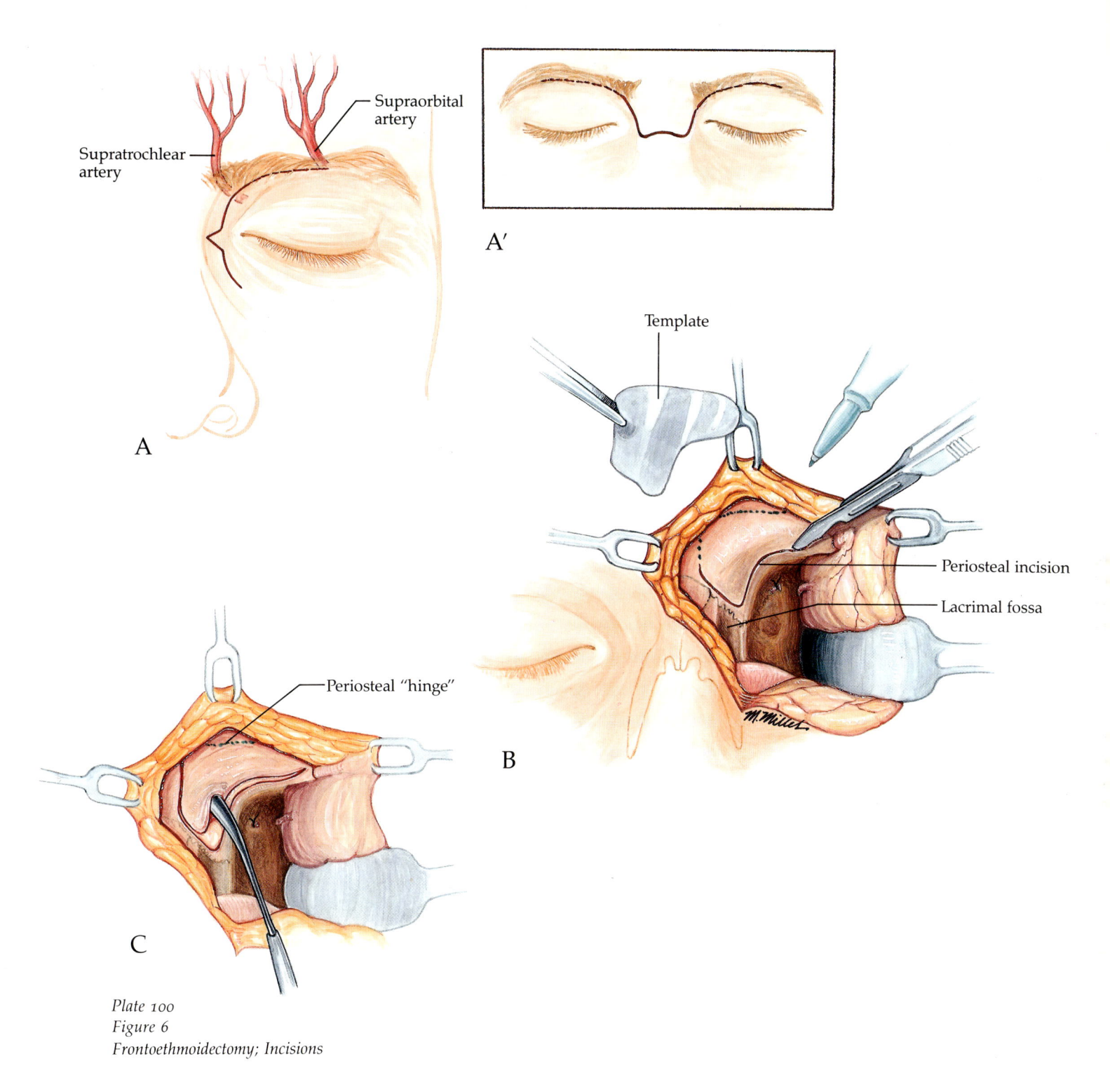

Plate 100
Figure 6
Frontoethmoidectomy; Incisions

of this incision. The incision extends down to the periosteum, and the plane above the periosteum is elevated to expose the anterior and lateral portions of the frontal ethmoid complex (Fig. 6B).

The Lynch incision is extended through the periosteum (Fig. 6B) with the expectation of leaving the osteoplastic flap attached medially and superiorly (Fig. 6C), where a periosteal hinge is maintained. If bilateral disease is present, the hinge area must be narrowed centrally or one unilateral attachment is chosen as the major blood supply, since the area of the superior portion of the frontal sinus would make too broad a bony attachment to the fracture. The Freer elevator is used to elevate the periosteum over the area of dissection for the ethmoidectomy (Fig. 6C).

Ethmoidotomy helps to provide orientation for the surgeon. The template, prepared in advance from a 6-foot Caldwell radiograph of the frontal sinus, is used to outline the bone flap on the periosteum using dots of brilliant green dye on an applicator. This dye should be used sparingly, as it will cause necrosis of the periosteum if *too much* is used. An oscillating saw is then used to enter the frontal sinus. Beveling the bone cuts is important, since perpendicular saw cuts that miss the frontal sinus will enter the anterior cranial compartment, and the bone flap will not sit as precisely at the completion of the procedure. Keep in mind that most templates slightly exaggerate the dimensions of the sinus. Care must be taken to ensure identification of the midline, especially for unilateral disease, and a midline cut extending the bone incision superiorly is also made (Fig. 6D).

The dissection is enlarged sufficiently so that a Gigli saw can be placed through the inferior and medial cuts. A Freer elevator is used to elevate the periosteal hinge. Using a small, malleable retractor to protect the periosteal hinge, the Gigli saw completes the bone incision, allowing superior and medial retraction of the osteoplastic flap (Fig. 6E). Retraction through this portion of the procedure can be frustrating because there is little stretch of the forehead skin laterally, and it is during this portion of the procedure that many surgeons wish they had planned a coronal approach. The cuts with the Gigli saw need not be carried completely through, as the narrowed bone pedicle can often be fractured with an osteotome to complete its removal. When using an osteotome, the broadest instrument that will fit should be chosen so that the force is spread out over a large area to help ensure that the osteoplastic flap is not fractured at sites other than the hinge. It may be difficult to fracture a bilateral osteoplastic flap because of its connection to the central septum. If necessary, divide the septum through the inferior portion of the ethmoidectomy, or pass the oscillating saw from the inferior aspect and carefully cut the lateral part of the septum, keeping the blade parallel to the plane of the forehead. Care must be taken not to incise, lacerate, or dehydrate the periosteal bridge because doing so will make a free graft out of the osteoplastic flap. This is probably the most important aspect of the procedure. Replacing a free graft in an infected area increases the risk of significant complication of flap or central nervous system infection substantially.

Plate 101

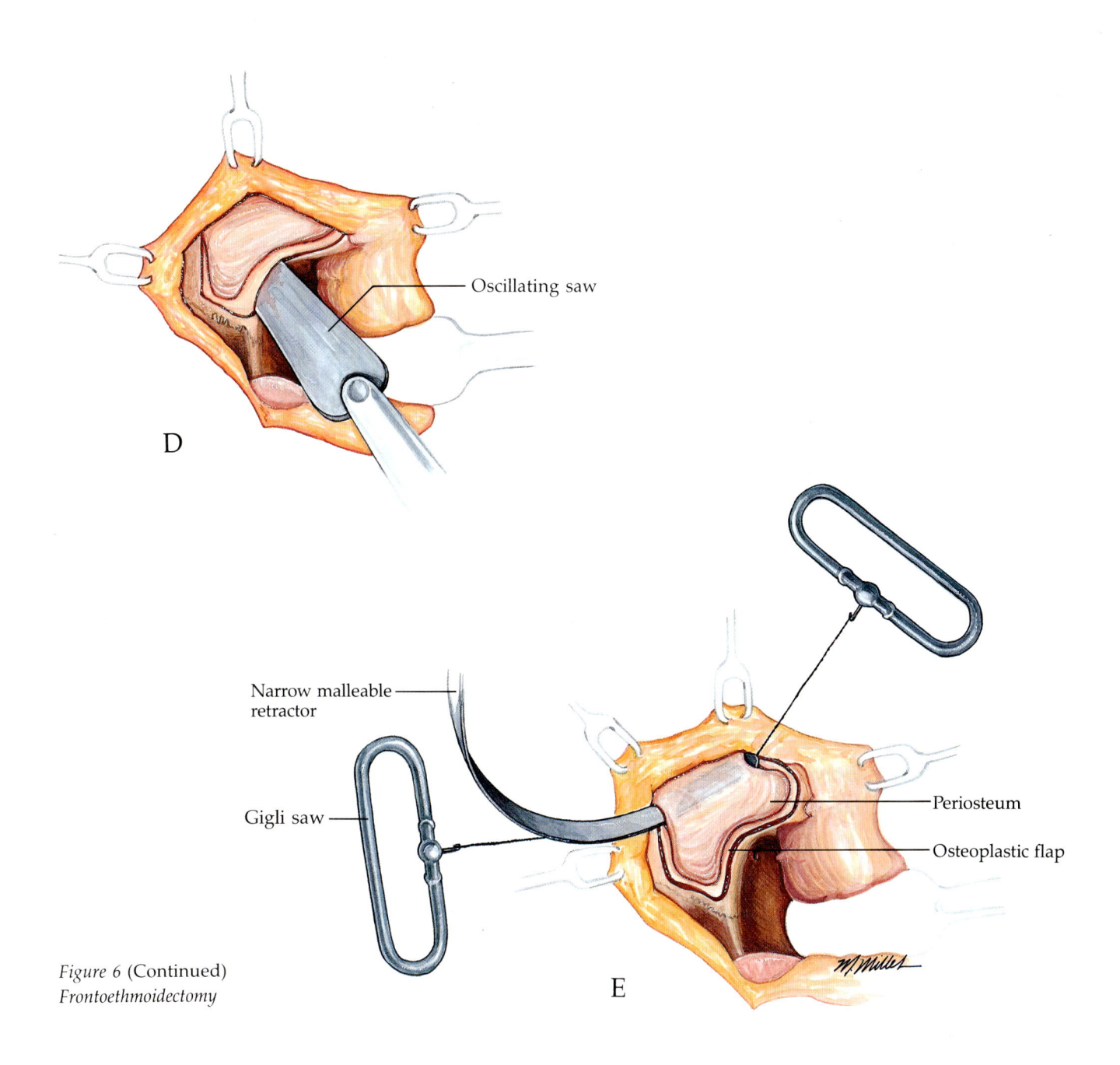

D — Oscillating saw

E — Narrow malleable retractor, Gigli saw, Periosteum, Osteoplastic flap

Figure 6 (Continued) Frontoethmoidectomy

233

The sinus is opened, and at this point a decision regarding the reversibility of the disease process must be made (Fig. 6F). This requires judgment, particularly with regard to marsupializing the frontal sinus into the nose through the ethmoidectomy. If irreversible disease is present, a bur is used to remove all mucosa from the frontal sinus (Fig. 6G). This is done down to the base of the sinus, where the remaining mucosa is incised in the axial plane and then reflected inferiorly so that it provides a complete seal resisting ingrowth of mucosa into the frontal sinus (Fig. 6H). Occasionally, a small mirror may be useful for looking into the superior and lateral recesses of the frontal sinus to ensure that all mucosal disease has been removed. Once sealed inferiorly, the sinus is packed with abdominal fat (see Osteoplastic Frontal Sinusectomy), and the osteoplastic flap is closed with wire sutures after placing small holes along the bone incision. Care is taken to turn the ends of the wire inward into drill holes, since the brow and medial canthal area are easily palpated by the patient. Remember to obtain samples of sinus mucosa and bone for routine anaerobic and fungal cultures and stains prior to closing the incision.

A standard external ethmoidectomy may be performed when the sinus disease is thought to be reversible (Fig. 6I). The path leading from the frontal sinus may be sigmoid in shape, which is a possible cause of failure of intranasal surgery. The frontal sinus recess should be enlarged anteriorly, as dissection of the posterior wall leads to the anterior cranial compartment and is not recommended. The use of a drill may be necessary to enlarge the bone compartment along the anterior aspect of the frontal sinus recess. Open all of the ethmoid air cells in this area, including the supraorbital ethmoids, which may be a site of residual disease. The anterior ethmoidal artery crosses just posterior to the upward and anterior swing of the frontal sinus recess. It should be identified and clipped laterally prior to initiation of the ethmoidectomy. It is probably best to obliterate the sinus with abdominal fat if it does not appear that the frontal sinus will remain ventilated as a result of the surgical approach. The Sewall septal mucosal flap can be used to maintain patency by relining the frontal sinus recess utilizing nasal mucosa.

The skin is closed in the standard fashion after replacing the osteoplastic flap, as described earlier. A small Penrose or rubberband drain is placed in the wound to be removed the following day. A light, compressive dressing can be placed over the incision.

Postoperative Care

Injury to the eye and anterior cranial contents is of immediate concern. Vision should be checked early in the postoperative setting. The eye needs to be inspected at least for light perception, even if a light compressive dressing has been placed over the wound. This can be done by placing a light on the inferior lid and having the patient respond to the presence of light. Discrete visual changes and range of motion can be checked as soon as the bandage is removed. Any unusual pain in the eye requires a complete eye examination.

Postoperative evaluation endoscopically is desirable and indispensable in the management of many patients. This obviates the need for a

Plate 102

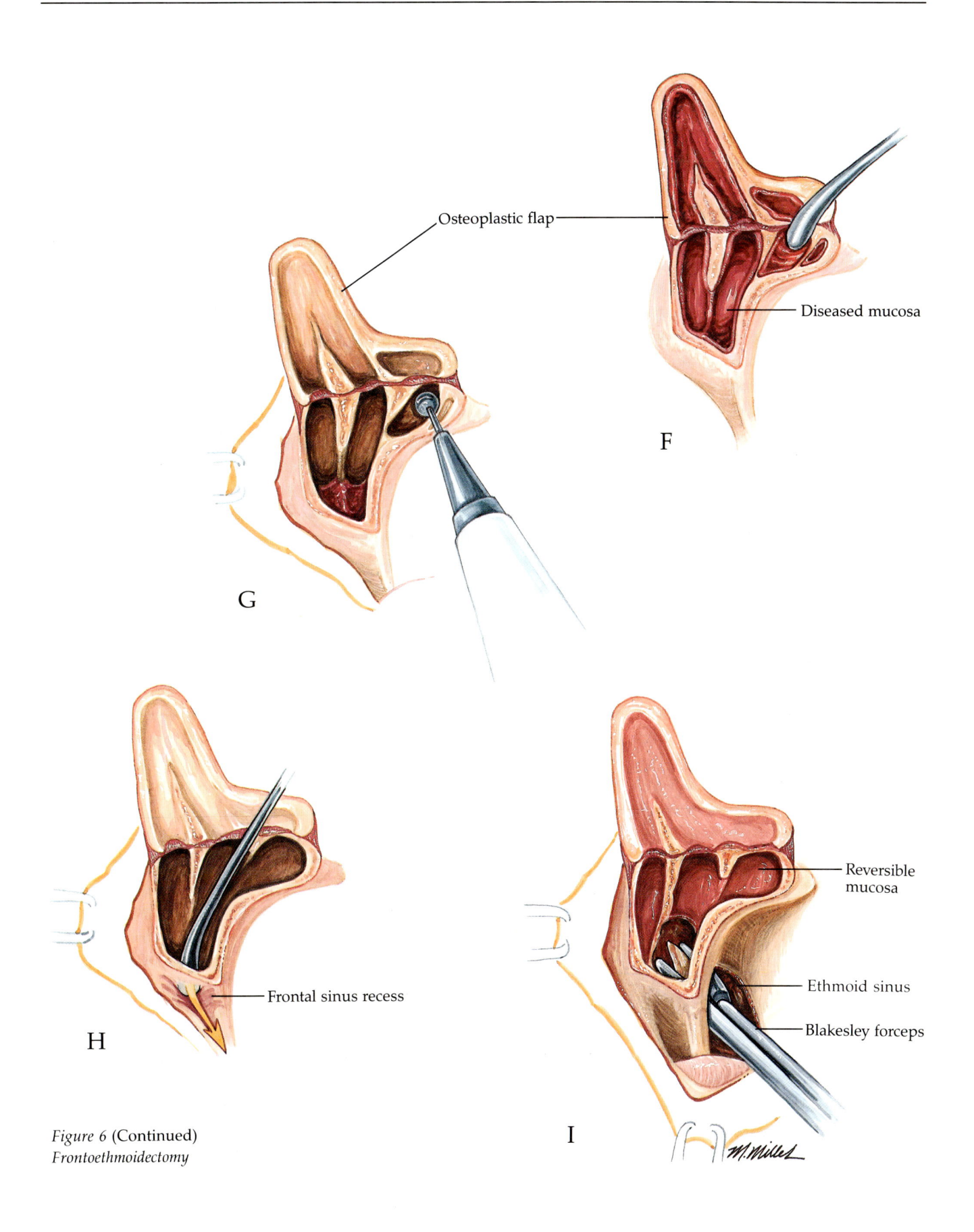

Osteoplastic flap

Diseased mucosa

F

G

Frontal sinus recess

H

Reversible mucosa

Ethmoid sinus

Blakesley forceps

I

Figure 6 (Continued)
Frontoethmoidectomy

mucosal flap to re-epithelize the frontal sinus recess. The patient is continued on a wide-spectrum antibiotic that includes coverage for anaerobes. A decision regarding further antibiotic coverage is made when culture results are available. The sutures may be removed early (4 to 5 days), since there is virtually no tension on the incision. The patient should be advised not to blow his or her nose, since any orbital or intracranial defect will permit the development of dramatic and acute postoperative encephalocele or ophthalmocele.

Risks, Complications, and Sequelae

The following problems can ensue after the procedure: (1) a cosmetically undesirable external scar; (2) anesthesia of the brow; (3) subluxation of the trochlea with diplopia; (4) ligation of the supraorbital and supratrochlear arteries; (5) recurrence or persistence of the sinusitis due to osteitis, allergic mucosal disease, synechia, or scarring in the ethmoid sinus; (6) intracranial or orbital entry causing direct injury and/or allowing infection to spread; (7) necrosis of the osteoplastic flap or infection with resultant cosmetic deformity; and (8) bleeding into the nose or orbit from the anterior ethmoidal artery.

Pearls and Pitfalls

Demand an excellent quality radiologic study: coronal computed tomography and a 6-foot Caldwell view for the template.

Prepare the abdomen even if you plan drainage through the ethmoid sinus.

Bevel the skin incision so as to miss hair roots and bevel the bone incision so as not to miss the sinus.

Preserve the periosteal hinge from laceration and desiccation.

Pitfalls include an attempt to obdurate too large an area of the sinus via this approach; finding an unsuspected malignancy; the occurrence of postoperative synechia in the ethmoid, obstructing the frontal sinus recess; missing diseased supraorbital ethmoid or agger nasi air cells; and forgetting to obtain culture specimens intraoperatively.

Loring W. Pratt, M.D.

OSTEOPLASTIC FRONTAL SINUSECTOMY

Indications

In 1972 Goodale, Holmes, and Montgomery introduced a method of treating chronic frontal sinusitis with an osteoplastic flap and implantation of a free fat graft harvested from the abdominal wall to fill the sinus. This operation has the advantage of effectively obliterating the cavity of the frontal sinus while maintaining the cosmetic appearance of the patient's brow. The procedure is a relatively simple technique and works well in most cases if the critical steps are carried out with precision.

Preoperative Considerations

Preoperative diagnosis of chronic purulent frontal sinusitis or mucocele of the frontal sinus is an indication for radical frontal sinus surgery.

Preoperative studies to establish this diagnosis should include x-ray films and/or computed tomographic scans, cultures for both aerobic and anaerobic organisms, complete blood studies, and a general physical, ophthalmologic, and neurologic evaluation of the patient.

Preoperative preparation includes x-ray studies of the frontal sinuses in the classic frontal sinus projection position, taken at a distance of 6 feet from the x-ray tube. This gives an image approximately the same size as the sinus itself. This film is then cut to make a template, which is the size and shape of the frontal sinus. It is accurately oriented over the sinus and provides a guide to mark the boundaries of the frontal sinuses prior to making incisions in the periosteum and the bone.

Operative Steps

The incision may be made either just above or just below the unshaved brow or it may be made in a coronal plane, 2 cm posterior to the hairline (Fig. 7A). If the brow incision is elected, the incision should be carried through the skin and subcutaneous tissues to and through the galea and the periosteum. This incision has the disadvantage of producing numbness of the forehead; it also leaves the patient with a life-long scar. The eyebrows should not be shaved, since sometimes they do not grow back. There is no need to shave the hair from this region, since it is easily cleaned during the preoperative skin preparation. In cases in which there are fistulous tracts and a scar will persist in this region in any event, the brow incision may be indicated, as it may be possible to remove some of the fistulous tracts by judicious placement of the incision.

If the patient is concerned about cosmesis and even a well-healed scar on the brow is undesirable, a coronal incision should be utilized. The incision should be made well behind the anterior border of the hairline, and in the male allowance should be made for the future possibility of a receding hairline with advancing age.

The incision should be made through the skin and galea and down to but not through the periosteum (Fig. 7B). Rapid achievement of hemostasis is facilitated by application of Cushing or Raney clips to the transected margins of the scalp and galea. The scalp should then be reflected to expose the region of the brow. As this dissection is deep to

Plate 103

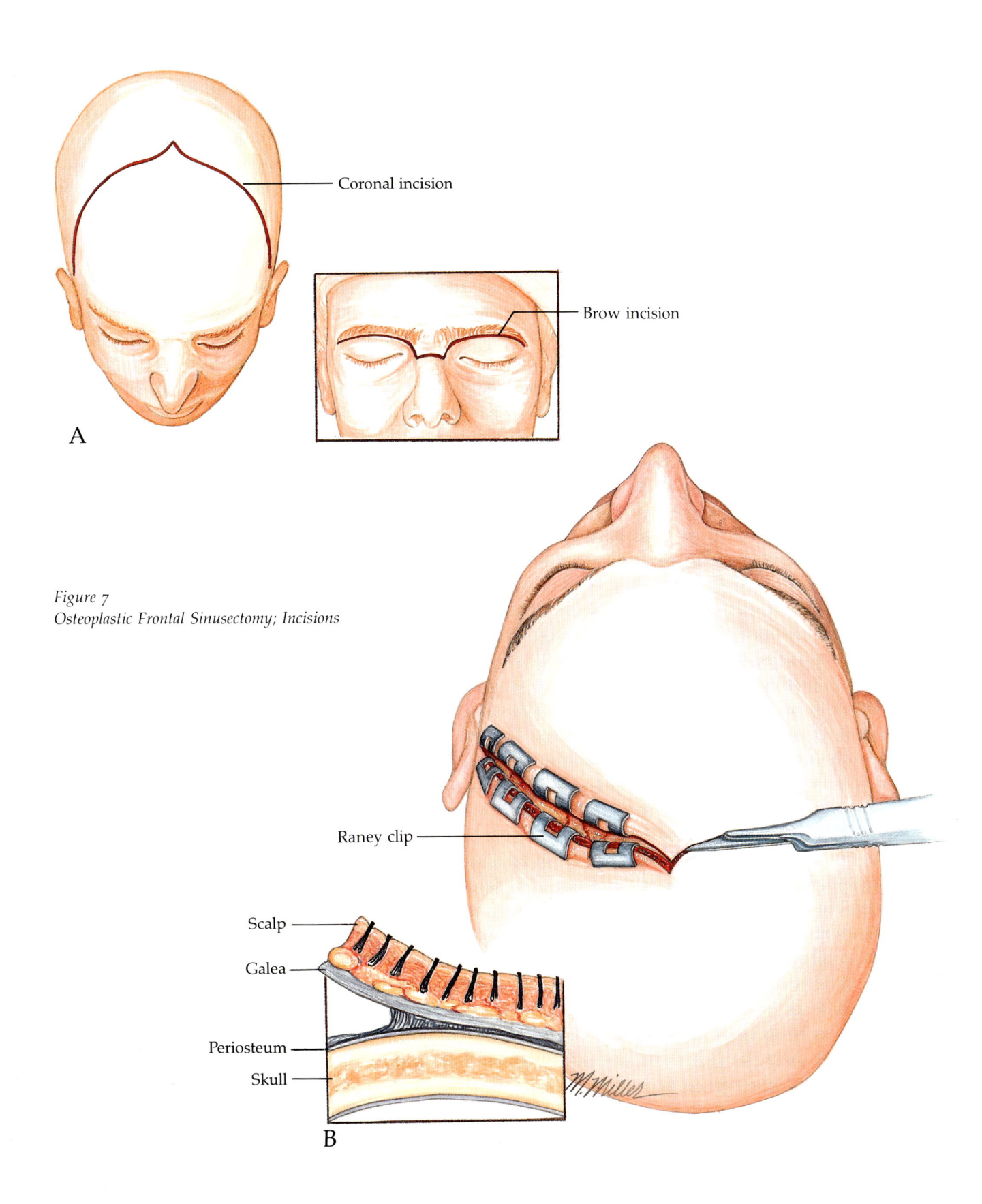

Coronal incision

Brow incision

A

Figure 7
Osteoplastic Frontal Sinusectomy; Incisions

Raney clip

Scalp
Galea
Periosteum
Skull

B

239

the sensory nerve supply of this region, there is little likelihood of any significant anesthesia or paresthesia of the brow or forehead. Elevation of the flap must extend sufficiently low to allow for application of the x-ray template of the frontal sinuses to the frontal bone, so that it may be positioned accurately (Fig. 7C). An arrow may be used to mark the midline of the frontal bone, and a pointer on the inferior border of the template can be aligned with this arrow. The supraorbital notches may be used to position the inferior border of the template.

Once the template is properly positioned, the periosteum may be marked with methylene blue, a marking pencil or other dye to indicate the upper margin and scalloping of the frontal sinus. The mark should not be made with a scalpel, as it is desirable to have intact periosteum over the region of the bone incision into the frontal sinus.

The periosteal incision should be made 1 cm above and lateral to the mark on the frontal bone (Fig. 7D). No incision should be made along the supraorbital margin of the frontal sinuses. A small amount of periosteum should be elevated above the margin of the sinus, and the lower flap of periosteum should be freed from the frontal bone and reflected inferiorly only to the extent necessary to allow the access required to make the bone incision (Fig. 7E).

Plate 104

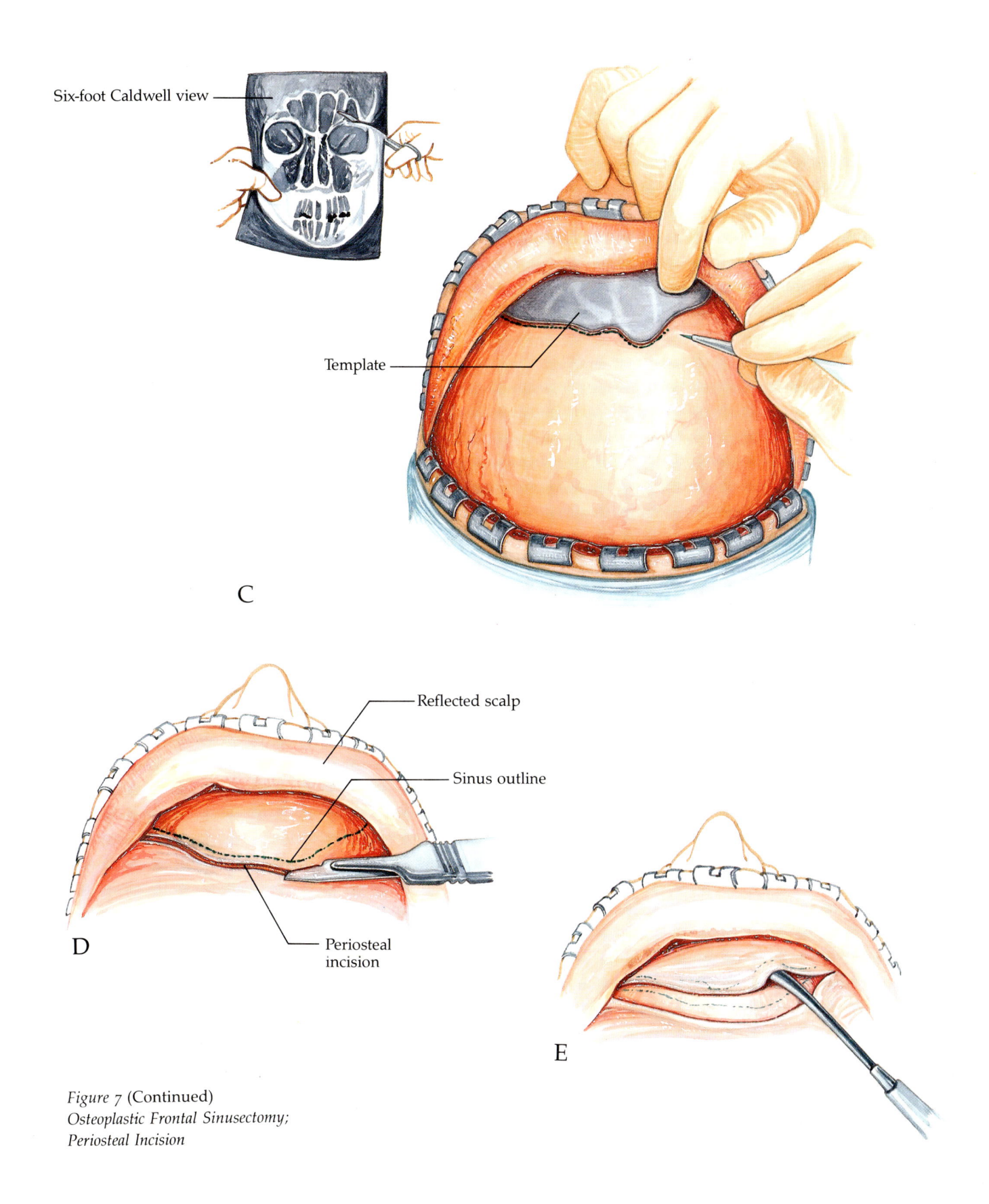

Six-foot Caldwell view

Template

C

Reflected scalp

Sinus outline

D

Periosteal incision

E

Figure 7 (Continued)
Osteoplastic Frontal Sinusectomy;
Periosteal Incision

The incision in the bone should be made with a reciprocating saw held with the blade at an angle of 10 degrees. It should be begun slightly peripheral to the mark on the frontal bone so that the blade enters the sinus as close as possible to its most distal extension, leaving a beveled portion of bone on which the bone flap may rest when it is replaced. Care must be taken in making the incision that the saw blade does not penetrate the inner table of the skull and injure or enter the meninges (Fig. 7F). When the lumen of the sinus is entered, there is often a gush of pus, and this should be smeared and cultured for both aerobic and anaerobic organisms. When the superior and lateral margins of the sinus have been freed and only attachment at the brow remains, an attempt should be made to pry the bone flap up and to fracture its inferior attachment (Fig. 7G). If this is not possible without using excessive force, a small incision in the periosteum of the brow must be made and a narrow chisel or saw blade introduced to help fracture the bone (Fig. 7H). Care should be taken to avoid injury to the supraorbital and trochlear nerves. Once the bone flap has been freed and elevated, it should be handled with care so as not to injure or divide the periosteal attachment at the inferior margin, as this is the only source of nourishment for the bone flap for the immediate future.

Plate 105

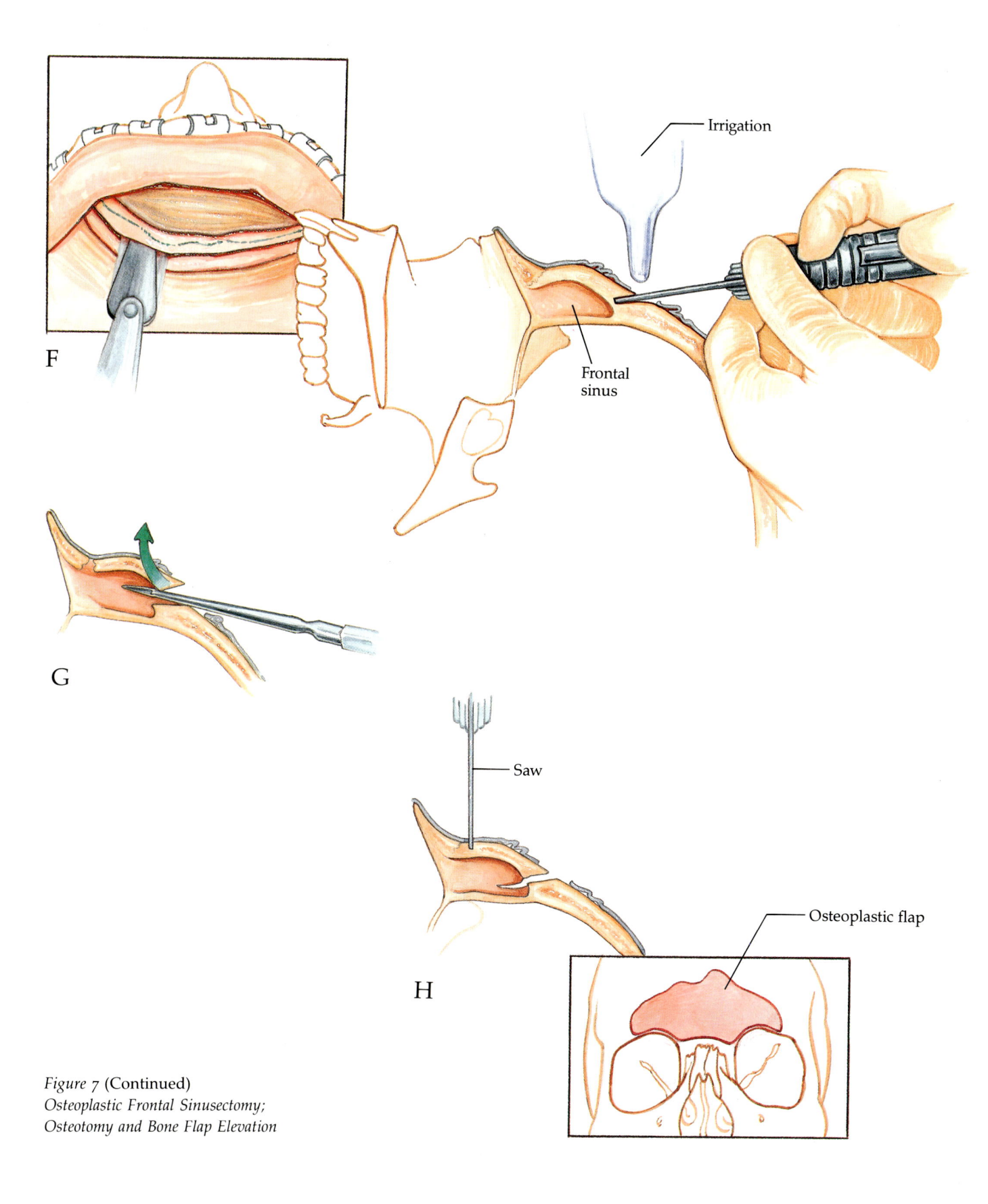

Figure 7 (Continued)
Osteoplastic Frontal Sinusectomy;
Osteotomy and Bone Flap Elevation

The inner surface of the bone flap must be cleaned of all mucosa (Fig. 7I). The mucosa surrounding the inner ostia of the nasofrontal ducts is inverted into the ducts (Fig. 7J). The bone surface is skived with a large olive bur in order to make certain that no remnant of mucosa is left attached (Fig. 7K). Once the bone has been adequately cleaned, it should be wrapped in a sponge soaked with normal saline and anchored to the patient and drapes in such a way that the periosteal pedicle cannot be disrupted and desiccation of the bone will be prevented. The posterior wall and all extensions of the frontal sinus must be cleaned of mucosa.

Any supraorbital ethmoid cells must also be saucerized and opened so that they are one with the cavity of the frontal sinus. Any material that is removed should be cultured for both aerobic and anaerobic organisms and sent for histopathologic study. Recesses of the sinus may be explored using otologic bone burs. The condition of the recesses and the completeness of mucosal removal may be better evaluated with the aid of the operating microscope. Particular attention should be paid to the margins of the bone incision to be certain that the bevel is maintained, so that the bone flap may be replaced with minimal residual deformity. If the bone edges are not level, or if there is a wide space between the bone edges when the flap is replaced, there will be a visible defect in the healed forehead, even though the coronal incision is used. A clean surface should be prepared so that there is a good bed for the fat graft.

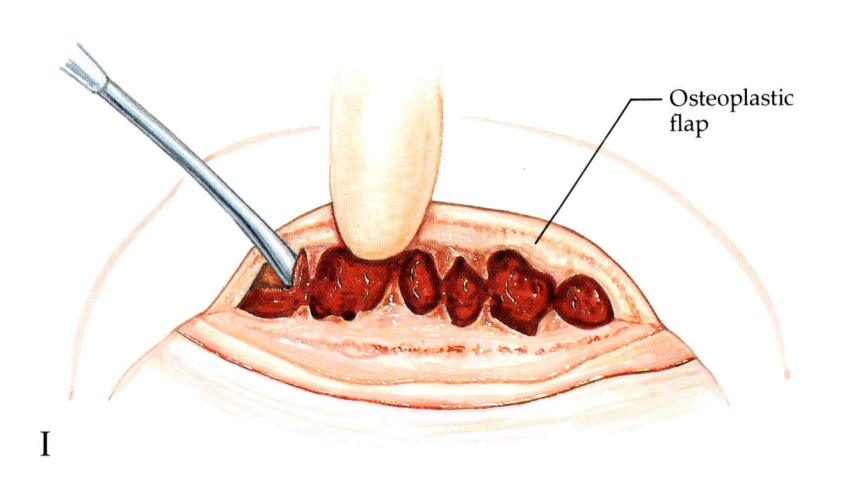

Plate 106

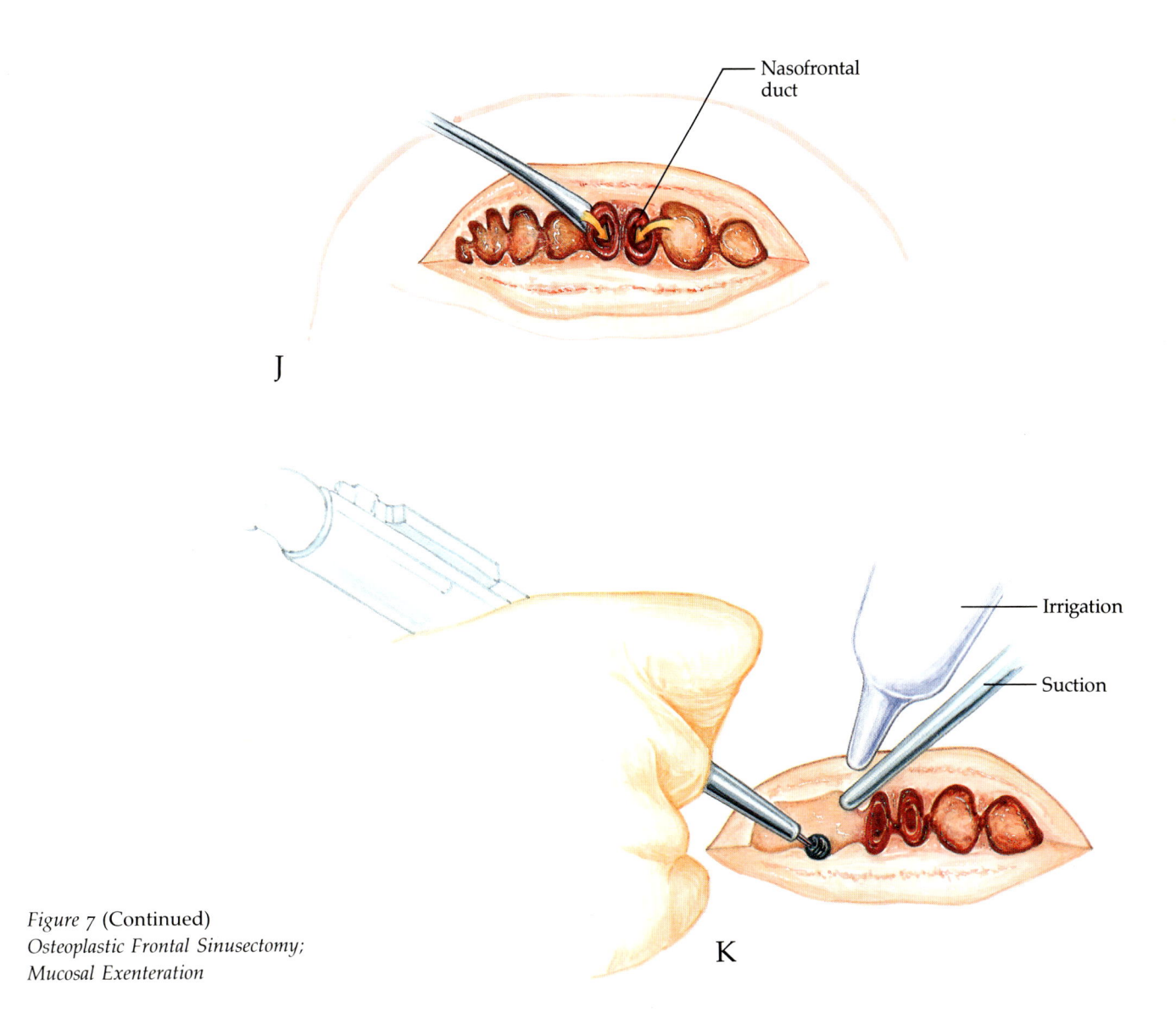

I — Osteoplastic flap

J — Nasofrontal duct

K — Irrigation / Suction

Figure 7 (Continued)
Osteoplastic Frontal Sinusectomy;
Mucosal Exenteration

Fat is harvested from the anterior abdominal wall through an incision whose placement would not mislead or confuse another surgeon subsequently in the event of suspected intra-abdominal disease. The fat should be obtained in a single piece, large enough to completely fill the cavity of the sinus (Fig. 7L). Although the cavity must be completely filled with fat, it must also be possible to replace the bone flap so that it lies flat in its beveled bed without any protrusion of fat. The bone edges must meet without interposed fat if healing is to take place quickly. The bone may be sutured in place and fixed with wire sutures (Figure 7M), but usually this is not necessary. If it is possible to get a good fit and hold the flap in place by closure of the periosteum with slowly absorbable sutures, this is most desirable (Fig. 7N), as wire sutures often show through the skin of the forehead when healing is complete. Shingling the bone incision and the more distal position of the periosteal incision reduce the likelihood that the bone incision will show through the scalp and skin of the forehead.

If any of the adjacent bone is soft or osteomyelitic, it should be removed with a margin of normal bone included to ensure that only healthy bone is left behind. This can often be accomplished effectively with a rongeur, as the "snap" of healthy bone is quite different from the soft mushy sensation obtained from the removal of diseased bone. If the posterior wall of the sinus is involved, it must be removed and good healthy bone obtained on all margins. The fat graft may be placed directly on dura mater.

The scalp may then be replaced, Raney clips removed one by one, and any persistent bleeding controlled with electrocautery or free ties. The incision should be closed by interrupted sutures in the galea, sutures in the scalp, and deep mattress sutures or staples in the skin (Fig. 7O). Placement of flat Silastic suction drains helps coapt the scalp to the bone and decreases the incidence of hematoma and seroma.

Nasal packing impregnated with antibiotic ointment should be applied to the nose to provide support for the inferior end of the nasofrontal duct region.

A light but firm compressive dressing over the frontal sinus and the area from which the scalp has been elevated is helpful in reducing the possibility of edema, hematoma, or dislocation of the flap of frontal bone.

Plate 107

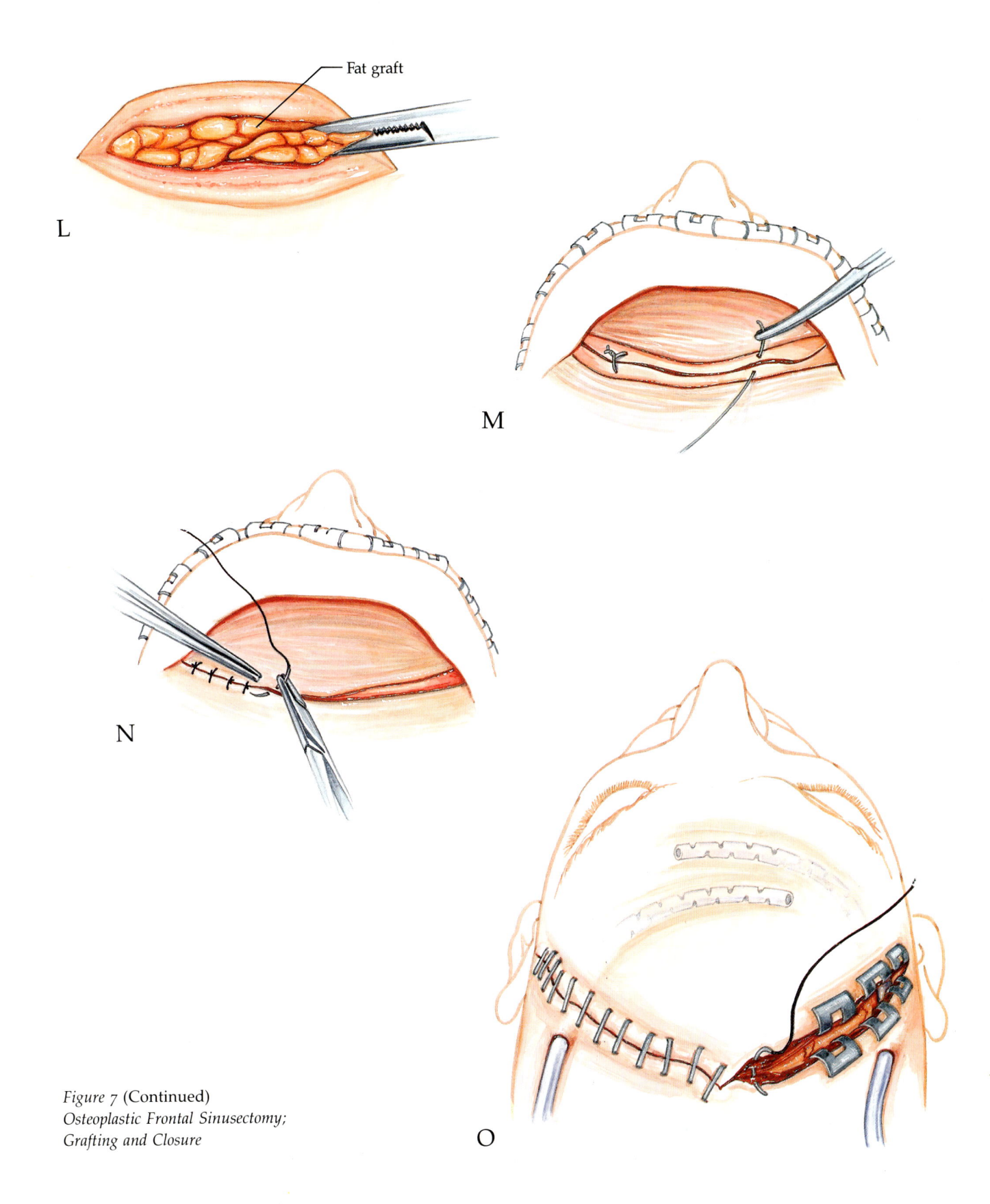

Fat graft

L

M

N

Figure 7 (Continued)
Osteoplastic Frontal Sinusectomy;
Grafting and Closure

O

247

FRONTAL SINUS ABLATION

If it is impractical to use the procedure as described above, a reasonable alternative may be collapse of the frontal sinus. In this procedure the entire outer wall of the frontal sinus is removed by a rongeur, and then the outer and lateral margins of the sinus are exenterated with cutting burs. As in the case of the osteoplastic procedure, it is necessary to remove all supraorbital ethmoid extensions to ensure the complete removal of the infected bone and sinus membrane and to obliterate the air space, which might become infected at a later date. The supraorbital ethmoid cells are meticulously exenterated. In some instances it is necessary to remove the posterior wall of the sinus, leaving the anterior fossa dura exposed (Fig. 7P). When the skin incision is closed, the skin is placed directly on the posterior wall of the sinus or on the dura mater, and it is held there with a pressure dressing. Drains are necessary in this procedure to prevent the accumulation of blood or serum or both under the flap. Residual mucosa may form mucoceles and provide the nidus for recurrent infections. The deformity produced by this operation is substantial (Fig. 7Q).

Distant foci of osteomyelitis that have located some distance from the frontal sinus by passage of septic emboli from the sinus through the diploic veins of Breschet must be removed. It may be necessary to make separate incisions to accomplish their complete exenteration.

Postoperative Care

Appropriate antibiotic coverage should be provided during and following surgery for these infections. The antibiotics should be continued postoperatively until it is clear that the infectious process has been eradicated.

The patient should be kept in semi-Fowler's position to reduce the venous stasis.

The patient should begin ambulation within 24 hours.

The compressive dressing should be used for at least a week to prevent the development of edema or hematoma or both and to provide fixation for the bone flap.

The nasal packing should be removed after 2 or 3 days and the nose cleaned thereafter with sterile suction tips and vasoconstrictor spray, as necessary.

If drains have been placed, they should be removed after 48 hours.

Risks, Complications, and Sequelae

Infection of the scalp or persistent infection of the sinus and bone of the skull are the most bothersome complications of frontal sinus osteoplastic sinusectomy. Fortunately they are not often seen. The most common infections seen in the immediate postoperative period are cellulitis of the brow, cellulitis and abscess of the orbit, or both. Persistent osteomyelitis of either the regional bone or distant areas of the skull is the most difficult to cure.

Intracranial infection resulting from spread of infection from the sinus, although rare, is a worrisome possibility. Such infections include meningitis, epidural abscess, arachnoiditis, subdural abscess, and brain abscess. These either may be contiguous infections and appear in the frontal lobe or may spread by vascular routes and appear in noncontiguous parts of the brain.

Plate 108

Skull

Dura mater

Nasal bone

P

Frontal sinus ablation defect

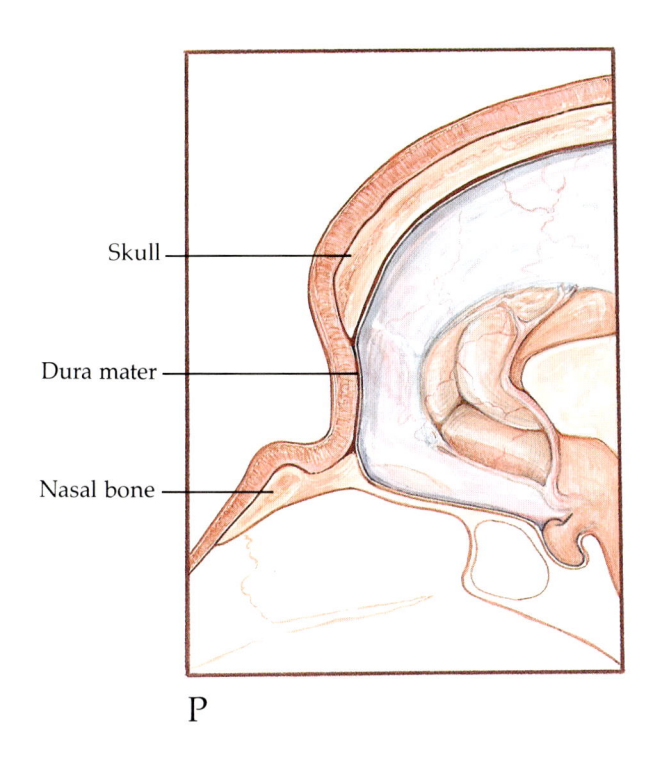

Q

Figure 7 (Continued) *Osteoplastic Frontal Sinusectomy; Frontal Sinus Ablation*

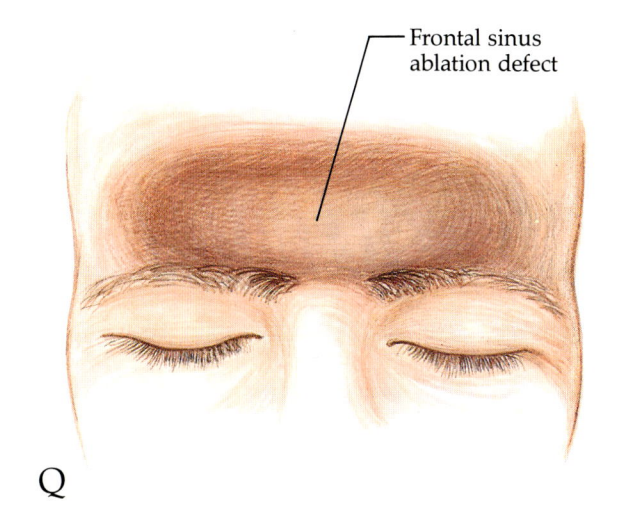

Hematogenous conditions associated with this procedure are septicemia, epidural hematoma, subdural hematoma, and diploic spread of infection to remote areas of the skull. Venous extension of the septic process to the cavernous sinus and thrombosis of the sagittal sinus may occur. Hematomas occur as part of the postoperative course if hemostasis is inadequate.

Neurologic sequelae include anesthesia of the brow, forehead, and scalp, superior oblique palsy, brain trauma, epidural abscess, meningitis, brain abscess involving the frontal lobe, and abscess of the brain in remote areas.

Orbital complications include loss of eyebrow hair (from shaving), edema of the upper lid, cellulitis of the upper lid, abscess of the lid, orbital cellulitis, and orbital abscess. These complications may lead to ophthalmoplegia and proptosis. Surgical dislocation of the trochlea may simulate a paralysis of the abducens nerve and give rise to diplopia.

Complications related directly to postoperative care include meningitis resulting from the dissemination of infection by irrigations or chemical meningitis due to extravasation of irrigating fluid. Erosion of the posterior table of the skull may result from the pressure of a drain, leading to intracranial extension of the infectious process or to the development of osteomyelitis of the skull.

Pearls and Pitfalls

Conduct a careful preoperative examination for neurologic abnormalities.

Photograph the forehead pre- and postoperatively.

Obtain a 6-foot x-ray film for making the template.

Clean all recesses of the sinus, and check the area with a microscope for any remaining disease.

Do not use pressure to irrigate the wound.

Never use an irrigant that is not well tolerated intrathecally (use normal saline).

Pressure dressings should be firm but not too tight, and special care should be taken that no pressure is placed on the globe of the eye.

When discussing informed consent, tell patient that he or she may have numbness of the forehead following the procedure.

John C. Price, M.D.

MIDFACIAL DEGLOVING APPROACH TO THE SINUSES

A description of the midfacial degloving approach was first published by Casson, Bonanno, and Converse in 1974. The method of rhinoplastic release of the nasal soft tissue when combined with bilateral anterior maxillary exposure provides a wide surgical approach to lesions beneath the midface without producing a visible facial scar. Access to lesions of the nasal cavity, nasal septum, maxillary, ethmoid, and sphenoid sinuses, nasopharynx, and clivus is excellent. Exposure and surgical facility are equal or superior to that of more traditional procedures, which require facial incisions. This approach may be combined with coronal, brow, temporal, and palatal incisions for extensive lesions and for those involving the skull base. The bilateral exposure allows immediate control of the internal maxillary arteries as needed. The approach is also of great advantage in removing very large lesions.

Indications

Casson's original report dealt primarily with the use of the midfacial degloving approach for repair of fractures and reconstructive procedures, including midfacial grafting and osteotomies with advancement and recession. It is an excellent approach for recontouring of the maxilla involved with fibrous dysplasia. In 1979, Conley and Price reported 26 cases of tumors managed by this method. In 1984, Sacks and Conley and colleagues reported a composite experience of 46 cases of inverted papilloma that were removed by the degloving approach. Terzian has combined this method with microsurgical technique to remove juvenile angiofibroma in 25 cases. Price, Holliday, and Kennedy and coworkers further elaborate on the usefulness of this technique applied in combination with a microsurgical approach for management of skull base tumors and fungal diseases of the sinuses.

The degloving approach has been used successfully in the management of the following benign sinonasal tumors: inverting papilloma, nasopharyngeal angiofibroma, salivary neoplasia, angioma, hemangiopericytoma, schwannoma, fibroma, chondroma, glioma, and chordoma. Certain low-grade malignancies, such as chondrosarcoma, mucoepidermoid carcinoma, acinic cell carcinoma, woodworker's adenocarcinoma of the ethmoid, carcinoma ex pleomorphic adenoma, and esthesioneuroblastoma, have also been removed. High-grade malignancies, including very limited anterior and inferior maxillary sinus tumors, carcinoma of the hard palate, and small nasal septal cancers, are also amenable to management with this approach.

Combination of the degloving approach with other incisions facilitates the removal of tumors of the skull base and larger lesions of the sinuses. Maniglia reports this procedure for total maxillectomy with orbital exenteration. It has been useful in the management of extensive benign conditions such as massive polypoid rhinosinusitis, large septal perforations, hereditary hemorrhagic telangiectasias, rhinoscleroma, and nasal sarcoidosis.

Candidates for this procedure should be carefully selected on the basis of both patient and pathologic indicators. The dominant patient consideration is avoidance of facial scar. This is most desirable in an adolescent, a child, or a public figure. Degloving may also avoid complications in patients prone to keloid formation and should be used in any patient who resists a necessary operation on the basis of a possible facial scar.

The inverting papilloma is the ideal pathologic lesion for the degloving approach. An en bloc excision of the lateral nasal wall can be readily accomplished, and extensions into the maxillary, ethmoid, and sphenoid sinuses are easily removed. Involvement of the cribriform plate is removed by frontal craniotomy and is repaired by pericranial flap technique. Management of frontal sinus involvement requires an additional incision.

The degloving approach should be considered a major alternative method for the resection of juvenile angiofibromas. Both internal maxillary arteries are easily accessible for ligation. Extensions into the pterygomaxillary space and cheek are readily managed, and transtemporal and frontal craniotomies allow control of nearly all lesions with dural extensions. Exposure of the maxillary, ethmoid, and sphenoid sinuses is superior to that gained through the transpalatal approach. Once medial maxillectomy and ethmoidectomy have been completed and the tumor has been removed, the pharyngobasilar fascia over the clivus is widely exposed and can be stripped and cauterized under direct control. The large sinonasal cavity that is established makes postoperative disease surveillance by anterior rhinoscopy simple. The lack of risk of oral nasal fistula and palatal dysfunction is also a significant advantage.

Exposure of the sphenoid and clivus is extensive and is superior to that provided by any surgical approach other than maxillectomy. It is therefore the ideal procedure for management of chordomas of the clivus.

Preoperative Considerations

General anesthesia is administered via oral intubation. The preformed curved endotracheal tube is secured to the chin in the midline. The patient is placed in the supine position with the head resting on folding towels to facilitate intraoperative positioning. Topical 4 percent cocaine solution on pledgets is applied intranasally as a vasoconstrictor and decongestant. The nose is then injected with 1 percent lidocaine with 1:100,000 epinephrine for local hemostasis, as for rhinoplasty. The buccogingival sulcus and the canine fossa are similarly infiltrated. Suture tarsorrhaphies or corneal protectors are placed bilaterally. A standard surgical scrub is carried out, and a head drape and a split sheet are then positioned. Illumination with a headlamp is essential: a light with a parabolic reflector is preferred, although fiberoptic illumination is adequate.

Operative Steps

A columellar transfixion incision is carried out, taking care that it extends the full length of the septum, from high in the tip area well onto the nasal floor and sweeping slightly posteriorly as the incision is completed. A double-ball retractor or an alar protector facilitates exposure inside the nasal tip (Fig. 8A). The intercartilaginous incisions are begun at the anteriormost extent of the transfixion incision. These incisions are carried laterally between the upper lateral cartilage tip and the lateral crus of the alar cartilage and are continued past the lateral margin of the upper lateral cartilages. The transfixion and intercartilaginous incisions effectively separate the nasal tip from the nasal dorsum (Fig. 8B). The incision is then extended around the piriform margin and nasal floor, passing the knife in one motion through the epithelium, soft tissue, and periosteum (Fig. 8C). This completes a circumvestibular release. Care should be taken to position this incision at the juncture of the vestibular skin and nasal mucosa. Placement too close to the external nasal skin will compromise and complicate the final closure. The extent of the disease may necessitate special considerations in designing the incisions. The nasal soft tissues are then widely elevated in the subperiosteal plane with either the curved Joseph knife or with fine Metzenbaum scissors. It is essential that this dissection be carried down to the juncture of the nasal bones with the frontal process of the maxilla. Care must be taken to separate all adhesions between the nasal skeleton and the overlying tissue so that complete elevation is possible (Fig. 8D).

Plate 109

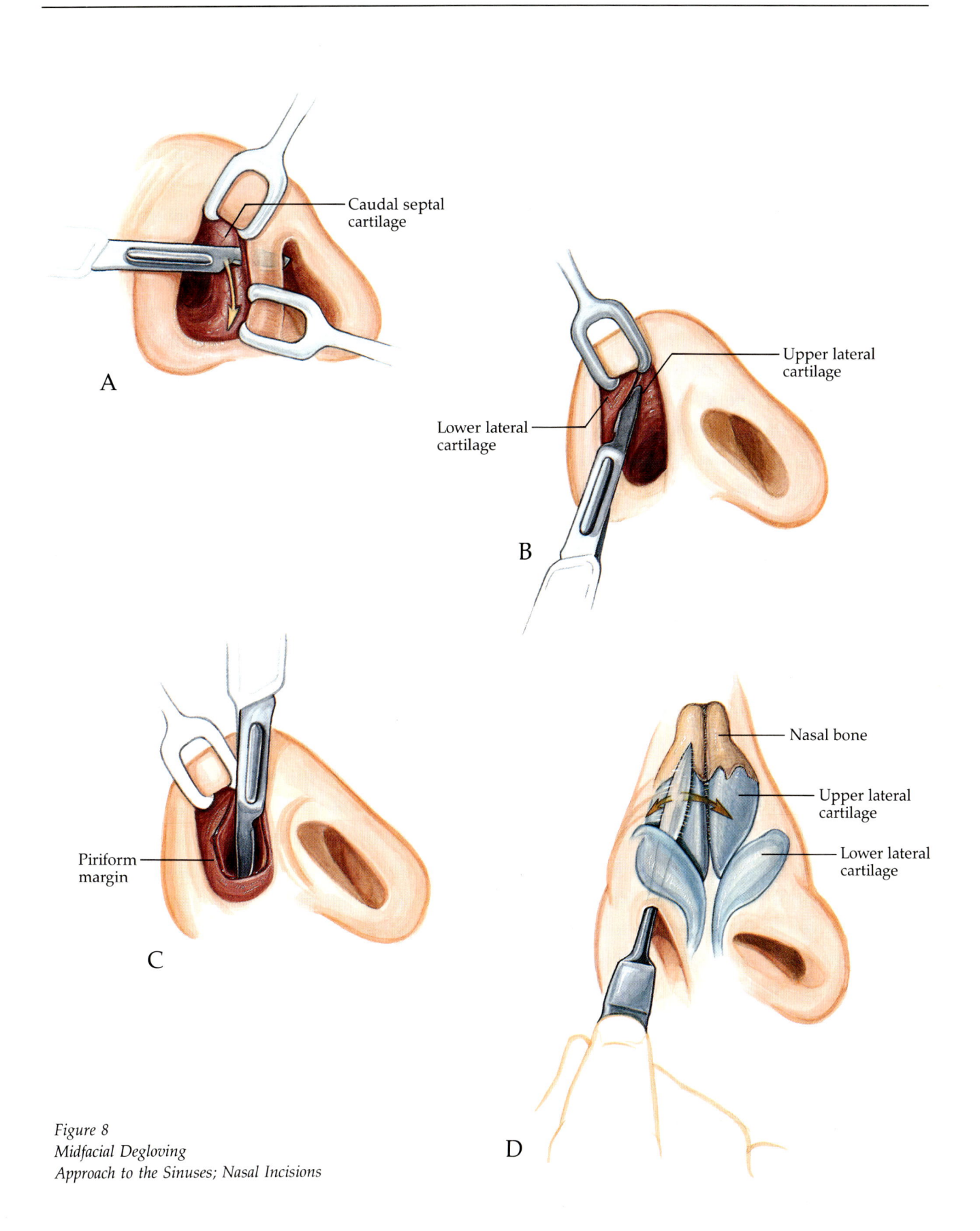

Figure 8
Midfacial Degloving
Approach to the Sinuses; Nasal Incisions

A — Caudal septal cartilage

B — Upper lateral cartilage; Lower lateral cartilage

C — Piriform margin

D — Nasal bone; Upper lateral cartilage; Lower lateral cartilage

255

The sublabial incision is made with a No. 15 blade and usually extends across the midline to just above the first molars (Fig. 8E). Unilateral extension of the incision can be carried beyond the maxillary tuberosity and onto the palate as necessary to gain access to the pterygomaxillary space for lateral control of tumors or for palatectomy or maxillectomy. The soft tissues over the anterior maxilla are elevated in the subperiosteal plane (Fig. 8F). This dissection is taken widely to expose the lateral limit of the anterior maxilla and the inferior orbital rim. The lateral surface of the maxilla and the pterygomaxillary space may also be exposed. Care is taken to identify and protect the infraorbital nerve and vessels. Dissection is carried well around this neurovascular bundle laterally up to the inferior orbital rim. The remaining soft tissue attachments to the anterior maxillary spine and nasal floor are separated using Metzenbaum scissors and working through the nasal incisions. Attempting to do this from the sublabial approach may result in two sets of incisions inside the nose and may compromise the soft tissue reconstruction or the tumor margin. The cheek

Plate 110

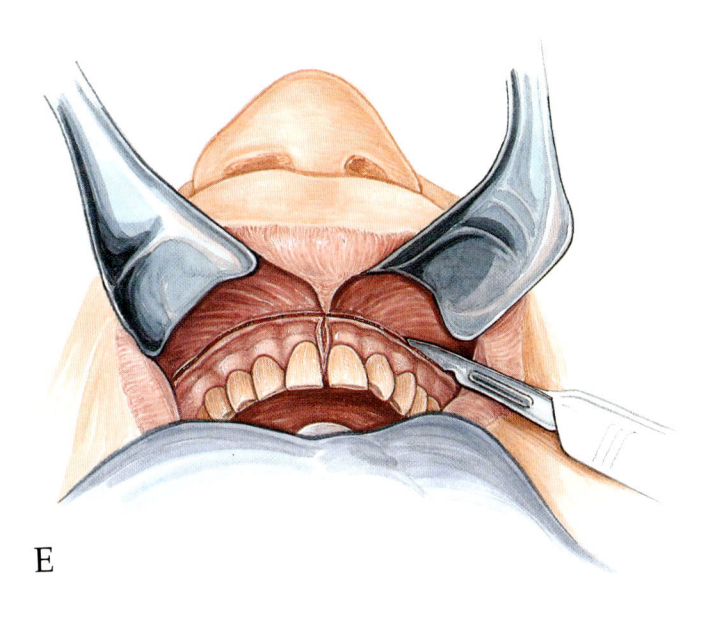

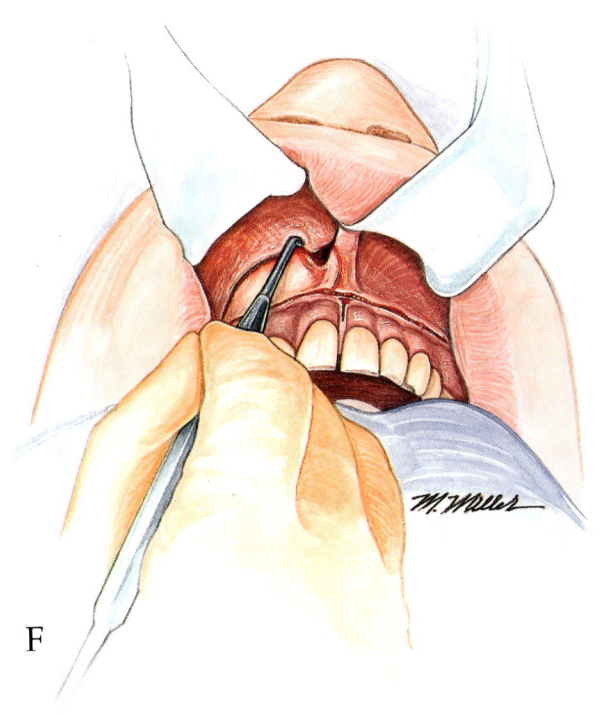

E

F

Figure 8 (Continued)
Midfacial Degloving
Approach to the Sinuses; Oral Incisions

and nasal soft tissues are retracted upward with Army-Navy or equivalent retractors. A residual adhesion of periosteum to bone becomes apparent between the nasal dorsal and maxillary tunnels (Fig. 8G). This is lysed by inserting one blade of the scissors into each tunnel and holding the scissors tightly against the bone as the tissue is sectioned. This final maneuver allows the facial soft tissues, the upper lip, the intact columella, and the nasal tip, including the alar cartilages to be retracted over the nose to the level of the medial canthus, thereby providing the final exposure (Fig. 8H). The superiorly and inferiorly based bipedicle flap allows preservation of additional nasal mucosa on the side of resection (Fig. 8I). Medium Richardson retractors or Jones antrostomy retractors are well suited for this task. Large Weitlaner self-retaining retractors are useful for maintaining exposure during microsurgical procedures.

Bone is then resected to expose and allow surgical removal of the lesion. Typically, Kerrison rongeurs are utilized to remove the entire anterior wall of the maxilla from its lateralmost extent well around the medial and lateral aspects of the infraorbital foramen and high onto the frontal process of the maxilla. Medial maxillectomy, complete ethmoidectomy, and sphenoidectomy are then accomplished in a sequential fashion. The entire nasal septum is then accessible and may be released and deflected by incising along the nasal floor ipsilateral to the medial maxillectomy, by separating the cartilage from the maxillary crest with a cartilage knife, and by elevating the mucoperiosteum from the contralateral nasal floor. The septum may be partially or totally resected, although it is usually possible to preserve a dorsal and caudal strip in order to provide tip support for preservation of nasal contour and function. The cribriform plate can then be brought into view by lowering the top of the head approximately 30 degrees and by angling the chin toward the surgeon 15 degrees. This allows careful inspection of the cribriform and fovea ethmoidale for residual disease, dural tears, or cerebrospinal fluid leakage. These steps may be duplicated as needed on the opposite side. The exposure is usually adequate for most nasal problems. Full access to the nasopharynx may require removal of the posterior wall of the maxillary antrum and of the heavy ascending process of the palatine bone. An otologic drill with a cutting bur greatly facilitates this maneuver. The greater palatine foramen is disrupted, and brisk bleeding is usually encountered from the palatine artery. Adequate suction and bipolar bayonet cautery forceps are necessary to control the bleeding. Access is thereby gained to the pterygoid muscles and plates, the posterior wall of the sphenoid sinus, the nasopharynx, and the base of the sphenoid (clivus). A drill with a large, coarse diamond bur may then be employed under microscopic control to resect the pterygoid plates and the clivus back to the optic nerve and chiasm and the dura over the pituitary and the posterior cranial fossa. This establishes the posterior limits of resection. The petrous apex is not accessible by this approach, being limited by the carotid arteries laterally and the optic nerve superiorly. The cribriform plate and anterior cranial fossa are the superior limits of dissection, although the cribriform may be safely removed when osteotomies are made through a bifrontal craniotomy. The lateral limit of the dissection is the

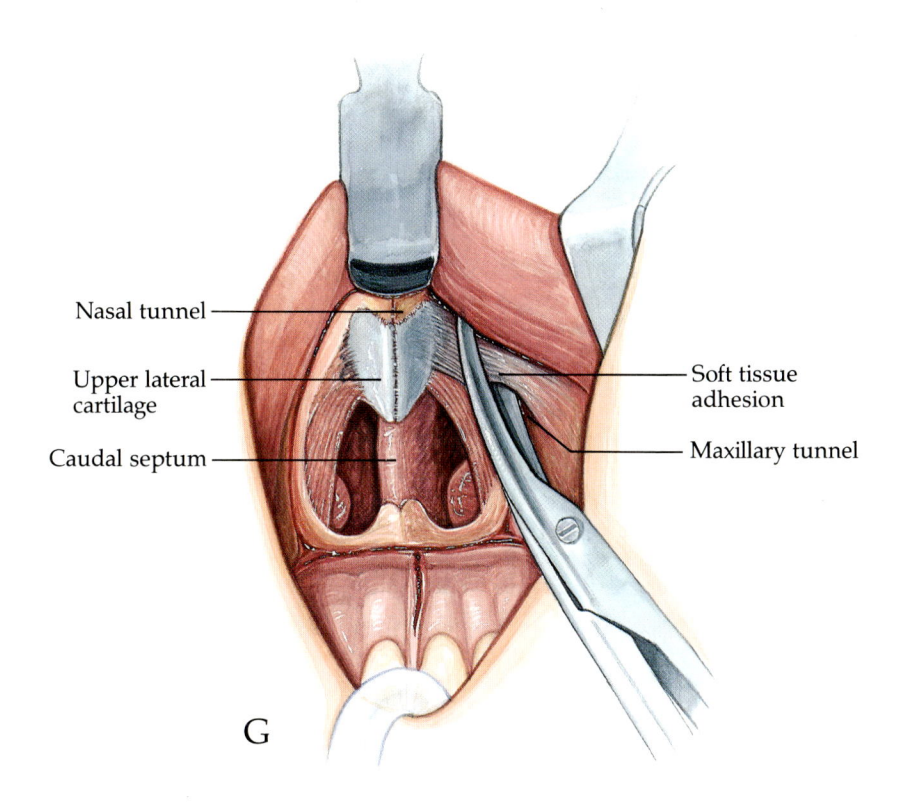

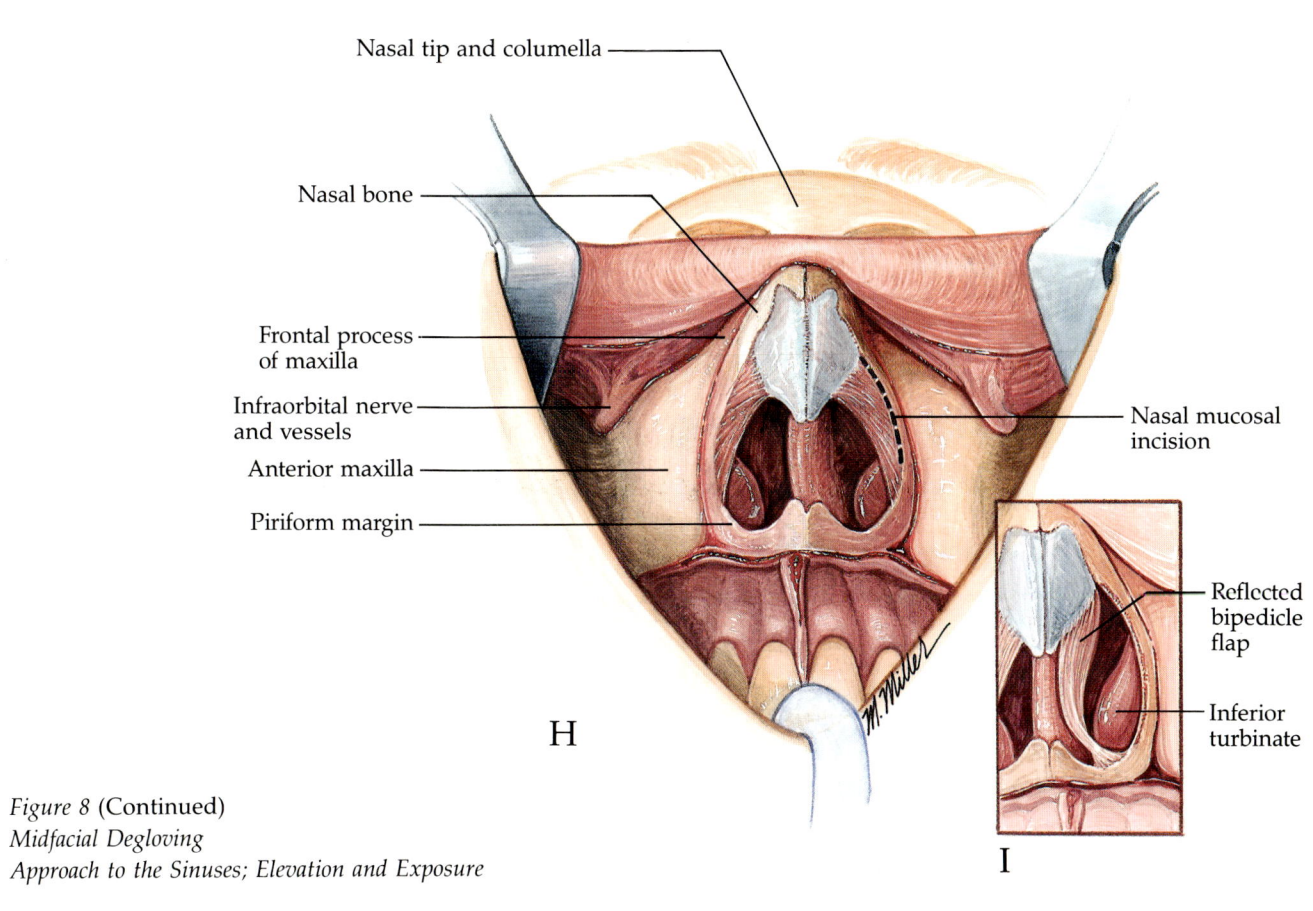

Plate 111

G — labels: Nasal tunnel, Upper lateral cartilage, Caudal septum, Soft tissue adhesion, Maxillary tunnel

H — labels: Nasal tip and columella, Nasal bone, Frontal process of maxilla, Infraorbital nerve and vessels, Anterior maxilla, Piriform margin, Nasal mucosal incision

I — labels: Reflected bipedicle flap, Inferior turbinate

Figure 8 (Continued)
Midfacial Degloving
Approach to the Sinuses; Elevation and Exposure

mandible anteriorly and the carotid arteries posteriorly. The inferior boundary is usually the palate. Palatectomy and inferior maxillectomy, however, may be easily done with this approach.

Bone spicules and rough surfaces should be carefully smoothed with a large diamond bur. Hemostasis is achieved initially by the application of a temporary packing saturated with 1 percent phenylephrine hydrochloride (Neo-Synephrine) solution or 1 ml of 1:1,000 epinephrine diluted in 10 ml of normal saline. This is removed, and any discrete bleeders are cauterized with the bipolar bayonet forceps. It may become necessary to pack areas of diffuse oozing with Gelfoam or Avitene. Split-thickness skin grafting in the cavity is employed only when additional protection and support for large dural defects are needed. In general, the presence of split-skin grafts inside the nasal cavity increases the problems with crusting and with fetid nasal odor; unless specifically indicated, they are undesirable. If the use of a graft is indicated, it is placed against the dura or pericranial flap, and a contoured Gelfilm support is placed against the keratinized surface. One half-inch antibiotic-saturated petrolatum gauze is then packed firmly in the cavity. Six to nine feet of gauze may be required on each side if a major resection is done. Packing is initially layered to be even with the anterior maxilla, and then the extra length is passed through the nostril.

The nasal tip is carefully repositioned with the transfixion suture of 3–0 chromic on a Keith needle (Fig. 8J). The sutures must be placed with extreme accuracy, as they determine the final healing position of the nose. The vestibular skin is then carefully sutured to the nasal mucosa with a minimum of three 4–0 polyglycolic acid sutures positioned in the intracartilaginous, piriform, and nasal floor areas (Fig. 8K). The midline of the sublabial incision (frenulum) is carefully approximated, and a one-layer closure incorporating the mucosa and periosteum is completed with running interlocking 3–0 polyglycolic acid suture (Fig. 8L). The skin is then carefully cleaned, dried, and prepared with benzoin and rhinoplastic taping, and splinting is applied to reduce facial edema.

Postoperative Care

Packing should be removed by twice daily advancements, beginning on the third or fourth postoperative day; antibiotic therapy is continued until all packing is removed. Crusting may present a significant early problem, but this should resolve in 2 to 3 months. Initially, meticulous care with frequent removal of the crust is required. Irrigation with physiologic saline by nasal syringe four times daily is essential while healing progresses and must start immediately. The cavity walls should be lined with healthy granulation tissue when the packing is removed; this tissue will then be covered by metaplastic epithelium.

Plate 112

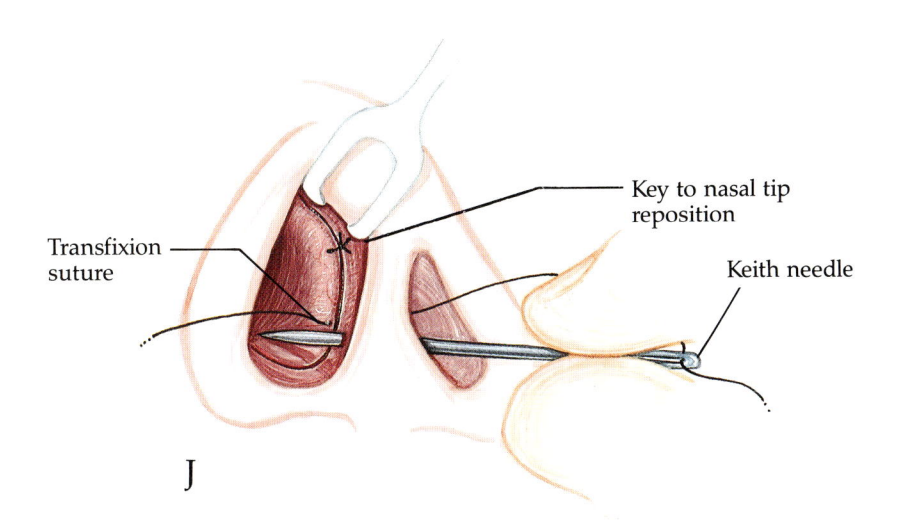

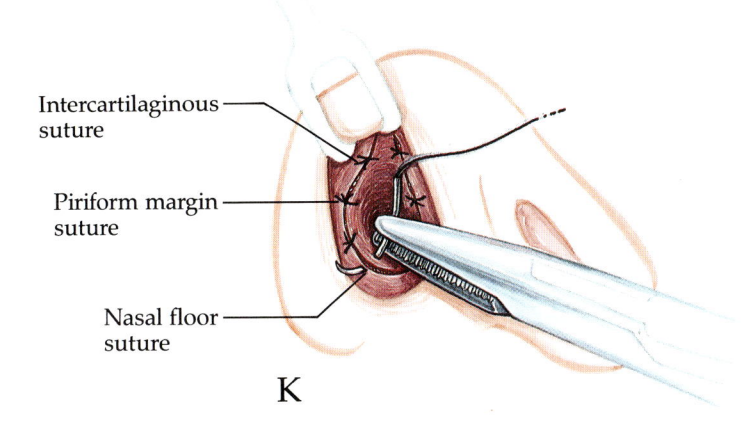

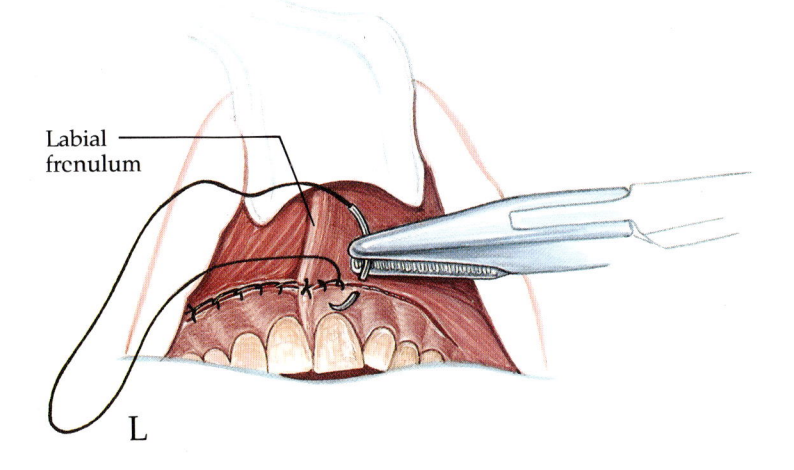

- Transfixion suture
- Key to nasal tip reposition
- Keith needle

J

- Intercartilaginous suture
- Piriform margin suture
- Nasal floor suture

K

- Labial frenulum

L

Figure 8 (Continued)
Midfacial Degloving
Approach to the Sinuses; Closure

Risks, Complications, and Sequelae

Moderate nasal crusting poses a problem during the first 3 months postoperatively; however, no cases of ozena have been reported. The most frequent complaint voiced by patients is that of infraorbital and dental numbness and paresthesias. This problem usually resolves within 3 to 6 months. Hemipalatal anesthesia may occur when resection of the greater palatine canal is required. This is a highly vascular area and operative bleeding can be considerable. Transfusion may be necessary. Dorsal nasal hematomas have been encountered in patients in whom unusual operative bleeding was a problem.

Hyperplastic collagen deposition has occurred beneath the flap (over the nose and maxilla), resulting in a "sneer" deformity. This was evident 6 weeks postoperatively and then slowly resolved. Vestibular stenosis has been reported. Vestibular narrowing resembling early stenosis is commonly seen during the phase of active collagen deposition, which occurs between 6 and 12 weeks postoperatively. This should uniformly resolve without treatment. Disturbance of facial growth centers in infants and young children has not been seen with degloving surgery. Epiphora and oroantral fistula have not been problems; however, these must be considered potential complications.

Pearls and Pitfalls

This is not an external rhinoplasty. No cutaneous incisions are made in the columella. The intact columella and the complete alar cartilage (including the medial and lateral crura) remain attached to the lip and facial soft tissues. The nasal septum and upper lateral cartilages are maintained in their normal positions.

The blood supply of the midfacial flap is derived from the facial, infraorbital, supratrochlear, and transverse facial vessels. This rich vascularity allows the addition of medial orbital, lateral nasal, or lip-splitting incisions, which are required by the extended exposure. Considerable blood loss can be markedly reduced by the use of dilute epinephrine in a local anesthetic solution.

Preservation of as much anterolateral mucosa as possible is desirable but should not interfere with adequate management of the disease process. The use of a bipedicle mucosal flap is recommended when it does not compromise resection margins.

The infraorbital canal, foramen, and neurovascular bundle can be freed by osteotomies along each side of the canal. Improved mobility of the flap and increased access to the orbits are thereby obtained.

Exposure of the nasofrontal duct may not be adequate; the pathologic process in this area may require the addition of a frontoethmoid incision or an entirely different approach.

Accurate positioning of the nasal tip and meticulous repair of the vestibule are critical to a reasonable cosmetic result and to avoiding vestibular stenosis. Proper taping and splinting decrease edema and the risk of dorsal nasal hematoma.

The nasal packing should remain in place for several days. This allows for epithelial healing of the vestibular incisions and stimulates rapid coverage of the resection bed with healthy granulation tissue. Once the packing is removed, any exposed bone can dramatically increase the amount of crusting and consequently increase the risk of significant osteitis. The use of a eucalyptus-based nasal emollient (such as Ponaris) three to four times daily following irrigations can significantly decrease the amount of crusting.

Nasal vestibular narrowing seen between 6 and 12 weeks following the operation does not necessarily represent stenosis. This is simply the active collagen deposition of normal scar formation and has uniformly resolved without treatment. Persistence of this condition beyond 6 months, however, may require the injection of deposteroids into the scar.

Suggested Reading

Allen GW, Siegel GJ. The sublabial approach for extensive nasal and sinus resection. Laryngoscope 1981; 91:1635–1640.

Casson PR, Bonanno PC, Converse JM. The midfacial degloving procedure. Plast Reconstr Surg 1974; 53:102–103.

Conley J, Price JC. Sublabial approach to the nasal and nasopharyngeal cavities. Am J Surg 1979; 138:615–618.

Maniglia AJ. Indications and techniques of midfacial degloving; A 15-year experience. Arch Otolaryngol Head Neck Surg 1986; 112:750–752.

Price JC. The midfacial degloving approach to the central skull base. Ear Nose Throat J 1986; 65:46–53.

Price JC, Holliday M, Kennedy D, et al. The versatile midfacial degloving approach. Laryngoscope 1986; 98:291–295.

Sacks ME, Conley J, Rabuzzi DD, et al. The degloving approach for total excision of inverted papilloma. Laryngoscope 1984; 94:1595–1598.

Terzian AE, Naconecy C. Juvenile nasopharyngeal angiofibroma; microsurgical approach in 25 cases as unique treatment. In: Myers EN, ed. New dimensions in otorhinolaryngology–head and neck surgery. Vol 2. New York: Elsevier, 1985:505–506.

John C. Price, M.D.
Wayne M. Koch, M.D.

MEDIAL MAXILLECTOMY

Indications

The exact procedure performed to remove tumors in the maxilla is determined by the oncologic aggressiveness of the lesion and its precise location. Medial maxillectomy is the procedure of choice for benign or low-grade malignant tumors involving the medial maxilla or lateral nasal cavity. Inverted papilloma is the most common of these lesions, which also include various minor salivary gland neoplasms. The ethmoid air cells are exposed in the standard medial maxillectomy procedure, but known tumor extension into the ethmoid sinus is an indication for extension of the procedure to include en bloc ethmoidectomy (see further on).

Preoperative Considerations

Physical examination with rigid Hopkins rod telescopes allows the surgeon to estimate the intranasal extent of lesions involving the medial maxilla as well as the status of the ostiomeatal complex. The status of the cranial nerves and extraocular mobility should be carefully noted. Exophthalmos or fullness of the malar region or canine fossa indicates an expansile lesion within the maxilla. Serous otitis on otoscopic examination may indicate nasopharyngeal involvement.

Modern radiographic studies have taken much of the guesswork out of preoperative planning for these cases. Conceptualization of the three-dimensional limits required for adequate tumor extirpation is greatly facilitated by axial and coronal computed tomographic studies, and axial, sagittal, and coronal magnetic resonance imaging. In addition to detection of tumor extent with these modalities, bone erosion, the presence of surrounding inflammation, and the degree of vascularity may be ascertained. Lesions with significant blush on computed tomographic scans with intravenous contrast material should be further investigated by arteriography. Embolization of major feeding vessels with Gelfoam at the time of arteriography may greatly reduce vascularity and thus blood loss at surgery. Surgery must follow the embolization within 24 hours in order to take advantage of this benefit; thereafter, the vessels reopen.

Intranasal biopsy may be performed on an outpatient basis in some cases. Once again, sinus endoscopic equipment is valuable in obtaining tissue from the area of interest. Radiographic studies should be obtained beforehand to assess the degree of vascularity and to rule out a direct communication with the central nervous system, as with an encephalocele. Only with a firm diagnosis based on a preoperative biopsy can surgical planning to limit resection to a medial maxillectomy be made with any degree of certainty. If histologic results are unobtainable, the patient must be prepared for a more extensive procedure and the decision made at sinusotomy at the outset of the resection.

A blood sample for typing and cross-matching should be sent to the blood bank in addition to the laboratory for routine preoperative studies.

Operative Steps

The midface degloving approach is an ideal approach for an unextended medial maxillectomy. Both orbits are protected by tarsorrhaphy, and the face is prepared and draped. A topical vasoconstrictor is placed in the nasal cavity on cotton pledgets, and local anesthetic with vasoconstrictor is injected into the planned incision sites.

After the incision is made, soft tissue is elevated off the anterior maxilla, exposing and preserving the infraorbital nerve. Care should be taken not to violate the orbital septum so as to avoid extrusion of fat. The nasal aperture is opened fully. If the histologic type of the tumor or its extent within the maxillary antrum is unknown, an anterior sinusotomy is performed. The bone is cut with a narrow chisel in an eggshell fashion approximately 1 cm inferior to the infraorbital foramen. The opening is widened with rongeurs to the floor of the antrum below, the infraorbital foramen above, the maxillary buttress laterally, and the lateral nasal wall medially (Fig. 9A). Sinus contents are inspected and biopsies taken for frozen section examination.

When sinusotomy is not required, bone cuts may be made with a chisel or sagittal saw from the superior nasal aperture laterally below the orbital rim and then inferiorly near the infraorbital foramen to meet a second horizontal cut at the level of the floor of the nose. If the patient is a child, care must be taken to ensure that the lower incision spares unerupted permanent teeth if at all possible. Posteriorly directed osteotomies are performed along the floor of the nose and the top of the middle meatus (Fig. 9B). The posterior maxillary sinus wall can be removed piecemeal if it is not involved with disease, exposing the pterygomaxillary fossa, including the internal maxillary artery and its branches. If possible, these should be identified and controlled at this point. Intranasal cuts along the floor and at the middle meatus are completed with curved Mayo scissors (Fig. 9C).

Plate 113

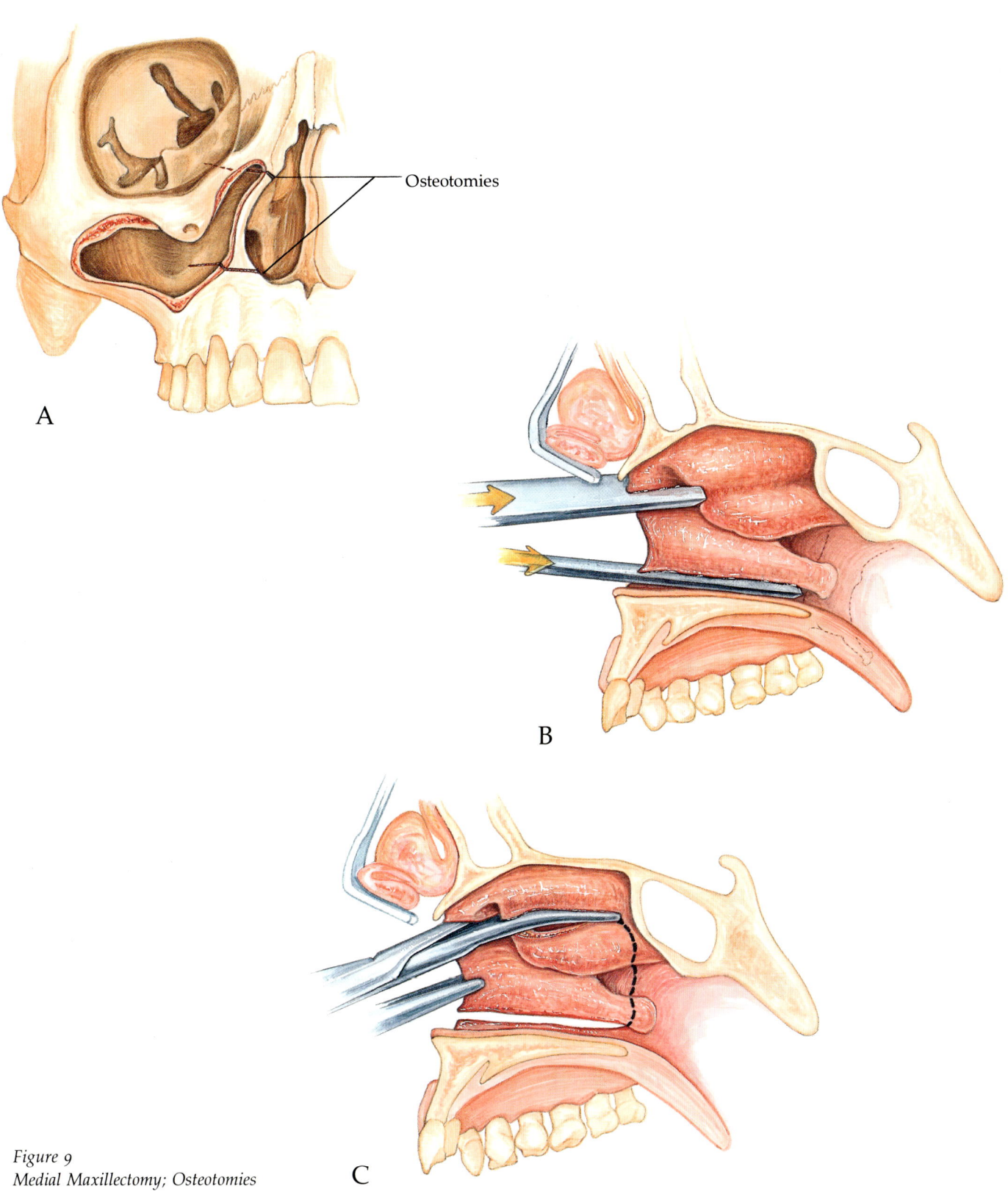

Osteotomies

A

B

C

Figure 9
Medial Maxillectomy; Osteotomies

Immediate control of hemorrhage is achieved by packing the cavity with a moist sponge followed by use of a bipolar electrocautery and suture ligature.

Exposed ethmoid air cells should be opened fully (Fig. 9D). Residual turbinate tissue is also removed (Fig. 9E). Special attention is given to the nasofrontal recess, which must be widely patent. Any bony rim separating the nasal floor from that of the maxillary antrum must be taken down. The surgical site is packed with gauze ribbon soaked in antibiotic ointment and placed to facilitate removal via the nares. Incisions are closed in layers.

Postoperative Care

Ice packs applied to the cheek help to control swelling in the immediate postoperative period. The patient may begin oral feeding and ambulation as soon after surgery as possible. Intravenous antibiotics should be maintained as long as the nose is packed. Packing is generally removed after 24 to 48 hours, depending on the vascularity of the tumor and the adequacy of intraoperative hemostasis. After packing has been removed, saline lavage or spray using a water pick is initiated to minimize crust accumulation. Crusts are removed periodically, assisted by endoscopic equipment. Sinus endoscopy also allows for removal of granulations from the nasofrontal recess during outpatient visits. A humidifier is useful to prevent excessive drying of the cavity.

Periodic examinations to rule out recurrent tumor are necessary; their frequency is based on the pathologic diagnosis. Computed tomographic scan, magnetic resonance imaging, and sinus endoscopy allow for careful monitoring and early detection of recurrence.

Risks, Complications, and Sequelae

Following the procedure, risks, complications, and sequelae include (1) numbness of cheek skin and teeth; (2) devitalized maxillary teeth; (3) nasal dryness and crusting; (4) frontal and ethmoid sinusitis; (5) conductive hearing loss due to eustachian tube dysfunction; (6) osteitis and sequestration of residual ethmoid bone spicules; (7) cerebrospinal fluid leak; and (8) meningitis.

Pearls and Pitfalls

The infraorbital nerve may undergo dehiscence along its course at the roof of the maxillary antrum. If this area is free of disease, it should not be disturbed in order to preserve sensation of the cheek.

Transantral ethmoidectomy should not extend above the level of the root of the medial turbinate so as to avoid entry into the cranial cavity. A stump of the turbinate should be left in place as a landmark.

Unipolar electrocautery should not be used in the posterior maxillary antrum, where conduction of the current can result in damage to the optic nerve. Bipolar cautery of small vessels and ligation of larger branches of the internal maxillary artery are preferred.

Medial Maxillectomy

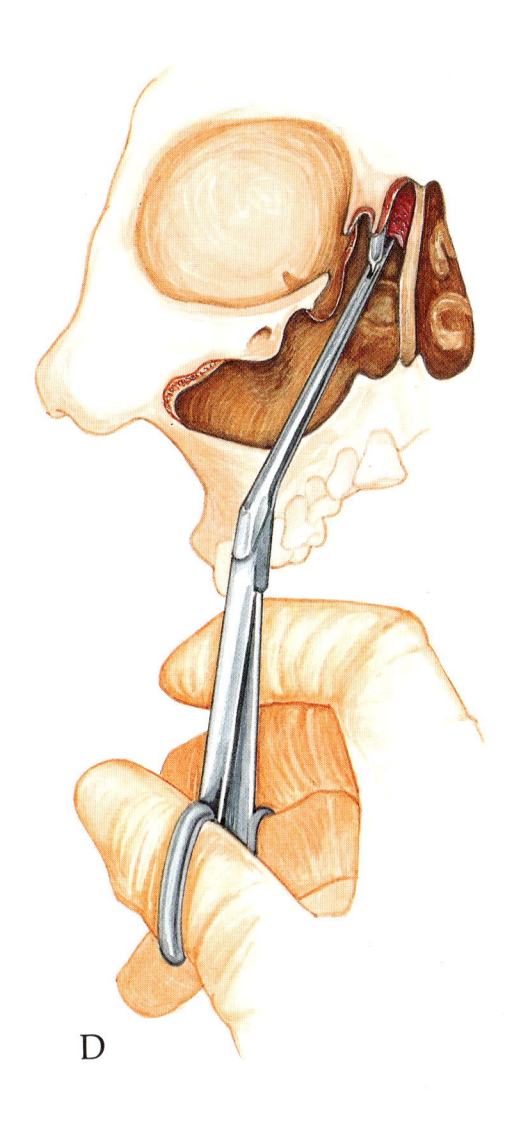

Plate 114
Figure 9 (Continued)
Medial Maxillectomy; Ethmoidectomy

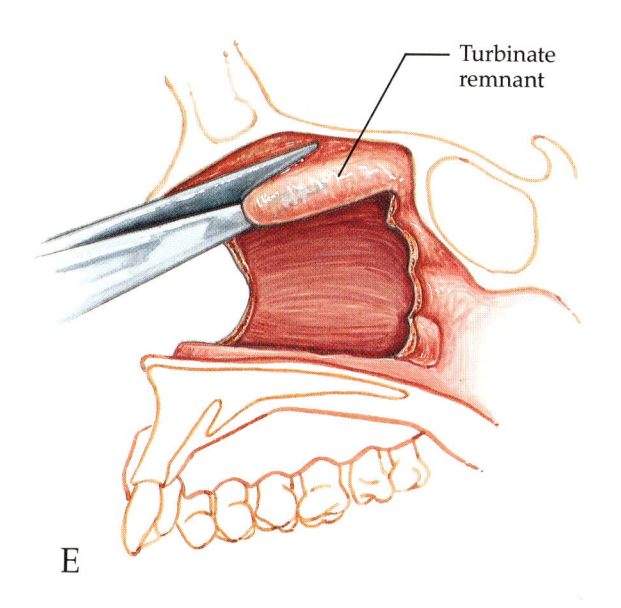

Excessive resection of the anterior maxillary sinus wall inferiorly endangers maxillary tooth roots.

Myringotomy and tube insertion may be required in the ipsilateral ear if the eustachian tube orifice is disturbed. Prophylactic tube insertion is indicated in cases in which postoperative otitis media is likely to occur.

Wayne M. Koch, M.D.
John C. Price, M.D.

LATERAL RHINOTOMY APPROACH TO THE SINUSES

Indications

Lateral rhinotomy was the standard approach to the medial maxilla, ethmoid sinus, and nasal cavity until the past decade, when it was replaced to some degree by the midfacial degloving approach (see page 251). Lateral rhinotomy has the obvious disadvantage of leaving a scar on the midface. However, a properly placed incision that heals without complications is cosmetically acceptable in most cases. Lateral rhinotomy allows access to the anterior ethmoid and frontal sinuses, which are not easily visualized via the degloving approach. It may also be chosen when there is a question of involvement of the soft tissue overlying the nasal dorsum and maxilla.

Operative Steps

A tarsorrhaphy stitch is placed, and the skin of the face is prepared and draped. The incision is marked parallel to the lower border of the eyebrow, then turning sharply downward at a point midway between the medial canthus and the dorsum of the nose. Here, the linear incision is broken by a W before it continues in the nasofacial sulcus and around the base of the nasal ala. A local anesthetic agent with vasoconstrictor (1 percent lidocaine with 1:100,000 epinephrine) is injected intradermally along the planned incision and into the mucosa of the nasal vestibule. Several superficial scratches made with the back of the scalpel perpendicular to the incision ensure that the skin can be accurately closed at the end of the procedure. The incision is then made beginning beneath the brow at an angle parallel to the hair fibers. It should be continued to the bone of the orbital rim in a single stroke. The W at the medial canthus may best be outlined with a No. 11 blade, and the incision completed to the alar base. The base is then released using an intranasal incision continuing superiorly along the piriform aperture (Fig. 10A). Hemostasis is achieved with electrocautery except at the angular vein, which should be ligated.

Periosteal elevators are used to raise soft tissue from the maxilla and nasal bone. The infraorbital nerve and lacrimal duct may be isolated and preserved, if possible allowing for adequate removal of diseased tissue (Fig. 10B).

When the resection is complete, the lateral rhinotomy incision is closed in layers, including three layers at the nasal aperture. If the medial canthal ligament was separated in the course of the procedure, it should be repositioned on the remaining nasal bone using a heavy, permanent suture. After the resection of all disease is completed, the incision is closed in layers—the mucosa of the nose and subcutaneous tissue with absorbable suture, and the epidermis with fine nylon suture.

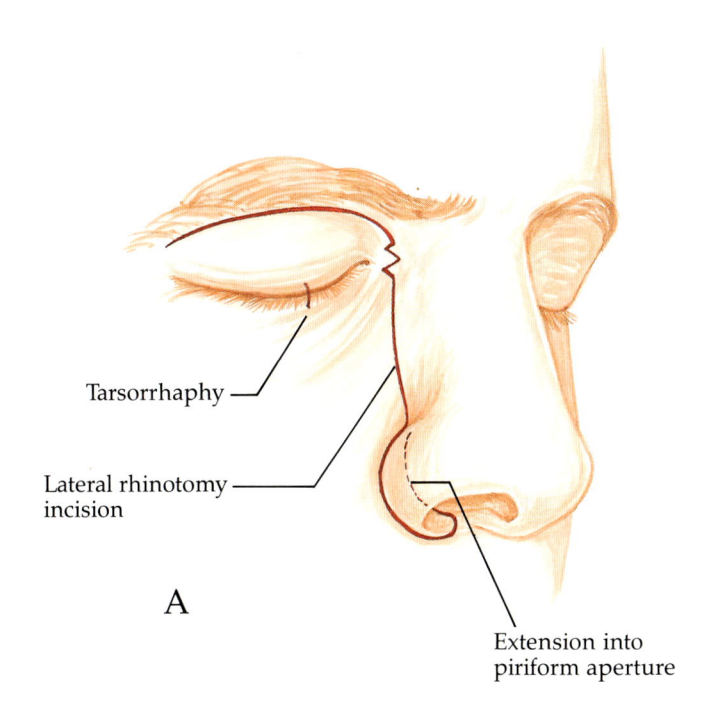

Plate 115

A

Tarsorrhaphy

Lateral rhinotomy incision

Extension into piriform aperture

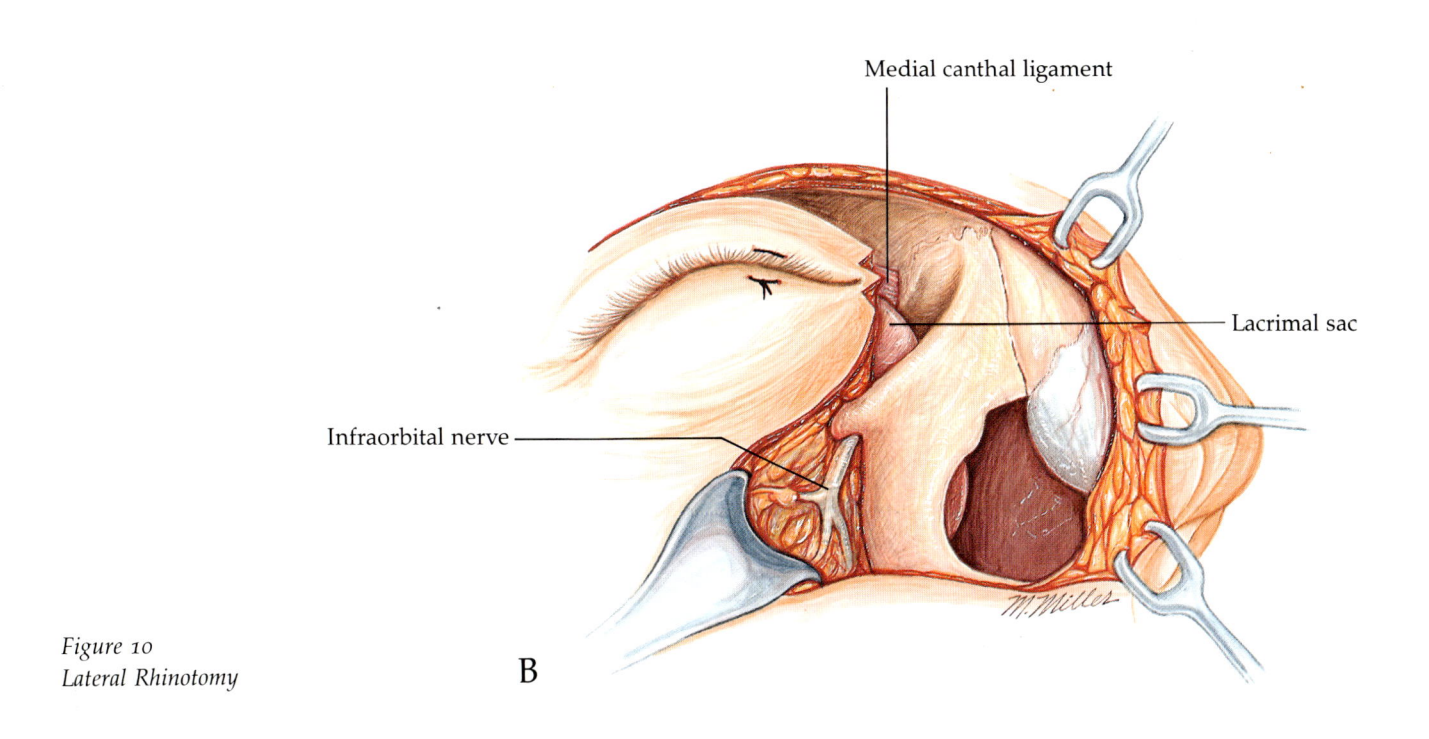

Medial canthal ligament

Lacrimal sac

Infraorbital nerve

Figure 10
Lateral Rhinotomy

B

271

Postoperative Care

The suture line is cleaned with peroxide and protected with antibiotic ointment. Skin sutures are removed after 5 days.

Risks, Complications, and Sequelae

The surgeon should be alert to the following risks, complications, and sequelae: (1) wound infection; (2) bleeding; (3) allergic reaction to local anesthetic agents; (4) hypertrophic scar or keloid formation with unacceptable cosmesis; (5) diplopia; (6) misplaced medial canthus with hypertelorism; and (7) webbing of the scar at the medial canthus with pseudohypertelorism.

Pearls and Pitfalls

A cross-hatch mark at the base of the alar lobule made prior to incision helps direct the alignment of skin edges at closure.

Improper angling of the incision beneath the eyebrow transects hair roots, causing hair loss.

Repositioning of the medial canthal ligament must be precise. Careful comparison with the contralateral eye to judge accuracy is required until satisfactory results are obtained. This often requires several "trial and error" attempts.

Wayne M. Koch, M.D.
John C. Price, M.D.

MEDIAL MAXILLECTOMY WITH EN BLOC ETHMOIDECTOMY

Indications

When a benign or low-grade malignant tumor involves the ethmoid air cells in addition to the maxillary antrum and lateral nasal wall, resection of the medial maxilla may be extended superiorly to include the ethmoid sinus, en bloc. This procedure is not sufficient when tumor extends to the skull base, orbit, or lateral maxilla. Involvement of the cribriform plate is an indication for craniofacial resection, and radical maxillectomy is required when the orbit or lateral antrum is invaded by tumor.

Preoperative Considerations

In addition to those discussed previously for medial maxillectomy, the patient undergoing en bloc ethmoidectomy is evaluated preoperatively by an ophthalmologist to assess visual acuity and extraocular muscular function. Informed consent must include discussion of the facial incision (lateral rhinotomy) and the additional risk to the optic nerve in the extended procedure.

Operative Steps

Lesions that extend high into the anterior ethmoid air cells or the nasofrontal recess are not easily reached via the midfacial degloving approach and require a lateral rhinotomy. The ipsilateral orbit is protected by tarsorrhaphy, and the face is prepared and draped. Cotton pledgets with topical vasoconstrictor are placed in the nasal cavity, and local anesthetic with vasoconstrictor is injected into the planned incisions. After the incision has been made and hemostasis has been achieved, soft tissue elevation in the subperiosteal plane opens the nasal aperture and extends laterally, sparing the infraorbital nerve. The medial canthal ligament is detached bluntly and the lacrimal apparatus elevated from the fossa. The orbital contents must be elevated bluntly off the lamina papyracea, leaving the periorbita intact. The globe may be gently retracted laterally using a slightly bent medium malleable retractor. The lacrimal duct may be transected sharply and the sac marsupialized by opening it vertically from the cut edge of the duct upward. The anterior and posterior ethmoidal arteries are identified and cauterized with bipolar current (see Fig. 12F) or ligated with silk suture or surgical clips. The nasal bone is then separated from the frontal process of the maxilla with an osteotome, as in a rhinoplasty procedure. Chisel cuts through the ethmoid labyrinth continue posteriorly across the orbital process of the palatine bone and the pterygoid process of the sphenoid sinus, approaching the optic foramen and orbital fissures (Fig. 11). The lamina papyracea is freed in its entirety with further chisel cuts inferiorly to the orbital floor and along the floor to the orbital rim. A sagittal saw is used to cut the anterior wall inferiorly, sparing the infraorbital nerve. An osteotomy along the nasal floor is performed, and the specimen may be removed en bloc using Mayo scissors to separate remaining soft tissue attachments. After bleeding has been controlled, the lacrimal sac is sewn open with a fine permanent suture to allow drainage of tears into the open surgical cavity. The medial canthus must be repositioned using a heavy, permanent suture. The cavity is packed and the incisions are closed in layers.

Postoperative Care

The postoperative care is the same as that for degloving and lateral rhinotomy.

Risks, Complications, and Sequelae

In addition to those listed in the section on medial maxillectomy, the following may occur after this procedure: (1) epiphora; (2) diplopia; (3) blindness; and (4) pseudohypertelorism.

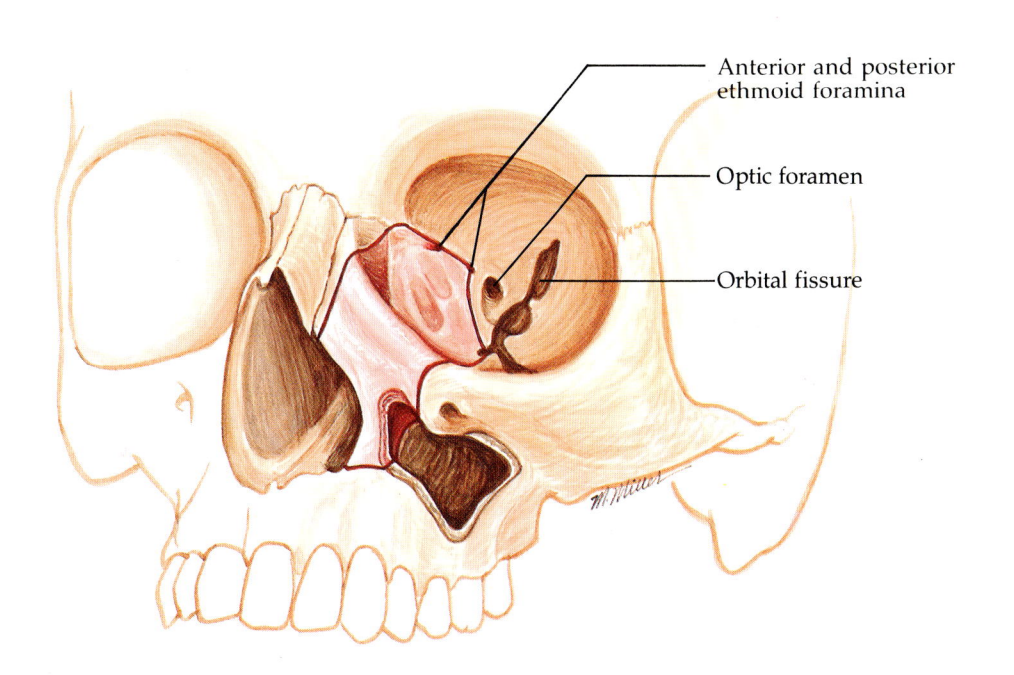

Plate 116
Figure 11
Medial Maxillectomy
with En Bloc Ethmoidectomy

Anterior and posterior ethmoid foramina

Optic foramen

Orbital fissure

Pearls and Pitfalls

A line joining the anterior and posterior ethmoidal arteries marks the floor of the anterior cranial fossa at the cribriform plate and, extended posteriorly, the location of the optic foramen. Osteotomies should not extend beyond this limit.

If the ipsilateral nasal bone has been removed in its entirety, the medial canthus may be fixed by suture extended to the nasal septum or opposite nasal bone. Care must be taken in positioning this structure to minimize epiphora, diplopia, and hypertelorism.

After the lacrimal sac is filleted, it is tacked open with permanent suture fixed to the periorbita. The duct and sac then will lie open in the defect of the nasal wall upon closure, allowing tears to enter the nasal cavity.

Wayne M. Koch, M.D.
John C. Price, M.D.

MAXILLECTOMY

Indications

All but the smallest, low-grade malignancies and benign lesions limited to the medial maxilla or lateral nasal wall require a surgical procedure more extensive than medial maxillectomy. The precise limits of the excision must be customized for the individual tumor; however, the goal in each case is the complete removal of neoplasm either with a margin of normal tissue (1.5 cm is suggested for malignant disease) or with an appropriate intact tumor barrier, such as periorbita, preferably en bloc. In general, total maxillectomy is indicated for advanced neoplasms of the antrum and ethmoid air cells. Extension to the hard palate or alveolus, the soft tissue of the cheek, the infratemporal fossa, the zygoma, or the pterygopalatine fossa requires that the procedure be modified. Tumor involvement of the middle fossa skull base or nasopharynx or massive bilateral maxillary disease or the presence of distant metastasis may change the scope of surgery required (for example, necessitating craniofacial resection) or limit the possibility of surgery with curative intent.

Preoperative Considerations

A complete physical examination, a radiographic evaluation (possibly with angiography and embolization), and a biopsy are performed preoperatively as discussed for medial maxillectomy. In addition, patients who are to undergo total maxillectomy should be seen in consultation by a prosthodontist. Dental impressions are taken and a prosthesis fashioned for placement at the close of the surgery. The status of the dentition remaining postoperatively is assessed in light of the potential need for adjuvant radiation therapy.

Ophthalmologic consultation is obtained to document baseline function, especially if removal of a significant portion of the orbital floor is contemplated. Informed consent should include a discussion of orbital exenteration if any chance of orbital involvement exists. Permission for a split-thickness skin graft is also obtained.

Maxillectomy

- Optional extension

A

Modified Dieffenbach-Weber-Fergusson incision

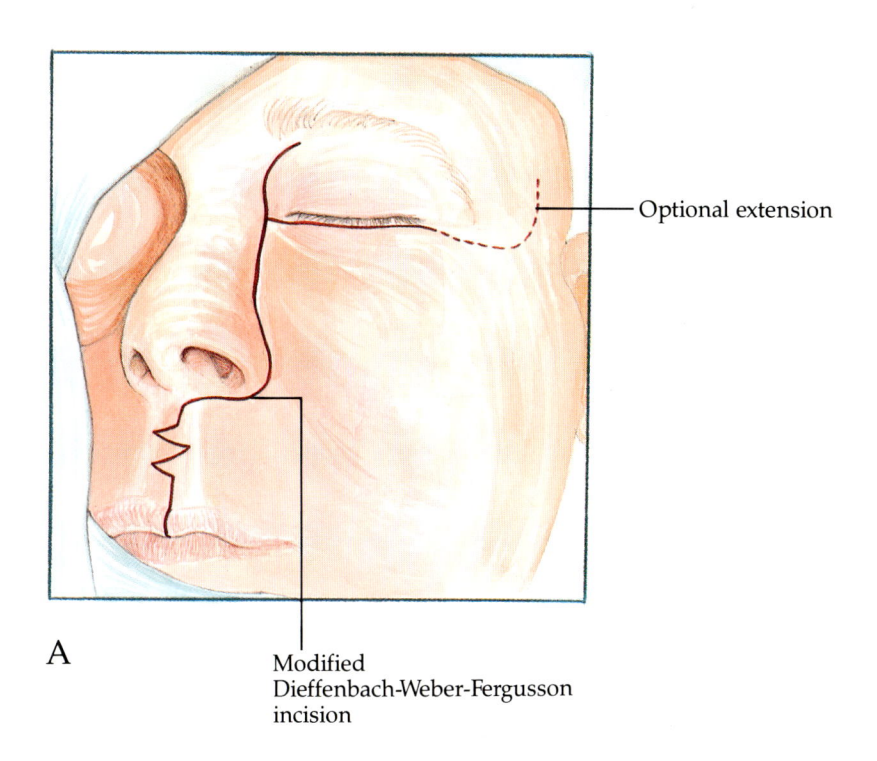

Plate 117
Figure 12
Maxillectomy; Incision

Operative Steps

A modification of the Dieffenbach-Weber-Fergusson incision (Fig. 12A) or a midfacial degloving approach is used. The facial incision has the advantage of ease of access to the soft tissue of the cheek, allowing flap elevation under direct scrutiny. This is useful in cases in which the anterior maxillary wall is eroded by disease, or palpation raises the question of soft-tissue invasion. A W placed in the incision at the philtrum prevents contraction from pulling the lip upward and interrupts the more noticeable linear scar.

The ipsilateral eye is protected by a tarsorrhaphy, and the incision is drawn on the skin and injected with epinephrine solution. The vertical portion of the incision in the nasofacial groove is completed with a single stroke carried down to the bone. The lip is held firmly on either side as the incision continues around the alar base and downward to the vermillion. After the W has been created through the full thickness of the dermis, the mucosa of the lip may be cut with a second linear stroke. Hemostatic control of the labial artery and angular vein is achieved, and the labiogingival incision is carried laterally to the hamulus. The skin of the lower lid is incised 2 mm below the lashes. At the lateral orbit, the orbital rim is identified bluntly, and a tunnel is created between the orbital septum and the orbicularis. After placing one blade in the tunnel and the other on the skin incision, a skin-muscle flap is created by a single scissors stroke, separating the muscle fibers just below the medial canthus.

The labial cheek flap is elevated laterally in the subperiosteal plane unless there is soft-tissue involvement by the tumor. The neurovascular bundle emanating from the infraorbital foramen is clamped, divided, and ligated (Fig. 12B). The periorbita is incised at the orbital rim immediately below the orbicularis oculi muscle fibers (Fig. 12C). Exposure of the orbital floor is achieved, avoiding penetration while elevating the periorbita from the orbital floor (Fig. 12D), and the globe is gently retracted upward (Fig. 12E). The lacrimal sac is elevated from its fossa, the duct transected, and the sac marsupialized. Depending on the superior extent of disease, the lamina papyracea is exposed and the ethmoidal arteries controlled (Fig. 12F) (see also Medial Maxillectomy with En Bloc Ethmoidectomy).

Figure 12 (Continued)
Maxillectomy; Exposure and Elevation of Orbital Contents

Plate 118

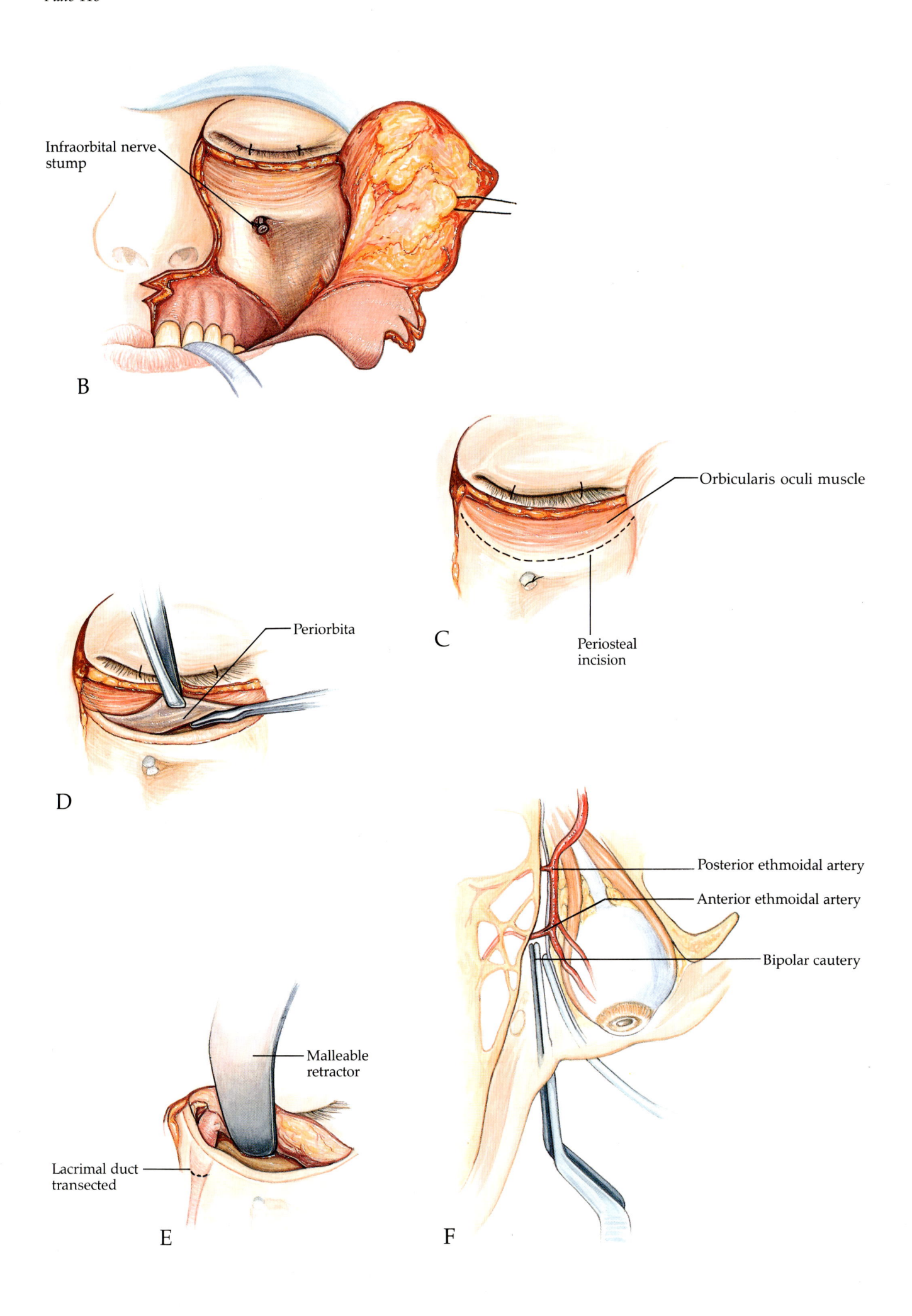

B
Infraorbital nerve stump

C
Orbicularis oculi muscle
Periosteal incision

D
Periorbita

E
Malleable retractor
Lacrimal duct transected

F
Posterior ethmoidal artery
Anterior ethmoidal artery
Bipolar cautery

Maxillectomy

Soft tissues of the nose are elevated medially, opening the piriform aperture. If a biopsy of the tumor has not been performed preoperatively, an anterior sinusotomy is done to obtain a specimen for frozen section examination. Appropriate bone cuts can then be made with a sagittal saw, chisel, or Gigli saw. Figures 12G and 12H demonstrate an example of the osteotomies for a total maxillectomy. The nasomaxillary process is cut from the nasal aperture to the orbital rim (Fig. 12I) and continued using a narrow osteotome posteriorly along the lamina papyracea, stopping short of the optic canal but entering the inferior orbital fissure if necessary (Fig. 12J). As much of the orbital floor is saved as is oncologically feasible in order to lend support to the globe. A vertical osteotomy from the orbital rim separates the specimen from the buttress of the zygoma (Fig. 12K).

Plate 119
Figure 12 (Continued)
Maxillectomy; Osteotomies

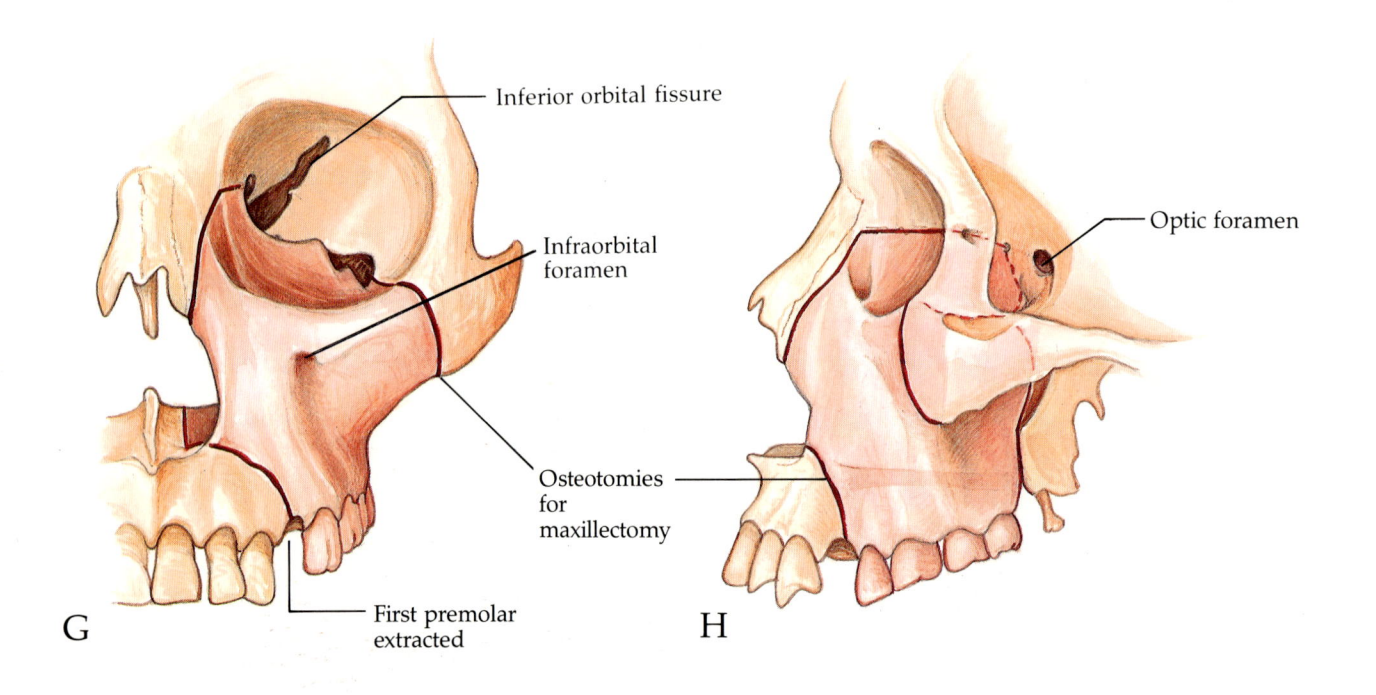

Plate 120

I

- Suction
- Irrigation
- Orbital contents retracted
- Nasomaxillary suture
- Osteotomy
- Lacrimal fossa
- Sagittal saw

J

- Narrow osteotome
- Anterior and posterior ethmoid foramina
- Optic canal
- Inferior orbital fissure

K

- Zygoma

Figure 12 (Continued)
Maxillectomy; Osteotomies

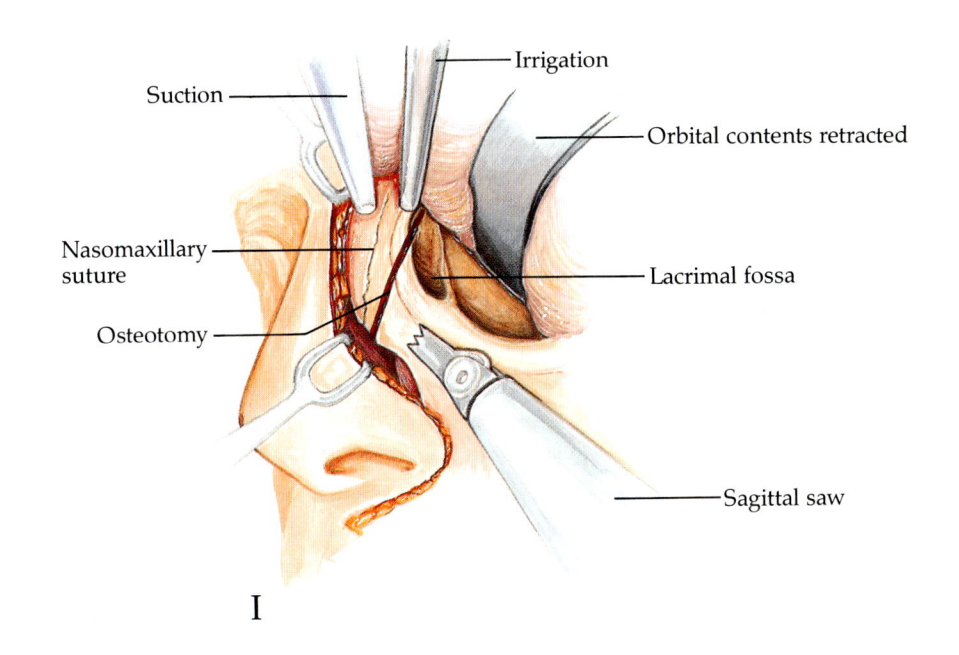

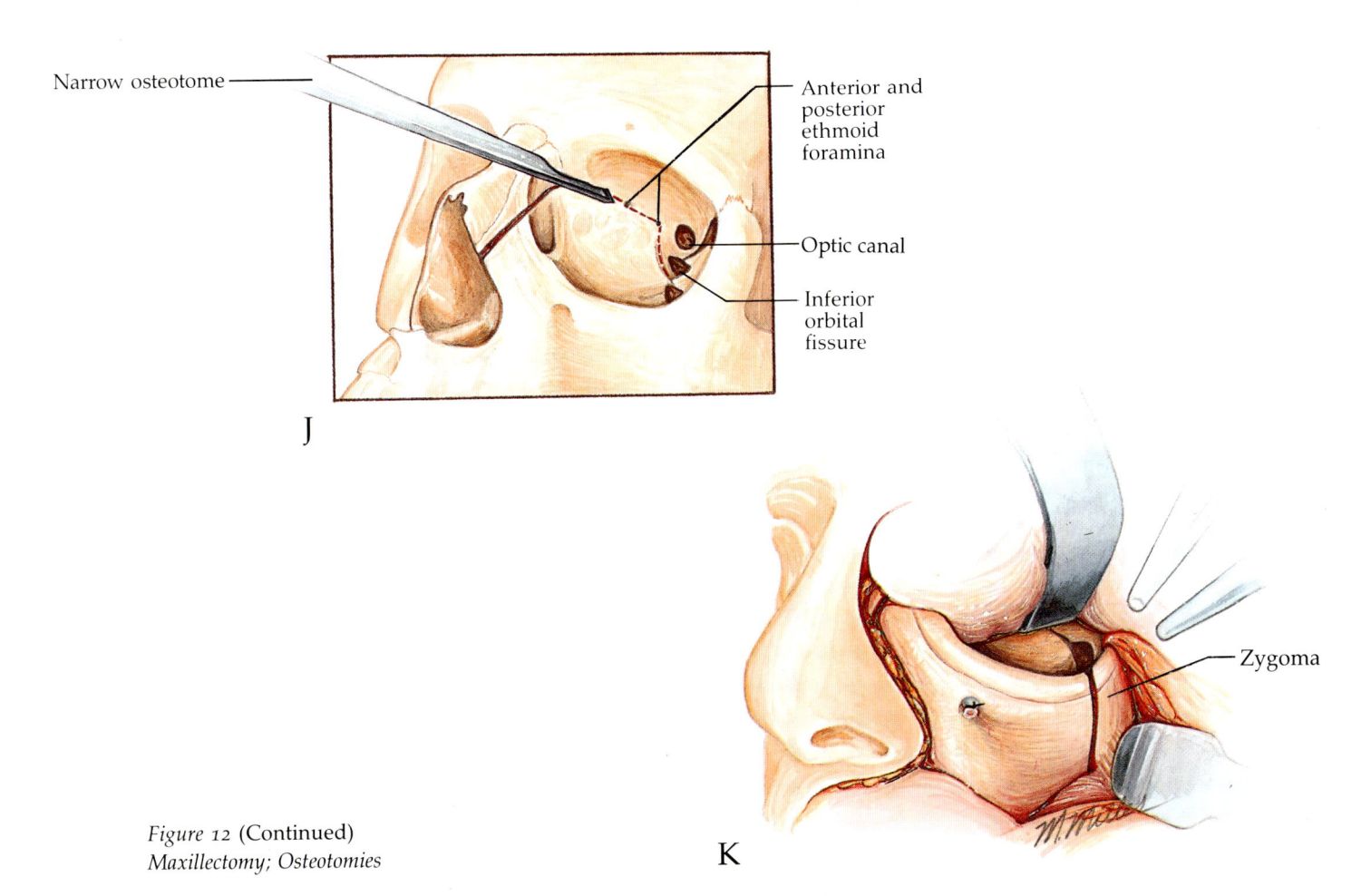

281

If the patient has maxillary teeth, the tooth that lies along the course of the medial osteotomy extending downward from the nasal aperture is extracted and the bone cut (Fig. 12L). Palatal incisions are made with electrocautery (Fig. 12M). If the palatal mucoperiosteum is not involved by tumor, it is helpful to place the soft tissue cuts so as to leave a flap that can be turned up to cover the cut bone surface, promoting more rapid healing. The junction of the hard and soft palates may be located by palpation and the floor of the nose entered bluntly by a right-angle clamp if a Gigli saw has been chosen for this portion of the procedure. Alternatively, palatal osteotomies may be made with the sagittal saw, as shown (Fig. 12N).

Plate 121

Piriform aperture

L

First premolar extracted

Palatal mucosal incisions

M

Sagittal saw

Figure 12 (Continued)
Maxillectomy; Palatal Osteotomies

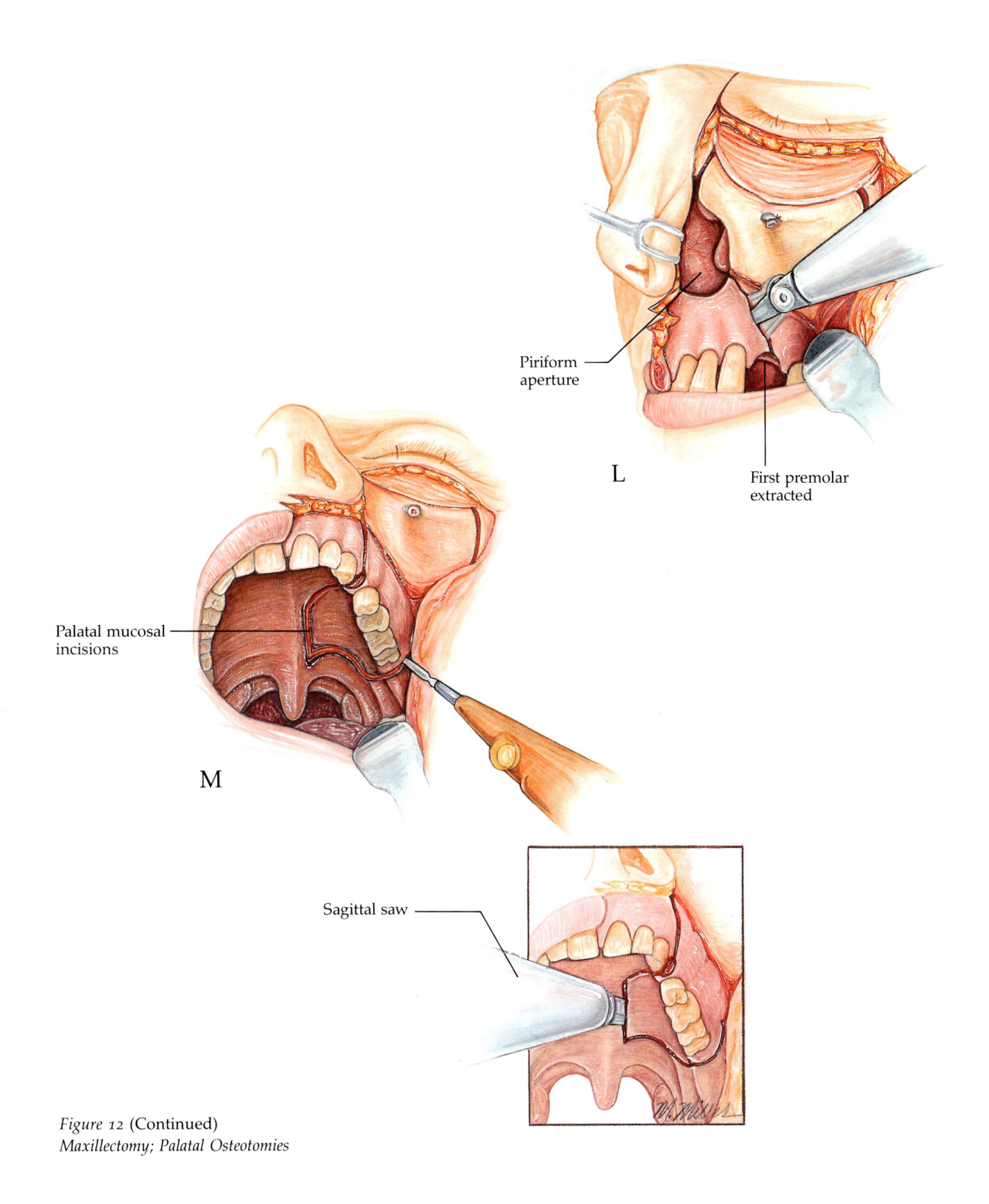

A broad, curved osteotome placed behind the hamulus and directed medially creates the final osteotomy, dividing the pterygoid plates (Figs. 12O and 12P). The specimen can now be rocked back and forth using large forceps. Soft tissue attachments in the nose and pterygoid muscles are freed with curved scissors (Fig. 12Q), and the specimen is removed. A moist gauze sponge is placed in the defect to control bleeding until the branches of the internal maxillary artery can be identified and ligated.

Plate 122

O

P

Curved osteotome

Final osteotomy with curved osteotome

Palatal osteotomy

Lateral pterygoid plate

Medial pterygoid plate

Hamulus

Q

Soft tissue attachments

Downward traction on specimen

Figure 12 (Continued)
Maxillectomy; Posterior Osteotomies and Specimen Removal

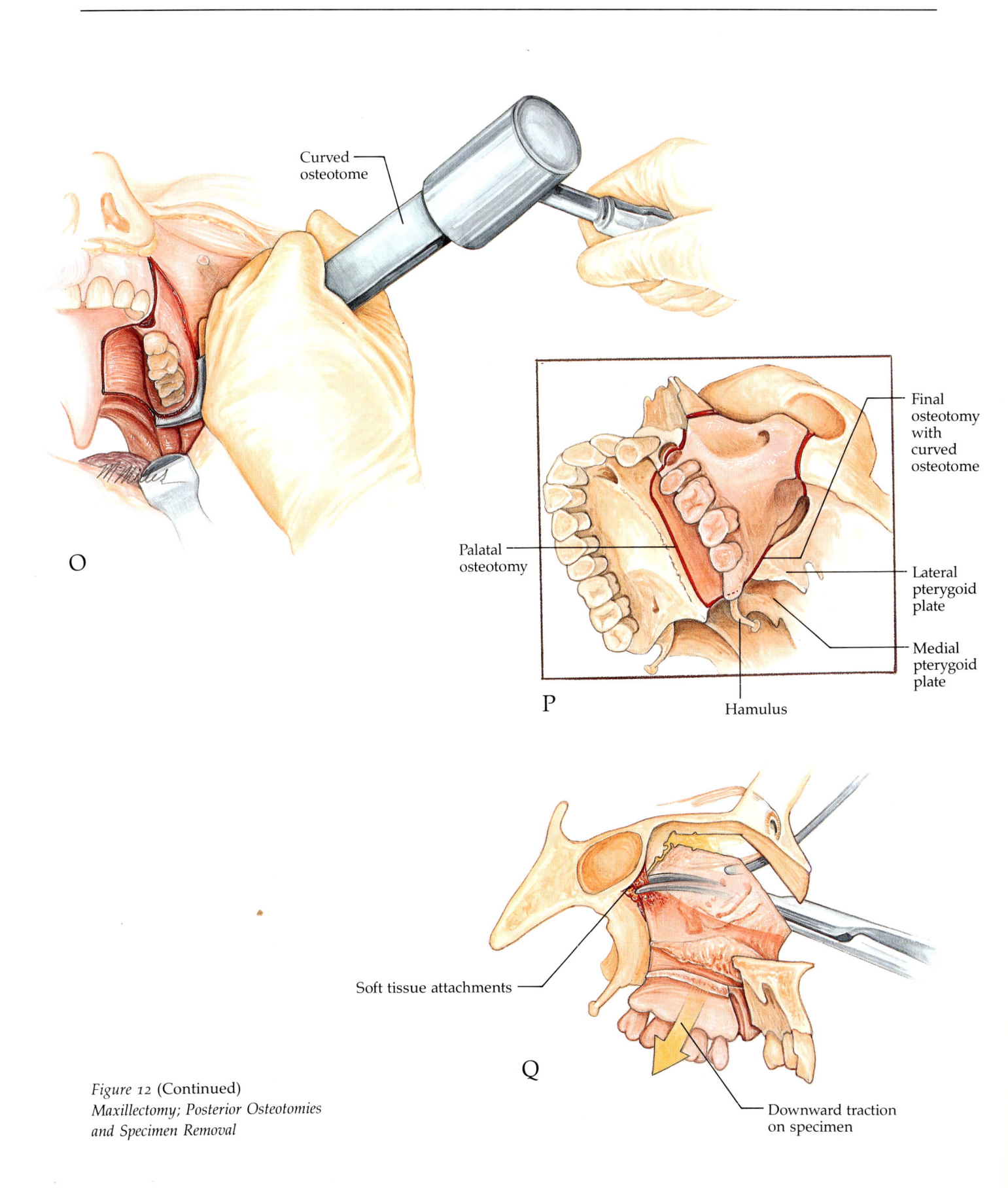

285

Rough bone edges are smoothed with a cutting bur or rongeurs (Fig. 12R), and the ethmoid mucosal fragments are cleared with special attention given to ensure patency of the nasofrontal recess. Margins may be improved by thinning bone at the attachments of the tumor to the skull base with a diamond bur. A split-thickness skin graft is harvested from the thigh, upper arm, or abdomen and sewn to the inside of the cheek flap (Fig. 12S). Several "pie-crust" perforations are made in the graft. The periorbita is closed if possible and the orbicularis oculi muscles are reapproximated at the medial canthus. If the medial canthus was displaced, it should be fixed with a permanent suture to remaining nasal skeletal structures. When a large portion of the orbital floor has been removed, the globe is supported by strips of temporalis fascia or fascia lata stitched to the remaining orbital bone. The palatal prosthesis is positioned and held in place by wires incorporated into the plastic that fit over remaining teeth or with wires that suspend it from the zygoma or alveolus bilaterally. A gauze strip saturated with antibiotic ointment is packed in the cavity and positioned to allow its removal from the nose (Fig. 12T). Incisions are closed in layers, taking special care to align the vermillion accurately (Fig. 12U).

Postoperative Care

The dental prosthesis is left in place for 5 to 7 days, after which it is removed for adjustment. The patient learns to position the prosthesis in the same way as a standard denture. Oral intake of food and fluid can begin as soon as the patient is awake and alert, and hospitalization is no longer required after removal of the packing 2 or 3 days postoperatively. The skin graft donor site is covered with a large, sterile-adhesive, clear plastic sheet (Opsite), which may be replaced if it becomes loosened or a significant collection of fluid occurs.

Risks, Complications, and Sequelae

In addition to those risks, complications, and sequelae discussed under medial maxillectomy, the following may be seen after this procedure: (1) enophthalmos; (2) loss of malar eminence; (3) infection of skin graft donor site; (4) blindness; (5) facial nerve injury; (6) difficulty chewing; (7) oronasal fistula; and (8) injury to the carotid artery with resultant carotid-cavernous sinus fistula, stroke, or death.

Plate 123

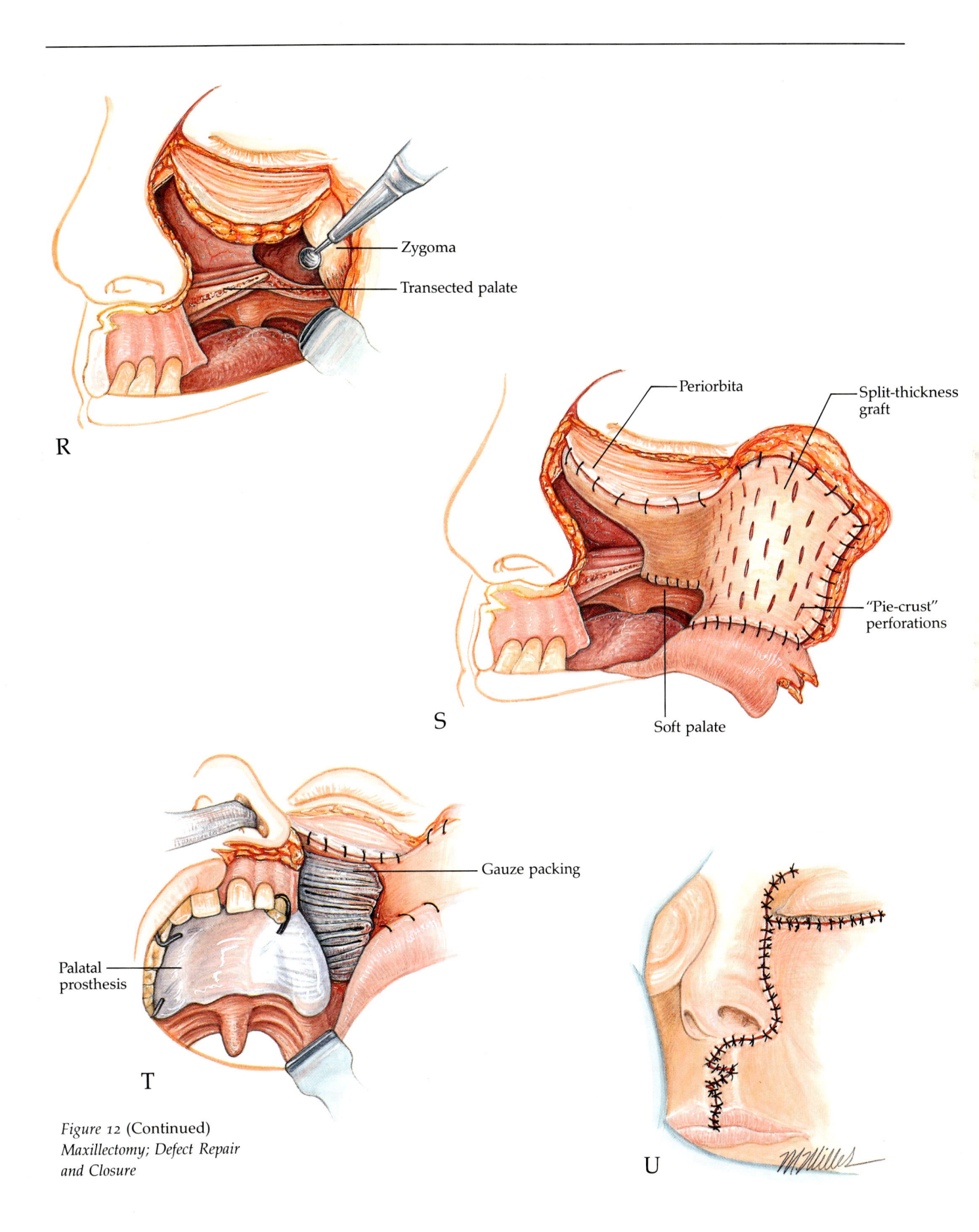

- Zygoma
- Transected palate

R

- Periorbita
- Split-thickness graft
- "Pie-crust" perforations
- Soft palate

S

- Gauze packing
- Palatal prosthesis

T

Figure 12 (Continued)
Maxillectomy; Defect Repair and Closure

U

287

Pearls and Pitfalls

Preservation of the malar eminence is desirable for maintenance of facial contour and position of the globe.

Osteotomy separating the pterygoid plates is directed lateral to medial in order to avoid injury to the skull base and internal carotid artery.

If the dental prosthesis is wired in place, a second general anesthetic may be required in order to remove it a week postoperatively. The use of a prosthesis, however, markedly reduces postoperative recovery time, allowing oral intake almost immediately. This is a significant improvement over alternative methods of bolstering packing in place with heavy suture.

Proper lip function is dependent on accurate reanastomosis of orbicularis oris fibers at closure.

Wayne M. Koch, M.D.
John C. Price, M.D.

RADICAL MAXILLECTOMY

Indications

Maxillectomy may be extended in several ways to permit complete extirpation of widespread disease. For example, when tumor erodes the lateral wall of the antrum or extends into the pterygopalatine fossa, the zygomatic buttress must be removed, giving the surgeon access to the infratemporal fossa and the skull base. The precise limits of resection depend on the pattern and extent of tumor growth.

Preoperative Considerations

These are the same as for maxillectomy.

Operative Steps

Operative steps are the same as for maxillectomy, with the following modifications

Removal of zygomatic buttress. Elevation of the cheek flap is carried laterally to the coronoid process and condyle. This may require lateral extension of the Dieffenbach-Weber-Fergusson incision (see Fig. 12A). The temporalis muscle is retracted posteriorly and a clamp passed deep to the zygomatic process either to pass the Gigli saw blade or as a guard for the sagittal saw. The zygomaticofrontal process is also cut with a saw or chisel (Fig. 13A). It may be necessary to support the dental prosthesis with a wire through the remaining zygomaticofrontal process at the time of closure.

Resection of orbital floor. Up to one-third of the orbital floor can be removed without the need for reconstruction to support the globe. Tumors that involve the entire roof of the antrum may necessitate complete removal of the floor, as shown in Figure 13A. Osteotomies within the orbit utilize the superior and inferior fissures. Prior to closure, the globe is supported with temporalis fascia or fascia lata.

Dissection of the pterygopalatine fossa. In addition to removal of the buttress, the coronoid process or the entire ascending ramus of the mandible may be removed or retracted after mandibulotomy. The lateral pterygoid muscle may be released from the inner table of the angle of the mandible and the medial pterygoid muscle from the temporomandibular joint capsule. The pterygoid plates are removed in their entirety, together with the main specimen, by an osteotomy separating them from the base of skull (Figs. 13B and 13C). It is useful to control the internal maxillary artery at this juncture as it passes deep to the ramus. Dissection of soft tissue to the skull base can be accomplished after the main specimen, including the maxilla and pterygoid plates, has been removed.

Resection of soft palate. If necessary to achieve free soft-tissue margins, the soft palate may be resected, but with severe morbidity. Function is sacrificed, resulting in nasopharyngeal reflux and hypernasal speech. Obturators are not very successful for rehabilitation of soft palate defects.

Postoperative Care

Postoperative care is the same as for maxillectomy.

Risks, Complications, and Sequelae

In addition to those complications listed for maxillectomy and medial maxillectomy, the following conditions may occur subsequent to this operation: (1) facial numbness now may include V1 distribution if the infratemporal fossa has been dissected; (2) trismus results from scarring and fibrosis of the pterygopalatine structures; and (3) failure of prosthetic rehabilitation, especially when the soft palate is resected.

Pearls and Pitfalls

Facial nerve injury is avoided by staying in a plane deep to the periosteum in the malar region and limiting the use of the unipolar cautery. If tumor has penetrated the periosteum, palsy of the seventh cranial nerve is likely.

When mandibulotomy is required, we favor minicompression plating for repair.

Plate 124

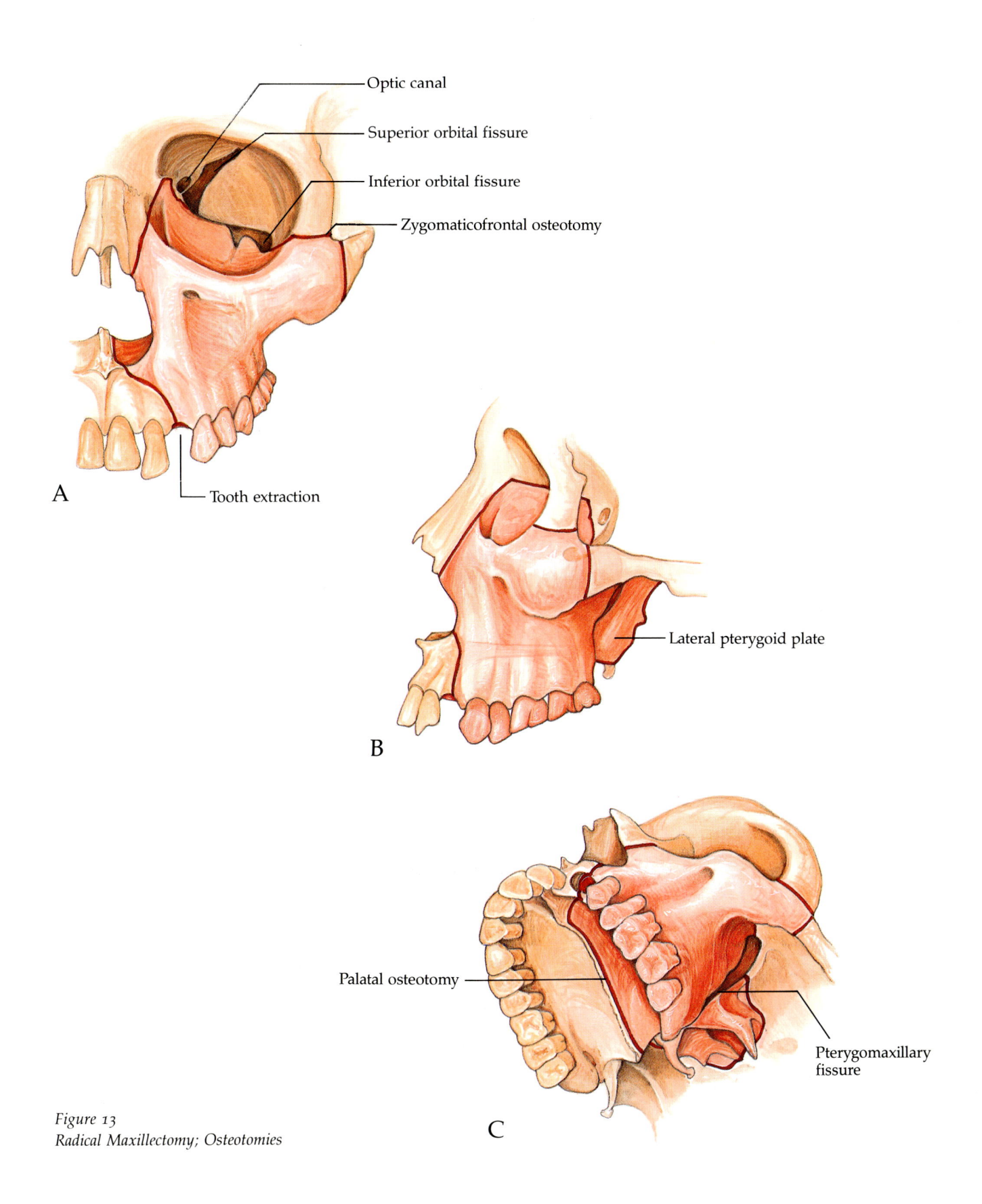

Figure 13
Radical Maxillectomy; Osteotomies

John C. Price, M.D.
Wayne M. Koch, M.D.

ORBITAL EXENTERATION

Indications

Malignant neoplasms that involve the periorbita or the orbit itself necessitate exploration of the orbit with possible exenteration. If the extent of involvement is uncertain, the periorbita may be biopsied without removing the globe (Figs. 14A to 14D). However, once the periorbita has been penetrated by tumor, the entire orbital contents must be removed in order to ensure adequate tumor extirpation.

Preoperative Considerations

Ophthalmologic consultation for documentation of baseline function of both the involved and the contralateral eye is obtained. Informed consent should include discussion of exenteration whenever tumor approaches the bony orbital walls, and especially when the walls are eroded.

Operative Steps

When tumor is noted to have penetrated the orbital floor and to be adherent to the periorbita (Fig. 14A), the orbital septum is incised (Fig. 14B) at the rim and the orbital contents are retracted, using several malleable retractors (Fig. 14C). If the inner surface of the periorbita does not evidence gross penetration by tumor, a small portion can be removed for frozen section analysis (Fig. 14D). If tumor has not penetrated the periorbita, the orbit may be preserved.

Plate 125

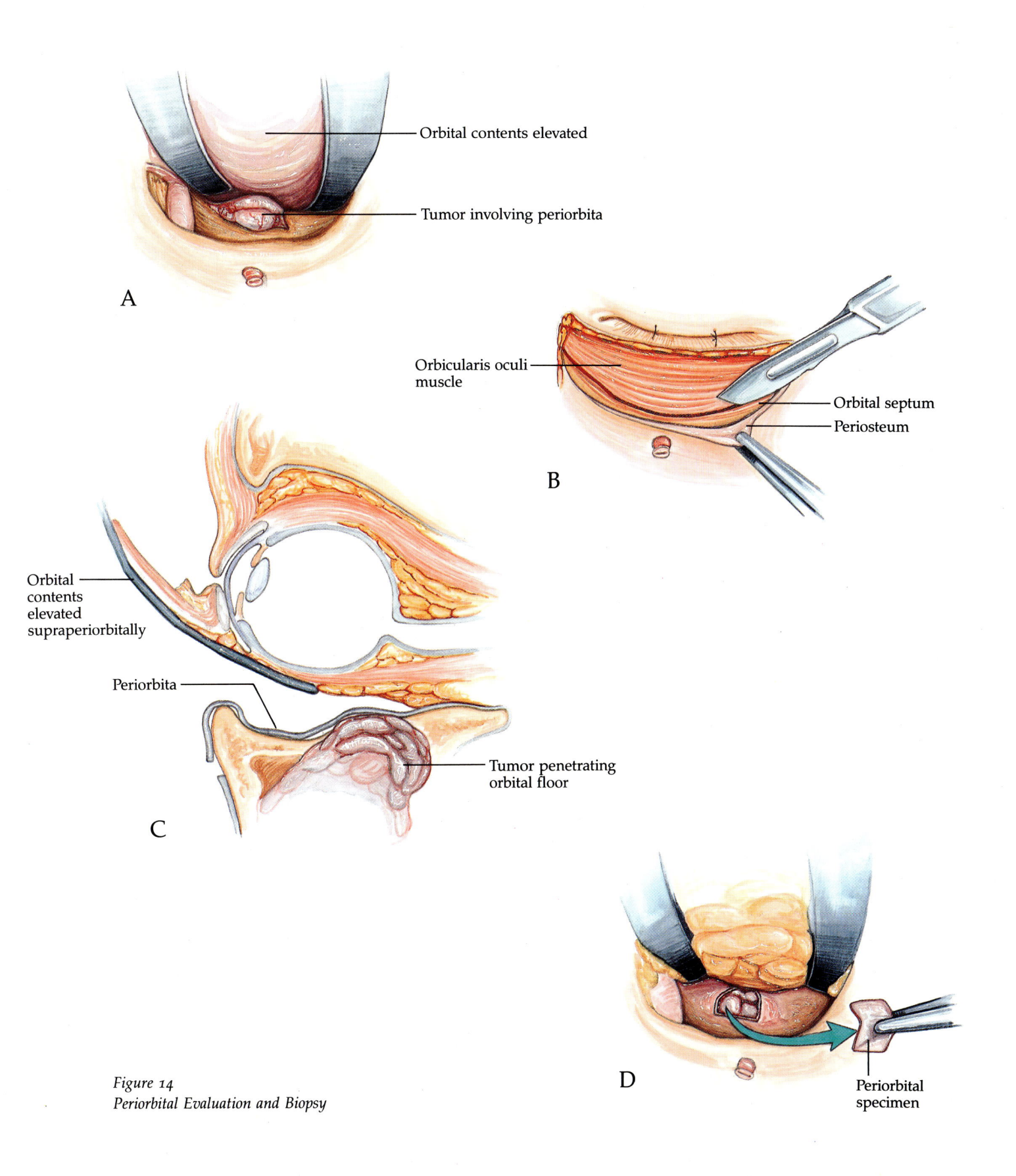

- Orbital contents elevated
- Tumor involving periorbita

A

- Orbicularis oculi muscle
- Orbital septum
- Periosteum

B

- Orbital contents elevated supraperiorbitally
- Periorbita
- Tumor penetrating orbital floor

C

- Periorbital specimen

D

Figure 14
Periorbital Evaluation and Biopsy

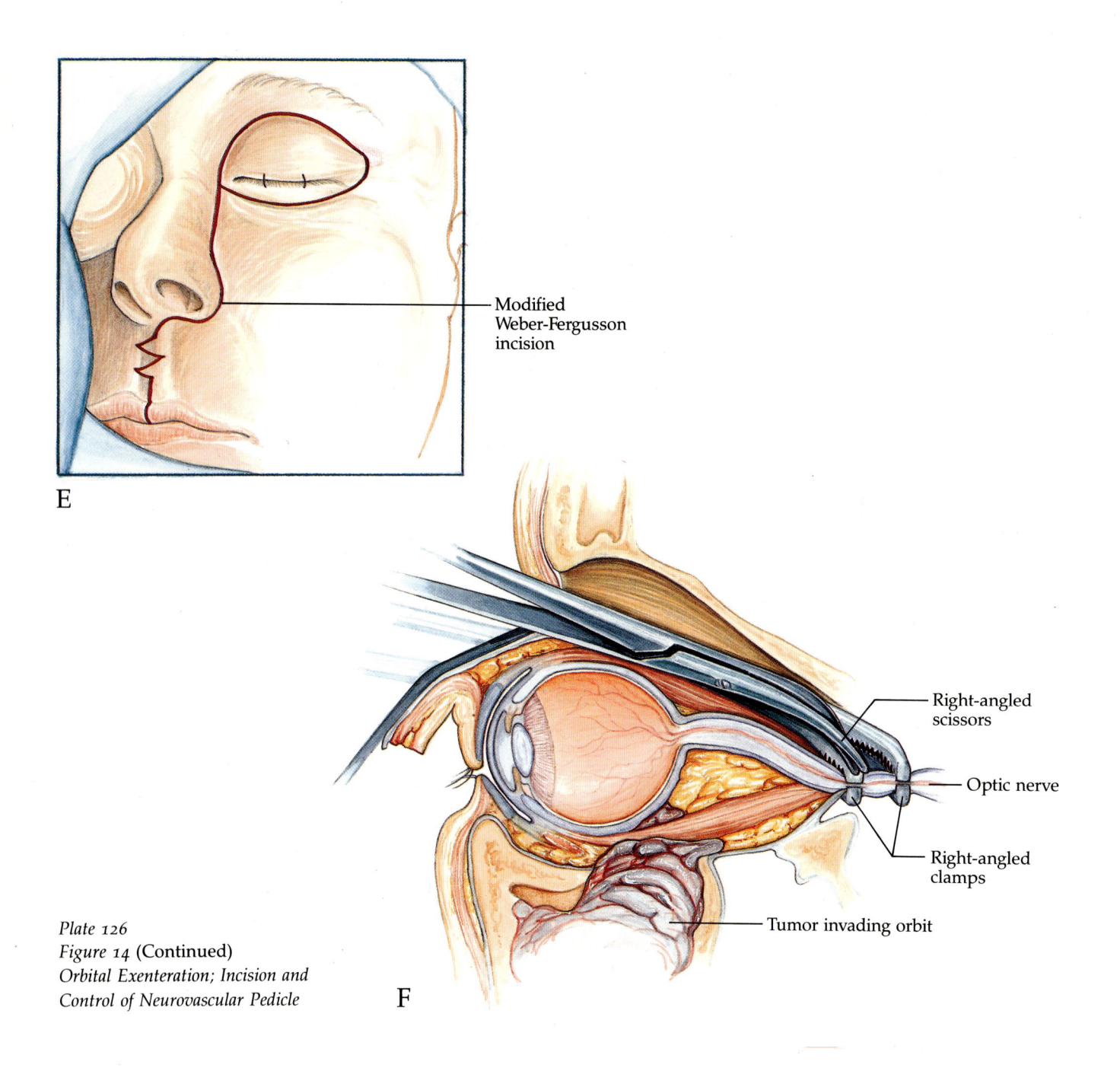

Orbital Exenteration

- Modified Weber-Fergusson incision

E

- Right-angled scissors
- Optic nerve
- Right-angled clamps
- Tumor invading orbit

Plate 126
Figure 14 (Continued)
Orbital Exenteration; Incision and Control of Neurovascular Pedicle

F

When computed tomographic or magnetic resonance imaging scans demonstrate clear orbital invasion and exenteration is definitely planned, the Weber-Fergusson incision is modified to incise along the superior orbital rim and below the eyelashes of the lower lid (Fig. 14E). Blunt dissection outside the periorbita exposes the anterior and posterior

Orbital Exenteration

G

Neurovascular pedicle

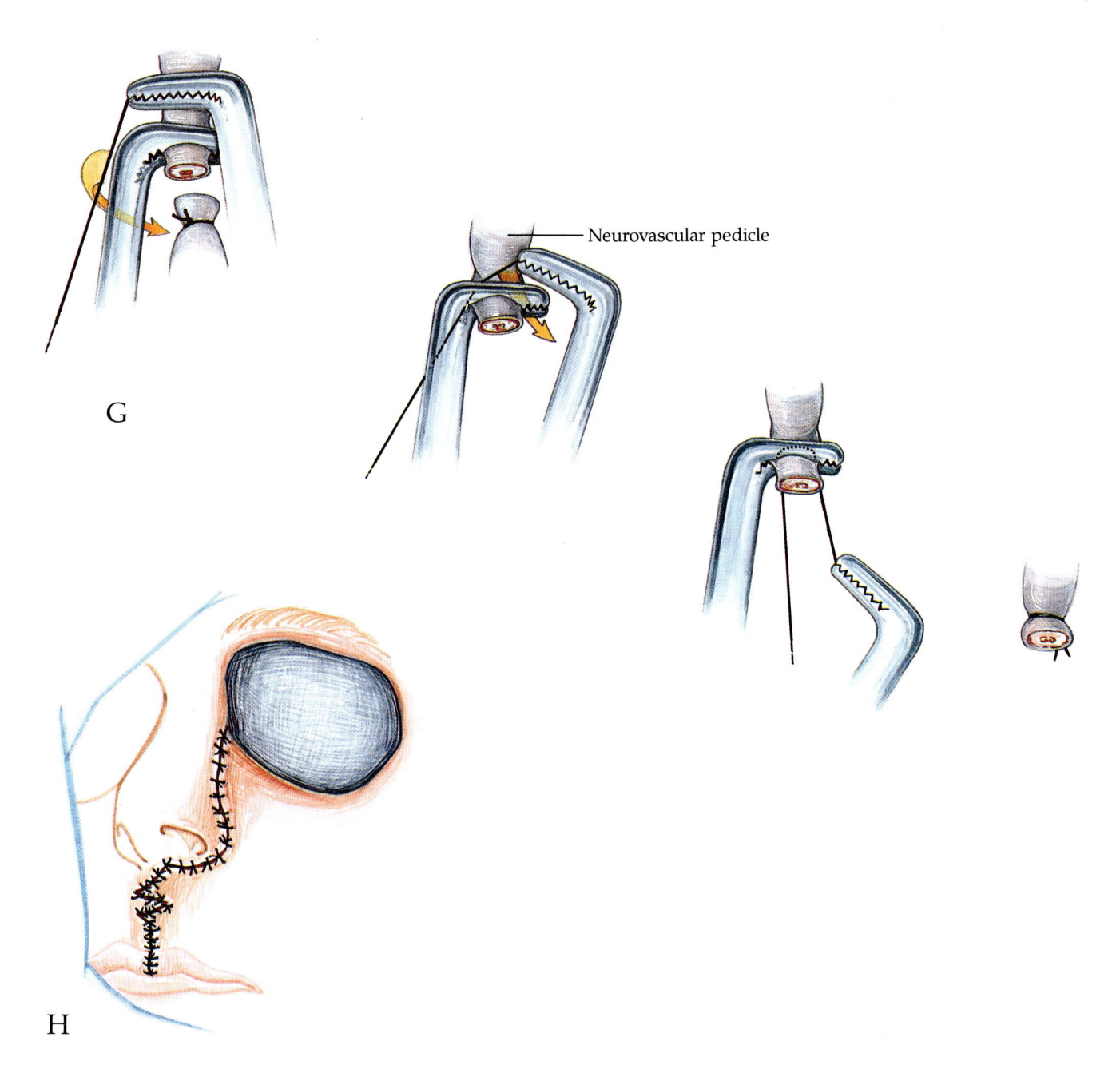

H

Plate 127
Figure 14 (Continued)
Orbital Exenteration; Ligation and Closure

ophthalmic arteries, which are ligated, and the optic nerve at the apex of the orbit. Two long right-angle clamps are placed on the neurovascular bundle and a right-angle scissors divides the nerve (Fig. 14F). Silk suture is passed around the proximal clamp and the pedicle is ligated (Fig. 14G). The orbit may be packed, along with the maxillary cavity at the close of the procedure (Fig. 14H).

Postoperative Care

After the packing has been removed, most patients initially choose to wear an eye patch over the orbital defect until after radiation therapy has been completed. A prosthesis that matches the skin color of the patient's cheek may be fabricated to fit the defect and is usually worn in conjunction with eyeglasses. Scar formation during healing and postoperative radiation will alter the size of the defect, so it is customary to postpone fabricating a prosthesis until the scarring process stabilizes (see section on Fabrication of an Orbital Prosthesis).

Risks, Complications, and Sequelae

These are the same as for radical maxillectomy, with increased concern for (1) bilateral blindness, (2) cerebrospinal fluid leak, (3) dural injury or herniation, and (4) meningitis.

Pearls and Pitfalls

Perineural involvement by tumor may result in tracking along the optic or trigeminal nerve roots into the cranial cavity. Tumors with a tendency toward perineural invasion necessitate following nerves proximally as far as possible and obtaining a margin at that point for frozen section analysis.

Upper and lower eyelids may be saved by incising skin parallel to the lashes and raising a skin-muscle flap superficial to the tarsal plates. The lids are then sewn shut at closure. This, however, prohibits direct inspection of the orbit postoperatively and is not of much benefit cosmetically.

Mark M. Miller, M.A.

FABRICATION OF AN ORBITAL PROSTHESIS

Indications

Following an orbital exenteration, an orbital prosthesis is the only cosmetic rehabilitation available to the patient because eyes and eyelids cannot be surgically reconstructed. Nonetheless, because an orbital prosthesis is structured around well-defined and static anatomic margins, an excellent cosmetic result is often achieved. An orbital prosthesis also serves to protect the orbital wound. Candidates for an orbital prosthesis should be at least 6 weeks postoperative with no residual edema. The wound should be free of crusting. If the wound has been grafted, the available central depth should be 2 cm or greater to allow for ocular clearance.

Procedure

All successful facial prostheses begin with good impression-taking techniques. The patient is placed in an upright sitting position with the head slightly tilted back. All exposed facial hair is coated lightly with petroleum jelly. The hair is covered with a nurse's bouffant, and the clothing is shielded with a protective drape. The orbital wound is thoroughly cleaned. If a maxillectomy has been performed in addition to the exenteration, the antral region must be carefully packed to occlude the choanae. It is rarely necessary to mold more than 2 to 2.5 cm of depth of the orbital wound; thus the deepest portions of the wound should be packed off. If the orbit is molded to its full depth, the alginate mold will almost certainly break during removal because of the extreme undercuts created by the superior and lateral orbital rims. As in molding a nasal defect, an irreversible hydrocolloid impression material is thoroughly spatulated with room temperature water to a relatively thin consistency and then applied to the superior margins of the orbital defect. Allowing the material to flow down the sides and into the wound lessens the chance of air entrapment. An impression is taken of the defect, the contralateral orbit, the nose, upper lip, and much of the forehead. This is to ensure availability of many facial landmarks when adjusting the position of the ocular. Before the first coat of material has solidified, a heavier layer of alginate is applied, with a thin layer of gauze being utilized between the two coats as a binder. It is important to reassure the patient by maintaining verbal and tactile communication during the molding process. Once the material is set, fast-set plaster bandages are layered upon the external surface of the impression for support. The room lights are dimmed and the patient is assisted to an upright position; the impression is carefully removed, paying specific attention to all undercuts.

Dental stone is mixed to a heavy consistency and slowly vibrated into the mold, allowing all air to escape from the lowest recesses and undercuts. As with a nasal defect cast, the stone should be poured up to but not over the highest point of the upturned mold. This creates a passage through which access is gained to the sculpture from the back. The cast is allowed to set, and then all edges and flashing are trimmed with a model trimmer or dental bur.

The plaster cast is prepared for sculpting by applying a thin layer of petroleum jelly to the defect area and then burnishing down a layer of aluminum foil as a separator between the clay sculpture and the plaster cast. This allows for easy removal of the sculpture during subsequent trial fittings. If the defect is large, an additional layer of dental bite wax is often melted over the aluminum foil to provide rigidity to the sculpture base.

After the ocular is delivered from the ocularist, three small depressions or "dimples" are drilled into its posterior surface using a fine bur. These concavities create corresponding convexities in the posterior plaster mold and thus serve as registration marks to align and lock in the position of the ocular during subsequent casting of the prosthesis. Sculpting should then proceed, with the patient present for immediate viewing of facial details. The orbital defect on the patient's cast is filled with sulfur-free modeling clay, leaving a depression for the placement of the ocular. Before sculpting proceeds, the ocular is positioned within the clay so that it corresponds to the position of the contralateral eye. Using the pupils as reference points, measurements are made of key anatomic relationships with calipers (Fig. 15A). These relationships include the distance from the midnasal bridge to the pupil, from the tip of the nose to the pupil, and from the corner of the mouth to the pupil. These measurements serve to facilitate the approximate placement of the ocular. Final position is determined by placing the crudely sculpted prosthesis on the patient and visually judging and adjusting the ocular accordingly. The decisive alignment is determined with respect to all spatial planes: right to left and superior to inferior, and the correct depth as referenced to the superior and inferior orbital rims, assuming the inferior rim has not been resected (Fig. 15B).

When the ocular is properly located and in primary gaze, sculpting proceeds with careful attention to details such as the appropriate thickness, shape, and character of the eyelids as well as the correct palpebral fissure width. The sculpture is occasionally removed from the cast and placed on the patient to judge its correctness. The evolving sculpture is occasionally refrigerated to enhance the firmness of the clay. Final skin texture is added with a fine bristle brush dipped in xylene or by pressing silicone patches of actual skin impressions into the surface of the clay.

Once the sculpting is complete, a dental stone mold is made of the anterior surface of the sculpted prosthesis, including at least a 3-cm margin of patient cast. Liquid separator is employed between all contacting plaster surfaces. If the sculpted prosthesis has been refrigerated, it must be allowed to warm to room temperature until all condensation has evaporated before mold making can commence.

Plate 128

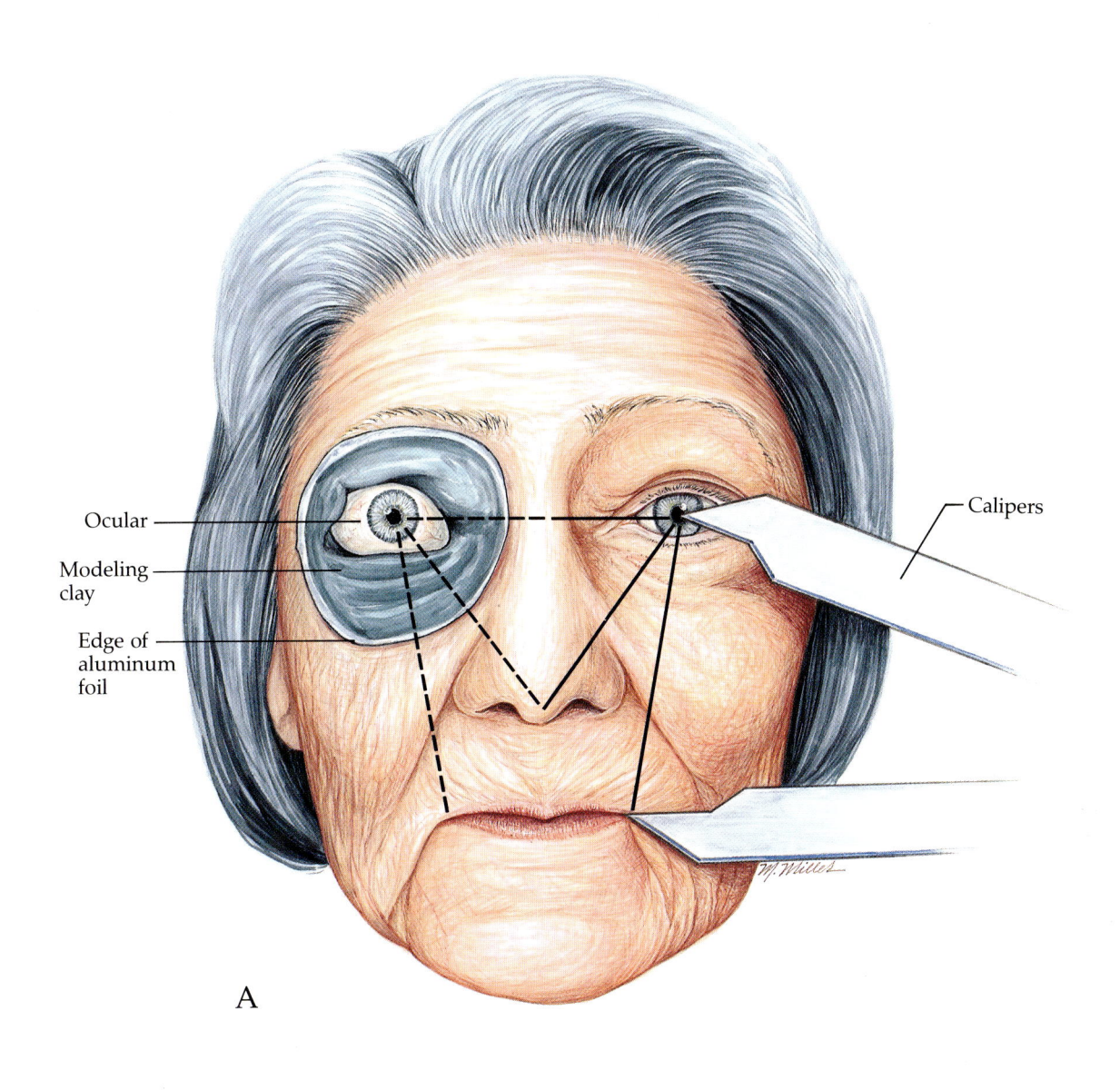

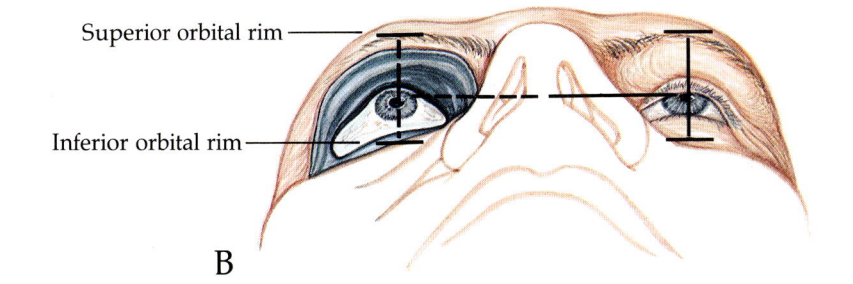

Ocular
Modeling clay
Edge of aluminum foil
Calipers

A

Superior orbital rim
Inferior orbital rim

B

Figure 15
Measurements for an Orbital Prosthesis

With the anterior mold set, sculpting proceeds through the back opening of the patient cast. The posterior surface of the ocular is carefully exposed by slowly removing bits of clay with a small dental elevator. Care is taken to avoid disturbing the position of the ocular. A 2- to 3-mm rim of clay is sculpted around the perimeter of the ocular (Fig. 15C). In the finished prosthesis, this rim will hold the ocular in place while allowing for its easy removal. Without a separator, a dental stone mold is made of the posterior surface of the patient cast, including the sculpted rim and posterior ocular surface. It is ensured that the three registration "dimples" previously drilled into the back of the ocular are completely filled with plaster. Once set, the anterior mold is removed and all clay discarded. With a dental bur, a 1-cm wide trough is drilled into the face of the anterior mold, circumferentially around the position of the prosthesis. This trough is connected to the outer edge of the mold with several radiating troughs (see Fig. 15E). As with the molds of the nasal prosthesis, these troughs allow for the escape of excess casting material when the molds are packed and clamped. The molds are then thoroughly cleaned of all clay residue and plaster dust using hot water and a mild detergent.

Once the molds are dry, the ocular is set in place using a small amount of prosthesis adhesive (Fig. 15D). The mold halves are packed with silicone dyed to the patient's skin color (see Fabrication of a Nasal Prosthesis in Chapter III, on the mixing of silicone skin color). Packing commences under the edge of the ocular and then proceeds to the rest of the orbital defect (Fig. 15E). Last, the surface of the anterior mold is "buttered" thoroughly with a coat of silicone. The mold halves are reapproximated, and excess silicone is extruded with hand pressure. Clamps are applied to the mold, and the prosthesis is allowed to cure.

Once it is cured, the prosthesis is carefully removed and trimmed of all excess flashing. The ocular is extracted from the back of the prosthesis and repolished. Eyelashes are added to the prosthesis in the following manner: A 2- to 3-mm deep slit is made in the upper eyelid using a scalpel and a No. 11 blade. This slit is made in a plane that will project the eyelashes forward, not downward. Thus the incision is not made parallel to the upper lid but rather in a plane approaching perpendicular to it. Short lengths of hair, matching the patient's in color and texture, are inserted into this slit with fine forceps. Once the hair is carefully arranged, it is glued in place with Adhesive A (Dow Corning Corporation, Midland, Michigan) thinned with xylene. When dry, the lashes are trimmed, if necessary. The prosthesis is gently washed with a mild detergent and warm water to remove any plaster or separator residue prior to extrinsic coloration.

With the patient present, surface coloration is applied in the same manner as with the nasal prosthesis, using a mixture of silicone base, xylene, and dry pigment (see Fabrication of a Nasal Prosthesis in Chapter III). With the prosthesis now complete, the patient's wound margins are cleaned with an alcohol sponge and the prosthesis is applied with an appropriate adhesive. Although adhesives are the most frequently used mode of prosthesis retention, osseointegrated titanium implants and mag-

Plate 129

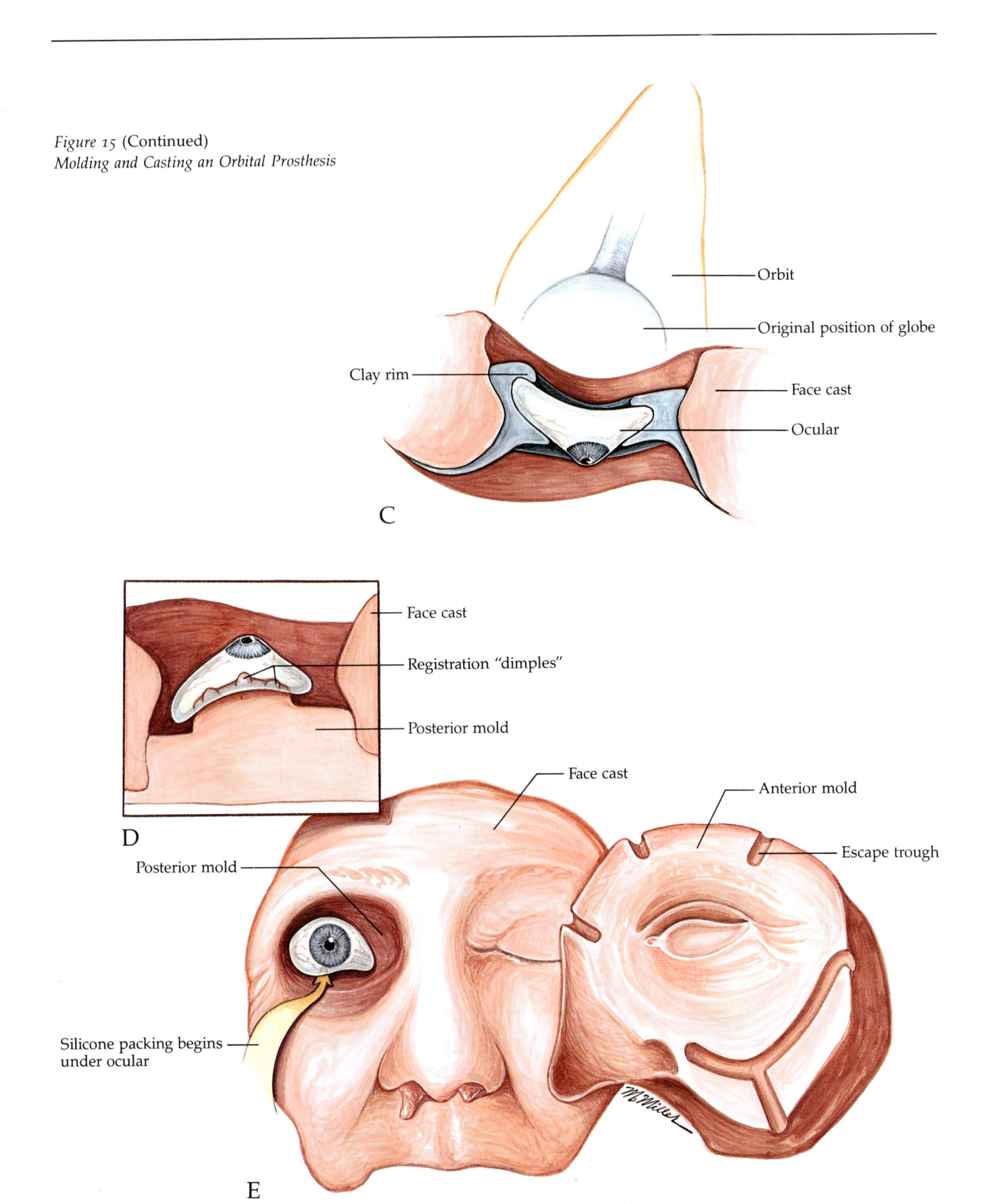

Figure 15 (Continued)
Molding and Casting an Orbital Prosthesis

301

nets also are currently being utilized for the retention of facial prostheses. Spectacles are often suggested for the patient for cosmetic enhancement. Upon completion of the placement of the prosthesis, the patient is thoroughly instructed on its proper care and maintenance.

Pearls and Pitfalls

An orbital prosthesis is one of the more difficult facial reconstructions to create successfully owing to the sensitivity with which human beings view another person's eyes. As the "windows to the soul," eyes may reveal emotions as well as states of health, mind, and awareness. When one eye is out of place spatially or out of gaze, this condition is quickly apparent to the observer, and the abnormal eye becomes a point of focus. The goal of the prosthetist is to diminish this tendency of the casual observer to focus on the abnormality of the reconstructed eye and orbit. This is accomplished by a concentrated effort to place the ocular correctly in relation to the contralateral natural eye and by the correct sculpting of the palpebral fissure. This cannot be overemphasized. Color flaws are minimal compared with the disturbing appearance of a misplaced or misshapen eye. The perfect placement is difficult to attain. However, the patient and the prosthetist will be satisfied only when the correct placement is achieved.

Suggested Reading

Albrektsson T, Brånemark P-I, Jacobsson M, Tjellström A. Present clinical applications of osseointegrated percutaneous implants. Plast Reconstr Surg 1987; 79:721–730.

Birnbach S, Herman GL. Coordinated intraoral and extraoral prostheses in the rehabilitation of the orofacial cancer patient. J Prosthet Dent 1987; 58:347.

Chalian VA, Drane JB, Standish SM. Maxillofacial prosthetics: Multidisciplinary practice. Baltimore: Williams & Wilkins, 1971:296.

Swartz B, Udagama A. Magnetic prostheses: An alternative fixation and orientation method. Plast Reconstr Surg 1982; 69:755.

Chapter V

THYROID AND PARATHYROIDS

Maria Allo, M.D.

THYROIDECTOMY

Anatomic Considerations

The thyroid gland is a bilobar structure interconnected by an isthmus (Fig. 1A). The apices of the lobes generally extend to the junction of the middle and lower thirds of the thyroid cartilage. The normal thyroid gland usually extends inferiorly to the level of the fifth or sixth tracheal ring. The isthmus connects the lower thirds of the lateral lobes at the level of the second or third tracheal rings. A communicating artery lies between the two superior thyroid arteries and runs along the cephalic border of the isthmus. The inferior thyroid veins are located at the lower border of the isthmus. If a pyramidal lobe is present, it is attached to the left side of the superior border of the thyroid. Blood supply to the thyroid gland includes two paired arteries and one unpaired artery. The superior thyroid arteries are branches of the external carotid artery and enter the gland at the superior pole. The inferior thyroid artery branches from the thyrocervical trunk and enters the gland at the midportion of the lobes laterally. Thyroidea ima, when present (approximately 30 percent of the time), derives from the brachiocephalic trunk. Venous drainage starts from a plexus on the surface of the gland in the trachea and generally enters the major draining vessels by way of three more or less well-developed paired veins. The superior thyroid vein and middle thyroid vein arise in the plexus and drain into the internal jugular vein. The inferior thyroid vein terminates in the brachiocephalic veins. There are subcapsular lymphatics that drain to superior deep cervical, pretracheal, paratracheal, retropharyngeal, and inferior deep cervical lymph nodes.

Two nerves, important in the innervation of the laryngeal muscles, are encountered within the field of dissection: the external laryngeal branch of the superior laryngeal nerve of the vagus nerve innervates the cricothyroid muscle and runs with the superior pole vessels until it deviates medially to enter the larynx. The recurrent laryngeal nerve branch of the vagus innervates all other intrinsic muscles of the larynx. The recurrent laryngeal nerve on the right arises from the right vagus nerve. As the vagus passes in front of the subclavian artery, it normally hooks below and behind the artery and ascends in the tracheoesophageal groove. The recurrent laryngeal nerve leaves the left vagus nerve at the aortic arch and hooks below the arch at the level of the ligamentum arteriosum; it then ascends to the right to the aortic arch in the tracheoesophageal groove. Once it enters the tracheoesophageal groove, the nerve is located medial to the corresponding lobe of the thyroid gland. At the level of the first or second tracheal ring, a sensory branch of the nerve travels to the laryngopharynx. It is of note that the nerve may be very tightly adherent to the ligament of Berry, and in particularly enlarged goiters it may be tented up to the surface of the gland. Most authors, however, feel that the nerve is virtually never embedded in normal gland surface. Further confounding the situation, it is unusual for the nerve to be identical in location on both the right and the left sides. Normally, before the nerve enters the larynx, it divides into two or more branches. However, the arrangement of fibers in these branches is highly variable. The nonrecurrent laryngeal nerve can be found in approximately 0.3 to 0.5 percent of patients and is usually on the right side.

Thyroidectomy

A — Superior thyroid vein; Superior thyroid artery; Middle thyroid vein; Inferior thyroid artery; Inferior thyroid vein

Superior thyroid artery; Intrathyroidal parathyroid vein; Inferior thyroid artery; Recurrent laryngeal nerve

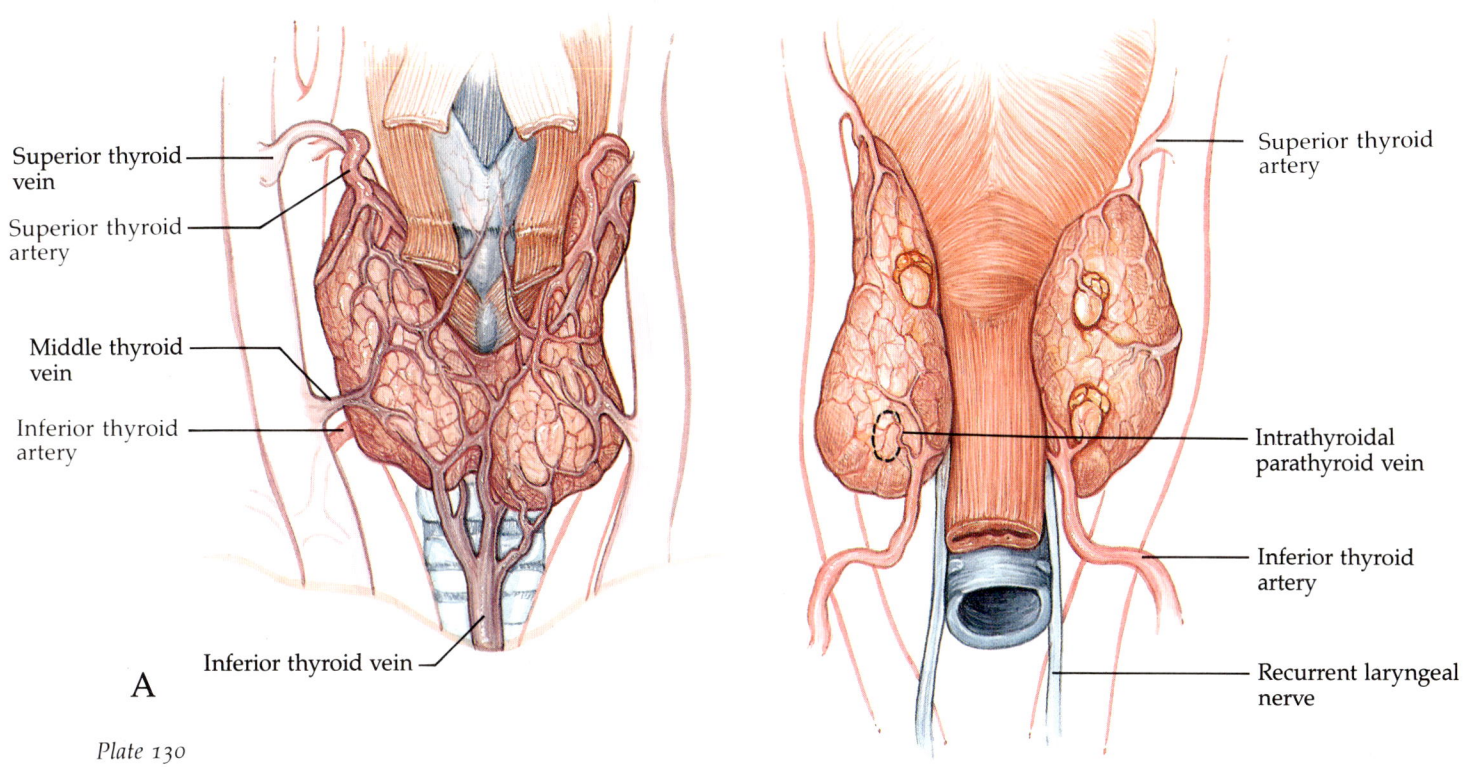

Plate 130
Figure 1
Thyroid Gland; Anatomy

Indications

Operations on the thyroid gland fall into two main categories: those to rule out or treat malignancy arising in solitary thyroid nodules, and operations to ablate large goiters. Patients with the latter condition may come to operation because of compressive symptoms, hyperfunction, or unacceptable disfigurement.

Preoperative Considerations

The diagnostic evaluation of the solitary thyroid nodule is accomplished most simply and most economically by fine needle aspiration cytology. Findings consistent with or suspicious for malignancy indicate the need for surgical intervention, usually total ipsilateral lobectomy to remove the dominant nodule leaving margins of uninvolved thyroid. In situations in which the cytologic findings are indeterminate, a thyroid scintigraphic scan with ^{99m}Tc, ^{131}I, or ^{123}I is helpful to determine the degree to which the nodule is functioning relative to the rest of the gland. In general a nodule with increased radionuclide uptake is benign; the incidence of malignancy in nodules that do not take up radioisotope is about 20 percent. Technetium-99m and ^{123}I deliver a lower radiation dose per study as compared with ^{131}I. The cost of ^{123}I, however, is significantly higher than that of ^{99m}Tc. Therefore, technetium should be used as the initial scanning agent. The vast majority of patients who undergo thyroid operations are biochemically euthyroid. Nevertheless, measurement of baseline thyroid function should be made prior to operation. Table 1 shows an algorithm for evaluation of the solitary thyroid nodule.

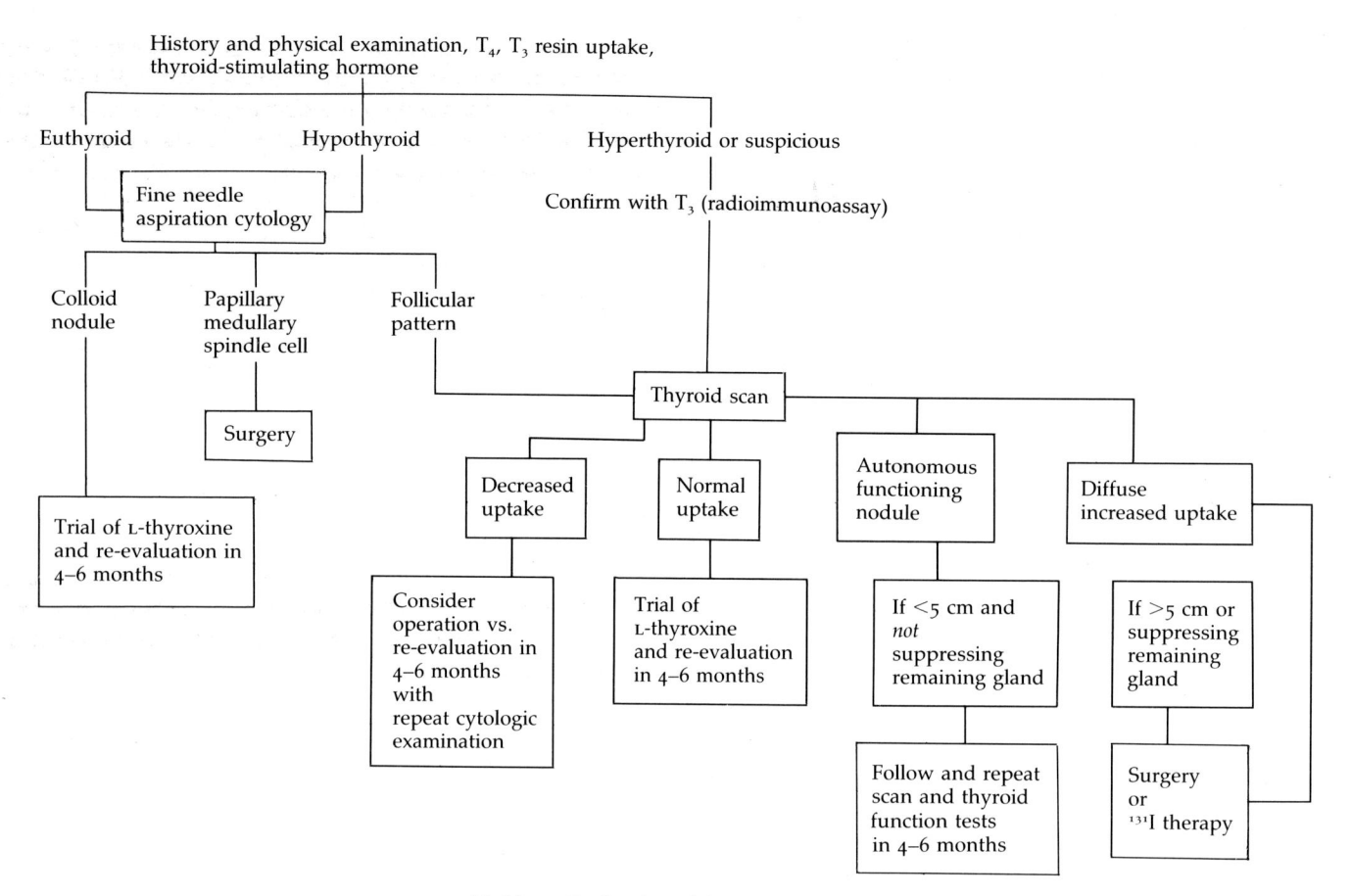

```
                History and physical examination, T₄, T₃ resin uptake,
                       thyroid-stimulating hormone
        ┌──────────────────────┼──────────────────────┐
   Euthyroid              Hypothyroid          Hyperthyroid or suspicious
        ├──────────────────────┤                      │
     ┌─────────────────┐                     Confirm with T₃ (radioimmunoassay)
     │  Fine needle    │
     │ aspiration cytology │
     └─────────────────┘
   ┌────┬─────────┬──────────┐
 Colloid  Papillary   Follicular
 nodule   medullary    pattern
          spindle cell
              │           │
          ┌───────┐       │
          │Surgery│       │
          └───────┘       │
                     ┌─────────────┐
  ┌──────────────┐   │ Thyroid scan│
  │Trial of L-thyroxine│ └─────────────┘
  │and re-evaluation in│  ┌────┬────┬────┬────┐
  │   4–6 months   │  Decreased  Normal  Autonomous  Diffuse
  └──────────────┘   uptake    uptake   functioning  increased uptake
                                         nodule
```

Table 1. *Evaluation of the solitary thyroid nodule.*

Large or obstructing goiters should be approached surgically after careful assessment of the degree to which the airway is compromised or large vessels are compressed. Substernal goiter is a nonmalignant cause of superior vena cava syndrome; facial swelling may be related to jugular compression. Plain chest films to look for substernal extension and tracheal deviation, and soft tissue films of the neck to look at the cervical airway, provide information helpful to the anesthesiologist. Baseline pulmonary function tests, including flow-volume loops, provide information as to the degree of extrinsic airway compromise due to the goiter. These measurements are particularly helpful in the patient with primary pulmonary disease that is complicated by goiter. An anesthesiologist comfortable with management of the difficult airway should assess the patient preoperatively. In some cases fiberoptic bronchoscopy or suspension laryngoscopy may be necessary to facilitate securing the airway prior to operation.

Patients who are thyrotoxic should always be rendered euthyroid prior to operation. Antithyroid medications (propylthiouracil or methimazole) should be administered for at least 7 to 10 days preoperatively, and normalization of thyroxine (T_4), triiodothyronine (T_3), and thyroid-

Thyroidectomy

Thyroidectomy; Incision

stimulating hormone (TSH) should be documented. β-Adrenergic blockers are helpful as adjuncts to control peripheral manifestations of thyrotoxicosis, including tremor, tachycardia, and arrhythmias, although in general, these symptoms rapidly improve as thyroid function normalizes. In the week immediately prior to operation, iodine drops may be given orally (as potassium iodide solution or sodium iodide). In the United States most patients with Graves' disease are treated with antithyroid drugs followed by ^{131}I ablation. Surgical management may be indicated in the presence of a large goiter, in women of childbearing age (including pregnant women whose disease cannot be controlled on doses of thiourea that are safe for the fetus), in patients with an aversion to radiation treatments, and in those who relapse following ^{131}I therapy or antithyroid medication. Subtotal resection is the usual operation of choice.

The usual blood loss during thyroidectomy or parathyroidectomy is less than 100 ml. Transfusion is rarely if ever indicated. The incidence of postoperative wound infection is considerably less than 1 percent. Unless there is a coexisting circumstance to indicate the use of perioperative antibiotics (e.g., the presence of a prosthetic heart valve, orthotic device, or vascular graft, immunosuppression following transplantation or chemotherapy, or the need for endocarditis prophylaxis), antibiotics are not administered.

Operative Steps

The patient is positioned in the supine position with the neck hyperextended (Fig. 1B). A rolled towel placed between the shoulder blades raises the shoulders and permits easy hyperextension. The head should be rested in such a way that the cervical spine is supported. A head ring is

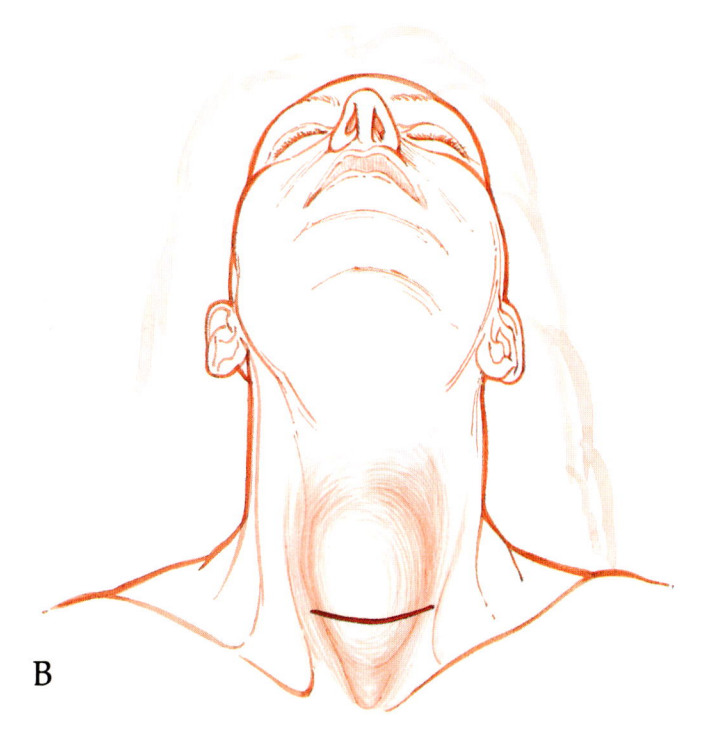

Plate 131
Figure 1 (Continued)
Thyroidectomy; Incision

B

sometimes helpful to permit hyperextension without causing the patient to hang by the cervical spine. Care is taken to locate the incision in a skin crease. Sometimes this does not result in an anatomically even incision; however, placement in the skin crease permits the scar to be well hidden. Although the traditional Kocher incision extended from ear to ear, this degree of exposure is not necessary. An incision extending from the two medial borders of the sternocleidomastoid, approximately one to two fingerbreadths above the sternal notch, provides adequate exposure (Fig. 1B). The incision is carried through the skin, the subcutaneum, and the platysma muscle. Flaps are raised to the sternal notch inferiorly and the thyroid cartilage superiorly in the plane between the platysma and the anterior cervical fascia. The strap muscles are separated at the midline and carefully dissected free from the thyroid and one another and reflected medially. It is not necessary to transect the strap muscles (Fig. 1C).

To raise the flaps, I prefer to use gentle dissection with the thumb rather than a knife (inset, Fig. 1C). If the initial dissection has been carried out carefully in the plane between the platysma muscle and the anterior cervical fascia, it is possible to raise the flaps bluntly with minimal blood loss. An occasional bleeding perforating vein can be controlled with electrocautery. Anterior jugular veins should be in view now within the anterior cervical fascia. These should remain intact. The fascia is incised at the midline (Fig. 1D). In cases in which there is a large goiter with tracheal deviation, the midline may not be in its obvious location with respect to surface landmarks. It is important to stay in the filmy areolar tissue at the midline in order to avoid bleeding from the strap muscles or severing the anterior jugular branches. The strap muscles are separated sharply. The assistant may pick up on the strap muscle while the surgeon applies gentle countertraction (Fig. 1E). The middle thyroid vein is not always present as a single, discrete, large structure, and frequently there are many branching veins in the space between the strap muscles and the carotid sheath. It is important to ligate these vessels carefully and to observe strict hemostasis, since the development of hematoma will make the definition of anatomic landmarks very difficult, and attempts to isolate these small vessels may result in inadvertent injury to the recurrent laryngeal nerve (Fig. 1F). Specific steps in proceeding with thyroidectomy depend on the anatomy of the specific gland being dissected. Whether the upper pole or lower pole is approached first or whether the isthmus is divided depends on which maneuvers are easiest to perform in the specific case. For example, in a patient with a relatively small, well-defined isthmus, division of the isthmus permits easily mobilization of the gland.

Plate 132

- Platysma muscle
- Areolar tissue
- Anterior jugular vein

C

- Superficial cervical fascia

D

- Sternohyoid muscle reflected laterally
- Thyroid gland

E

- Middle thyroid vein
- Carotid artery

F

Figure 1 (Continued)
Thyroidectomy; Flap Elevation and Lateral Gland Mobilization

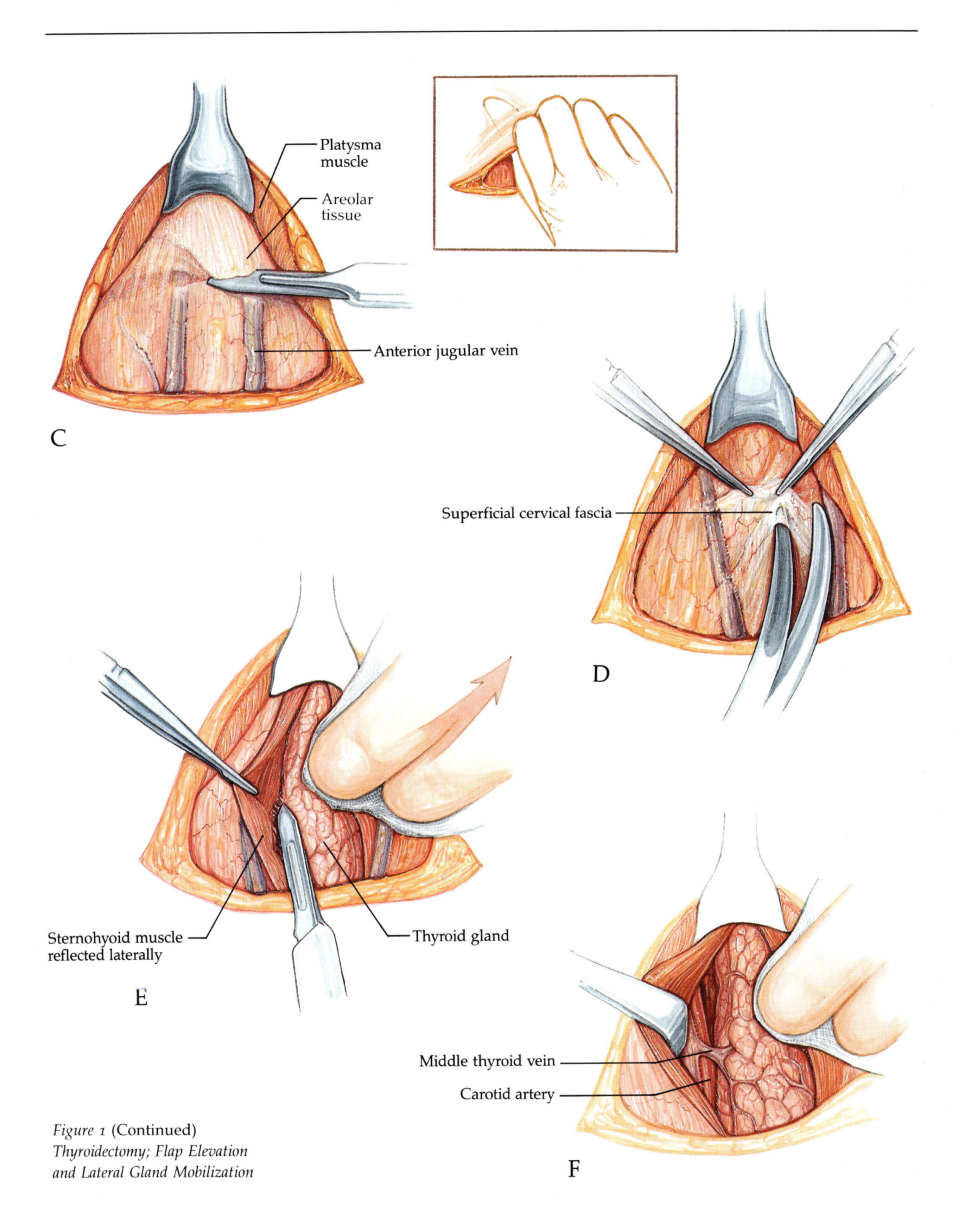

309

This, however, is not the case in a patient with a diffuse goiter and significant isthmic thickening. The inferior pole vessels should be clamped as they enter the thyroid gland in order to expose the trachea inferiorly (Fig. 1G). The upper isthmus should then be freed using sharp and blunt dissection (Fig. 1H). Beware of small vessels running along the medial border of the upper pole from the upper isthmus. The pyramidal lobe, when present, usually arises from the left side of the thyroid gland. This should be carefully dissected off the laryngeal musculature without disrupting the muscles. This can usually be done by carefully lifting the gland with forceps and dissecting in the plane between the thyroid capsule and the muscle. Small perforator vessels may be present that can be cauterized or ligated. A residual thyroglossal tract should be followed cephalad until it becomes fibrotic, and then it should be ligated. The isthmus may then be divided between clamps (Fig. 1I). Clamps should be placed so that the curves are parallel to one another. The remnants should be suture ligated. When ligating the isthmus, care should be taken to include the capsule of the thyroid within the suture so that adequate hemostasis can be achieved. Prior to the dissection of the upper pole vessels, the cricothyroid space should be defined and the upper pole separated from the larynx in the laryngeal musculature (Fig. 1J). Care

Plate 133

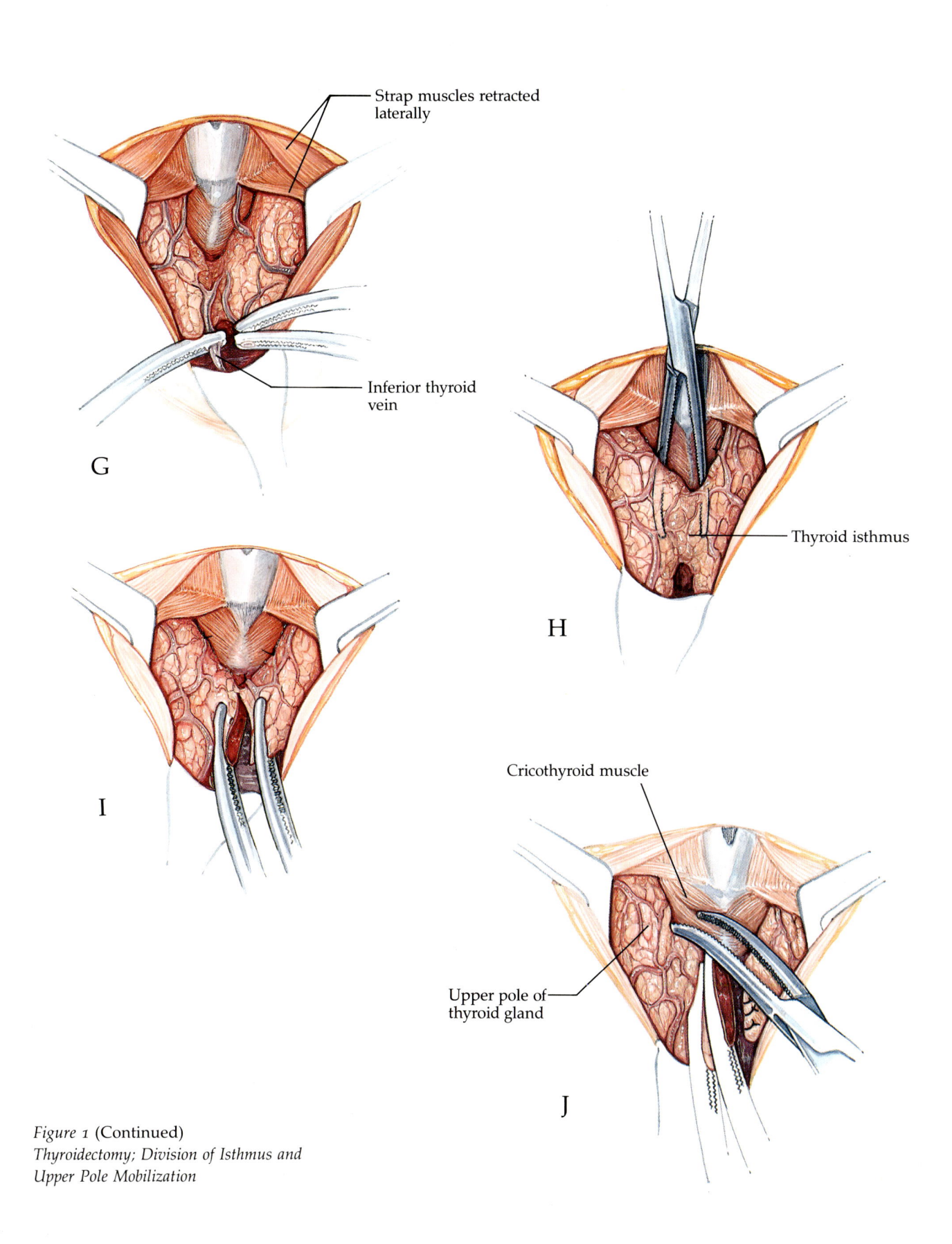

G — Strap muscles retracted laterally; Inferior thyroid vein

H — Thyroid isthmus

I

J — Cricothyroid muscle; Upper pole of thyroid gland

Figure 1 (Continued)
Thyroidectomy; Division of Isthmus and Upper Pole Mobilization

should be taken to dissect muscle fibers laterally from the upper pole so that the vessels may be isolated and individually clamped, divided, and ligated with silk ligatures (Fig. 1K). One normally finds a substantial superior thyroid artery and multiple (usually four or five) superior thyroid veins entering at the level of the upper pole (Fig. 1L). It is probably not advisable to clamp the entire upper pole and divide it between clamps for two reasons: (1) a remnant of upper pole thyroid tissue may be left behind, and (2) injury may occur to the external branch of the superior laryngeal nerve. Generally, by isolating the vessels as they enter the thyroid gland, the individual vessels that are being ligated can be clearly identified. Frequently the nerve can be seen coursing medially toward the cricothyroid muscle and thereby be spared injury (Fig. 1M). The parathyroids virtually always exist in a plane separate from the thyroid gland. Occasionally one will find "intrathyroidal" parathyroids that are truly intrathyroidal. It is unusual for all four parathyroids to be truly intrathyroidal. The risks of permanent hypoparathyroidism are generally related to inability to identify any parathyroids. Those parathyroid glands located on the surfaces of the thyroid gland generally lie in a separate plane from the thyroid and can be preserved without leaving thyroid tissue behind. One can lift the areolar tissue just above the parathyroid gland with fine forceps. The parathyroid gland generally pops out as the areolar tissue is divided and can be isolated on its vascular pedicle, usually a branch of the inferior thyroid artery, and dissected free of the thyroid tissue. The gland can be reflected medially once the isthmus has been divided and the upper pole vessels ligated. The recurrent laryngeal nerve should be identified coursing in the tracheoesophageal groove, and normally the parathyroids come into view. Their usual location is not on the surface of the thyroid gland but actually adjacent to the recurrent laryngeal nerve just above and below the junction of the recurrent nerve and the inferior thyroid artery. Any residual small venous branches of the inferior thyroid vein should be clamped as they enter the capsule of the thyroid gland and then divided and ligated with silk ties. Although this may seem a tedious procedure, careful hemostasis avoids subsequent injury to the recurrent nerve that may result from chasing a bleeder that may have retracted into the tracheoesophageal groove. Electrocautery of these lateral vessels should be avoided adjacent to the nerve, because nerve injuries can occur from heat generated by the electrocautery immediately adjacent to the recurrent nerve. Once the lateral vessels have been divided and ligated, the gland can be tipped farther medially. With the nerve in view, the remaining attachments to the ligament of Berry may be severed (Fig. 1N). Small bleeding points on the trachea can be cauterized, since this is well out of the way of the recurrent laryngeal nerve.

Plate 134

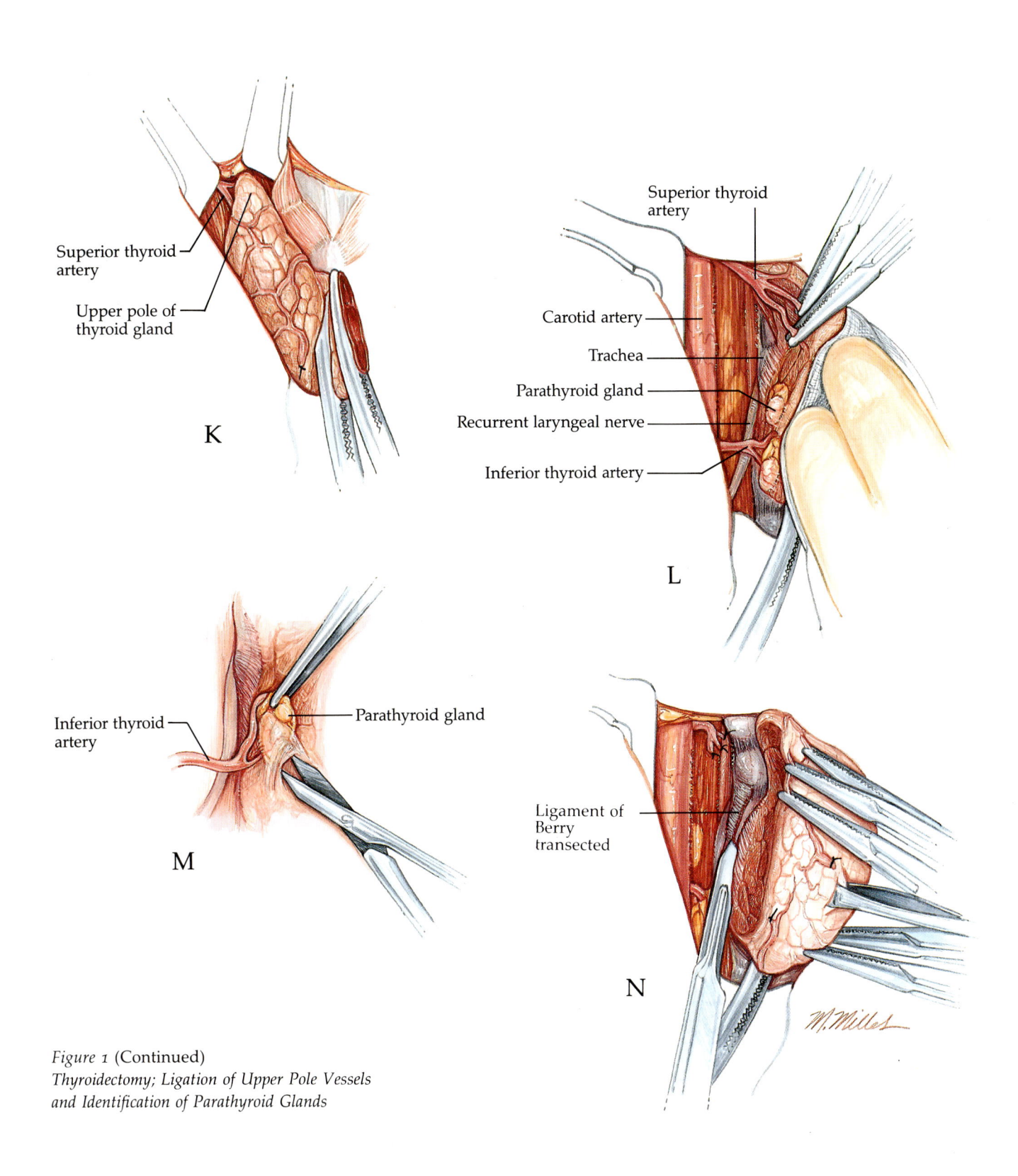

K

L
Superior thyroid artery
Carotid artery
Trachea
Parathyroid gland
Recurrent laryngeal nerve
Inferior thyroid artery

Superior thyroid artery
Upper pole of thyroid gland

M
Inferior thyroid artery
Parathyroid gland

N
Ligament of Berry transected

Figure 1 (Continued)
Thyroidectomy; Ligation of Upper Pole Vessels and Identification of Parathyroid Glands

313

Remnants should be left laterally if subtotal thyroidectomy is performed (Figs. 1O and 1P). The inferior thyroid artery should be spared as it enters the remnant and clamps applied along the medial border of the tissue to be left. The ideal size of the remnant is a subject of some controversy. About 2 g per side is usually ample. Resection should be more generous in children with Graves' disease to avoid recurrence of hyperthyroidism.

The strap muscles are reapproximated with 4–0 Vicryl or Dexon (Fig. 1Q). Next approximate the platysma with absorbable suture. I prefer fine nylon suture, usually 6–0, to approximate the skin (Fig. 1R). In situations in which there is a very large goiter with much residual dead space or mediastinal extension of goiter, a small, closed suction drain may be used and can be brought out through a separate stab incision. I do not routinely use drains for thyroid or parathyroid operations.

Postoperative Care

The majority of patients undergoing thyroidectomy are ready for discharge within 24 to 48 hours of operation. Postoperative observation should be directed toward avoidance of airway compromise and recognition of hypocalcemia.

Risks, Complications, and Sequelae

Stridor immediately following extubation suggests vocal cord injury. Direct laryngoscopy at the time of extubation does not entirely rule out vocal cord injury but allows assessment of arytenoid movement and the presence of edema. Stridor developing in the recovery room after uneventful extubation may suggest impending airway obstruction from bleeding into the operative site. The fact that minimal drainage is produced or the absence of external bleeding does not rule out postoperative hematoma. This is a true postoperative emergency. A high index of suspicion is important, since initial presentation of the hematoma may be very subtle (e.g., high pitching of the patient's voice, a sense of impending doom on the part of the patient, small decreases in blood oxygen saturation). Initial treatment is to reopen the surgical site. Evacuation of the hematoma relieves the airway distress. Emergency intubation may be difficult, and failed attempts may exacerbate the respiratory problems. The best prevention of this complication is meticulous hemostasis prior to closure.

Hypocalcemia requiring intervention should be a rare occurrence. Nevertheless, transient drops in blood calcium levels commonly occur after successful parathyroidectomy and after operations for Graves' disease. Usually the nadir level of serum calcium occurs 24 to 36 hours postoperatively, although levels may continue to drop for as long as 3 or 4 days after operation. Blood calcium levels should be measured at least every 12 hours until they are stabilized. Symptoms of perioral or peripheral numbness, tetany, or a positive Trousseau's sign are indications for treatment. Oral calcium supplements of 2 to 3 g of elemental calcium per day abort mild symptoms. Moderate or severe symptoms may require a continuous infusion of calcium gluconate (usually 1 to 2 g in 100 to 200 ml of saline over 6 hours) in addition to oral supplements. Patients who have difficulty absorbing oral calcium may need vitamin D supple-

Plate 135

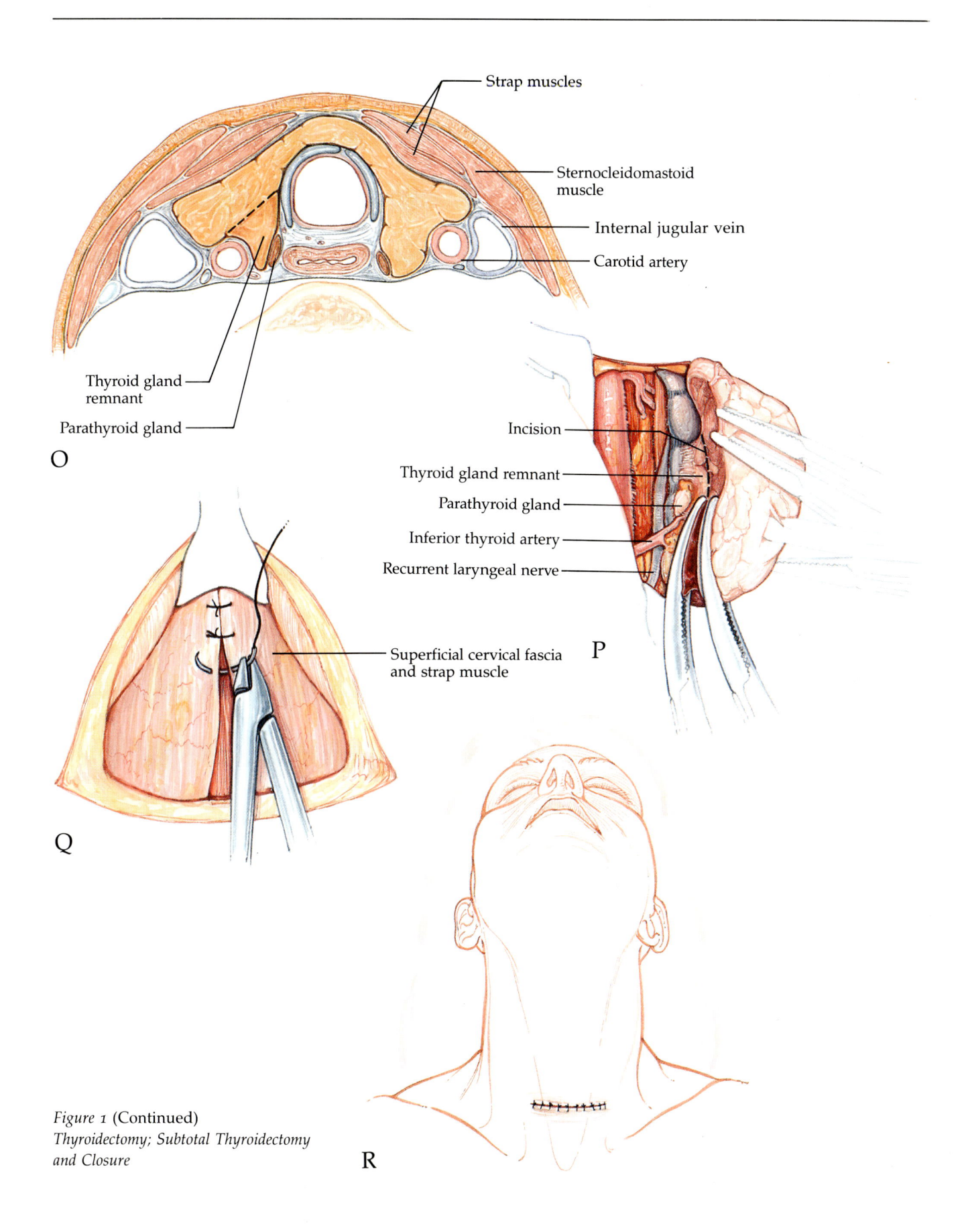

- Strap muscles
- Sternocleidomastoid muscle
- Internal jugular vein
- Carotid artery
- Thyroid gland remnant
- Parathyroid gland

O

- Incision
- Thyroid gland remnant
- Parathyroid gland
- Inferior thyroid artery
- Recurrent laryngeal nerve

- Superficial cervical fascia and strap muscle

P

Q

R

Figure 1 (Continued)
Thyroidectomy; Subtotal Thyroidectomy and Closure

ments to facilitate absorption. 1,25(OH)$_2$D$_3$ (Rocaltrol), 0.25 to 0.5 µg daily, provides rapid onset, short-acting supplementation.

Patients with well-differentiated thyroid carcinoma and those who have undergone total thyroidectomy should receive L-thyroxine orally for life. L-thyroxine is preferable to animal thyroid extracts because these latter preparations have a relatively high level of triiodothyronine compared with L-thyroxine and may result in iatrogenic T$_3$ toxicosis when administered in amounts adequate to suppress TSH. Patients with thyroid cancer who are to receive radioactive iodine as adjunctive therapy or postoperative scanning to look for metastatic disease should not receive L-thyroxine replacement until after scanning and/or treatment, since successful uptake of ^{131}I requires TSH stimulation of any residual iodine and tissue for maximal uptake.

Pearls and Pitfalls

Failure to dissect the sternothyroid muscle completely off the thyroid gland makes mobilization of the gland difficult and provokes unnecessary blood loss.

Visualization of the recurrent laryngeal nerve does not guarantee that injury will not occur. Be aware of the entire course of the nerve within the operative field. Also be aware of the rare (but not unheard of) possibility of a nonrecurrent laryngeal nerve, especially on the right side.

Do not use electrocautery to control bleeding from vessels directly adjacent to the recurrent laryngeal nerves. The heat transmitted may result in injury.

Be sure that the upper pole vessels are reliably ligated. Transient cessation of bleeding from an escaped vessel is usually just that (transient). Resumption of bleeding can result in obstructing hematoma.

Suggested Reading

Hunt PS, Poole M, Reeve TS. A reappraisal of the surgical anatomy of the thyroid and parathyroid glands. Br J Surg 1968; 55:63–66.

Kaplan EL, ed. Surgery of the thyroid and parathyroid glands. New York: Churchill Livingstone, 1983.

Roudebush CP, Astens GT, DeGroot LJ. Natural history of radiation induced thyroid cancer. Arch Intern Med 1978; 138:1631–1634.

Maria Allo, M.D.

PARATHYROIDECTOMY

Anatomic Considerations

The parathyroid glands are normally located within a 1-cm circle whose center point is the intersection of the inferior thyroid artery and the recurrent laryngeal nerve. About 80 percent of parathyroids are found in this circle. Missing lower glands are frequently found along the thymic tract and can extend anywhere from the level of the hyoid bone, to the carotid sheath, to down into the mediastinum. The missing upper glands generally are found medial and posterior in the tracheoesophageal groove. It is extremely important to note that the recurrent nerve may be over, around, or in a location otherwise very closely adherent to the parathyroids; for this reason great care must be taken to dissect the parathyroid to its vascular pedicle prior to removal of an adenoma or biopsy of a normal gland.

Indications and Preoperative Considerations

The first parathyroid operation was done in the early 1920s at a time when measurement of serum calcium concentration was difficult and measurement of parathyroid hormone was impossible. Patients undergoing surgery then had bone and renal manifestations of hyperparathyroidism that are rarely, if ever, seen today. Most patients with hyperparathyroidism diagnosed since the 1960s come to medical attention for other reasons or are found to be hypercalcemic when calcium level is measured as part of a panel of automated blood chemistries. Less commonly, patients present with kidney stones, and hyperparathyroidism is identified as an etiologic factor. It is unusual to find patients today with significant bone disease as the presenting symptom of hyperparathyroidism.

Evaluation should include documentation of hypercalcemia over several measurements, elevation of parathyroid hormone levels, decreased serum phosphate levels, and hypercalciuria. Patients with equivocal findings or with other identifiable etiologies for their hypercalcemia should undergo more extensive testing prior to neck exploration. Except in the uncommon setting of malignant hypercalcemia (serum calcium > 15 mg per deciliter), parathyroidectomy is an elective procedure and should be deferred until diagnosis has been definitely confirmed.

Operative Steps

The technique for parathyroidectomy entails a meticulous search for the normal and abnormal glands in a methodical manner that takes into account the most likely locations. The initial approach is identical to that for thyroidectomy. The same incision is used, and it extends through the skin, subcutaneum, and platysma muscle. The strap muscles are separated at the midline and reflected laterally. It is of crucial importance to dissect the sternothyroid muscle from the surface of the thyroid gland down to the prevertebral fascia. This allows the thyroid to be rolled medially with minimal or no disruption of its blood supply. A large middle thyroid vein that impedes medial mobilization of the thyroid may be divided and ligated. Maintenance of the blood supply to the thyroid gland permits selective venous sampling in the event of unsuccessful neck exploration.

Successful parathyroidectomy requires the ability to recognize normal and abnormal parathyroid tissue (and successfully distinguish it from fat, lymph nodes, or thyroid nodules); meticulous care in dissecting the glands from adjacent structures, particularly the recurrent laryngeal nerve and its branches; and methodical exploration of the areas in which glands may be found. Eighty percent of parathyroid glands are found in a 1-cm circle whose center point is the intersection of the recurrent laryngeal nerve and the inferior thyroid artery. The parathyroid glands lie in close proximity to the thyroid but are invested in areolar connective tissue within a separate and dissectable plane (Fig. 2A). Most people (85 to 90 percent) have four glands. Additional glands (most often a fifth gland) are found about 10 percent of the time. In patients with multiple endocrine neoplasia (MEN) I syndrome, about 25 percent have more than four glands. Ectopic superior parathyroids may be found along the tracheoesophageal groove with decreasing frequency as one moves cephalad from their most frequent location just above the junction of the recurrent laryngeal nerve and the inferior thyroid artery. About 4 percent of upper glands lie inferior to this intersection, thus mimicking an inferior gland. About 1 percent of upper glands are found within the carotid sheath. Upper glands in the carotid sheath usually lie in the level of the intersection of the recurrent laryngeal nerve and the inferior thyroid artery. About 1 to 2 in 1,000 glands are truly intrathyroidal, that is, entirely surrounded by encapsulated thyroid tissue. These are virtually always upper glands, which is not surprising, since the upper parathyroids derive embryologically from the fourth branchial pouch and migrate with thyroid tissue.

Ectopic lower glands can be found anywhere along the embryologic path of migration of the thymus. Most are near the lower pole of the thyroid within 1 cm below the intersection of the recurrent laryngeal nerve and the inferior thyroid artery. Most inferior glands not found in this location are adjacent to thymic remnant, and careful cervical thyroidectomy may be rewarded by delivery of a previously unnoticed adenoma. Much less commonly, lower parathyroid glands may be found "dropped off" in the area between the thyroid cartilage and the thymic remnant along the path of embryologic migration. (The lower parathyroid glands derive from the third branchial pouch endoderm and migrate with thymic anlage.) About 2 to 3 percent of lower glands are found in the anterior mediastinum, of which about 90 percent are within or near the mediastinal thymus and 10 percent are not in direct proximity to the thymus gland.

Adenoma is treated by total removal of the tumor (Fig. 2B). Subtotal (3 or $3\frac{1}{2}$ glands) resection should only be done in cases of proven hyperplasia. No tissue should be removed until all glands have been visualized. In symptomatic patients with MEN I syndrome, generous ($3\frac{1}{2}$ glands) resection should be done; patients with MEN II syndrome often have asymmetric hyperplasia but rarely have clinically significant or symptomatic hyperparathyroidism. Enlarged glands may be removed in hypercalcemic MEN II syndrome patients, but unlike in the case of the MEN I syndrome patient, 3 or $3\frac{1}{2}$ gland resection should be avoided. Histologic confirmation can be made by taking a small biopsy of parathyroid tissue. Care should be taken to preserve the vascular pedicle to the gland. If the

Plate 136

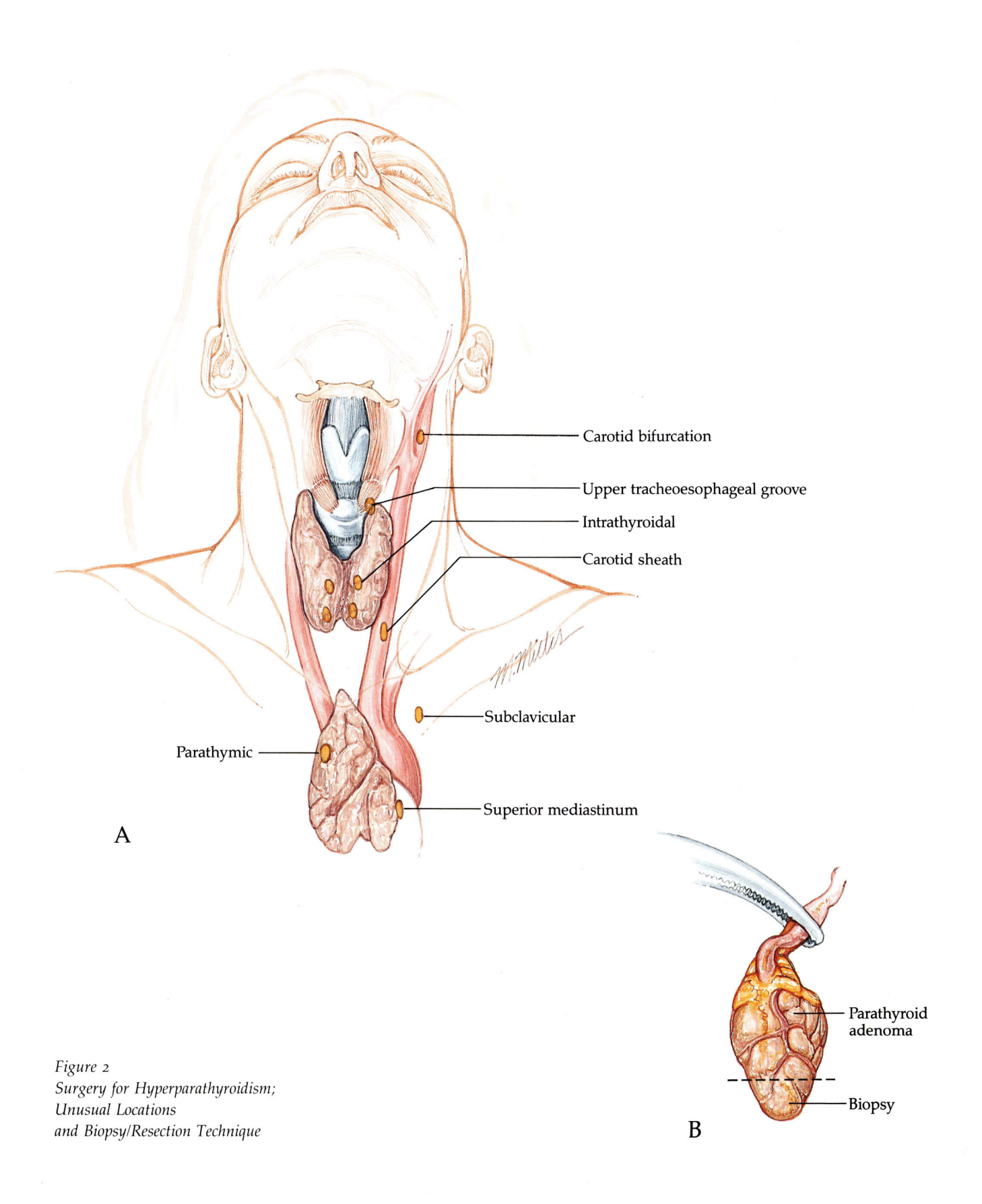

- Carotid bifurcation
- Upper tracheoesophageal groove
- Intrathyroidal
- Carotid sheath
- Subclavicular
- Parathymic
- Superior mediastinum

A

- Parathyroid adenoma
- Biopsy

B

Figure 2
Surgery for Hyperparathyroidism;
Unusual Locations
and Biopsy/Resection Technique

adenoma is not found in the neck, the operation should be terminated, and localization studies should be done before mediastinal exploration is undertaken.

Postoperative Care

The postoperative management of parathyroidectomy is the same as for thyroidectomy.

Risks, Complications, and Sequelae

The operative risks and postoperative complications are similar to those of thyroidectomy.

Patients operated on for primary hyperparathyroidism caused by solitary adenoma rarely have recurrences. Hypercalcemia occurring immediately following operation usually indicates inadequate operation. Hypercalcemia occurring months after operation in patients whose calcium level had normalized for at least 1 month postoperatively warrants evaluation for causes of hypercalcemia other than primary hyperparathyroidism, once serum parathyroid hormone level has been documented to be in the normal range.

Pearls and Pitfalls

See this section under Thyroidectomy.

Attention to the *entire* course of the recurrent laryngeal nerve cannot be overemphasized. Look for the nerve as you look for upper glands deep in the tracheoesophageal groove.

Occasionally one encounters "kissing parathyroids" (upper and lower glands in very close proximity just above and below the inferior thyroid artery). Be sure to dissect each to its vascular pedicle so as not to assume the pair to be a single gland or a small adenoma.

Be patient in your dissection of adenomas. Rupture of the capsule with spillage may result in autotransplantation of the tumor. Often adenomas are larger than they appear initially and pop out as the areolar tissue enveloping them is dissected. Frequently the recurrent laryngeal nerve or its branches may be adherent to the investing connective tissue. A major cause of recurrent or persistent disease is not failure to find the adenoma but failure to remove it completely.

There is a definite learning curve involved in successful identification of parathyroids. During thyroid and other operations in this region, use the opportunity to identify normal parathyroids.

If you have any doubt about having removed all normal parathyroid tissue, transplant a small amount of tissue (proved by biopsy to be parathyroid) into the forearm or another accessible location. *Do not transplant adenoma.*

Do not remove any parathyroid tissue until the adenoma is found. Never remove normal glands (except a tiny biopsy specimen for positive identification as parathyroid tissue) if no adenoma is found.

Sternotomy should not be done at the time of initial exploration unless there is clear documentation that the adenoma is in the mediastinum.

Localization studies may be very misleading. Often patients with large adenomas and biochemically apparent disease do not have their tumors visualized preoperatively. Or not uncommonly, the same alleged adenoma is seen in different locations or not visualized at all by simultaneously performed localizing techniques.

Patients with MEN-associated hyperparathyroidism have asymmetric hyperplasia. The natural history and severity of the disease are highly variable, depending on the specific syndrome and the family history. Recurrences are not uncommon after operation. Unless you are particularly experienced in managing these patients, they should be referred to a center familiar with the idiosyncrasies of this uncommon form of the disease.

Primary hyperparathyroidism is very uncommon in prepubertal children. Familial hypercalcemic hypocalciuria, MEN syndromes, and other unusual alterations in calcium metabolism should be investigated before proceeding with surgery.

Suggested Reading

Kaplan EL, Bartlett S, Sugemoto J, Fredland A. Postoperative hypocalcemia—its relation to different operative techniques. The deleterious effect of excessive use of parathyroid biopsy. Surgery 1982; 92:827–834.

Scholz DA, Purnell DC. Asymptomatic primary hyperparathyroidism: 10 year prospective study. Mayo Clin Proc 1981; 56:473–478. *Results of a 10-year study looking at what happens to people with asymptomatic but biochemically evident primary hyperparathyroidism.*

Wang CA. Surgery of the parathyroid glands. Adv Sur 1966; 5:109–127.

Wells SA, Gunnells JC, Shelburne JD, et al. Transplantation of the parathyroid gland in man: Clinical indications and results. Surgery 1982; 78:827–834.

Chapter VI

SALIVARY GLANDS

Michael E. Johns, M.D.
Wayne M. Koch, M.D.

SUBMANDIBULAR GLAND EXCISION

Indications   Indications for submandibular gland excision include (1) neoplasm or mass in the gland (the incidence of malignancy is higher than in the parotid gland, approaching 50 percent); (2) chronic or recurrent acute sialoadenitis requiring repeated courses of antibiotics, glandular dysfunction, history of abscess in the submandibular, or sublingual space involvement; (3) recurrent or intractable sialolithiasis with resultant sialoadenitis (more common in the submandibular than in the parotid gland); and (4) sialorrhea, or drooling (controversial).

Preoperative Considerations

Excision of the submandibular gland is best done with the patient under general anesthesia, and routine preoperative medical evaluation is required. The healthy patient may be admitted to the hospital on the morning of surgery. The typical hospital stay is for a single postoperative day. In cases of acute sialoadenitis, it is desirable to wait for 4 to 6 weeks after the resolution of inflammation prior to excision.

A firm mass in the submandibular region should be assessed by bimanual palpation, taking note of possible lymphatic adenopathy adjacent to the gland or stones within Wharton's duct or the hilus of the gland. A helpful physical diagnostic sign is that masses within the submandibular gland cannot be "rolled" over the mandible, whereas a lymph node may be more mobile. The presence and nature of glandular secretions should be noted. In addition, a fine needle aspiration of the mass should be performed. Adjacent nodes may contain squamous carcinoma, alerting the surgeon to the need for careful work-up to identify the primary focus of malignancy. Salivary neoplasms within the submandibular gland are malignant in 50 percent of cases. This information is important in planning the surgical approach to the gland.

Modern computed tomography and magnetic resonance imaging are useful in assessing the nature and extent of submandibular disease. Both coronal and axial views should be obtained. The presence of calculi, cystic degeneration, extension beyond the capsule of the gland, and adjacent adenopathy may be discerned. Although these studies have replaced the sialogram for routine examination of the gland, infusion of the ductal system with contrast medium may be useful in demonstrating constriction of the duct or intraductal stones. However, the submandibular sialogram is somewhat difficult to perform because of the small ductal orifice. The risk of overinjection and attendant patient discomfort does not justify the routine use of this procedure. For suspected tumors, delineation of the ductal system does not aid in surgical decision making. Most important, any imaging study should be requested only if it will make a difference in how you treat the patient. In general, small masses in the gland or ductal stones are treated by excision of the gland, and the computed tomographic or magnetic resonance imaging scan would not alter patient management.

Informed patient consent is obtained, accompanied by discussion of potential damage to the marginal mandibular branch of the facial nerve as well as the lingual and hypoglossal nerves. In cases of proven or highly suspicious malignancy, the possible need for neck dissection and resection of nerves, of a mandibular segment, and/or of the floor of the mouth with appropriate reconstruction measures is discussed.

Prophylactic antibiotics are not generally required, although preoperative antibiotics are continued when surgery is performed in the setting of acute infection.

Operative Steps

General anesthesia without neuromuscular blockade is performed. A curvilinear incision is planned within or parallel to the skin creases of the neck, located 3 to 4 cm below the inferior border of the mandible, from the anterior edge of the sternocleidomastoid muscle curving anteriorly 5 to 6 cm (Fig. 1A). The planned incision may be injected superficially with a local anesthetic containing vasoconstrictor for hemostasis. The initial incision is carried through the platysma (except in cases of known malignancy), and subplatysmal flaps are raised superiorly over the mandibular ramus and inferiorly below the hyoid bone. The facial vein can be identified and ligated at the incision site and the superior flap elevated deep to the vein (Fig. 1B). Since the marginal mandibular nerve is superficial to the vein, the nerve will be protected in this way. When malignancy is suspected, the capsule of the gland and the surrounding soft tissue are included in the resection. The marginal mandibular nerve may now occasionally be visualized within the fascia overlying the gland. If it is not immediately apparent, it may be sought, spreading the fascia bluntly with a fine clamp in the direction of the nerve, parallel to the mandible. When the nerve is located, it is dissected along the extent of the incision and reflected superiorly with the flaps. An alternate method is to transect the facial vein and reflect it superiorly with the skin flap. If there is no malignancy, the fascia overlying the gland may be incised inferiorly and elevated, joining the flap superiorly. This maneuver allows the marginal nerve to be included in the elevated flap.

The facial vein and artery are located near the superior border of the gland as they course toward the mandible. Dissection is continued anteriorly along the inferior border of the mandible. Multiple smaller arteries and veins are located within soft tissue and should be ligated or cauterized with bipolar current. Blunt dissection inferiorly frees the gland from the digastric muscle (Fig. 1C). The facial artery is again encountered and transected posterolaterally near its origin at the external carotid artery just above the posterior belly of the digastric muscle (Fig. 1D). Caution must be exercised to avoid injuring the hypoglossal nerve at this stage, although it courses inferior to the digastric muscle.

Plate 137

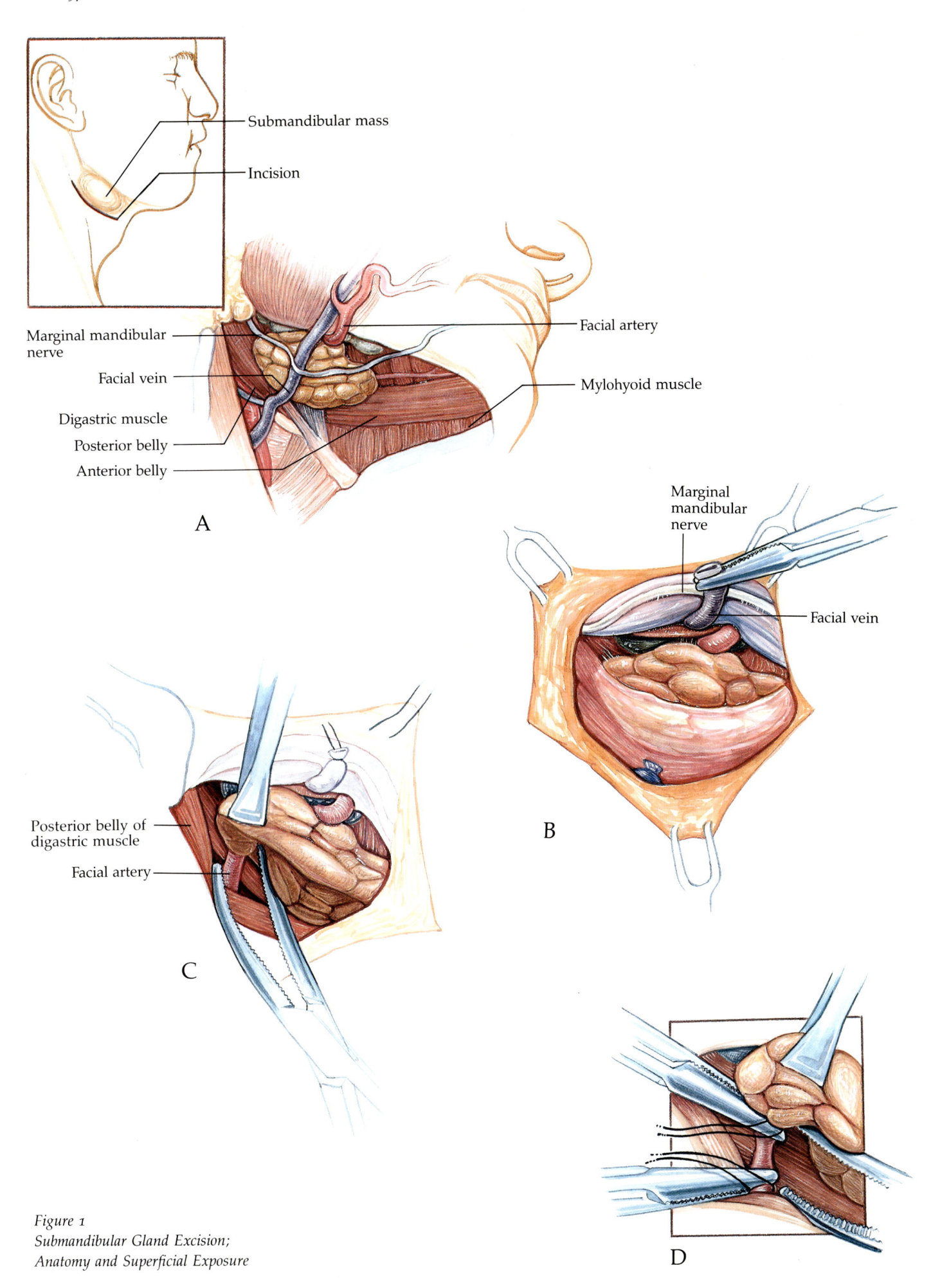

- Submandibular mass
- Incision

A
- Marginal mandibular nerve
- Facial vein
- Digastric muscle
- Posterior belly
- Anterior belly
- Facial artery
- Mylohyoid muscle

B
- Marginal mandibular nerve
- Facial vein

C
- Posterior belly of digastric muscle
- Facial artery

D

Figure 1
Submandibular Gland Excision;
Anatomy and Superficial Exposure

327

At the anterior border of the gland, the submental fat is dissected to the depth of the mylohyoid muscle and reflected posteriorly with the superficial portion of the gland that overlies the muscle. Lateral retraction on the gland allows for identification of the posterolateral border of this muscle. A retractor is inserted to pull the free edge of the mylohyoid muscle medially, exposing the floor of the submandibular triangle consisting of the hyoglossus muscle with overlying fat and fascia (Fig. 1E). Three important structures course within this fascia: the hypoglossal nerve, the lingual nerve, and Wharton's duct. Gentle downward traction on the gland permits easy visualization of the lingual nerve arching downward, with its lowest point midway along the gland. Here branches of the nerve go to and from the submandibular parasympathetic ganglion on the superior aspect of the gland (Fig. 1F). The duct is often surrounded by glandular tissue and thus may be difficult to identify at first. It begins inferior to the lingual nerve, passing deep to the nerve as it goes anterosuperiorly to the frenula. The hypoglossal nerve lies inferior to the gland and duct posteriorly. It courses superomedially, accompanied by the ranine vein, and enters the tongue musculature. When all structures have been identified, the lingual nerve branches are ligated near the gland (Fig. 1G). The duct is ligated as high as it can be clearly visualized (Fig. 1H). Gland and contiguous soft tissue may then be removed. The wound is inspected for hemostasis, a rubber ribbon drain is inserted deep to the platysma, and the wound is closed in layers.

In the context of malignancy, nodal disease may be present along the facial and jugular veins and there may be local invasion of surrounding soft tissues, nerves, or skin. Excision including a safe margin of normal tissue may require resection of the lingual, hypoglossal, or marginal mandibular nerves, the floor of the mouth mucosa, the tongue musculature, and the mandible or skin. The marginal mandibular nerve may pass directly over or around facial vein nodes, and judgment must be exercised in each case as to the feasibility of preserving it by dissection from such nodes. Radical neck dissection may be incorporated with this procedure as indicated.

Plate 138

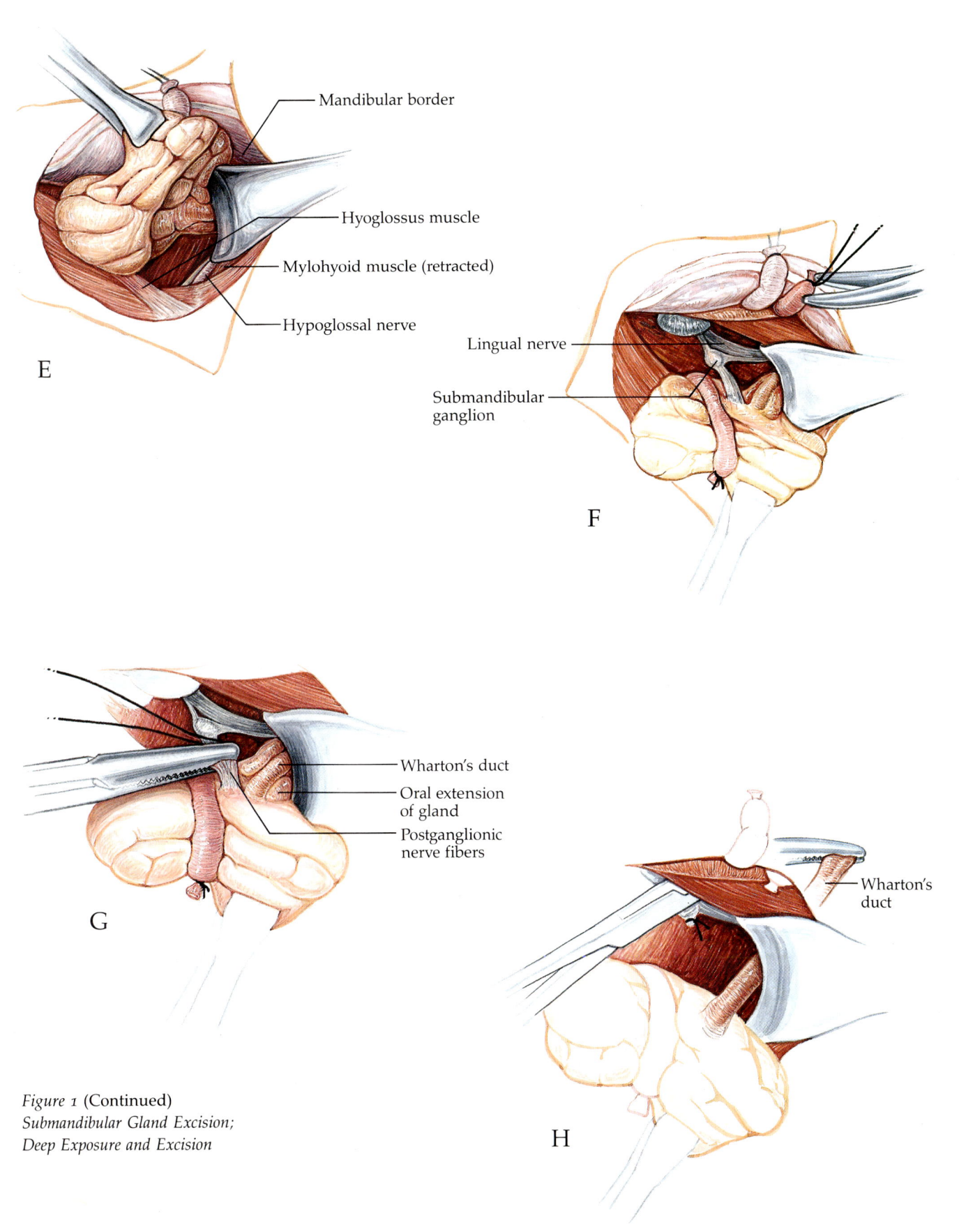

- Mandibular border
- Hyoglossus muscle
- Mylohyoid muscle (retracted)
- Hypoglossal nerve

E

- Lingual nerve
- Submandibular ganglion

F

- Wharton's duct
- Oral extension of gland
- Postganglionic nerve fibers

G

- Wharton's duct

H

Figure 1 (Continued)
*Submandibular Gland Excision;
Deep Exposure and Excision*

329

Risks, Complications, and Sequelae

Complications of submandibular gland excision are few. The most common postoperative finding is marginal mandibular weakness. This paresis often occurs when the nerve is dissected from underlying adenopathy. Weakness also may occur from persistent traction on the upper flap. Complete return of function is the rule but may require several months. Loss of lingual and hypoglossal nerve function is rare unless these nerves are included in the resection.

Pearls and Pitfalls

Avoid infiltrating local anesthetic superior to the skin incision so as not to block conduction of impulses from instruments and the nerve stimulator, which alert one to the location of the marginal mandibular nerve.

The best means of preserving the marginal mandibular nerve is its positive identification and elevation after dissection of the nerve with the surrounding fascia. Placement of the skin incision well below the mandible flap, elevations deep to the platysma including the fascia overlying the gland when possible, and transection of facial vein below the gland with reflection of the vessel stump are all measures aimed at nerve preservation.

Posterior dissection and reflection of the superficial portion of the submandibular gland from the mylohyoid muscle are essential before the posterior margin of this muscle can be identified and then retracted anteriorly. This maneuver is critical to the identification of the duct and its neighbors, the lingual and hypoglossal nerves.

When a sialolith is present within the duct, an effort is made to push it posteroinferiorly, including it in the specimen. Failing this, an intraoral incision over the stone in the floor of mouth may be required to remove it.

There is no place for unipolar cautery in submandibular gland excision. Important neural structures are nearby at every point of the procedure.

Michael E. Johns, M.D.

PAROTIDECTOMY

Indications

Indications for parotidectomy are a mass or lesion in the parotid gland, metastasis to or great likelihood of metastasis to the parotid gland, recurrent sialadenitis that is refractory to medical management, and a parotid duct stone.

Preoperative Considerations

The patient is admitted to the hospital on the day of surgery. The length of stay is commonly one or two nights.

A general anesthetic technique without paralysis is preferred. The patient is positioned in the supine position, with the head at the top of the table and the entire body positioned as far to the same side of the table as the parotid gland to be operated on. The head is then turned to the opposite side, and a small shoulder roll is placed under the shoulder to extend the neck and face. Rotating the table 10 to 15 degrees away from the operating surgeon facilitates the dissection. The head rests on a sponge donut.

The endotracheal tube is positioned in the corner of the mouth opposite the surgical field, and all tape used to secure the tube is kept off the operative half of the face. An ophthalmic ointment is placed in each eye. The eyelid on the operative side is either sutured closed or a small piece of tape is applied only to the medial half of the lid to prevent eye exposure during surgery but allow easy monitoring of the orbicularis oculi muscle during facial nerve dissection.

The incision site and facial flap are then injected with 1:100,000 lidocaine with epinephrine to achieve vasoconstriction and minimize small vessel bleeding during the incision and elevation of the flap. This should be done prior to preparing and draping the patient in order to allow adequate time for vasoconstriction to occur. The sideburn hair and the hair over the occipital area are pulled back and held out of the operative field using 2-inch masking tape.

The patient is then prepared with an appropriate antiseptic solution to include the hemiface and neck on the operative side. This includes the pinna and the mastoid region. The external auditory canal is lightly packed with a 1-inch wide strip of gauze covered with petroleum jelly to prevent blood from clotting on the tympanic membrane.

Draping is accomplished with towels and an adhesive plastic drape. The towels are placed just along the hairline from the midforehead posteriorly and above the zygoma; along the postauricular hairline down along the trapezius muscle; horizontally across the neck; and last just beyond the midline of the face. This last towel is folded longitudinally in quarters so it covers the endotracheal tube and midline of the opposite side of the face but does not obstruct visualization of the operative side of the facial muscles. Towel clips are used to secure the posteriorly positioned towels. The anteriorly placed towel is secured by the adhesive plastic barrier. It is my preference to have the plastic barrier start just anterior to the pinna and in front of the incision line. This eliminates the necessity to cut through the plastic drape and put up with the curling edges of plastic through the rest of the procedure. Most important, the plastic drape serves as a window to the face and secures the anterior midline drape in the field. The remainder of the body is draped using a split head sheet, and appropriate barriers are used to protect the assistant surgeons from contamination.

Operative Steps

SUPRANEURAL PAROTIDECTOMY

The incision is outlined as seen in Figure 2A. It can be extended up into the hairline or more anteriorly along the horizontal cervical portion of the incision, depending on the extent of the surgery needed. In general, an incision that starts just along a line where the helix of the pinna attaches to the side of the face extends inferiorly just behind the free edge of the tragus and down along the line of attachment of the lobule of the pinna. It curves gently into a horizontal crease in the neck anteriorly to a level approximately at the greater cornu of the hyoid bone. The incision can be shortened or lengthened, depending on the exposure needed. The portion of the incision that extends from the lobule over the mastoid tip and into the neck need not curve far posteriorly, only just under the lobule. If taken too far back, it will create a "finger" of the flap, which may turn cyanotic and adds nothing to the exposure. The cervical portion of the incision should be just behind the anteromedial border of the sternocleidomastoid muscle, as it is here that the tail of the parotid gland must be freed from its fascial attachment to the muscle.

The skin flap is sharply dissected in a plane just above the superficial parotid fascia. As the flap is dissected anteriorly, care is taken to avoid peripheral branches of the nerve as they emerge from the gland. A thick flap minimizes the chance for future onset of Frey's syndrome. Successful and rapid identification of the main trunk of the facial nerve depends upon familiarity with important anatomic landmarks and wide exposure. The tail of the parotid gland is dissected free from the sternocleidomastoid muscle, the mastoid tip, and the auricular cartilage. This is accomplished by incising the sternocleidomastoid-parotid fascia along the anteromedial edge of the sternocleidomastoid muscle (Fig. 2B) and then using blunt and sharp dissection (Fig. 2C). A plane is established between the anterior edge of the sternocleidomastoid muscle and the tail of the parotid gland. This plane is created from just below the mastoid attachment of the sternocleidomastoid muscle down to the posterior facial vein. The facial vein is left intact, as the facial nerve courses over the vein, and the vein need not be ligated to remove the superficial lobe. Moreover, the cervical and frequently a marginal branch of the facial nerve are in close proximity, and if care is not taken, these small branches may be injured. Ligation of this vein also may contribute to venous congestion of the gland and increase the amount of venous and capillary bleeding.

Plate 139

A — Incision; Tragal cartilage; Parotid tumor; Duct; Masseter muscle; Cranial nerve VII (branch); Digastric muscle; Sternocleidomastoid muscle; Posterior facial vein

B — Parotid tumor; Marginal branch of cranial nerve VII; Great auricular nerve; Sternocleidomastoid parotid fascia

C — Sternocleidomastoid muscle; Cervical branch of cranial nerve VII; Posterior facial vein

Figure 2
Parotidectomy;
Incision and Parotid Tail Dissection

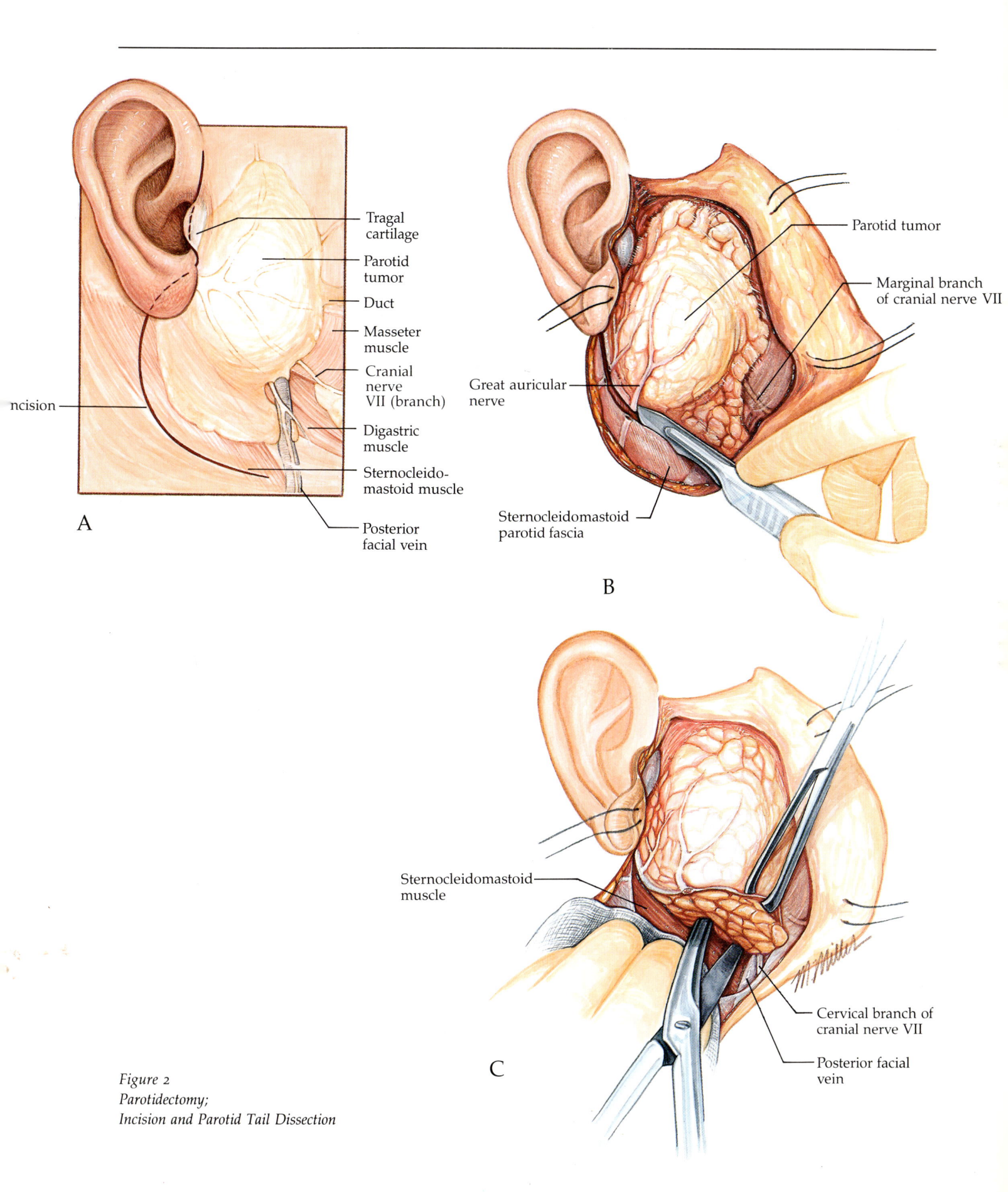

The digastric muscle is usually seen as this tail of the parotid gland is elevated and the above-mentioned plane is developed (see Fig. 2D). This is an important anatomic landmark, since the facial nerve exits the stylomastoid foramen on a plane at or just below the attachment of the digastric muscle in the digastric groove of the mastoid tip.

Once the tail of the parotid gland is elevated, a second plane in the pretragal space is developed using a hemostat for blunt dissection. This is accomplished by placing the tip of a hemostat just anterior to the tragus and opening it progressively deeper parallel to the facial nerve (antero-posterior) (Fig. 2D). This exposes the tragal pointer and opens a plane from the zygoma superiorly to just above the styloid process inferiorly. The tympanic bone should be identified.

The pretragal and tail portions of the parotid gland are now mobilized leaving a narrow "bridge" of parotid and fascia attached to the mastoid tip (Fig. 2E). With the knowledge that the facial nerve is about 1.0 cm deep to the tip of the tragal pointer (lying just anterior and inferior to the tip), 6 to 8 mm below the end of the tympanomastoid suture (the tympanomastoid suture line is an easily palpated groove separating the mastoid tip from the tympanic portion of the temporal bone), and just above and on the same plane as the attachment of the digastric muscle in the digastric groove, the surgeon can predict where the facial nerve sits in this narrow bridge of tissue. Using this anatomic knowledge, a hemostat is passed above the level of the facial nerve over the mastoid tip, creating a tunnel between the tail and pretragal planes. A No. 15 blade is then used to incise the parotid fascial attachments down to the hemostat (Figs. 2F and 2G). The importance of adequate exposure, especially elevation of the tail from the underlying musculature, cannot be overemphasized. Wide exposure of the operative field will prevent the surgeon from "working in a hole" and allow visualization of all pertinent landmarks required for rapid identification of the main nerve trunk. The tympanomastoid suture line can now be easily palpated, and if the above steps are done properly, there is a 5 to 10 mm wide bridge of soft tissue at the inferior

Plate 140

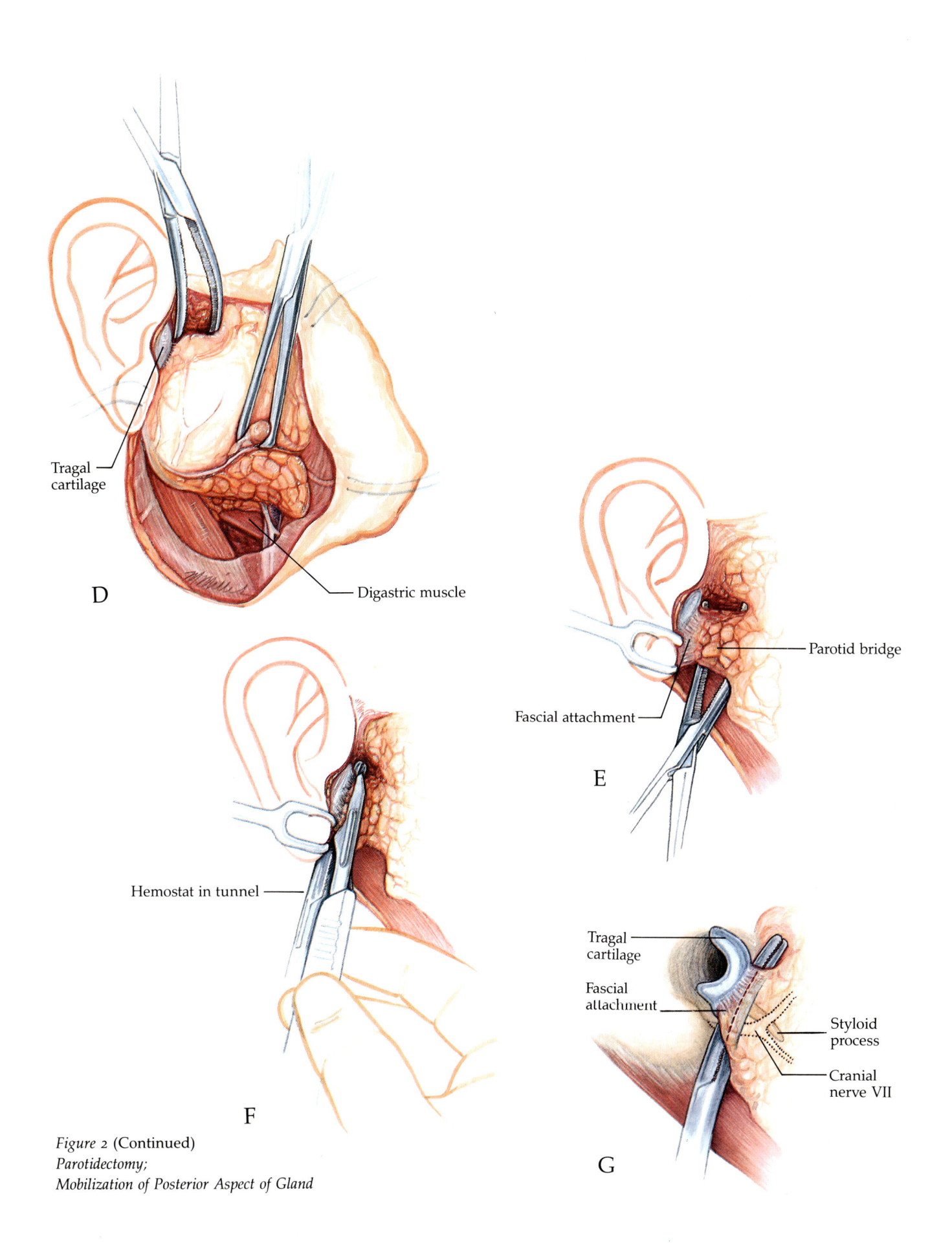

D
Tragal cartilage
Digastric muscle

E
Parotid bridge
Fascial attachment

F
Hemostat in tunnel

G
Tragal cartilage
Fascial attachment
Styloid process
Cranial nerve VII

Figure 2 (Continued)
Parotidectomy;
Mobilization of Posterior Aspect of Gland

level of the tympanomastoid suture line that is bluntly dissected with a fine pointed hemostat in order to identify the facial nerve. The hemostat is gently opened in the direction of the facial nerve, slowly teasing the soft tissues apart until the facial nerve is visualized (Fig. 2H). It should be kept in mind that the facial nerve is relatively deep in relation to the surface plane, as it exits the stylomastoid canal but ascends through the parotid tissue quite steeply to a midglandular level, where it takes a more horizontal course. In difficult situations, a nerve stimulator may be used for confirmation of the location of the nerve, but it should be used sparingly to avoid nerve injury. Once the nerve trunk is identified, the individual branches are followed peripherally, the parotid gland being progressively separated from the nerve from a superior to an inferior direction. This is accomplished by sliding a small pointed hemostat in a plane just on top of the nerve for a small distance, lifting the hemostat off the nerve, and then gently spreading open the tips to create a small tunnel in which the nerve can be seen. Using a No. 12 surgical blade, the parotid tissue is incised in a plane parallel to the nerve (Fig. 2I). The technique is slide, lift, spread, and then cut in a horizontal plane parallel to the visible nerve. The cut is always made from the safe visible tunnel to the next safe plane above. The nerve is followed to the periphery of the gland using this technique. Once a branch is exposed completely, the surgeon returns to the origin of the major division he or she is working on, identifies the next branch takeoff, and follows it to the periphery. This is accomplished in succession until all branches have been exposed and the superficial portion of the gland is removed in a single bloc (Fig. 2J).

If the goal of the procedure is now complete (i.e., removal of tumor mass in the tail or supraneural parotid), the wound is irrigated with saline and hemostasis secured. The wound is irrigated once again, and then the main trunk of the facial nerve is examined for its integrity and stimulated at 0.5 mA while the face is observed by the assistant and anesthesiologist, who confirm that all branches of the nerve are causing contraction of all parts of the facial musculature. Each branch is then examined and followed to the periphery in a similar fashion to ensure its continuity. If any portion of the nerve is not stimulating, careful inspection of the branch using the microscope if necessary is imperative. A suture may be seen to be encompassing the nerve or an actual separation of the nerve may be found that requires microsurgical repair.

Plate 141

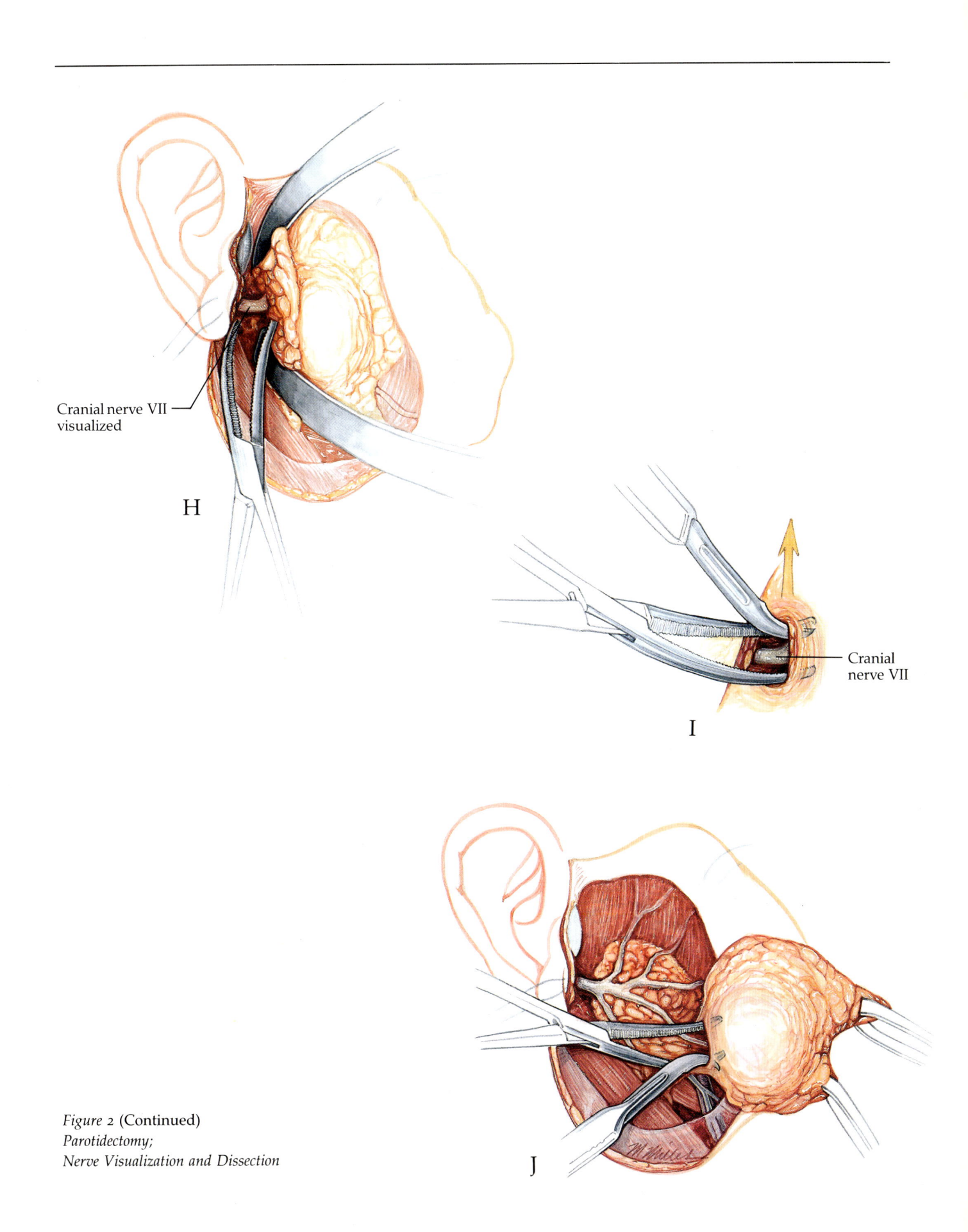

Cranial nerve VII visualized

H

Cranial nerve VII

I

Figure 2 (Continued)
Parotidectomy;
Nerve Visualization and Dissection

J

TOTAL PAROTIDECTOMY

A total parotidectomy, strictly speaking, is a misnomer. Removal of all parotid tissue is nearly impossible and is usually not necessary. The concept of a total parotidectomy is that of removal of parotid tissue, both medial and lateral to the facial nerve with the accompanying tumor. The particular technique employed may differ, depending upon the location of the tumor. If the tumor is confined to the deep lobe, the superficial lobe does not, by definition, need to be removed. However, in most cases, identification of the nerve is accomplished most easily by a superficial parotidectomy. After the nerve is satisfactorily exposed it is freed up over the tumor and the mass is removed using careful blunt dissection from beneath the nerve (Figs. 2K and 2L). This maneuver may result in some postoperative weakness, but if the surgeon avoids undue tension and stretching of the nerve, function will return. Some deep lobe tumors are dumbbell in configuration, with the isthmus or waist being found at the stylomandibular ligament. When this situation occurs, further exposure to the portion of the gland medial to the facial nerve is required.

It is apparent that for difficult parotid tumors, the surgeon and patient must be prepared for a variety of approaches to ensure their complete removal.

CLOSURE

A 7-mm flat silicone drain with bulb suction device is inserted into the wound bed just above the free border of the sternocleidomastoid muscle and below the marginal division of the seventh nerve (Fig. 2M). It is inserted through a separate stab incision made just in front of but in the same line as the cervical portion of the incision. A short portion of drain (about 5 cm) is carefully placed in the wound so that it does not contact the facial nerve.

The skin flap is then carefully replaced and aligned. Care must be taken to ensure that the lobule of the ear is precisely reapproximated. The subcutaneous tissues are reapproximated with 4–0 absorbable sutures and the skin with 5–0 Prolene. A dressing is rarely utilized.

RETROGRADE DISSECTION OF THE NERVE

If the main trunk of the facial nerve cannot be located using the above technique, one of the peripheral branches must be found and followed retrograde to the main trunk. The cervical branch may be found coursing along the posterior facial vein. The marginal mandibular branch passes over the vein in close proximity. The buccal branch is usually found within millimeters of Stensen's duct. The duct may be found as it passes over the masseter muscle on the line between the upper lip and the tragus. The temporal branch is located where the hairline crosses the zygomatic arch. The nerve stimulator may be useful in confirming these peripheral branches.

FACIAL NERVE RESECTION AND GRAFTS

If a malignant tumor is invading a peripheral branch of the facial nerve, that portion of the nerve should be resected and grafted. We currently advise a microscopic epineural suture technique using 10–0 monofilament

Plate 142

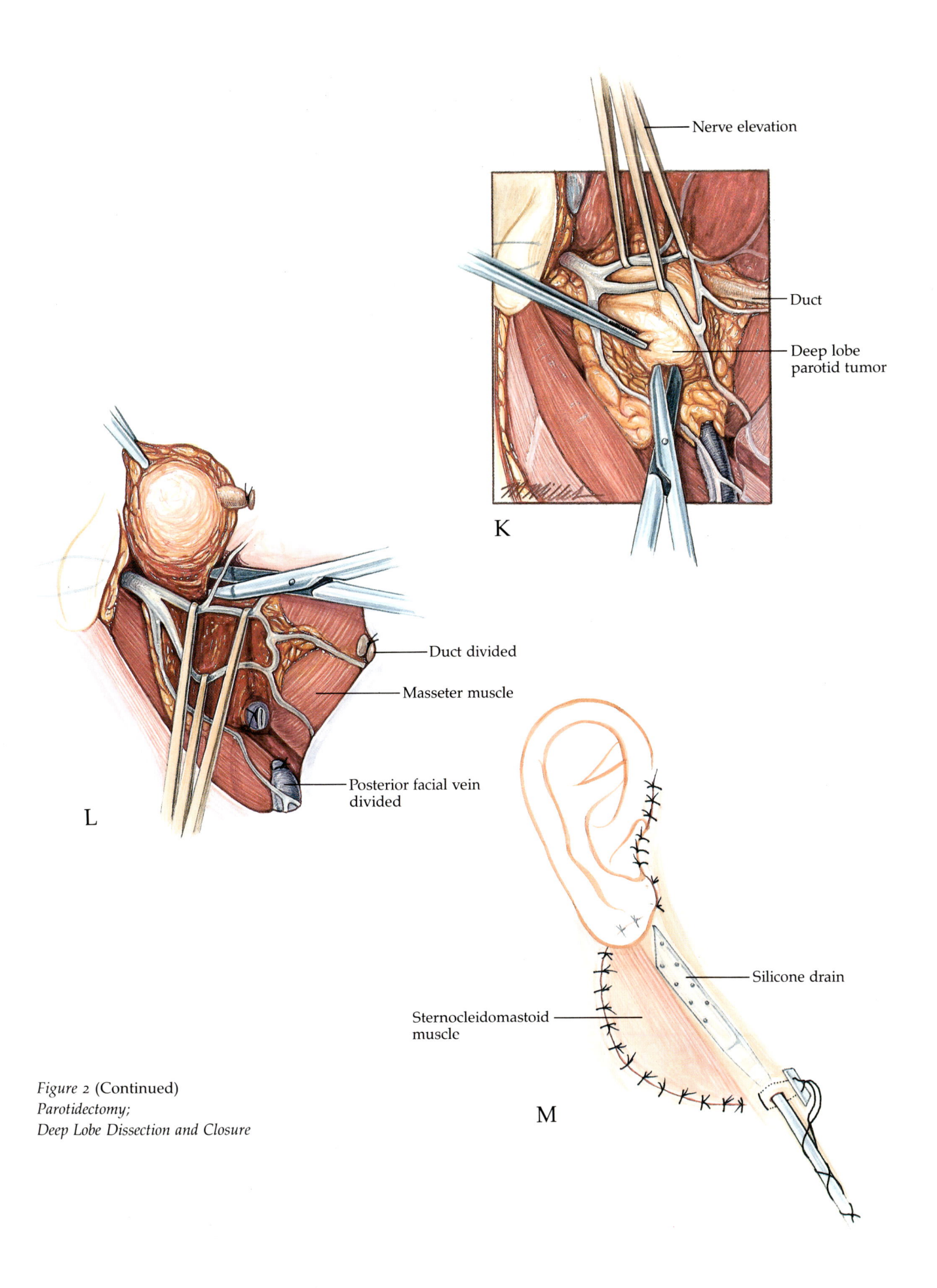

Nerve elevation

Duct

Deep lobe parotid tumor

K

Duct divided

Masseter muscle

Posterior facial vein divided

L

Silicone drain

Sternocleidomastoid muscle

M

Figure 2 (Continued)
Parotidectomy;
Deep Lobe Dissection and Closure

nylon. The nerve graft may be harvested from the neck using the great auricular nerve or sural nerve, which gives a large donor nerve length. Important factors for success include a close match of nerve and graft diameter, sharp nerve transection, and a tension-free anastomosis. Surrounding the nerve with a protective sleeve of vein, gel film, or other material may also be beneficial in protecting the graft and discouraging neuroma formation. If the tumor involves the main trunk, the nerve must be followed proximally until frozen section diagnosis of a tumor-free margin is confirmed. The mastoid tip may be removed with an osteotome or rongeur to allow a more complete exploration of the foramen. Temporal bone exploration may be required, and both the patient and the surgeon should be prepared for this eventuality. If the nerve is transected in the temporal bone and all branches are transected, a cable graft should be developed such that the branches to the eye and the mouth are reinnervated. The principles of microscopic nerve grafting are utilized as described previously. Sutures are not necessarily required in the temporal portion as long as tension is avoided.

Postoperative Care

The incision site is cleaned with hydrogen peroxide and cotton swabs twice a day. The drain is removed on the first postoperative day in most cases. Sutures are removed on the fifth postoperative day.

Risks, Complications, and Sequelae

Complications of parotid surgery may be divided into early and delayed. Common immediate or early complications are partial or complete paralysis of all or some of the branches of the facial nerve. If extensive dissection was performed around particular branches, some loss of function is not unusual. However, complete loss of function of all branches is a potentially serious complication. For this reason, stimulation of the nerve at the termination of the procedure confirms function and nerve integrity; if some branches are not functional, a careful inspection will confirm anatomic integrity. The surgeon must be confident at the termination of the procedure that he or she has a clear understanding of the status of the dissected nerve. If marked loss of function is noted in the immediate postoperative period and there is no question as to the continuity and integrity of the facial nerve, the operating surgeon may wish to consider steroid therapy. The use of steroids in facial paralysis remains controversial; however, it is generally agreed that if steroids are used, they should be given immediately. The initial dose is in the range of 60 to 80 mg of prednisone or an equivalent dose of a comparable steroid preparation. This is maintained for 5 to 7 days and then tapered over a total course of 10 days. The intent is to reduce nerve edema in both the extra- and intratemporal portions of the nerve.

A relatively common complication is postoperative salivary fistula or sialocele formation. Since some parotid tissue inevitably persists following parotid surgery, the potential for a salivary fistula is always present. A fistula or sialocele occurs when the flap fails to seal over the remaining parotid tissue, and saliva develops underneath the flap or drains into the neck. Elimination of the fistula requires complete evacuation of salivary contents from beneath the flap and application of continual extrinsic pressure to overcome the secretory pressure of the remaining tissue. This may require repeated aspirations and application of a compression dressing on a daily basis until the complication has cleared. Atropine-like drugs may be of some benefit to counteract salivary stimulation. If compressive dressings are used, one must take care to protect the ear so as to avoid necrosis of the soft tissue surrounding it.

Hematoma formation is also a potential complication. If a hematoma does occur, re-exploration of the wound is required. Of course, with the facial nerve being exposed, extreme care must be exercised to avoid injury to the nerve.

The most common long-term complication is that of gustatory sweating or Frey's syndrome. This occurs when inappropriate autonomic reinnervation of the skin develops from the innervation to the remaining transected gland. The postganglionic secretosympathetic motor parasympathetics of the parotid gland reinnervate the postganglionic fibers in the skin. With Frey's syndrome, the patient has sweating and/or flushing in the skin overlying the remaining parotid gland prior to or during meals. The incidence of this syndrome is high, estimated to be 35 to 60 percent of postparotidectomy patients. A surgeon must make the patient aware of this potential complication so that if it occurs, the patient will not be alarmed. Medical therapy has included use of topical scopolamine and glycopyrrolate. Surgical intervention includes placement of a dermal graft or muscle between the remaining parotid gland and the skin to prevent reinnervation. Tympanic neurectomy has also been used to interrupt parasympathetic supply to the remaining gland.

Sequelae of this operation are short and long term. Stiffness of the soft tissues overlying the operative site and mild trismus are common and last for a few weeks. Hypoesthesia of the operative site resolves within a few months. Hypoesthesia of the pinna improves over 6 to 8 months but rarely recovers fully.

Pearls and Pitfalls

Any mass that lies on or above an imaginary line from the mastoid tip to the angle of the mandible should be considered a parotid tumor unless proved otherwise.

Most mass lesions are in the tail of the parotid (90 percent) and 90 percent of tumors are benign.

Those tumors sitting below the zygoma and anterior to the tragus are more likely to sit deep to the facial nerve than lesions in the tail of parotid gland.

In the majority of parotid tumors (90 percent of which are in the tail and usually smaller than 3 cm), no diagnostic tests (computed tomography, magnetic resonance imaging, or fine needle aspiration) are indicated, as the parotidectomy will result in the definitive histopathologic diagnosis and curative therapy. Imaging gives the surgeon no more information than that gained from physical examination. These examinations should be considered and used with recurrent tumors, with large tumors, when the clinical picture does not fit together, or if there is a medical reason to avoid surgery if at all possible.

Raise a thick parotid flap just above the parotid fascia in order to minimize the chance of the patient's developing postoperative Frey's syndrome.

In the previously unoperated parotid, the facial nerve monitor is not used to identify the facial nerve; rather, reliable anatomic landmarks are employed. The nerve stimulator is set at 0.5 mA and pretested on muscle; it is used to check the stimulation ability of the facial nerve at the conclusion of the procedure and to confirm the integrity of all facial nerve branches.

I have found the use of loupes to be helpful during dissection of the facial nerve. The operating microscope may be used, but I find it cumbersome and the field of vision quite small; the loupes provide more than adequate magnification and much greater freedom of movement. The microscope is used for nerve grafting and anastomosis.

Peter W. Orobello, Jr., M.D.

EXCISION OF FIRST BRANCHIAL CLEFT CYST

First branchial cleft anomalies may be divided into two groups according to the Work classification: type I and type II, respectively. Type I is considered a first cleft ectodermal defect and is a duplication anomaly of the membranous external auditory canal. The cysts in this case are located anterior and inferior to the pinna and are associated with the parotid gland. The fistulous tract from the cyst extends superiorly and then turns anteriorly and parallels the external auditory canal. In its course, it may be intimately associated with the facial nerve.

Controversy exists with regard to type II first branchial cleft cysts. They are thought to be first cleft and perhaps second arch defects involving both ectoderm and mesoderm. They represent duplication anomalies of the external auditory canal and the pinna. The cysts from this anomaly are present in the submandibular triangle anterior to the sternocleidomastoid muscle. Similar to the type I cysts, the fistulous tract extends superiorly; however, in the type II anomaly, there is more intimate association with the facial nerve in the parotid gland (Fig. 3A).

Indications

The presence of a first branchial cleft anomaly does not constitute an indication for surgery. Surgery is indicated in cases in which the cysts have been subject to recurrent infection requiring antibiotics. The cyst may have undergone excision and drainage for what appears to be an abscess in the neck. The patient may occasionally have drainage from the ear; palpation of the cyst may express material into the anteroinferior portion of the external auditory canal near the bony cartilaginous junction.

Preoperative Considerations

The technique for excision essentially involves a superficial parotidectomy, and the patient should be counseled for that procedure. Antibiotics should be started preoperatively by mouth or intravenously at the time of operation. Patients are admitted to the hospital after surgery and most typically remain one night.

There are no diagnostic tests indicated in the management of this lesion. The most definitive information is obtained at the time of surgery. A computed tomographic or magnetic resonance imaging scan may be used in cases of very large branchial cleft cysts or in which the diagnosis is questioned because of a peculiarity in the clinical picture.

In small children the use of magnification in order to separate the fistulous tract from the facial nerve is helpful. Although the operating microscope may be used, the use of operating loupes with a 2.5 magnification is ideal for this purpose.

Operative Steps

General anesthesia without paralysis is required. The patient is placed supine on the table in a slight reverse Trendelenburg position. The endotracheal tube is placed on the side opposite that of the cyst. The head is also turned slightly away from this side. The patient should be draped so that the entire hemiface on the side of the surgery can be visualized to facilitate monitoring of the facial nerve.

The incision is the same as that used for parotidectomy, with the exception that it is placed on the posterior surface of the tragus and then into the preauricular crease. The incision site should be injected with 1 percent lidocaine with 1:100,000 epinephrine in order to achieve vasoconstriction. The entire region of the hemiface may then be scrubbed with a preparation solution of choice. An adhesive plastic drape may be used to secure the operative site, and the surgical towels are placed around the perimeter of the dissecting field.

The skin incision in the preauricular and tragal areas can be made with a microsharp eye knife or a straight Beaver blade. The portion of the incision that extends into the neck may be performed using a No. 15 scalpel blade. The plane of dissection should be just above the superficial parotid fascia. The flap may be elevated with either a scalpel or facelift scissors.

The parotid gland is released from the sternocleidomastoid muscle, mastoid tip, the auricular cartilage, and the upper neck contents to the posterior facial vein. The posterior facial vein should be preserved as an important landmark, since the cervical and marginal mandibular branches of the facial nerve lie superficial and in close proximity to the vein. The next important landmark is the digastric muscle, which marks the plane of the stylomastoid foramen. The tragal pointer is identified. The facial nerve lies approximately 1.0 cm deep to the tip of this pointer and 6 mm below the end of the tympanomastoid suture line. Once the facial nerve is identified, dissection is carried along the nerve with a small curved hemostat and a No. 15 blade. Tissue superficial to the nerve is mobilized with the hemostat to protect the nerve and is incised. Dissection of the parotid gland away from the facial nerve should be carried forward to the point where the cyst and fistulous tract can be well visualized. Once this is accomplished, the cyst and tract may be removed. The course of the fistula may be found to interdigitate with the branches of the facial nerve (Fig. 3B). A number of patterns have been noted by various surgeons. It is important not to violate the cyst wall in order to avoid spillage. It may become difficult to distinguish tract from facial nerve as the tract is dissected superiorly. The tract should be perpendicular around the lower divisions of the facial nerve. It may parallel the branches in the upper divisions. Magnification is recommended for this reason. Injection of methylene blue into the fistulous tract may assist with this process, care being taken not to apply too much pressure or inject too great a volume lest extravasation of the methylene blue occur. Once the fistula is followed through its origin at the external auditory canal, the end is amputated (Fig. 3C) and a 3–0 to 4–0 Dexon pursestring suture is used to invert the stump into the external auditory canal (Fig. 3D).

The wound is irrigated with an antibiotic solution and a 7-mm flat Silastic suction drain is placed along the free border of the sternocleidomastoid muscle well below the marginal division of the seventh nerve. The skin flap is carefully replaced and aligned and a subcutaneous closure carried out using 4–0 polyglycolic acid suture. Skin closure is achieved using a 6–0 fast absorbing running interlocking suture or a 4–0 monofilament nylon running subcuticular stitch.

Plate 143

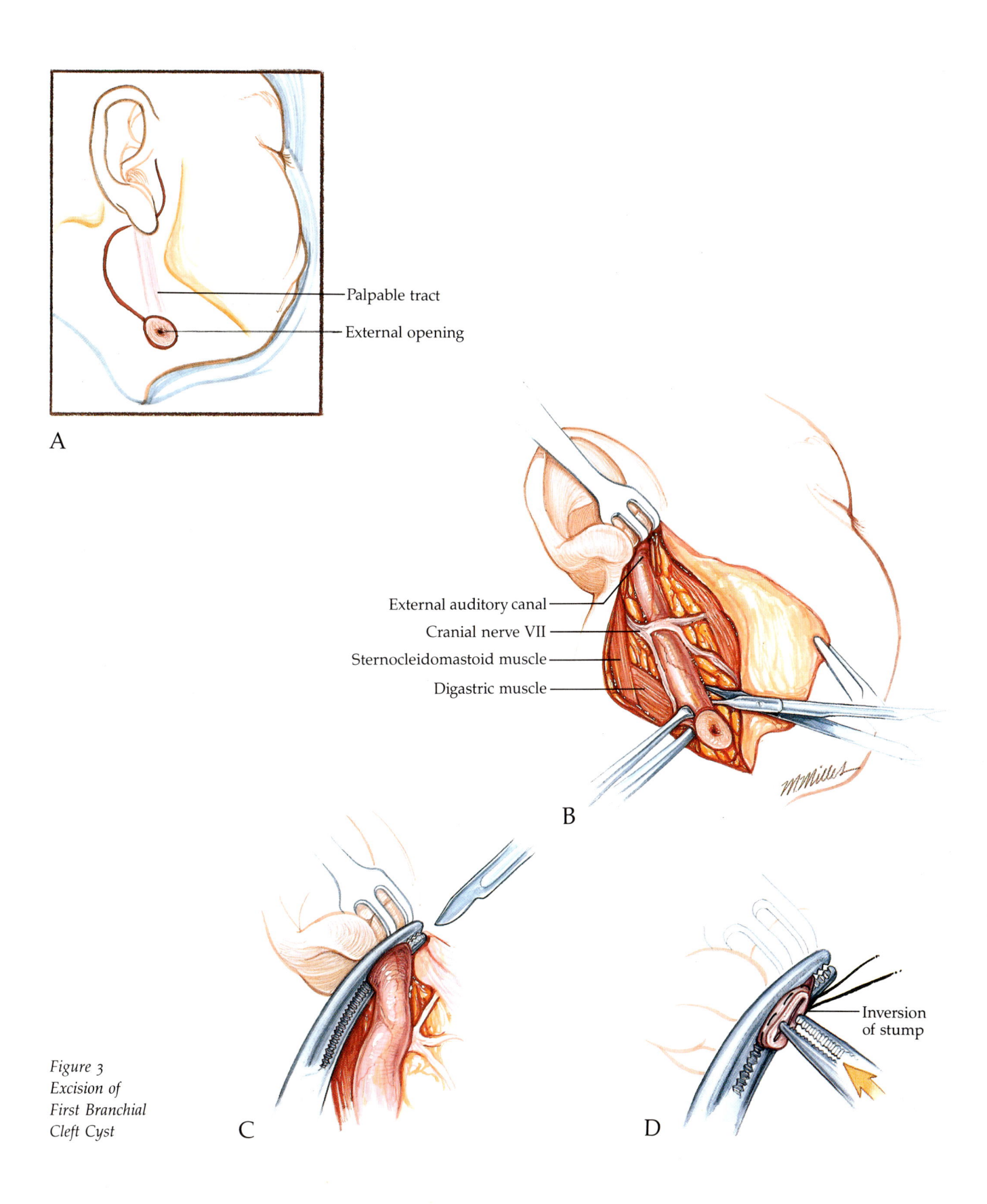

- Palpable tract
- External opening

A

External auditory canal
Cranial nerve VII
Sternocleidomastoid muscle
Digastric muscle

B

Figure 3
Excision of
First Branchial
Cleft Cyst

C

Inversion of stump

D

345

Postoperative Care

The drain can be removed the morning following surgery in most cases. If there is excessive drainage (>15 ml in 24 hours), consider continuing use of the drain for another 12 to 24 hours. Patients should be placed on intravenous antibiotics at the time of surgery. The antibiotics should be continued by mouth for 7 to 10 days. Suture line care is performed by using peroxide cleansing with a Q-tip and a light coating of antibiotic ointment two to three times per day. This is continued for 7 to 10 days.

Risks, Complications, and Sequelae

The risks and complications for surgical excision of first branchial cleft cyst are similar to those for superficial parotidectomy. These include anesthetic reaction, bleeding, infection, and scar formation, as in any surgery. There may be increased risk of wound infection, as most of these cysts have been infected on numerous occasions. The risk to the facial nerve centers around the marginal mandibular nerve, which may be injured in the lower part of the dissection and appears to be the branch at greatest risk. The zygomatic branch may be injured in the course of elevating the flap as a result of its superficial course in children. Transection of the great auricular nerve may result in neuroma formation with a tender spot over the sternomastoid muscle just below the mastoid tip. Some degree of Frey's syndrome has occurred in nearly all cases; clinical manifestations may be minimized by elevating a thick flap. The risks of recurrence of this process are quite low when excision is adequate.

Pearls and Pitfalls

Positioning of the patient and exposure are of paramount importance.

Meticulous hemostasis using monopolar cautery and bipolar cautery is essential.

The strategy of the operation should be directed toward the identification of the facial nerve and dissection of the parotid substance anteriorly so that maximal visualization of the cyst and fistula tract can be obtained.

Dissection of the fistulous tract from the facial nerve should be carried out using 2.5× operating loupes.

The fistulous tract must be tracked superiorly to its origin. The tract may become quite thin as it nears the external auditory canal. A small lacrimal probe or a No. 24 gauge wire can serve as a sounding device to help identify the tract.

The use of antibiotics remains controversial; it is the author's opinion that these wounds should be considered clean contaminated wounds.

Antibiotic and saline solution is used to irrigate the wound.

Douglas E. Mattox, M.D.

EXCISION OF PARAPHARYNGEAL SPACE TUMORS

Anatomy

The parapharyngeal space is a potential space having the shape of an inverted pyramid with the base resting on the inferior surfaces of the temporal and sphenoid bones and the apex at the greater cornu of the hyoid bone. The lateral boundary is formed by the pterygoid muscle, ramus of the mandible, and posterior belly of the digastric muscle. The posterior boundary is formed by the vertebral column and paravertebral muscles. The medial boundary is composed of the superior pharyngeal constrictor, the tonsillar pillars, and the soft palate. Only the medial boundary is soft and distensible; therefore most tumors of the parapharyngeal space manifest as a bulge within the soft palate or lateral pharyngeal wall.

The parapharyngeal space is divided into anterior and posterior components by the styloid process and the attached styloid musculature. The anterior (prestyloid) compartment contains the deep lobe of the parotid, the internal maxillary artery, and the inferior alveolar, lingual, and auriculotemporal nerves. The retrostyloid space includes the internal carotid artery, the internal jugular vein, cranial nerves IX, X, XI, and XII, and the cervical sympathetic chain.

Parapharyngeal space extensions of parotid tumors have been referred to as "dumbbell" and "round" tumors. Patey and Thackeray described dumbbell tumors arising from the deep lobe of the parotid and extending through the stylomandibular tunnel. This stylomandibular tunnel is formed by the base of the skull, the ramus mandible, the styloid process, and the stylomandibular ligament. They noted that tumors originating in this portion of the deep lobe of the parotid gland may send an extension through the stylomandibular tunnel into the parapharyngeal space. The central portion of these tumors is constricted by the stylomandibular ligament and styloid process; hence they are called dumbbell tumors. Only about 12 percent of parotid tumors originate in the deep lobe and less than 5 percent actually extend through the stylomandibular tunnel to involve the parapharyngeal space. Sixty percent of tumors arising in minor salivary glands in the palate are malignant. However, the majority of these tumors are adenoid cystic carcinomas. Mucoepidermoid carcinoma and adenocarcinoma are the next most common varieties. Tumors originating from the stylomandibular projection of the deep lobe produce both an internal and an external mass.

Work and Hybels described round tumors originating from an extension of the retromandibular portion of the gland in contrast to the tumors originating in the stylomandibular extension of the gland (see Fig. 4A). Tumors originating from the inferior extension of the retromandibular portion are not constricted, grow in a round shape, and have little or no external mass. Round tumors may also originate from minor salivary glands of the palate. Neurogenic tumors of the parapharyngeal space appear similar to round tumors.

It has also been suggested that some pharyngeal space tumors may arise from ectopic salivary tissue within lymph nodes of the parapharyngeal space. Warrington and coworkers noted that there are no anatomic connections with the deep lobe of the parotid gland in several cases. In fact five of these tumors arose medial to the superior constrictor muscle, making it impossible for them to have arisen from the deep lobe. These tumors were also histologically inconsistent with minor salivary glands of the palate in that only serous acini were found in the mass, whereas minor salivary glands generally contain mixed serous and mucous acini.

Round tumors can generally be removed through an inframandibular approach. Dumbbell tumors require dissection of the parotid gland, division of the stylomandibular ligament, and fracture of the styloid process in order to release the central constriction around the tumor.

Pathology

The majority of parapharyngeal space tumors are benign lesions and are almost equally divided between salivary gland tumors (benign mixed tumors) and tumors of neurogenic origin (neurilemomas and paragangliomas). Other benign lesions that can occur in this area include meningioma, neurofibroma, hypertrophic lymph nodes, and lipomas and mesenchymal tumors.

Approximately 15 to 30 percent of parapharyngeal space tumors are malignant. These are almost all of salivary gland origin; adenoid cystic carcinoma and malignant mixed tumors are the most common. These salivary tumors can arise either from the deep lobe of the parotid gland or from minor salivary glands in the soft palate. Less commonly occurring malignant histologic types include squamous cell carcinoma of the parotid gland or metastatic squamous cell carcinoma, carcinoid tumors, lymphoma, and rhabdomyosarcoma.

Neurilemomas can arise from any of the last four cranial nerves or from the parasympathetic nerves. However, the vast majority of these tumors arise from the vagus nerve. These tumors can be classified on the basis of the neural elements from which they arise: (1) nerve sheath tumors (neurilemoma, neurofibroma, malignant schwannoma); (2) ganglion cell tumors (ganglioneuroma, sympathicoblastoma); (3) paraganglion cell tumors (paraganglioma); and (4) secondary neurogenous tumors (meningioma, meningiosarcoma). These tumors rarely produce symptoms in the nerve of origin or in other cranial nerves and usually present as a mass in the oral cavity or upper lateral neck. The majority of neurogenic tumors are benign and do not produce obvious deficits in their nerve of origin. Cranial nerve deficits suggest malignant change, which occurs in 10 percent of neurofibromas and less than 1 percent of schwannomas.

Signs, Symptoms, and Evaluation

The majority of patients with parapharyngeal space tumors present with either an intraoral or a neck mass.

The pharyngeal or palatal mucosa is usually smooth and without superficial ulceration, because these lesions are anatomically lateral to the superior constrictor muscle.

Bilateral palpation and ballottement of the tumor mass should give the examiner an appreciation of whether the tumor is attached to the deep side of the parotid gland or is separate from it. The mass should also be examined for expansile pulsations and auscultated for bruits to exclude a carotid aneurysm or vascular tumor.

Less common presenting symptoms include dyspnea, dysphasia, or a foreign body sensation in the throat caused by the mass and size of the lesion. Occasionally a patient develops serous otitis media and conductive hearing loss from obstruction of the cartilaginous portion of the eustachian tube.

Initial evaluation of parapharyngeal space masses should be with a contrast-enhanced computed tomographic scan. The presence of a radiolucent line between the tumor and the parotid gland indicates that the tumor does not arise from the deep lobe of the parotid. If the contrast-enhanced scan is suggestive of a highly vascular mass, arteriography with preoperative embolization is indicated.

The contrast computed tomographic scan will also demonstrate the direction and degree of displacement of the great vessels by the tumor. In general, benign mixed tumors displace the carotid artery posteriorly, but neurilemomas have a variable relationship to the carotid artery, depending on the nerve of origin. Arteriography should be reserved for tumors that are extraparotid and enhance on computed tomography, for extremely large tumors, or when there is suspicion of malignant neoplasm with vascular invasion.

Although there is a great temptation to biopsy these masses, this practice is hazardous and should be discouraged. Transcervical biopsy only obscures the planes and landmarks when the mass is definitively removed. Transoral biopsy is unsafe because of the potential for seeding of benign mixed tumor in the palatal wound. Furthermore, intraoral carotid artery hemorrhage can occur from direct injury of the vessel during the biopsy or from infection of the wound from salivary contamination. Such intraoral carotid hemorrhages are extremely difficult to manage. Last, in the absence of signs of malignancy (erosion of bone, cranial nerve deficits, erosion of mucosa, or palpable cervical lymphadenopathy), the histologic type of the tumor is unimportant, since the definitive treatment is removal of the mass. If there are signs of malignancy, a transpalatal or computed tomographic controlled transcervical fine needle biopsy may provide important information for surgical planning.

Sialography is of no use in the evaluation of deep lobe masses.

Preoperative Considerations

Postoperative recovery from removal of salivary gland lesions of the parapharyngeal space is rapid. However, if the lesion proves to be neurogenic, the patient will suffer some disability related to the sacrifice of the corresponding cranial nerve(s). Therefore, it is very important preoperatively to attempt to identify any subtle asymmetries in cranial nerve function and to prepare the patient for the prolonged recovery and extensive rehabilitation needed for cranial nerve deficits. This should include a thorough explanation of the impact of loss of lower cranial nerves on swallowing, aspiration, and speech.

The majority of the dissection is carried through avascular planes and therefore hemorrhage during the procedure is usually not a great problem. However, vascular injury is possible, and the patient should be typed and screened for two units of blood. The exceptions to this rule are paragangliomas. These patients require preoperative arteriography and embolization.

The patient is placed supine on the operating table with the head turned away from the surgeon. Anterior subluxation of the mandible can be accomplished much more easily if there are no tubes or airways in the mouth. Therefore the patient should have nasal intubation. The temperature probes and stethoscope should all be placed in alternative sites (not in the mouth or nose).

The procedure can be performed with the contents of most basic neck sets. A sagittal saw should be available in the rare instances in which a mandibular split is needed. Exposure is also improved by a large self-retaining retractor such as a Fisch infratemporal fossa retractor.

The drapes should leave the entire side of the face exposed under a plastic self-adherent drape to allow observation of facial function during the dissection of the facial nerve. A temporary tarsorrhaphy can be used to prevent the eye from opening beneath the drapes.

Although intraoral removal of round tumors has been described, this practice should be discouraged. Specific dangers of the transoral approach include increased chance of subtotal removal of the tumor or rupture of the tumor because of limited exposure available; the risk of damage to the internal carotid artery, which is extraordinarily difficult to control transorally; increased risk of infection because of salivary contamination of the wound; and increased risk of injury to the facial nerve.

Operative Steps

For the purposes of this discussion, it is assumed that the tumor is a "round" tumor, of either salivary or neural origin within the parapharyngeal space (Fig. 4A). Dumbbell tumors of the deep lobe of the parotid gland are discussed in the section on Parotidectomy. These lesions, totally medial to the mandible, present no risk to the main trunk or bifurcation of the facial nerve; therefore a formal facial nerve dissection is not required.

The skin incision extends from near the midline above the hyoid bone around the angle of the mandible to the mastoid tip. The inferior portion of the incision should follow a natural skin crease (Fig. 4B). The greater auricular nerve is identified and divided. The skin flaps should be elevated in the subplatysmal plane, and the superficial layer of the deep cervical fascia is identified. Beneath the anterior flap the fascia of the capsule over the submandibular gland should be identified as well as the anterior facial vein. The marginal mandibular branch of the facial nerve should be identified and preserved. The nerve is found superficial to the facial veins in the loose areolar tissue over the submandibular gland. The nerves should be mobilized anteriorly and posteriorly and then reflected up with the skin flap. The anterior facial vein can be ligated and sutured to the skin flap to protect the marginal mandibular nerve (Fig. 4C). Excision of the submandibular gland may be useful in some large tumors but is not routinely performed.

The posterior skin flap is elevated over the sternocleidomastoid muscle. The spinal accessory nerve should be positively identified, either at the posterior border of the sternocleidomastoid muscle or on the medial side as it enters the muscle. The sternocleidomastoid muscle is then elevated from the underlying carotid sheath from the carotid bifurcation to the mastoid tip. The carotid sheath is opened, and all neurovascular structures within it are identified, including the internal jugular vein, the

Plate 144

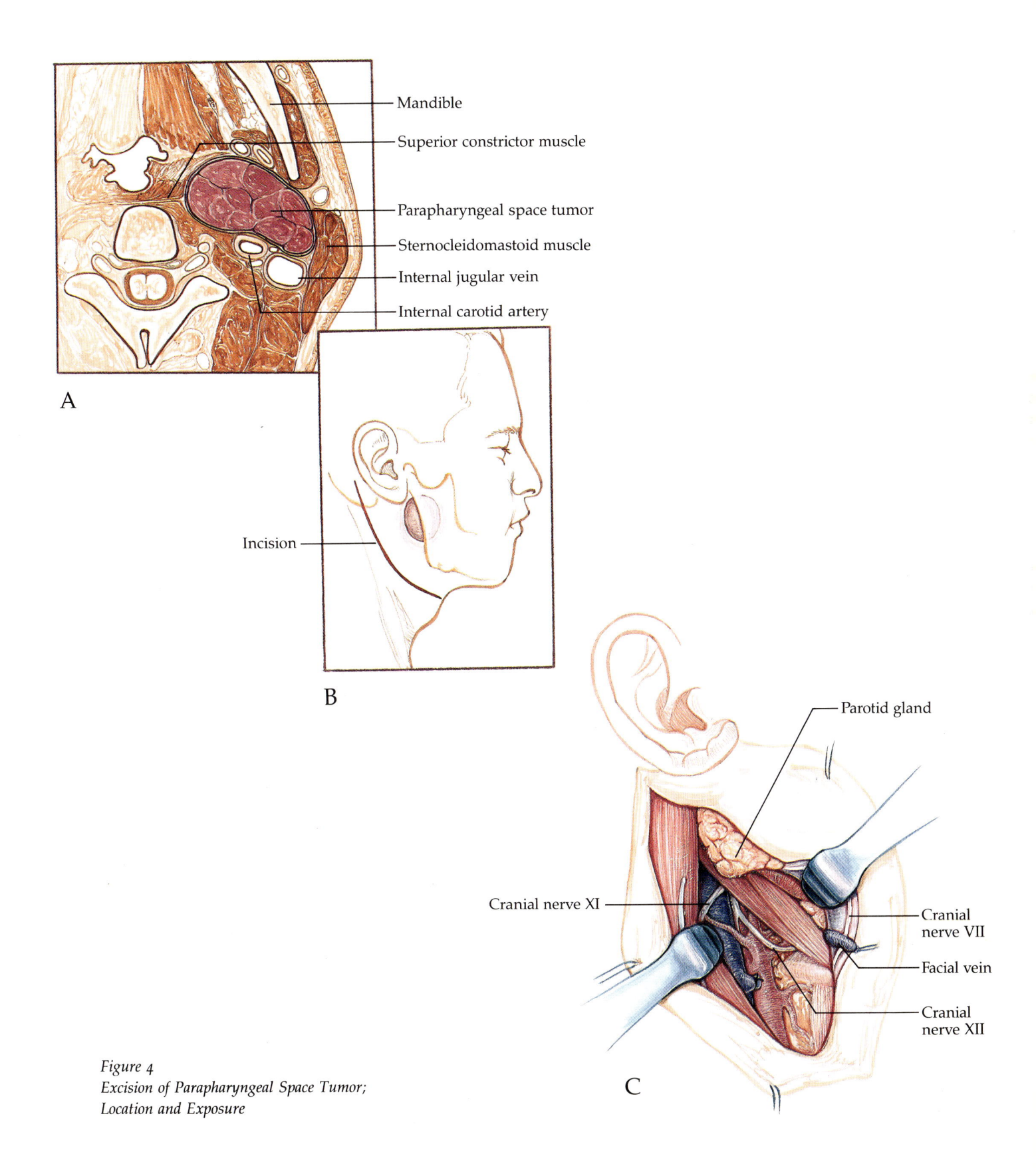

- Mandible
- Superior constrictor muscle
- Parapharyngeal space tumor
- Sternocleidomastoid muscle
- Internal jugular vein
- Internal carotid artery

A

Incision

B

- Parotid gland
- Cranial nerve XI
- Cranial nerve VII
- Facial vein
- Cranial nerve XII

C

Figure 4
Excision of Parapharyngeal Space Tumor; Location and Exposure

351

carotid bifurcation, the internal and external carotid arteries, the vagus nerve, and the sympathetic trunk. The hypoglossal nerve should be identified as it crosses lateral to the carotid arteries just above the bifurcation.

The lingual, facial, and distal external carotid arteries may need to be ligated and divided. The common facial vein is transected and tied.

The digastric and stylohyoid muscles are identified, and after all neurovascular structures have been identified and protected, the central portion of the posterior belly of the digastric and stylohyoid muscles is divided (Fig. 4D). Additional space and relaxation of the mandible can be obtained by dividing the stylomandibular ligament and styloglossal muscle. The styloid process can be removed with bone cutting forceps.

With firm anterior retraction of the mandible, either by an assistant or with a self-retaining retractor, the posteroinferior portion of the tumor is exposed. This anterior subluxation of the mandible is more difficult to perform if an endotracheal tube, oral airway, or other obstructive device passes between the incisors.

The tumor is removed with a combination of sharp and blunt dissection through the loose areolar tissues surrounding it. The actual tumor capsule is not exposed or violated (Fig. 4E). Blunt finger dissection can be used to mobilize the medial and superior portions of the tumor (Fig. 4F), and eventually the tumor is retracted inferiorly behind the posterior margin of the mandible (Fig. 4F). Attention must always be paid to the internal carotid artery, which frequently develops some spasm during the dissection, making it less obvious and easy to injure. Furthermore, in elderly individuals the internal carotid may become tortuous, with one or more loops before it enters the base of the skull.

If the mass proves to be a neurilemoma, the corresponding cranial nerve should be identified below the tumor and above the tumor as well, although this may be difficult before the lower end of the nerve is divided and the tumor mobilized. Other cranial nerves must be identified, mobilized away from the tumor, and protected so that only one neural deficit occurs from the surgery.

A small minority of tumors (10 percent) require mandibulotomy for adequate exposure and removal of the tumor. The mandibulotomy may be performed either at the angle (Fig. 4G) or in the paramedian position medial to the mental nerve. It should be performed in a stair-step fashion (Fig. 4G) and holes drilled for secure fixation. Division of the stylomandibular ligament is important; it allows adequate anterior and lateral reflection of the mandible in order to fully expose the tumor. The mandible is repaired with either wiring or compression plating. Accurate realignment of the mandibular segments leads to rapid inferior dental nerve regeneration.

Resection of malignant tumors may require inclusion of the facial nerve, masseter muscle, ramus of the mandible, pterygoid plates, and skull base and temporal bone.

If transoral biopsy or attempted excision has been performed in the past, the resection must include removal of the mucosa around the biopsy site and the deeper tissues of the palate en bloc with the tumor in order to decrease the recurrence rate from tumor seeding from the previous biopsy.

Plate 145

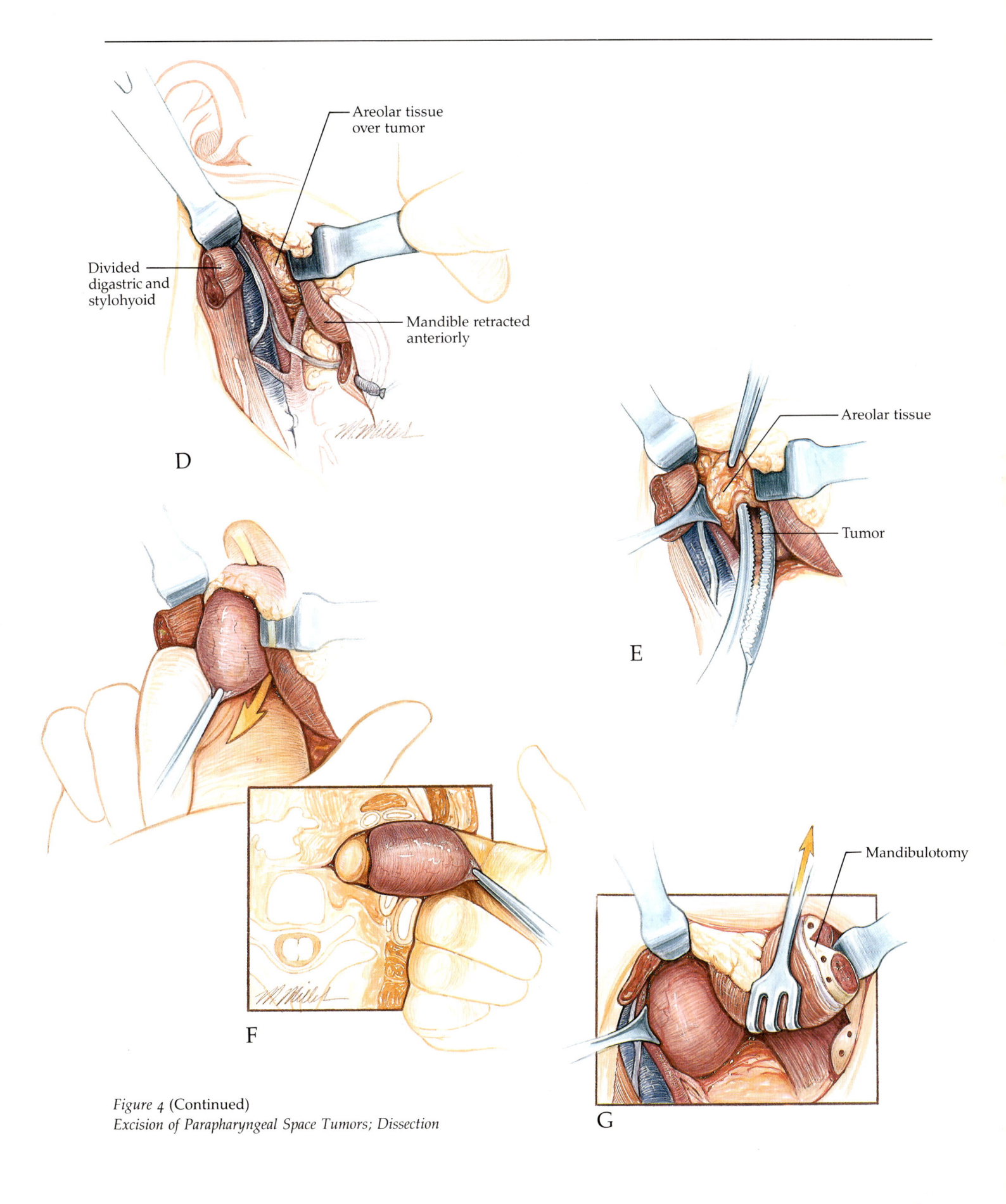

- Areolar tissue over tumor
- Divided digastric and stylohyoid
- Mandible retracted anteriorly

D

- Areolar tissue
- Tumor

E

F

- Mandibulotomy

G

Figure 4 (Continued)
Excision of Parapharyngeal Space Tumors; Dissection

353

Before closure, the wound is irrigated and examined for adequate hemostasis. A suction drain is placed in the wound. Suction obliterates any dead space in the wound as the lateral pharyngeal tissues resume their normal anatomic position. The digastric muscle is reapproximated, and the wound is closed in layers.

Postoperative Care

Tracheostomy is not routinely used in these patients. However, they do need to be watched carefully for signs of expanding hematoma, which could compromise the airway.

All cranial nerves should be checked immediately after surgery, including fiberoptic laryngoscopy to check vocal cord function. If the cranial nerves are intact and the oral mucosa has remained intact, alimentation can be started as soon as the patient wishes. If there are cranial nerve deficits, it is wise to delay eating until the immediate postoperative discomfort and swelling have resolved. These patients should be watched carefully for signs of aspiration pneumonia, which can develop even from aspiration of saliva before alimentation has been started. Early intervention by a swallowing therapist before inappropriate habits have developed will speed recovery in these cases.

Drains are removed on the second or third day as soon as drain output is minimal. Sutures are removed between the seventh and tenth days.

Risks, Complications, and Sequelae

Regardless of the histologic type of the tumor, the marginal mandibular nerve, and cranial nerves IX, X, XI, and XII are at risk during this procedure. Paralysis may develop in one or more of these nerves from the retraction and exposure needed to remove the tumor.

The risk of recurrence of pleomorphic adenoma of the parapharyngeal space seems to be less than for the same histologic type in the superficial lobe, probably because the encapsulation of the tumor in the parapharyngeal space is more dense. Conversely, the odds of recurrence for malignant lesions of the parapharyngeal space are greater than for the same histologic type found in the parotid gland.

Secondary rehabilitative measures for lower cranial nerve deficits include Teflon vocal cord injections, laryngoplasty with Silastic or cartilage implants, and central Z-plasty of the tongue to provide neurotization of the paralyzed hemitongue.

Pearls and Pitfalls

Extensive bone destruction on computed tomographic scan suggests a malignant lesion that may require extended resection, if it is operable.

A malignant lesion that is adherent to and invasive in the adjacent structures will be evident on initial exposure of the tumor. At this time a biopsy specimen for frozen section examination can be obtained. If the lesion is deemed unresectable, the incision can be closed with negligible morbidity to the patient from the procedure.

The postoperative morbidity from vagal section may be very serious in elderly patients. In this instance, exploration of the tumor and biopsy without sacrifice of the nerve may be the wisest course of action.

An intraoral approach is condemned because it is fraught with dangers of hemorrhage, subtotal resection of tumor, airway obstruction, false aneurysms of the carotid artery, and thrombosis of the internal jugular vein.

Suggested Reading

Batsakis JG. Tumors of the head and neck. Baltimore: Williams & Wilkins, 1974.

Conley JJ, Clairmont AA. Tumors of the parapharyngeal space. South Med J 1978; 71:543–546.

Patey DH, Thackeray AC. The pathological anatomy and treatment of parotid tumors with retropharyngeal extension (dumbbell-dumbbell tumors). Br J Surg 1957; 44:352–358.

Shoss MN, Donovan DT, Alford BR. Tumors of the parapharyngeal space. Arch Otolaryngol Head Neck Surg 1985; 111:753–757.

Som PM, Biller HF, Lawson W. Tumors of the parapharyngeal space: Preoperative evaluation diagnosis and surgical approaches. Ann Otol Rhinol Laryngol 1981; 90(Suppl 8):3–15.

Warrington G, Emery PJ, Gregory MM, Harrison DFN. Pleomorphic salivary gland adenomas of the pharyngeal space. J Laryngol Otol 1981; 95:205–218.

Work WP, Hybels RL. Study of tumors of the parapharyngeal space. Laryngoscope 1974; 84:1748–1754.

Chapter VII

THE NECK

Glenn E. Peters, M.D.

EXCISION OF SECOND AND THIRD BRANCHIAL CLEFT CYSTS

The branchial apparatus forms during the fourth week of embryonic development and consists of five branchial arches separated by four external clefts and four internal pouches. The second arch soon begins to overgrow the third and fourth arches, resulting in formation of the cervical sinus of His, which is an ectoderm-lined cavity. Incomplete obliteration of the cervical sinus of His may give rise to the formation of branchial cleft anomalies, including cysts, sinus tracts, and fistulas.

The most commonly encountered branchial cleft anomalies in the neck arise from the second and third branchial clefts, in that order of frequency. A fourth branchial cleft cyst has been conjectured but has yet to be proved clinically. These clefts typically present as soft, mobile swellings along the anterior border of the sternocleidomastoid muscle and deep to the platysma. The second branchial cleft cyst is found along the upper to middle one-third of the sternocleidomastoid muscle, and the third branchial cleft cyst along the middle to lower one-third. An external opening from a fistula or sinus tract also may be present in these locations.

The location of a fistulous tract differs, depending on the cleft of origin. Anomalies from the second branchial cleft (fistula and sinus tracts) ascend along the carotid sheath and pass between the internal and external carotid arteries superior to both the glossopharyngeal and hypoglossal nerves. The fistula terminates in the tonsillar fossa, where an internal opening may be present (Fig. 1A). Fistulas and sinus tracts of third cleft origin ascend along the common carotid artery and pass posterior to the internal carotid artery. The tract passes superior to the hypoglossal nerve, superficial to the vagus nerve, and inferior to the glossopharyngeal nerve. It pierces the thyrohyoid membrane, and the internal opening is in the piriform sinus (Fig. 1B).

Indications

The differential diagnosis of a mass in the anterior cervical triangle includes inflammatory lymphadenopathy, primary neoplastic processes, malignancy metastatic to cervical lymph nodes, and congenital anomalies. Careful evaluation, including history, physical examination, and radiographic studies, is essential for making a correct diagnosis. A soft, mobile mass along the anterior border of the sternocleidomastoid muscle in a patient without obvious pathology in the upper aerodigestive tract or thyroid gland is the key physical finding. A computed tomographic scan will demonstrate a cystic lesion in the appropriate location. Fine needle aspiration biopsy will most likely produce fluid containing keratin debris or exfoliated squamous cells without cytologic evidence of malignancy.

Indications for surgical excision include airway compression, dysphagia, recurrent infection, persistently draining fistula, unacceptable cosmetic appearance, and the need to confirm the diagnosis.

Plate 146

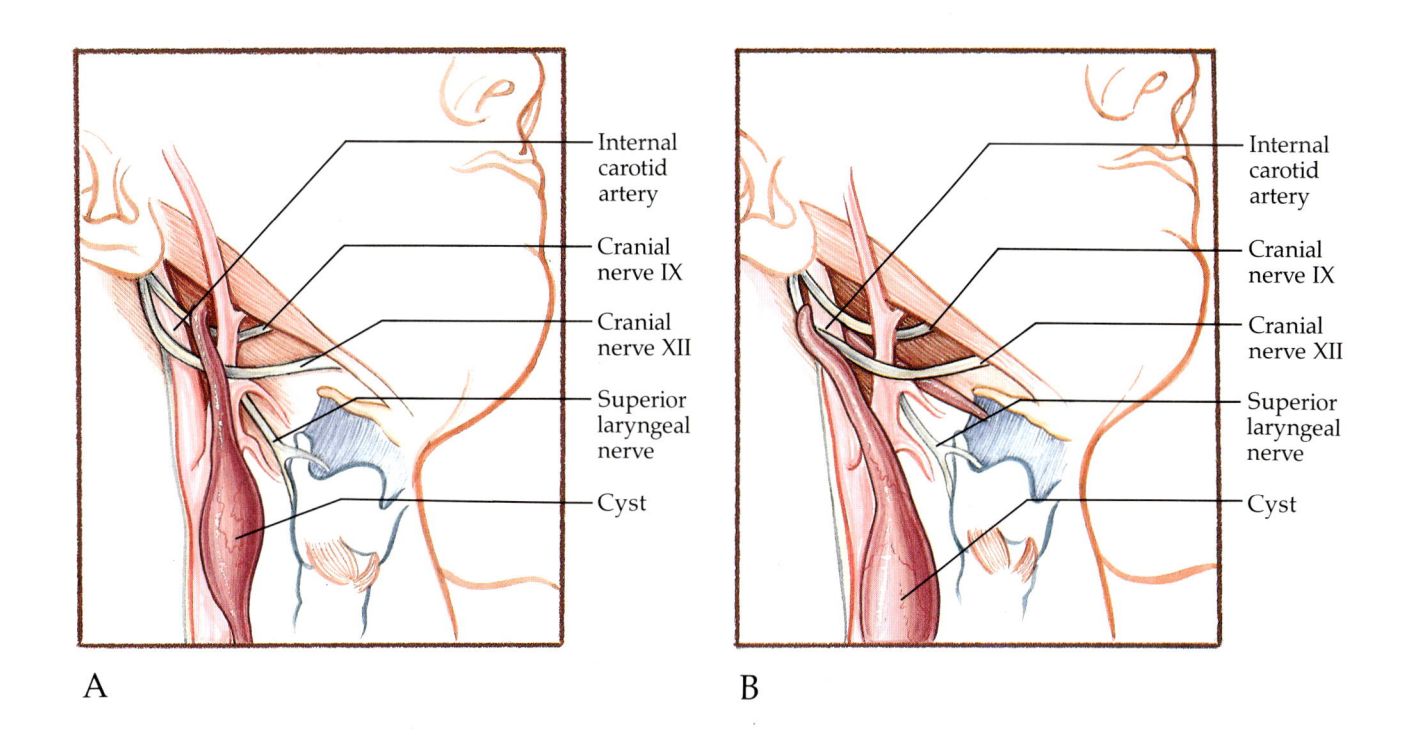

A

B

Figure 1
Excision of
Second and Third Branchial Cleft Cyst;
Anatomy

Preoperative Considerations

The operation for excision of branchial cleft cysts should be done when no infection or inflammatory changes are present in the cyst. If the cyst becomes infected, as is sometimes seen with concomitant upper respiratory tract infections, the patient should be placed on antibiotics and the procedure delayed until the cyst has become quiescent. Incision and drainage of an infected cyst should be avoided if possible.

The patient is positioned in the supine position, and the neck is extended by placing the shoulders on a small folded sheet. A general anesthetic is administered through an oral endotracheal tube. The surgical field is prepared and draped from the lower border of the mandible to the clavicle.

Operative Steps

The preferred incision is horizontal and oriented in a natural skin crease. It should be placed over the cyst (Fig. 1C). If an external opening is present, this should be excised with a horizontally oriented ellipse. Multiple horizontal incisions may be required, particularly if it is necessary to dissect the fistula tract superiorly to its junction with the pharynx. These "stepladder" incisions provide a better cosmetic result than a single oblique incision along the anterior border of the sternocleidomastoid muscle. The skin incisions are carried through the platysma muscle, and superior and inferior flaps are developed in the subplatysmal plane. Wide exposure is desirable to facilitate identification and preservation of important neural and vascular structures.

Initially the cyst is mobilized from the anterior border and medial surface of the sternocleidomastoid muscle (Fig. 1D). Care must be taken to avoid injury to the spinal accessory nerve, which enters the medial surface of the sternocleidomastoid muscle in its upper one-third. Medially the cyst (or fistula) is mobilized in the area of the carotid sheath (Fig. 1E).

The fistulous tract, if present, is identified, and this is further dissected superiorly in the area of the carotid bifurcation. The hypoglossal nerve and ansa hypoglossi are identified and preserved. There are several veins in the area of the hypoglossal nerve; these should be accurately controlled, as bothersome bleeding and blind clamping may result in injury to the nerve. Dissection in this area is facilitated by mobilizing the posterior belly of the digastric muscle and retracting it superiorly (Fig. 1F).

Plate 147

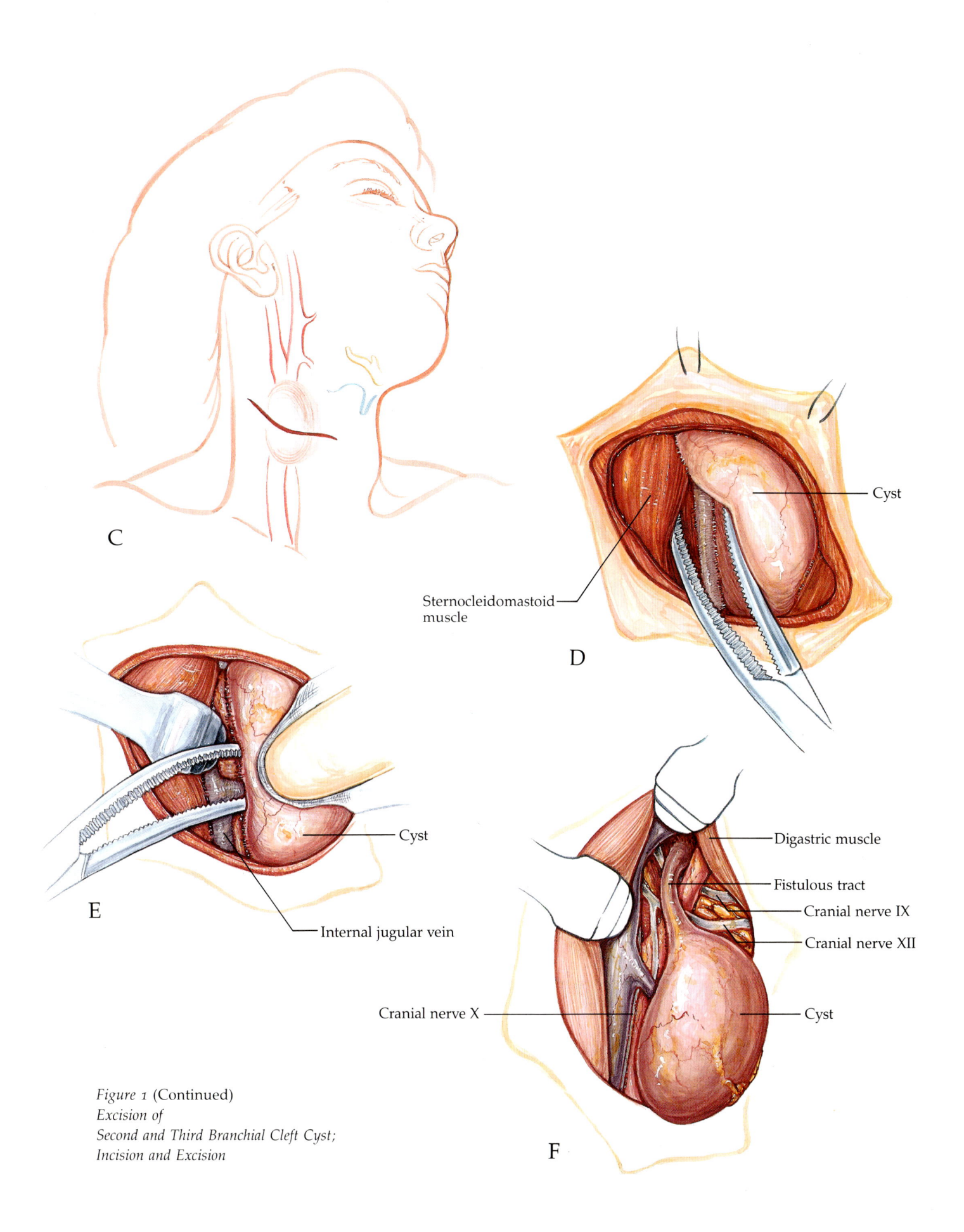

C

D
Sternocleidomastoid muscle
Cyst

E
Cyst
Internal jugular vein

F
Digastric muscle
Fistulous tract
Cranial nerve IX
Cranial nerve XII
Cranial nerve X
Cyst

Figure 1 (Continued)
Excision of
Second and Third Branchial Cleft Cyst;
Incision and Excision

After the tract is mobilized in the region of the carotid bifurcation, it can be traced on to the pharynx (Fig. 1G). A second cleft tract passes between the internal and external carotid arteries above both the hypoglossal and glossopharyngeal nerves. A third cleft anomaly lies posterolateral to the internal carotid artery. It is superficial to the vagus nerve and passes over the hypoglossal nerve. The tract then lies medial to the carotid artery system as it extends toward the thyrohyoid membrane. Once inside the thyrohyoid membrane, the tract terminates in the lateral aspect of the piriform sinus. Meticulous dissection allows identification and preservation of these structures while the tract is mobilized.

The final step in the dissection is to free the tract from the lateral aspect of the pharynx. It may be necessary to resect a small portion of the mucosa in the tonsillar fossa (second cleft) or piriform sinus (third cleft), particularly if an internal opening is present.

The pharyngeal defect is closed in a layered fashion with absorbable sutures (Fig. 1H). The pharyngeal mucosa is inverted into the pharynx. The wound is irrigated and reinspected for bleeding. A small silicone-Silastic suction drainage catheter is placed in the wound deep to the platysma muscle. The platysma is approximated with absorbable sutures, and the skin is closed with fine nylon sutures or skin staples.

Postoperative Care

Closed suction wound drainage is maintained until the output is less than 20 ml per 24-hour period. Early patient ambulation is encouraged. The diet can be advanced as tolerated, as the entrance into the pharynx should be small and not at risk of development of a fistula. The wound is cared for with twice daily cleanings and antibacterial ointment applications.

Risks, Complications, and Sequelae

Problems associated with the procedure include bleeding; wound infection; neural injuries, including injuries of the facial, vagus, glossopharyngeal, hypoglossal, superior laryngeal, and spinal accessory nerves; injury to the carotid artery; recurrence of the cyst; anesthetic complications; and perioperative death.

Pearls and Pitfalls

Complete excision of the cyst and fistula tract is necessary to prevent recurrence.

Avoid operation on an acutely inflamed or infected lesion. Avoid incision and drainage if possible. Recurrent infections or previous drainage causes scarring and makes dissection more difficult.

Surgery in neonates is best deferred until age 3 or 4 years unless problems with recurrent infection or aerodigestive tract compression occur.

G

Plate 148
Figure 1 (Continued)
Excision of
Second and Third Branchial Cleft Cyst;
Excision

— Fistulous tract
— External carotid artery

Superior pharyngeal constrictor muscle

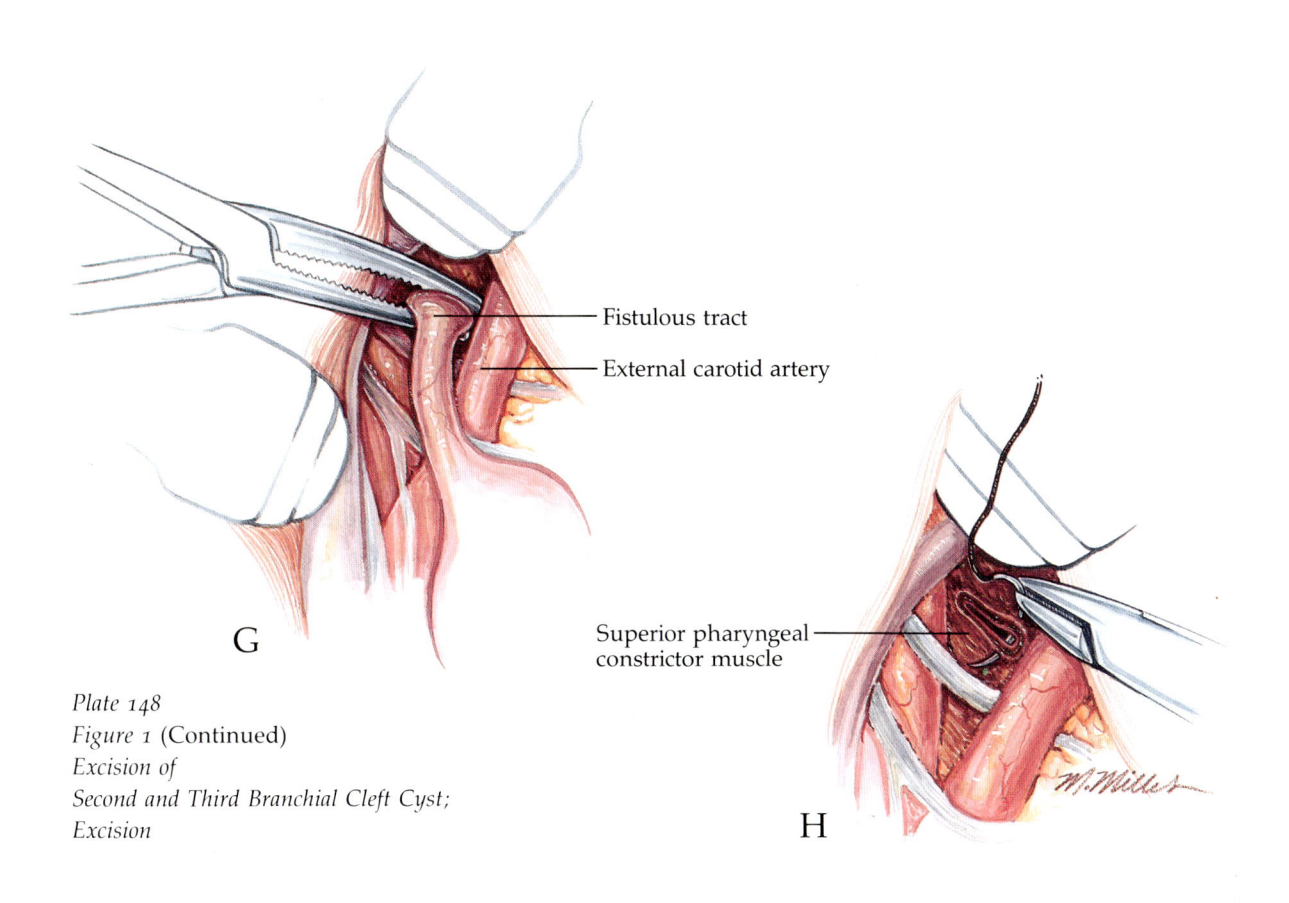

H

Suggested Reading

Albers CS. Congenital sinuses and fistulas of the neck and pharynx. In: Maloney WH, ed. Otolaryngology IV. New York: Harper & Row, 1975.

Chandler RA, Mitchell B. Branchial cleft cysts, sinuses, and fistulas. Otolaryngol Clin North Am 1981; 14:175–186.

Davies J. Embryology and anatomy of the head and neck. Embryology of the face, palate, nose, and paranasal sinuses. In: Paparella MM, Shumrick DA, eds. Otolaryngology. Philadelphia: WB Saunders, 1973.

Proctor B, Proctor C. Congenital lesions of the head and neck. Otolaryngol Clin North Am 1970; 3:221–248.

Simpson R. Lateral cervical cysts and fistulas. Laryngoscope 1969; 79:30–59.

Glenn E. Peters, M.D.

EXCISION OF THYROGLOSSAL DUCT CYST

A thyroglossal duct may persist at any point along a tract corresponding to the descent of the primitive thyroid anlage, from the foramen cecum to the thyroid gland. Generally this duct disappears during embryonic development; however, if the duct persists, it may give rise to thyroglossal duct cysts (Fig. 2A).

The thyroglossal duct lies in close association with the body of the hyoid bone. The duct not only passes on the bone's anterior surface but also dips behind its inferior border to rest against its posterior surface, and it may even penetrate the hyoid bone. Therefore, it is essential to remove the central portion of the hyoid bone to prevent recurrent disease.

The thyroglossal duct cyst generally presents as a soft, mobile mass in the anterior neck, close to but not necessarily in the midline. The cyst may become infected and manifest as a draining fistula. Evaluation includes a detailed patient history and physical examination with careful palpation of the neck and thyroid gland. Special studies include ultrasonography, computed tomographic scanning, radionuclide scans, and needle aspiration biopsy.

Indications

The surgical procedure as outlined by Sistrunk is used for anterior neck masses near the midline thought to be thyroglossal duct cysts. This approach provides exposure of the medial compartment of the neck from the thyroid isthmus to the base of the tongue. Resection of the body of the hyoid bone is easily accomplished.

Preoperative Considerations

A short course of perioperative antibiotics is indicated, since the pharynx may be entered through the mucosa of the tongue base. The patient is positioned in the supine position with the neck extended by placing a small folded sheet under the shoulders. The surgical preparation should extend from the mouth to below the clavicles. The draping should provide exposure of the entire anterior neck from the chin to the sternal notch.

Operative Steps

The choice of incision varies with the location of the cyst and the presence of a draining fistula or sinus tract. For a cyst located anterior to the thyroid cartilage or thyrohyoid membrane, a simple horizontal incision may be used (Fig. 2B). The incision should be oriented in a skin fold at the level of the thyrohyoid membrane and should extend to the anterior border of the sternocleidomastoid muscle. Low-lying cysts may necessitate the use of multiple stepladder incisions (Fig. 2C). If a sinus tract is present, it should be excised using a horizontal elliptic incision (Fig. 2D).

Superior and inferior skin flaps are elevated deep to the platysma and anterior to the sternohyoid muscles. These flaps are elevated to expose the thyroid isthmus inferiorly and the body of the hyoid bone superiorly. The cyst can be seen between the medial borders of the sternohyoid muscles.

Plate 149

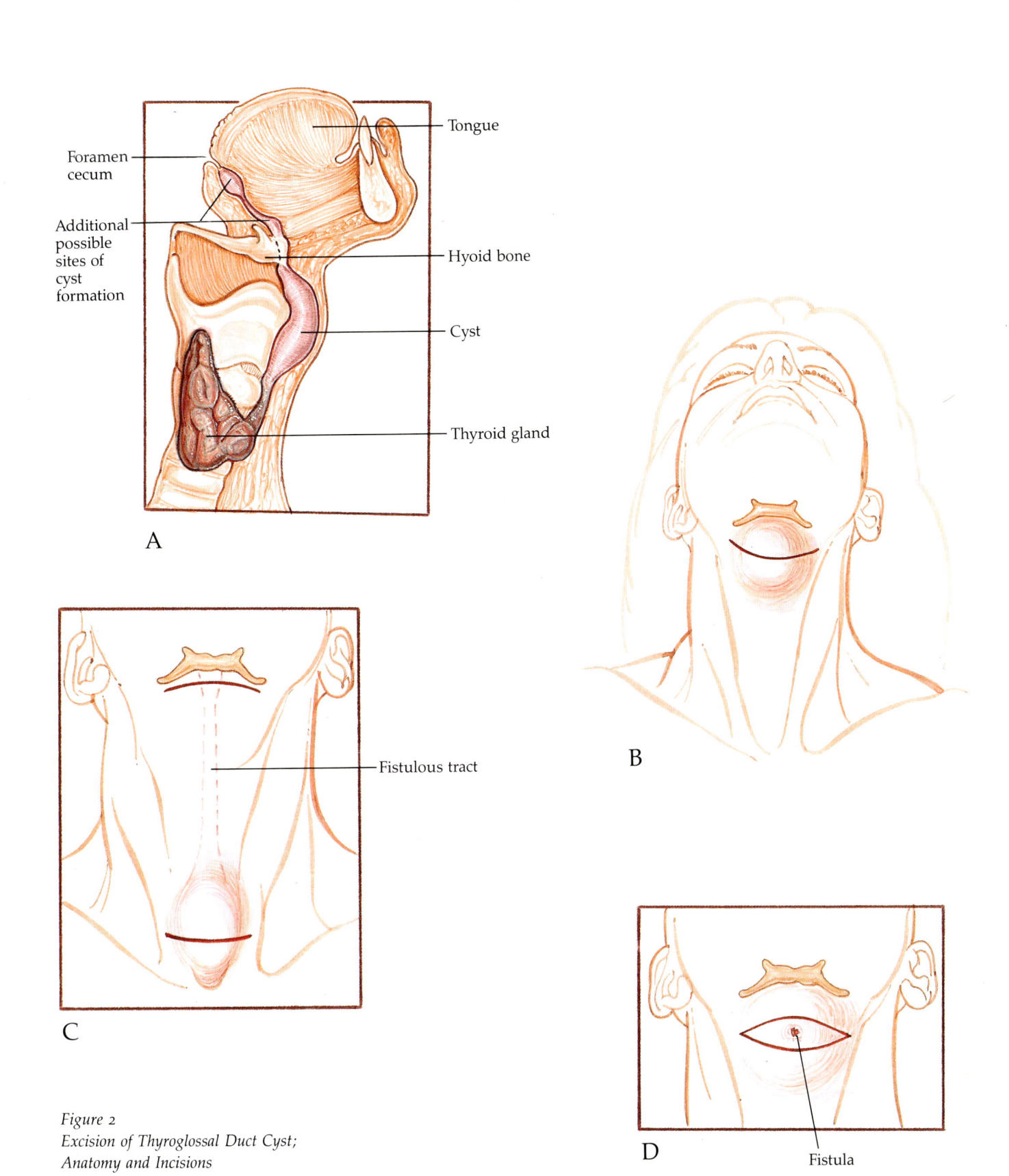

Figure 2
Excision of Thyroglossal Duct Cyst;
Anatomy and Incisions

365

The superficial layer of the deep cervical fascia is incised, and the sternohyoid muscles are elevated off the cyst and the thyroid cartilage (Fig. 2E). The muscle bellies are retracted laterally to fully expose the cyst and the pyramidal lobe if present. As the muscles are retracted laterally, the cyst is fully mobilized on its lateral aspect (Fig. 2F).

The inferior pole of the cyst is fully mobilized. If there is an attachment between the inferior border of the cyst and the pyramidal lobe or isthmus, it is divided between clamps and tied (Fig. 2G). The cyst is dissected superiorly, freeing it from the anterior surface of the larynx and the thyrohyoid membrane. This leaves the cyst attached to the inferior border of the hyoid bone.

Plate 150

E

- Platysma
- Superficial layer of deep cervical fascia
- Sternohyoid muscle

F

- Sternohyoid muscle retracted
- Cyst

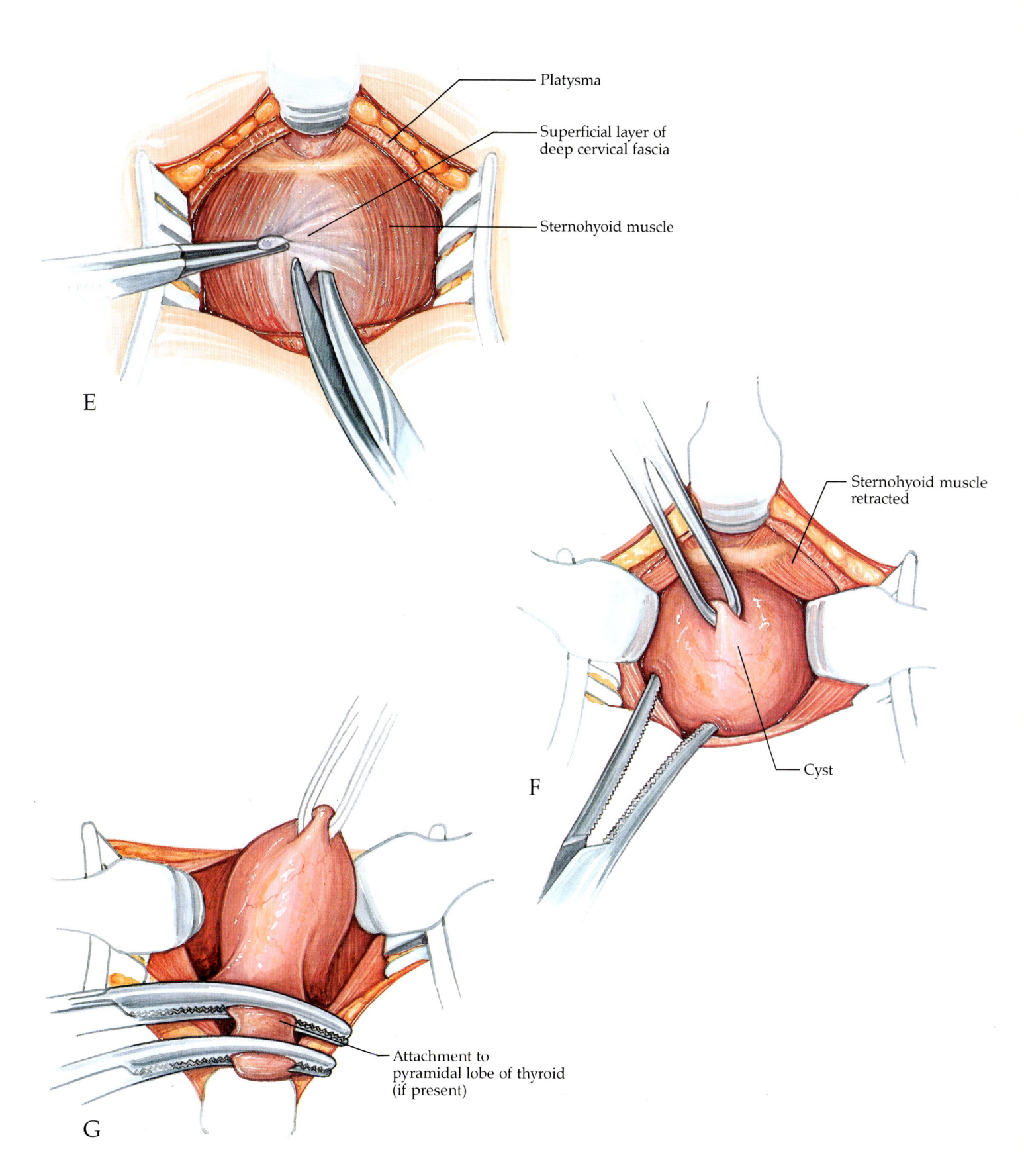

G

- Attachment to pyramidal lobe of thyroid (if present)

Figure 2 (Continued)
Excision of Thyroglossal Duct Cyst;
Mobilization of Cyst

367

The medial portions of the upper ends of the sternohyoid muscles are detached from the body of the hyoid bone. Similarly, the mylohyoid muscle is detached from the superior border (Fig. 2H). A Mixter clamp is passed underneath the lesser cornua of the hyoid bone to free these areas from underlying soft tissue (Fig. 2I). A bone cutter is then used to divide the hyoid bone just medial to each lesser cornu (Fig. 2J). In such a manner the body of the hyoid bone is mobilized and remains attached to the cyst.

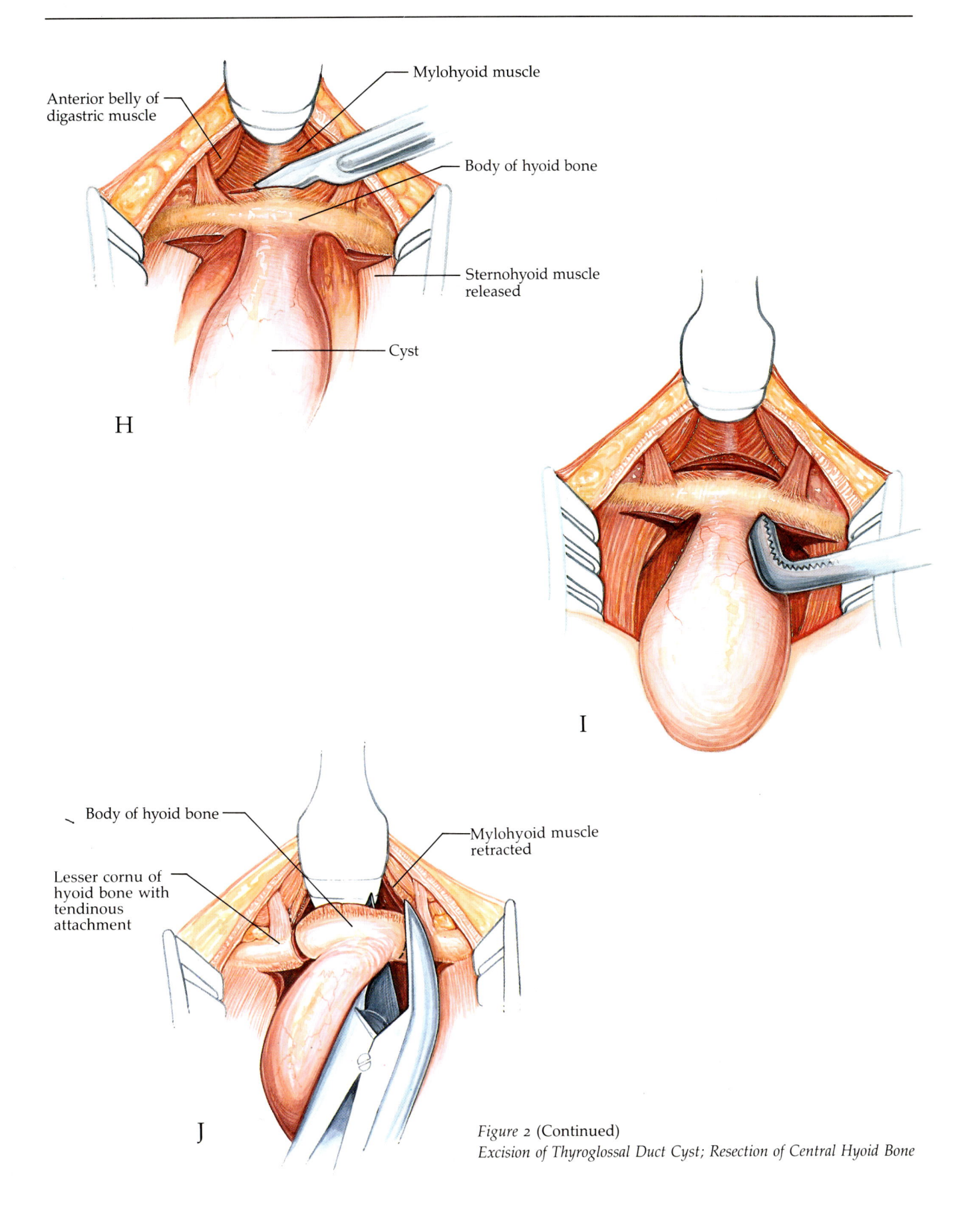

Plate 151

- Anterior belly of digastric muscle
- Mylohyoid muscle
- Body of hyoid bone
- Sternohyoid muscle released
- Cyst

H

I

- Body of hyoid bone
- Lesser cornu of hyoid bone with tendinous attachment
- Mylohyoid muscle retracted

J

Figure 2 (Continued)
Excision of Thyroglossal Duct Cyst; Resection of Central Hyoid Bone

Further soft tissue dissection proceeds through the suprahyoid muscles in the tongue base. A core of tissue is removed surrounding the suspected path of the thyroglossal duct (Fig. 2K). (Often an actual duct or tract is not seen above the hyoid bone.) This dissection is carried to the area of the foramen cecum in the tongue base. The pedicle of tissue deep to the mucosa of the tongue can be clamped and tied. The surgeon's finger inserted through the mouth may help to locate the proximal limit of the tract (Fig. 2L).

Plate 152

- Tongue base
- Resected tongue base musculature surrounding tract

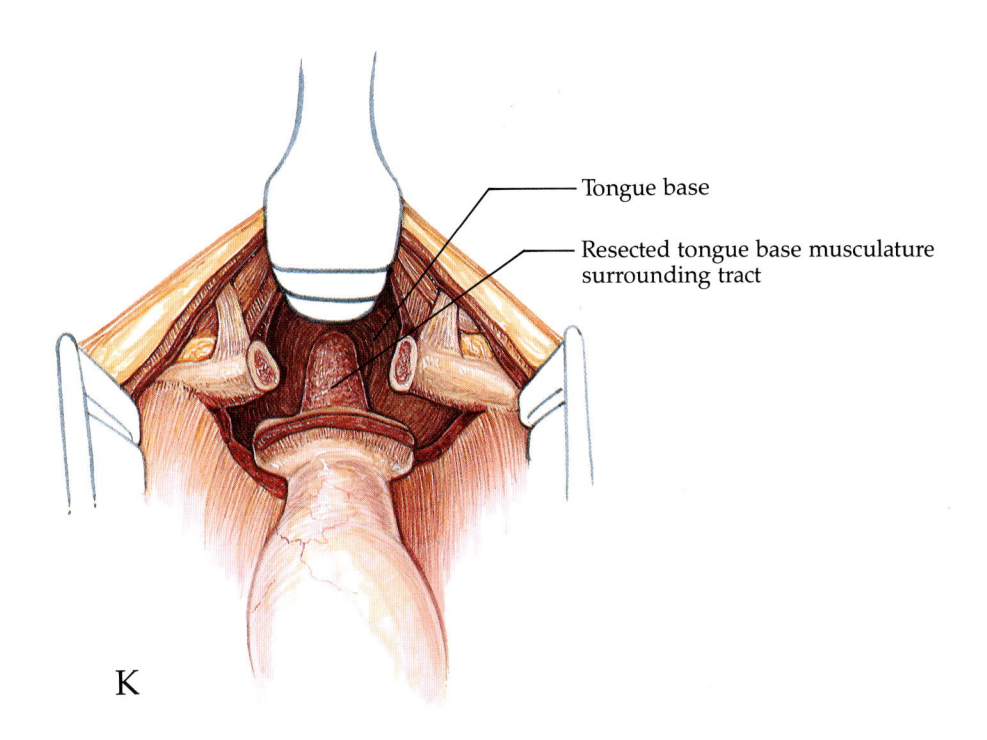

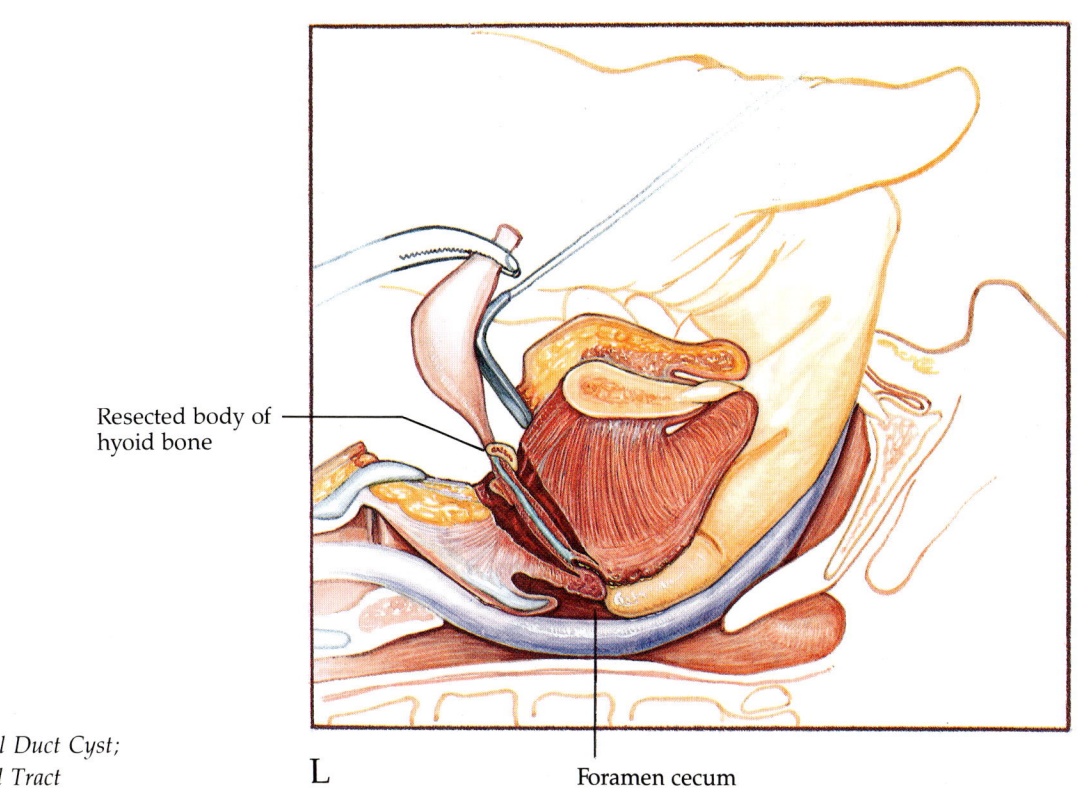

K

- Resected body of hyoid bone
- Foramen cecum

Figure 2 (Continued)
Excision of Thyroglossal Duct Cyst; Resection of Suprahyoid Tract

L

371

Plate 153

Hypopharyngeal mucosa

M

Mylohyoid muscle

Sternohyoid muscle

N

O

Figure 2 (Continued)
Excision of Thyroglossal Duct Cyst; Closure

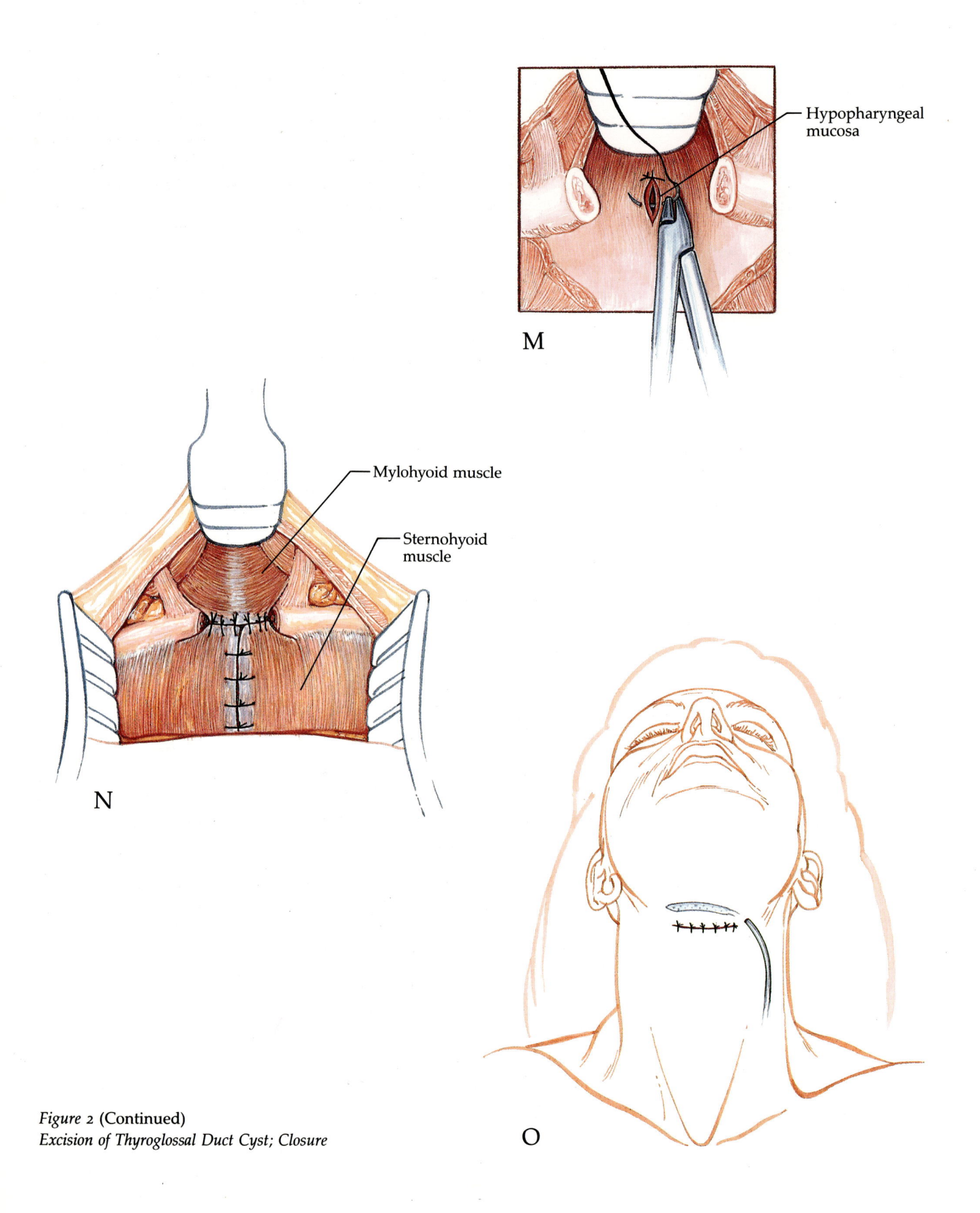

If the pharynx is entered through the tongue base, the mucosa should be closed in a layered fashion, inverting the mucosal edges into the pharynx (Fig. 2M). The mylohyoid muscles are sutured to the sternohyoid muscles in the area of the body of the hyoid bone (Fig. 2N). The medial borders of the sternohyoid muscles are loosely approximated (Fig. 2N). Flat silicone-Silastic suction catheters are placed between the strap muscles and platysma to prevent fluid accumulation under the skin flaps (Fig. 2O). The incision is closed in the standard layered fashion.

Postoperative Care

Early patient ambulation is encouraged. The patient's diet may be advanced as tolerated if the oropharynx was not entered. Otherwise, the patient can be fed through a nasal feeding tube for several days postoperatively. Closed suction wound drainage should continue until the output is less than 20 ml per 24-hour period.

Risks, Complications, and Sequelae

Risks, complications, and sequelae encountered with this procedure are a scar on the neck, which may produce a cosmetic problem, wound infection, bleeding and hematoma formation, injury to the hypoglossal nerves, airway obstruction requiring tracheotomy, injury to the internal branch of the superior laryngeal nerve, and recurrence of the cyst.

Pearls and Pitfalls

The incidence of recurrence is greatly reduced by removal of the central portion of the hyoid bone.

Damage to the hypoglossal nerve can be prevented by avoiding dissection lateral to the lesser cornu of the hyoid bone. Creation of a tunnel underneath the hyoid with the Mixter clamp also helps to avoid hypoglossal injury.

Surgery on large or recurrent lesions may produce airway obstruction, which may necessitate tracheotomy or result in injury to the internal branch of the superior laryngeal nerve as it enters the thyrohyoid membrane.

There is a low incidence of carcinoma arising in thyroglossal duct cysts. This usually is thyroid papillary carcinoma. If the malignancy is confined to the cyst, no further surgery is indicated provided the thyroid gland is normal on palpation and thyroid scanning, and no cervical adenopathy is noted.

Suggested Reading

Sistrunk WE. The surgical treatment of cysts of the thyroglossal tract. Ann Surg 1920; 71:121.

Glenn E. Peters, M.D.

FINE NEEDLE ASPIRATION BIOPSY

The evaluation of a mass in the head and neck area involves a careful history, physical examination, and assessment of tissue obtained from biopsies of the mass and other suspicious mucosal lesions. The fine needle aspiration biopsy has greatly facilitated the procurement of tissue useful in arriving at a diagnosis. The technique is safe, simple to perform, and has a low incidence of contaminating tissues surrounding the mass. When used in conjunction with modern radiologic techniques, the fine needle aspiration biopsy allows sampling of deep-seated lesions that were reached previously only by open biopsy.

Indications

Indications for fine needle aspiration biopsy include (1) biopsy of cervical lymph nodes in patients known to have squamous cell carcinoma of the upper aerodigestive tract, either previously treated or as yet untreated; (2) biopsy of salivary masses; (3) biopsy of thyroid nodules; (4) evaluation of enlarged nodes or suspicious nodes when no lesions are noted in the upper aerodigestive tract; (5) aspiration of cystic lesions; and (6) biopsy of masses in the infratemporal fossa, parapharyngeal space, and retropharyngeal space.

Preoperative Considerations

Handling tissue samples is greatly facilitated by having the cytopathology technician or cytopathologist present at the time of the biopsy. The diagnostic adequacy of the specimen can be assessed immediately after the sample is obtained, and the need for additional biopsies can be determined.

The patient is seated comfortably in the examination chair with the head supported by the head rest. The patient's head is positioned so that it is facing in the direction opposite the side of the neck mass. The overlying skin is prepared with alcohol or an iodine-containing solution. A small wheal of local anesthesia is infiltrated into the overlying skin using 1 percent lidocaine. (The use of a local anesthetic may be optional in some patients.)

Equipment consists of a 20-cc syringe loaded into a syringe holder with a $1\frac{1}{2}''$ 20- or 22-gauge needle placed on the end of the syringe. One cubic centimeter of air is aspirated into the syringe.

Operative Steps

The neck mass is immobilized between the thumb and index finger of the left hand, and the syringe holder is held in the right hand. The needle is advanced into the immobilized neck mass, and the position of the needle is confirmed. Suction is applied to the syringe by withdrawing the handle on the syringe holder (Fig. 3A). After full negative pressure is achieved, multiple passes of the needle are made in the mass, making certain that the tip of the needle remains fully within the mass at all times (Fig. 3B).

The sample consists of cells aspirated into the barrel of the needle. A small amount may be just visible in the distal part of the needle hub. It is desirable to have a mixture of cells without contamination by a large amount of blood. After the specimen is obtained, all suction is released from the syringe *prior* to removing the tip of the needle from the mass. The needle is withdrawn from the neck without any suction applied, thus reducing the possibility of seeding along the needle tract.

Plate 154

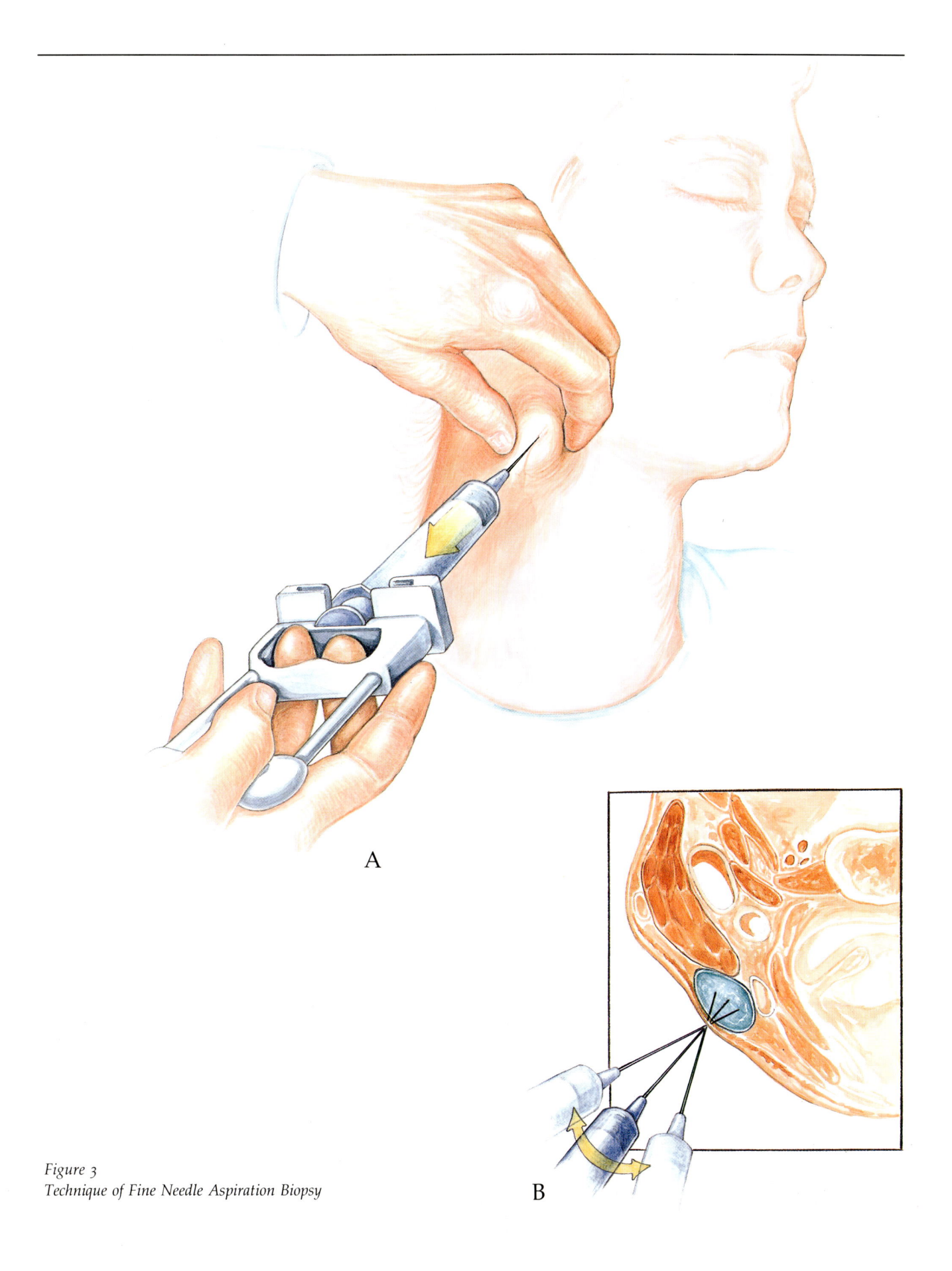

Figure 3
Technique of Fine Needle Aspiration Biopsy

375

The syringe is removed from the holder, and the contents of the needle are evacuated onto clean glass slides. The needle is also washed by aspirating Hank's solution for the preparation of a cell block. Standard cytologic smears are made. The smears can be immersed in 95 percent alcohol or stained immediately for determining the adequacy of the specimen. The procedure should be repeated if an adequate specimen is not obtained.

Postoperative Care

Following removal of the needle, gentle pressure is applied to the puncture site for several minutes. A small adhesive strip can be placed on the site prior to discharging the patient.

Risks, Complications, and Sequelae

Problems that may be attendant upon this procedure include seeding the needle tract with malignant cells. However, this has not proved to be the case in large series as long as proper technique is observed. Injury to major vascular structures, resulting in a hematoma, also may occur. This can be controlled with pressure on the puncture site. Other associated complications are injury to the cranial nerves in the neck and local infection at the puncture site.

Pearls and Pitfalls

The diagnostic accuracy of the fine needle aspiration biopsy depends largely on two variables: (1) the skill of the person performing the biopsy, and (2) the experience of the pathologist interpreting the results.

Diagnostic accuracy should approach 85 to 95 percent.

The fine needle aspiration biopsy interpretation carries a high degree of specificity but only a moderately good sensitivity.

False-positive diagnosis of malignancy is rare.

Precise tissue classification is limited in some circumstances. The technique falls short in the following situations:
1. Classifying lymphoma in cervical nodes.
2. Classifying sarcomas.
3. Classifying certain salivary neoplasms.
4. Differentiating follicular adenoma from follicular carcinoma in a thyroid nodule.
5. Classifying malignant small cell neoplasms such as melanoma, lymphoma, adenocarcinoma, or poorly differentiated carcinomas.

A false-negative diagnosis may result in 15 to 20 percent of cases. A nonmalignant result must not mislead the clinician.

Although fine needle aspiration biopsy has eliminated the need for many open biopsies, some situations may require larger amounts of tissue for clarification, particularly if immunohistochemical stains, immunofluorescent stains, or electron microscopy is needed.

Glenn E. Peters, M.D.
John C. Price, M.D.
Michael E. Johns, M.D.

CERVICAL LYMPHADENECTOMY

Malignant tumors of the upper aerodigestive tract, salivary glands, and skin of the scalp, face, and neck tend to metastasize initially to the lymph nodes of the neck. It has been shown that predictable patterns of lymphatic spread exist for all areas in the head and neck. Furthermore, the presence of metastatic cancer in cervical nodes is detrimental to patient survival and represents a stronger negative prognostic factor than increased size of the primary lesion.

Crile's landmark treatise in 1906 described the en bloc technique for cervical lymphadenectomy. This was modified by Martin into the standard radical neck dissection, which involved removal of all node-bearing tissues in the anterior and posterior cervical triangles with sacrifice of the spinal accessory nerve, sternocleidomastoid muscle, and jugular vein. Beahrs, Bocca, and Ballantyne developed modifications of the radical neck dissection that allow conservation of these structures.

There is little standardization in the current literature concerning definitions for the various modifications of the cervical lymphadenectomy. In this atlas the following terms are used:

1. The radical neck dissection is the standard en bloc technique as described by Crile and modified by Martin that involves removal of the sternocleidomastoid muscle, jugular vein, and spinal accessory nerve.
2. The modified neck dissection is a variation of the radical neck dissection in which the spinal accessory nerve and the jugular vein are preserved either separately or together.
3. The functional neck dissection as described by Bocca is a complete cervical lymphadenectomy in which the spinal accessory nerve, sternocleidomastoid muscle, and jugular vein are all preserved.
4. The supraomohyoid dissection removes the lymphatics of levels I, II, and III, preserving all other structures.

Indications

There is little doubt that a "therapeutic" neck dissection is indicated when clinically evident nodal metastases are present in the neck, and radical neck dissection is generally the procedure of choice. The spinal accessory nerve may be preserved if there is no disease in the upper jugular nodes or the nodes in the spinal accessory chain. Considerable controversy exists, however, about the role of "elective" neck dissection in the management of the clinically negative neck. This discussion of the technical aspects of the radical neck dissection and its modifications does not emphasize the philosophic considerations concerning the management of the clinically negative neck, as they are beyond the scope of this atlas.

The radical neck dissection is performed when clinically positive nodes are present, both in the first echelon and in distal nodal groups. The operation is done when node dissection is a necessary part of the procedure for resection of the primary lesion in which the neck is entered surgically, as in the commando procedure. Surgical salvage of local or regional failure following curative radiation therapy should be done with the radical neck dissection procedure. Elective node dissection also may be done utilizing radical neck dissection if there is a sufficiently high risk (usually greater than 25 percent) of occult metastases.

Sacrifice of the spinal accessory nerve imposes profound functional deficits on the patient. These include shoulder drop, pain in the area of the glenohumeral joint, and weakness with limited movement in the shoulder due to loss of trapezius muscle function. The decision to preserve the accessory nerve must be made on an oncologically sound basis. Modifying the radical neck dissection to allow for conservation of the nerve can be done when there is no nodal involvement in the upper jugular chain (level II) or in the spinal accessory chain.

The work of Lindberg, Feind, Tanner, Sharpe, and others has shown that the distribution of pathologically involved nodes varies, depending on the site of the primary lesion. Specifically, these authors point to the infrequency of metastases to the posterior triangle group of nodes. Additionally, Fletcher and colleagues have shown that microscopic disease in the neck can be adequately controlled with radiation therapy. These findings have resulted in the development of several modifications of Martin's radical neck dissection procedure, wherein the spinal accessory nerve, sternocleidomastoid muscle, and jugular vein can be preserved.

A modified or functional neck dissection can be utilized as a "staging" procedure for elective management when clinical findings are negative and there is greater than a 25 percent chance of occult metastases from the primary lesion. Modified neck dissection can be utilized in situations in which findings are negative, but the neck must be entered for control of the primary lesion. Modified neck dissections also are used for bilateral procedures and for differentiated thyroid carcinomas with neck metastases. Postoperative radiation therapy is generally a necessary adjunct in cases in which modified neck dissections are performed.

Preoperative Considerations

Two to four units of packed red blood cells are typed, screened, and held in reserve; transfusion is utilized depending on the amount of intraoperative blood loss. In the majority of cases in which neck dissection is performed alone, transfusion is unnecessary. Perioperative antibiotics are mandatory if the pharynx or oral cavity is to be entered as a part of the operation. General anesthesia is administered through an oral endotracheal tube for standard neck dissections; alternately, a nasal tube or a preliminary tracheotomy may be used, as dictated by the location of the primary lesion. The patient is placed on the operating table in the supine position. A small folded sheet is placed under the shoulders to achieve adequate extension of the neck. (A Mayfield head rest may be used. This allows the operating surgeons to stand closer to the surgical field.) A standard surgical scrub using an iodine-containing solution is done. The area prepared extends from the patient's eyebrows to the nipples, including the posterior (dorsal) surface of the neck. The head and neck field is draped with folded half sheets that are sutured or stapled to the patient. The method of draping as outlined by Martin has proved to be the most successful in that the endotracheal tube is fixed to the head drape and can be moved with the patient's head during the operation. The remainder of the patient's body is covered with standard sterile sheets. It may be necessary to expand the operative field to include the chest and abdomen, depending on reconstructive plans.

Operative Steps

THE RADICAL NECK DISSECTION

The skin incisions are made depending on the site of the primary cancer. The options include the modified Schobinger (our preference), the "half-H," the anterior apron, and the McFee (Figs. 4A to 4D). Skin flaps are usually elevated in the subplatysmal plane, unless large neck masses with soft tissue extension necessitate resection of the platysma. The superior flap is elevated to the inferior border of the mandibular body, staying lateral to the tail of the parotid gland. After this flap is elevated, the

Plate 155

A Modified Schobinger

B Half-H

C Anterior apron

D McFee

Figure 4
Radical Neck Dissection; Incisions

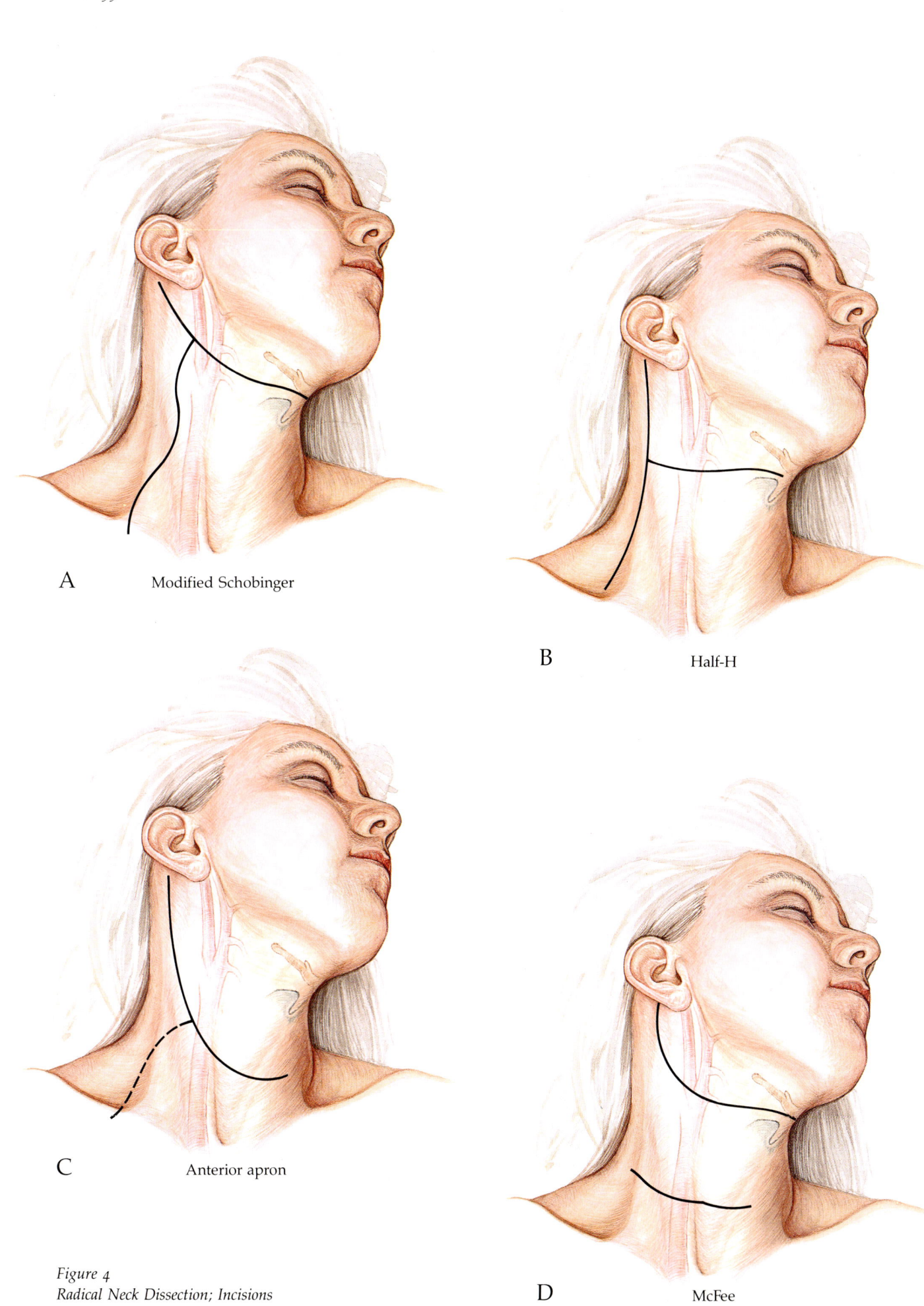

superficial layer of the deep cervical fascia is dissected upward off the capsule of the submandibular gland, thereby including the marginal mandibular branch of the facial nerve. This layer of fascia is then secured to the superior flap by using one of the ties placed on the anterior facial vein (Fig. 4F). (Alternately, the marginal mandibular nerve can be carefully dissected from surrounding soft tissue and suspended by the ligatures placed on the anterior facial vein.) The flaps are elevated to the strap muscles and the midline medially and to the level of the clavicle inferiorly. The posterior flap is elevated to the anterior border of the trapezius muscle (Fig. 4E). The skin flaps are then sutured either to the drapes or to the patient's skin.

INFERIOR DISSECTION. The sternal and clavicular heads of the sternocleidomastoid muscle are divided by placing upward traction on the belly of the muscle with a sponge and cutting the insertions with a No. 10 blade (Fig. 4G). This incision is done cautiously and in multiple layers because the carotid sheath and its contents lie immediately deep to the muscle. Alternately, the muscle can be separated from the underlying carotid sheath by gentle dissection with a blunt Kelly clamp. The insertions can then be cut with an electrocautery unit. Once the muscle in-

Plate 156

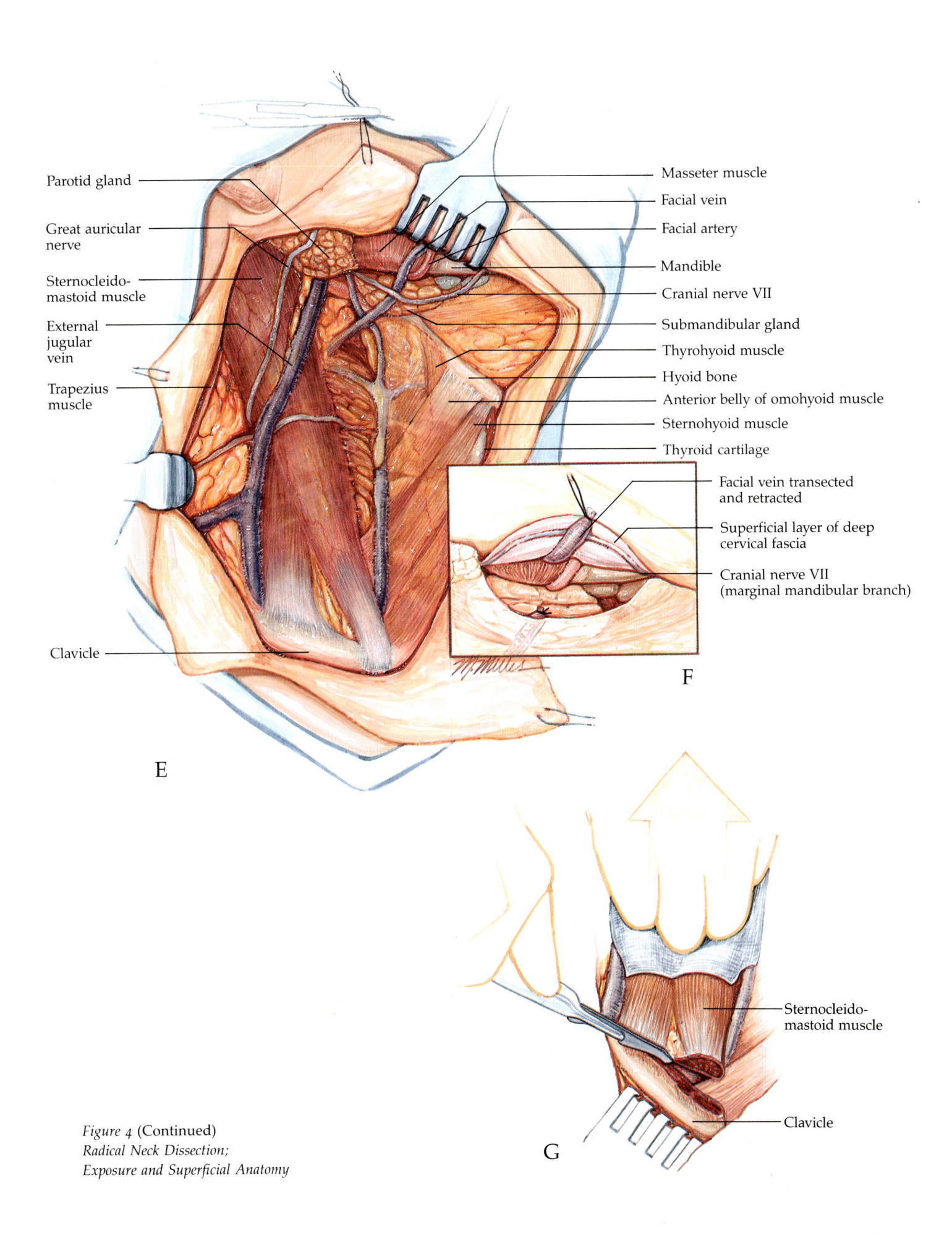

Figure 4 (Continued)
Radical Neck Dissection;
Exposure and Superficial Anatomy

sertions are divided, the soft tissue overlying the sternothyroid muscle is separated from the posterior border of the muscle. By retracting the sternothyroid medially, the carotid sheath is identified. The carotid sheath is opened with Metzenbaum scissors (Fig. 4H), and the jugular vein is bluntly dissected from surrounding soft tissue. The surgeon should avoid the use of Mixter clamps or the use of undue force on the vein with forceps because damage to the vein may result in severe hemorrhage in an area where bleeding can be difficult to control. A large inadvertent venotomy also may result in a life-threatening air embolism. A blunt Kelly clamp makes an ideal dissecting instrument. An adequate length of vein should be exposed to allow easy passage of clamps. Prior to clamping the vein, the vagus nerve and the carotid artery are visually identified to make certain that they are not included in the clamps (Fig. 4I).

Four Kelly clamps are applied to the lower aspect of the jugular vein (Fig. 4J). The vein is cut between the middle two clamps. Both ends of the vein are doubly ligated with 2–0 silk ties and 3–0 silk suture ligatures, as illustrated (Fig. 4K). Alternately, four free 2–0 silk ties may be passed and tied around the vein prior to its transection, but care must be taken not to "saw" through the vein with these ties.

Plate 157

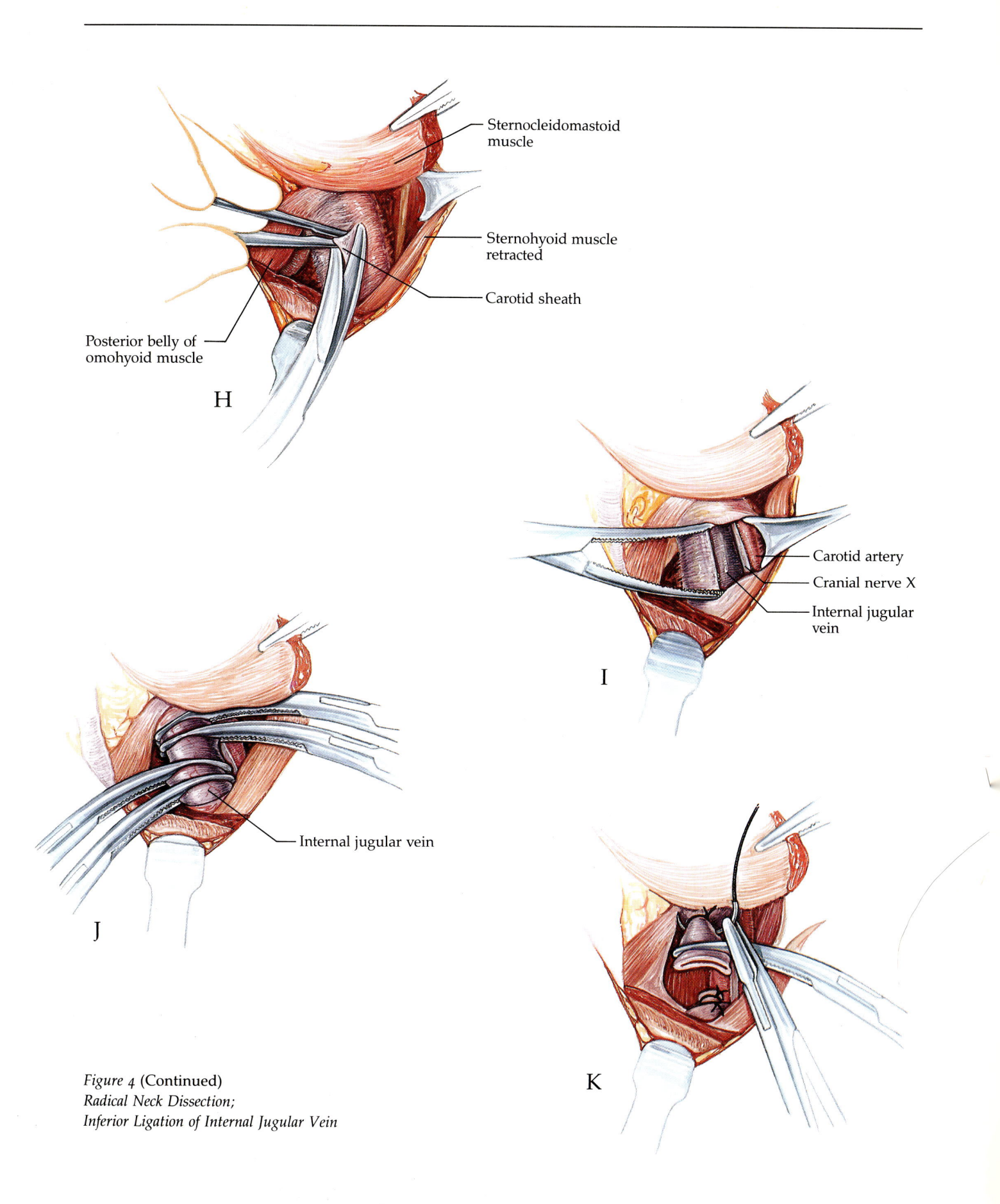

Sternocleidomastoid muscle

Sternohyoid muscle retracted

Carotid sheath

Posterior belly of omohyoid muscle

H

Carotid artery
Cranial nerve X
Internal jugular vein

I

Internal jugular vein

J

K

Figure 4 (Continued)
Radical Neck Dissection;
Inferior Ligation of Internal Jugular Vein

385

The fibrofatty tissue in the supraclavicular area is retracted with a sponge and incised sharply in sequential layers using a No. 10 blade (Fig. 4L). The external jugular vein is encountered in this area and is controlled with clamps and ties. The omohyoid muscle is identified and is divided between clamps (Fig. 4M). The division of the fibrofatty tissue extends from the jugular vein to the anterior border of the trapezius muscle. Soft tissue is divided, working toward the deep layer of the deep cervical fascia that overlies the phrenic nerve, brachial plexus, and posterior (motor) branches from the cervical plexus. As dissection approaches this fascial layer, continued cephalad traction with a sponge causes a release of the soft tissues just above the fascia. Preservation of this fascia facilitates avoidance of injury to the above-mentioned nerves. The transverse cervical artery and vein are encountered above the deep fascia; they may be preserved or ligated, depending on the preference of the surgeon.

On the left side the thoracic duct is often large and easily injured during the dissection. If the duct is transected, it must be clearly identified and ligated to avoid a chylous fistula. The pedicle of tissue in the area of the stump of the jugular vein lying between the phrenic nerve and the vagus nerve should always be divided between clamps and the cut ends tied. Although the thoracic duct is located in the left side of the neck, chyle leaks may also develop in the right side from failure to control the accessory lymphatic duct adequately.

Plate 158

Clavicle

Internal jugular vein

Phrenic nerve

L

Transverse cervical artery

Subclavian vein

Posterior belly of omohyoid muscle

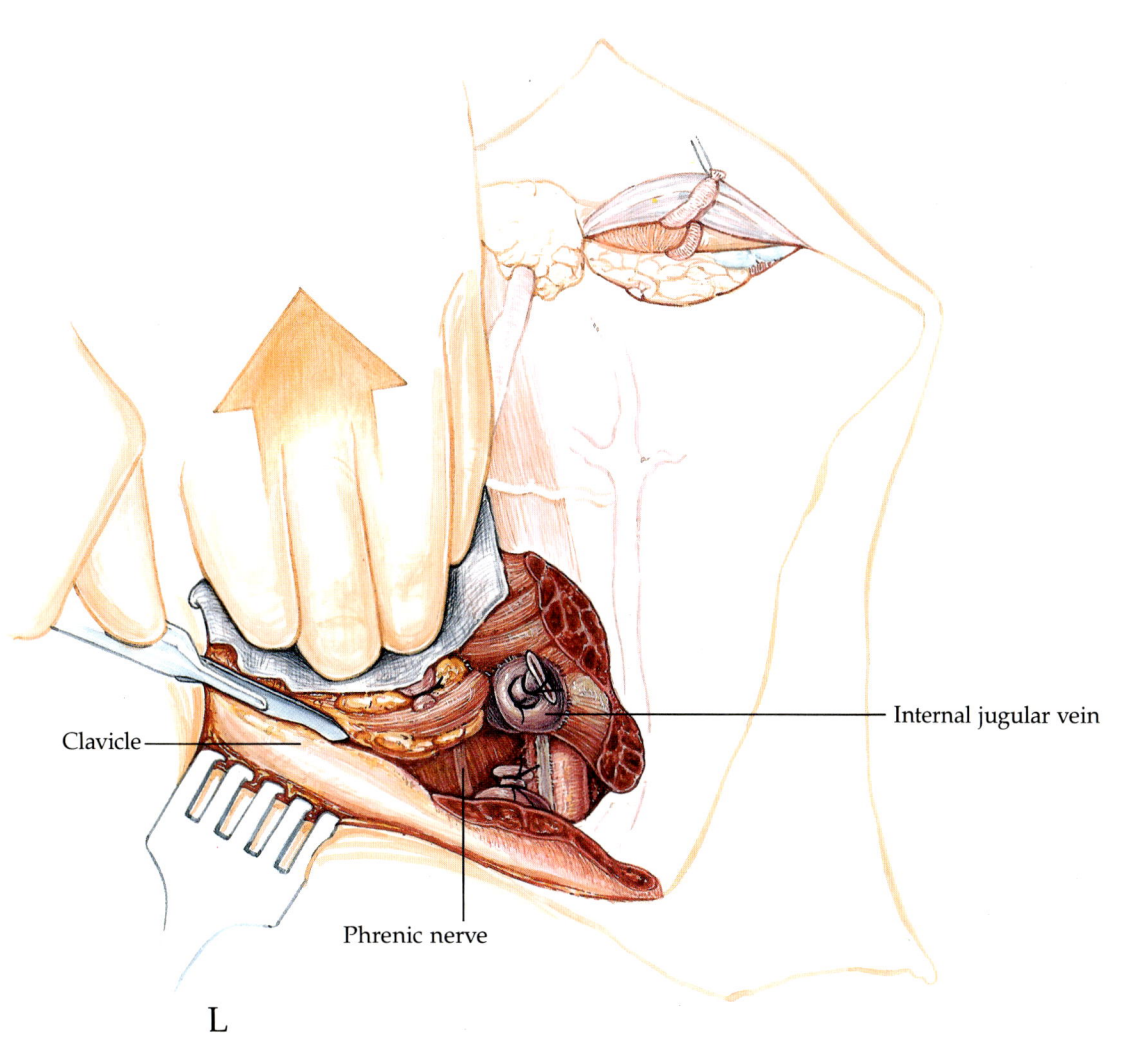

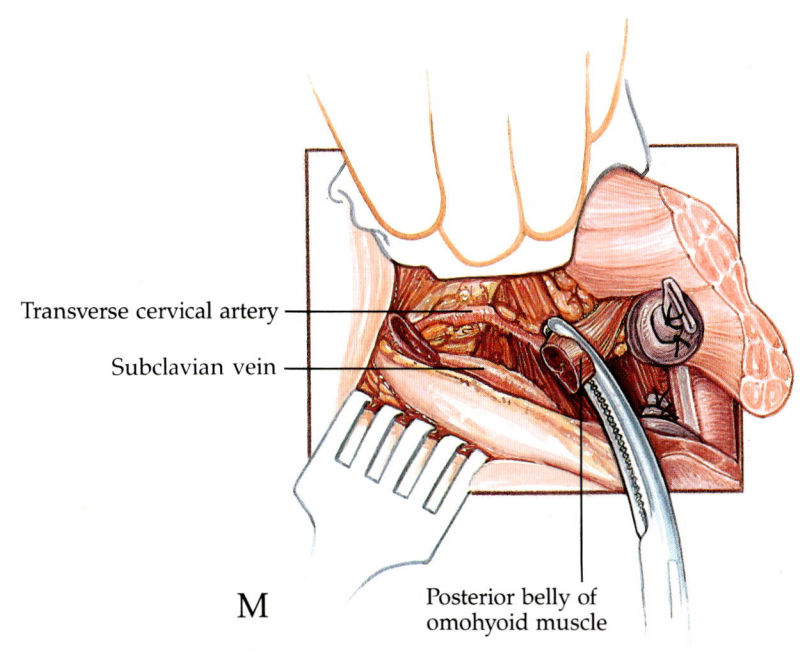

M

Figure 4 (Continued)
Radical Neck Dissection; Inferior Dissection

POSTERIOR DISSECTION. The posterior margin of the neck dissection is defined as the anterior border of the trapezius muscle. This muscle is delineated by sharp knife dissection from the level of the clavicle upward to its junction with the mastoid tip (Fig. 4N). The sternocleidomastoid muscle is divided along the anterior border of the trapezius and is freed from its mastoid insertion as part of the posterior dissection (Fig. 4O).

Plate 159

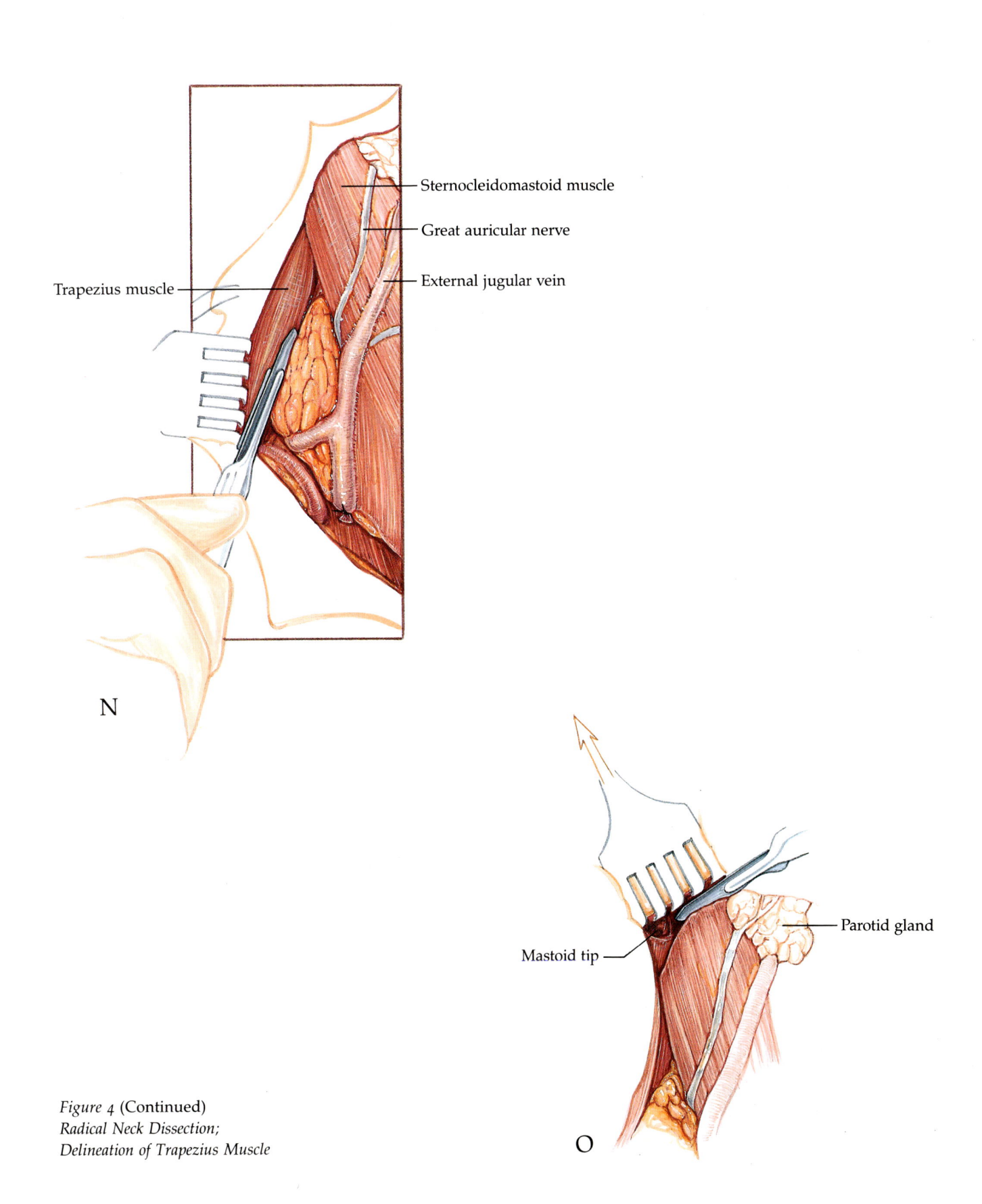

- Sternocleidomastoid muscle
- Great auricular nerve
- Trapezius muscle
- External jugular vein

N

Mastoid tip
Parotid gland

O

Figure 4 (Continued)
Radical Neck Dissection;
Delineation of Trapezius Muscle

Four Kocher clamps are placed on the posterior margin of the neck contents anterior to the border of the trapezius muscle. The clamps are used to provide traction on the posterior neck contents as they are sharply separated from the deep layer of the deep cervical fascia. Accurate dissection above this fascial layer allows preservation of the posterior (motor) branches of the cervical plexus, thereby preserving the innervation to the levator scapulae, splenius capitis, and scalene muscles. This dissection is taken upward and medially to the level of the cervical plexus (Fig. 4P). Each of the anterior (sensory) branches of the cervical plexus is divided. The carotid sheath is thereby approached from the posterior direction. It is important to use the belly of the knife blade during this part of the dissection in order to avoid inadvertent injury to the great vessels in the neck (Fig. 4Q).

P

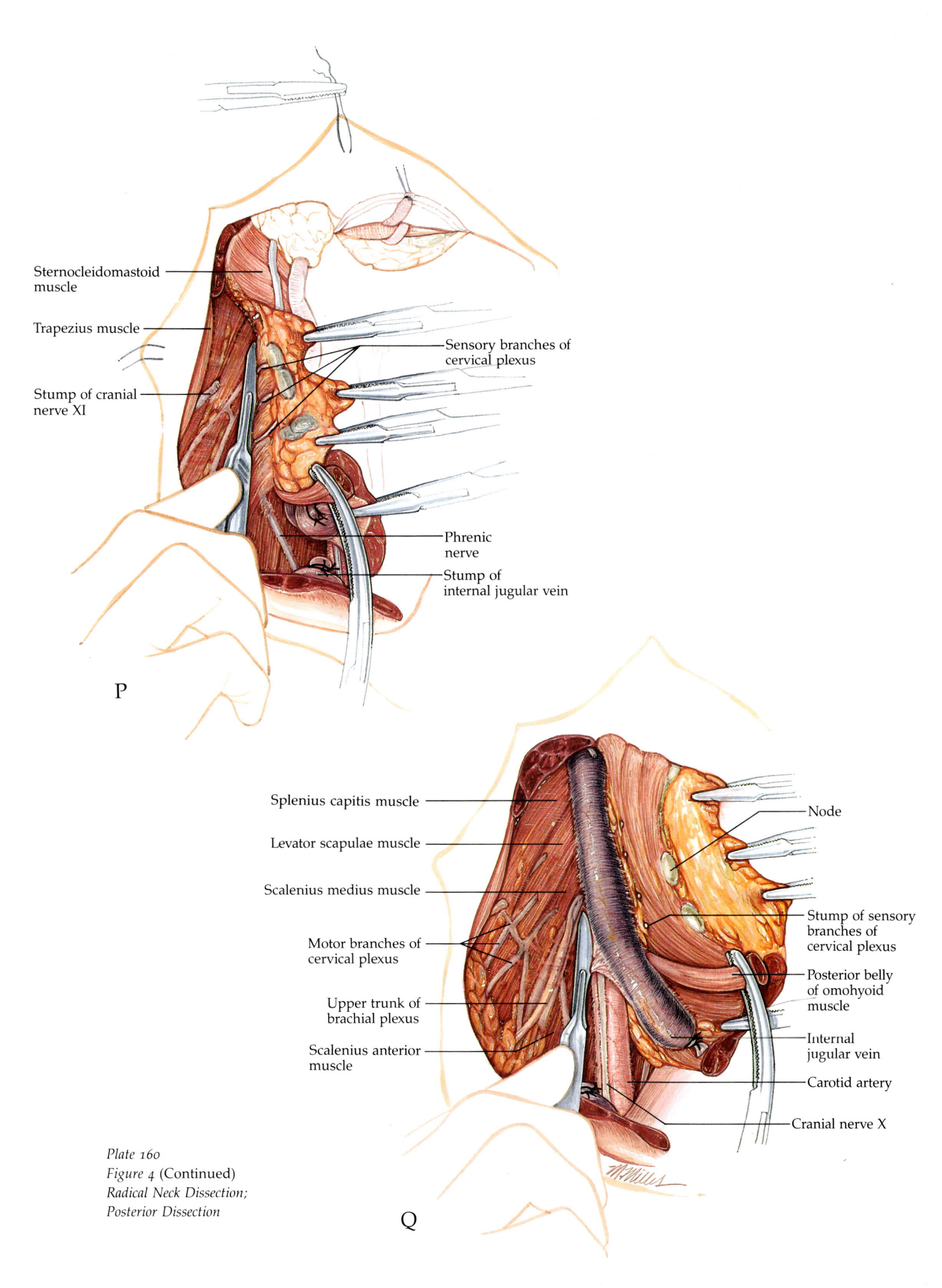

- Sternocleidomastoid muscle
- Trapezius muscle
- Stump of cranial nerve XI
- Sensory branches of cervical plexus
- Phrenic nerve
- Stump of internal jugular vein

Q

- Splenius capitis muscle
- Levator scapulae muscle
- Scalenius medius muscle
- Motor branches of cervical plexus
- Upper trunk of brachial plexus
- Scalenius anterior muscle
- Node
- Stump of sensory branches of cervical plexus
- Posterior belly of omohyoid muscle
- Internal jugular vein
- Carotid artery
- Cranial nerve X

Plate 160
Figure 4 (Continued)
Radical Neck Dissection;
Posterior Dissection

The remaining fibers of the sternocleidomastoid muscle are detached from the mastoid tip. The posterior belly of the digastric muscle is identified as it emerges from the mastoid tip. A tunnel is developed along the lateral surface of the posterior belly of the digastric muscle, deep to the tail of the parotid gland (Fig. 4R). The tail of the parotid gland is then divided, and the posterior facial vein is controlled as it is encountered.

Once the inferior border of the digastric muscle is delineated, a retractor (Army-Navy or Richardson) is placed underneath the posterior belly and is used to elevate this muscle superiorly. The jugular vein is then identified underneath the posterior belly of the digastric muscle. In dissecting the vein from the surrounding soft tissue, the proximal end of the spinal accessory nerve is cut. All soft tissue along the jugular vein in the area of the skull base and jugular foramen should be dissected inferiorly and incorporated in the specimen. The jugular vein is divided between four Kelly clamps, and the cut ends are tied and suture-ligated (Fig. 4S).

Once the jugular vein is divided superiorly, the specimen can be rolled forward and the soft tissue division continued. The vagus nerve and carotid artery are clearly defined and separated from the vein and surrounding soft tissues using careful knife dissection. The hypoglossal nerve is identified above the carotid bifurcation as it crosses lateral to the external carotid artery. The twelfth cranial nerve is traced forward to the point where it passes medial to the posterior belly of the digastric muscle. In the area of the hypoglossal nerve are several large veins, including the lingual vein and veins draining the pharyngeal plexus. Failure to ligate these veins may result in bothersome venous bleeding, the control of which risks injury to the twelfth nerve. The ansa hypoglossi is divided as it separates from the main trunk of the hypoglossal nerve. The ansa hypoglossi may be preserved if tumor considerations permit.

Plate 161

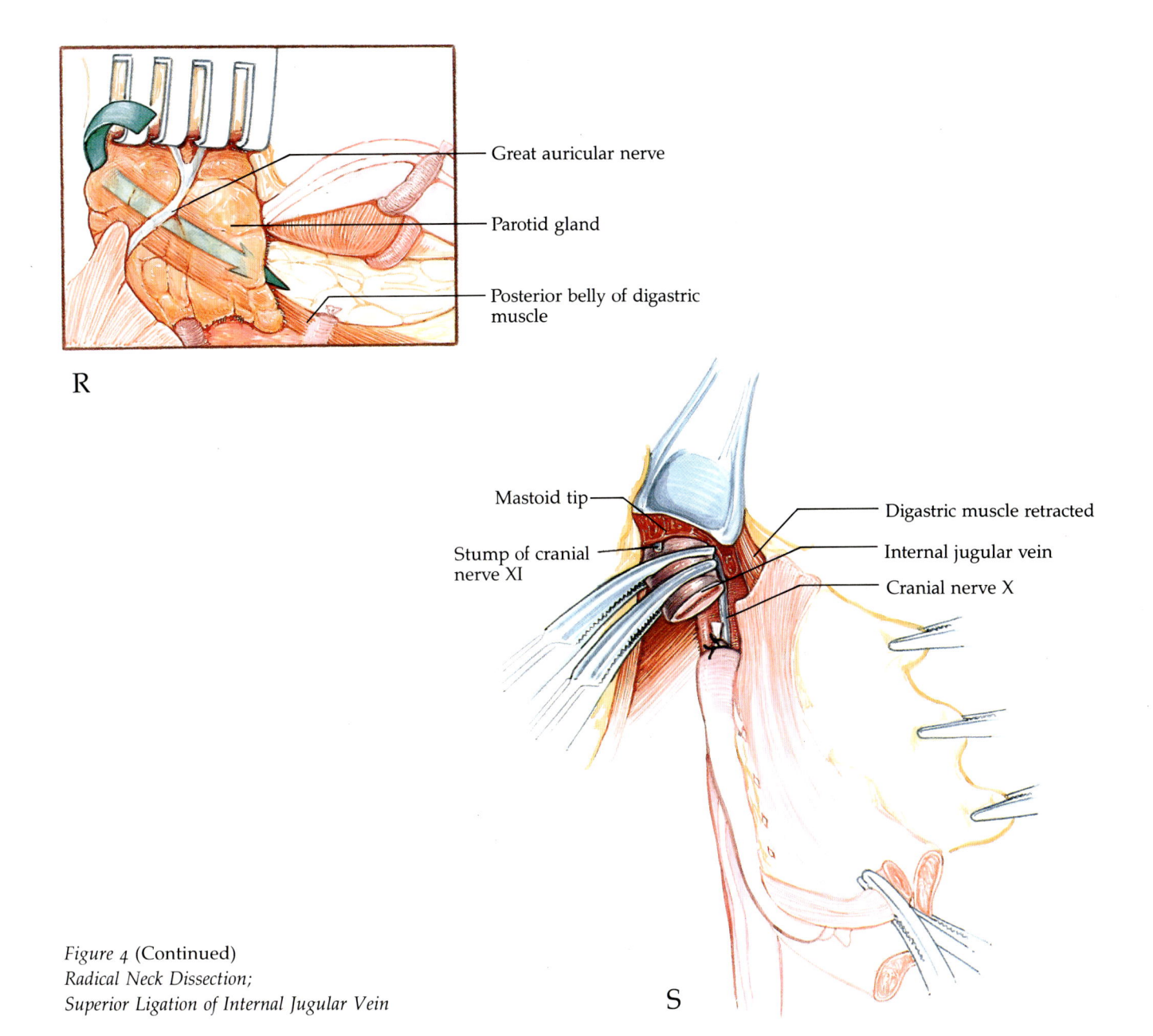

- Great auricular nerve
- Parotid gland
- Posterior belly of digastric muscle

R

- Mastoid tip
- Stump of cranial nerve XI
- Digastric muscle retracted
- Internal jugular vein
- Cranial nerve X

Figure 4 (Continued)
Radical Neck Dissection;
Superior Ligation of Internal Jugular Vein

S

ANTERIOR DISSECTION. Soft tissue along the anterior (medial) border of the anterior belly of the omohyoid muscle is divided using either a knife or a scissors. This is facilitated by placing downward traction on the omohyoid muscle (Fig. 4T). This dissection is carried up to the level of the hyoid bone, at which point the insertion of the anterior belly of the omohyoid muscle is divided. This leaves the specimen connected to the submandibular and submental triangle contents (Fig. 4U).

SUPERIOR DISSECTION. The fibrofatty tissues are incised along the anterior belly of the contralateral digastric muscle and swept inferiorly and posteriorly from the central portion of the mylohyoid muscle. The anterior belly of the ipsilateral digastric muscle is cleaned, leaving the submental contents attached to the contents of the submandibular triangle (Fig. 4V).

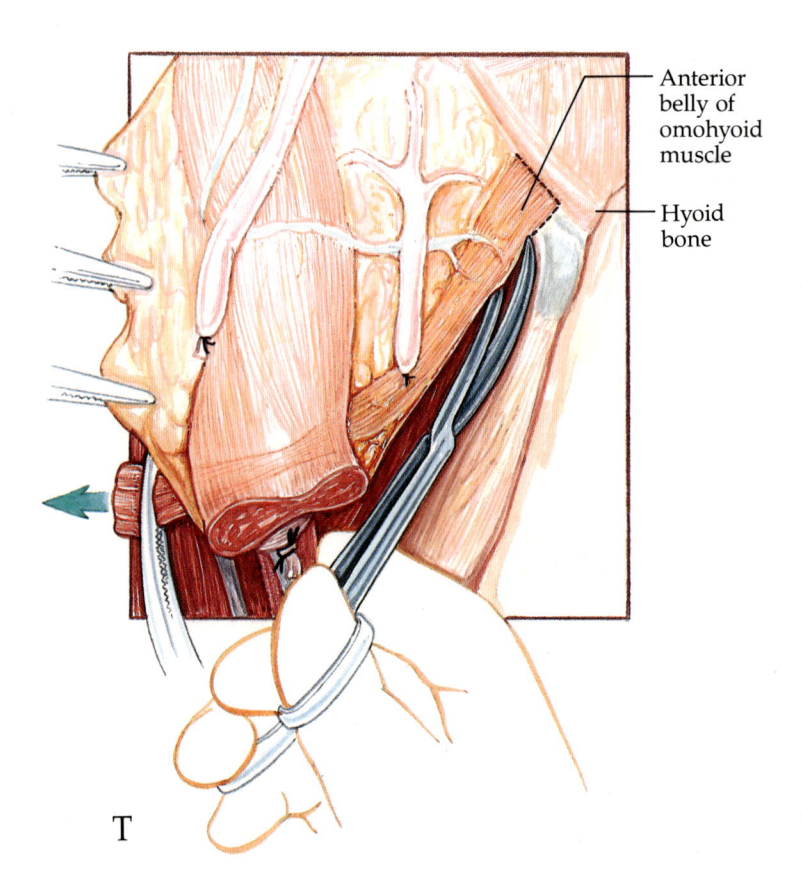

Plate 162
Figure 4 (Continued)
Radical Neck Dissection;
Anterior Dissection

Plate 163

- Transected parotid gland
- Cranial nerve XII
- Cranial nerve X
- Phrenic nerve
- Cranial nerve XI
- Tissue block

U

- Anterior belly of digastric muscle
- Mylohyoid muscle
- Contralateral digastric muscle
- Submental triangle fat and nodes

V

Figure 4 (Continued)
Radical Neck Dissection;
Submental Triangle Dissection

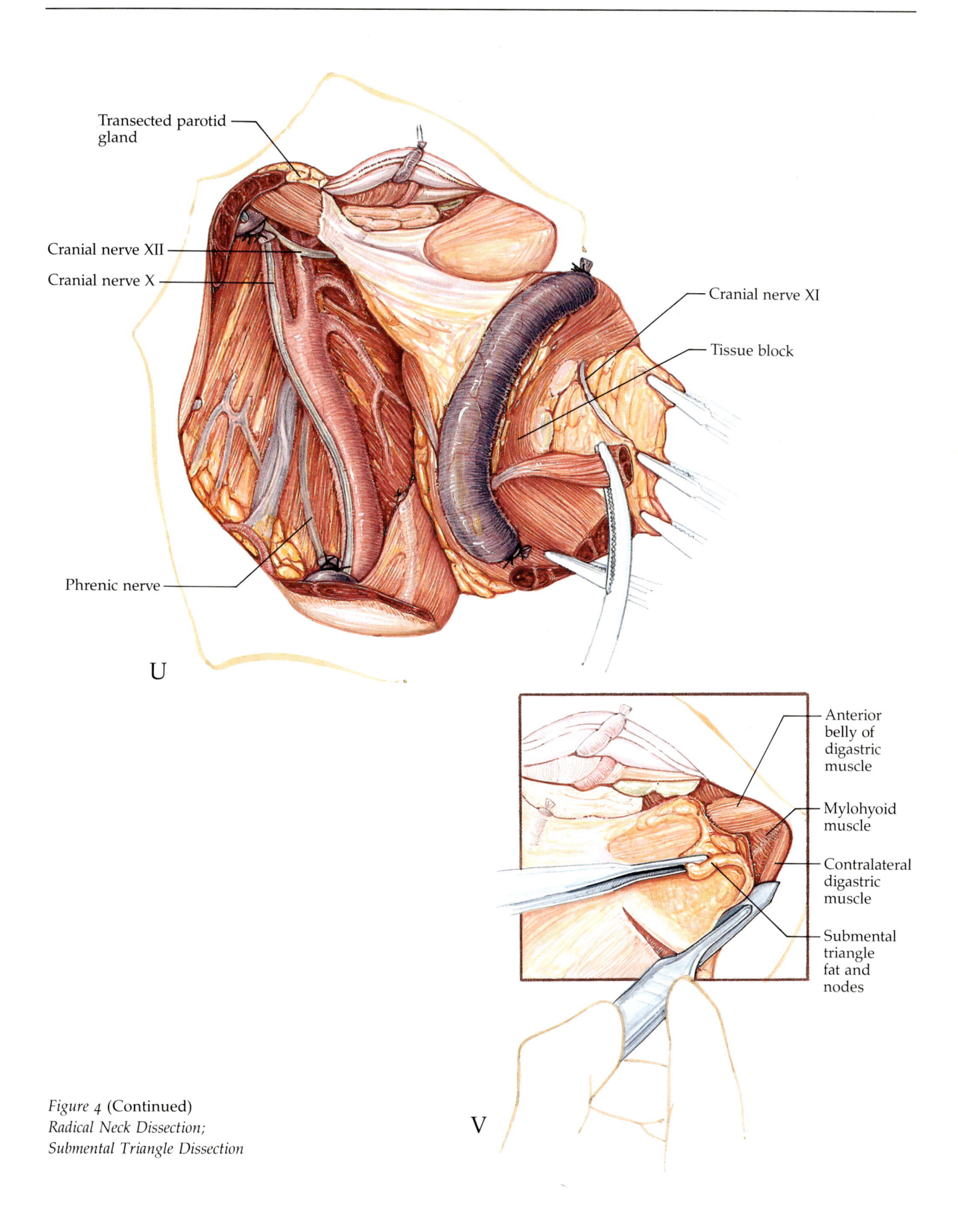

395

Both the anterior and posterior bellies of the digastric muscle are delineated, and the submandibular gland is elevated from the floor of the submandibular triangle, facilitating the identification of the hypoglossal nerve. Inferior traction is then placed on the specimen, and the soft tissues are separated from the inferior border of the mandibular body. The posterior border of the mylohyoid muscle is identified and an Army-Navy retractor placed underneath it for traction. The lingual nerve, submandibular ganglion, and postganglionic parasympathetic fibers to the submandibular gland are identified. The secretomotor fibers from the ganglion are divided between clamps and tied in order to control accompanying small veins (Fig. 4W). The submandibular duct is identified deep to the cut nerve fibers (Fig. 4X). This is also taken between clamps and tied. The oral extension of the submandibular gland is dissected posteriorly. Posterior and downward traction on the submandibular triangle contents allows identification of the facial artery at the superior border of the posterior belly of the digastric muscle. This vessel is clamped, divided, and ligated (Fig. 4Y). The remaining soft tissue attachments are cut, and the neck specimen is removed.

Plate 164

- Mylohyoid muscle retracted anteriorly
- Lingual nerve
- Submandibular ganglion
- Submandibular duct
- Postganglionic fibers to gland
- Submandibular gland
- Facial artery

W

X
- Submandibular duct

- Facial artery
- Mylohyoid muscle
- Digastric tendon

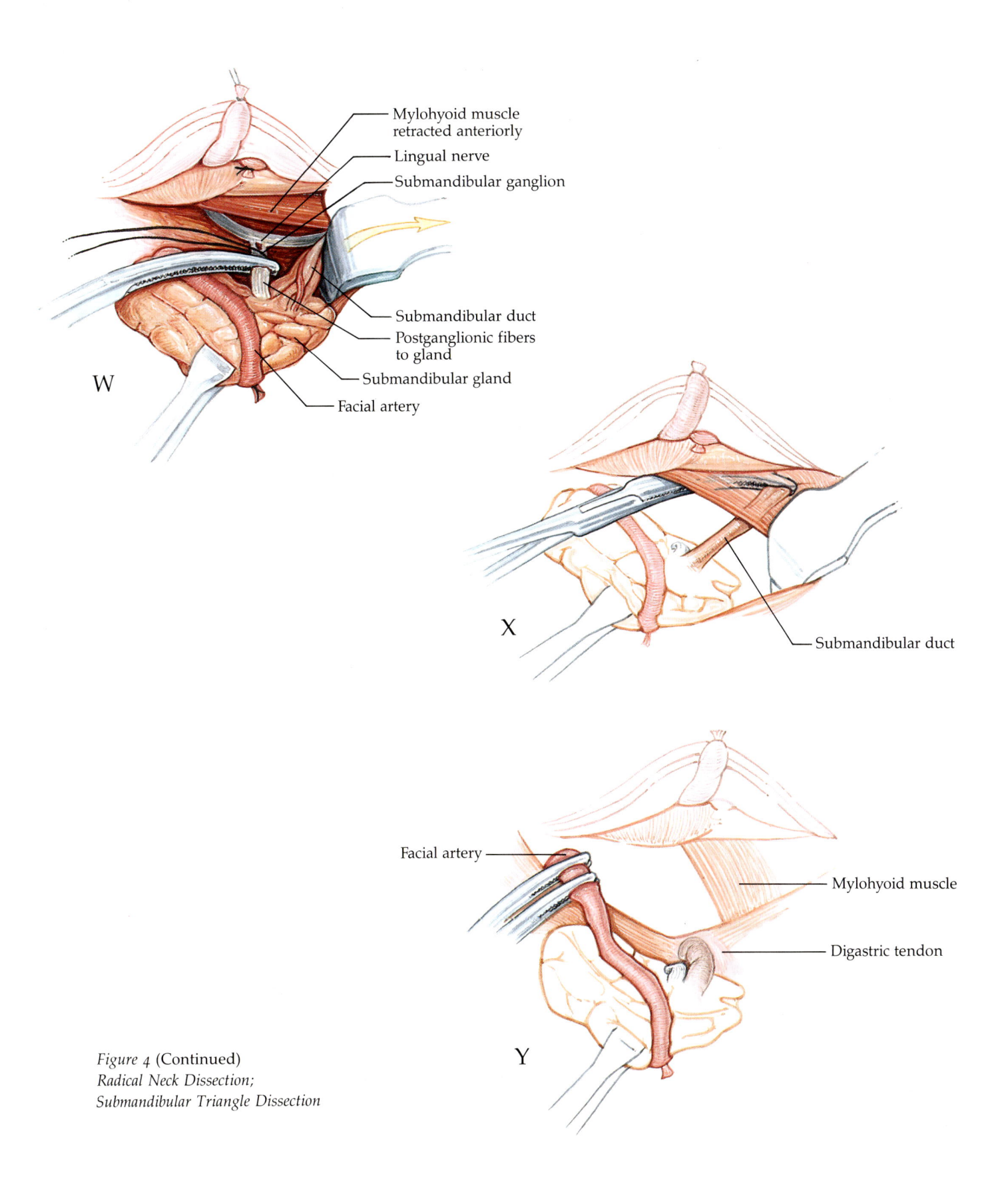

Y

Figure 4 (Continued)
*Radical Neck Dissection;
Submandibular Triangle Dissection*

CLOSURE. Meticulous hemostasis is obtained, and the wound is irrigated with sterile saline. Flat silicone-Silastic suction catheter drains (Jackson-Pratt) are placed into the wound through separate stab incisions in the lower flaps. The drains are secured in the wound away from the carotid artery, cranial nerves, and skin or mucosal suture lines.

The skin incisions are closed in layers. The platysma is closed with absorbable sutures in an airtight fashion. The skin is accurately reapproximated with stainless steel surgical staples or permanent sutures (Fig. 4Z).

Plate 165

Flat silicone closed suction drain

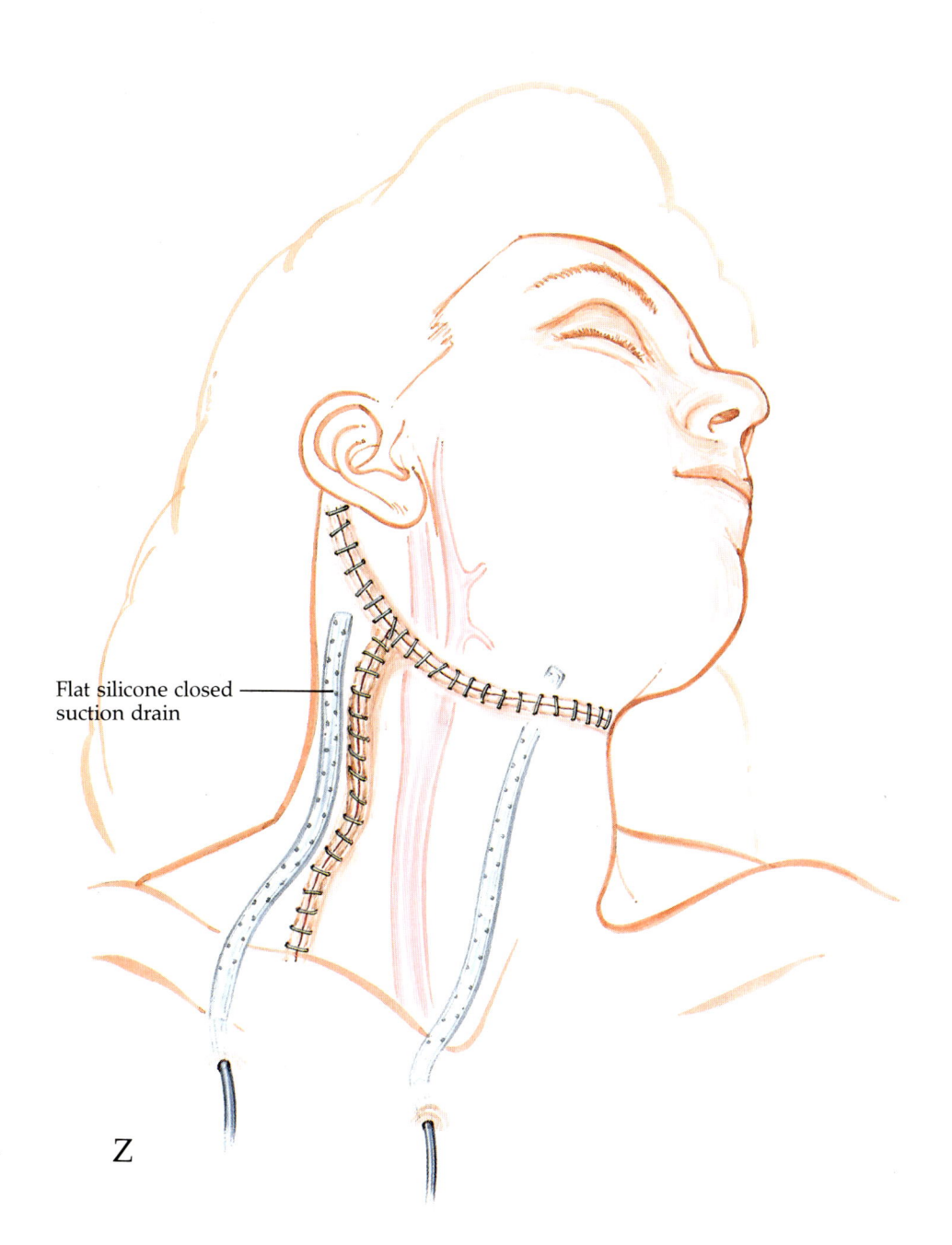

Figure 4 (Continued)
Radical Neck Dissection; Closure

Z

THE MODIFIED NECK DISSECTION

TECHNIQUE FOR PRESERVING THE SPINAL ACCESSORY NERVE. Following elevation of the posterior flap to the anterior border of the trapezius muscle, the spinal accessory nerve is identified. The most consistent area to locate the nerve is at the anterior border of the trapezius muscle. The surgeon identifies an imaginary intersection between the anterior border of the trapezius muscle and the clavicle and then measures approximately 2 fingerbreadths or 4 cm above this intersection. The spinal accessory nerve typically is found entering the undersurface of the muscle at that point (Fig. 5A).

The nerve is dissected free from the fibrofatty tissue of the posterior triangle. The nerve is thus traced to the posterior border of the sternocleidomastoid muscle.

The nerve then is dissected through the belly of the sternocleidomastoid muscle. A tunnel is developed above the nerve trunk, and then the overlying muscle fibers are divided (Fig. 5B). The entire sternocleidomastoid muscle is divided lateral to the nerve. Care is taken to avoid undue disruption of the soft tissue lymphatics in level II.

Once the nerve is traced through the anterior border of the sternocleidomastoid muscle, the main nerve trunk is seen extending toward the posterior belly of the digastric muscle. Here the nerve lies in close proximity to the upper end of the jugular vein. Careful dissection in this area will free the main nerve trunk from the surrounding soft tissues and jugular vein (Fig. 5C).

After soft tissue and muscle are divided lateral to the main nerve trunk, the branches supplying the sternocleidomastoid muscle are readily apparent. A vessel loop or nerve hook is passed beneath the main nerve trunk and used to gently elevate it off the muscle belly as the motor branches to the sternocleidomastoid muscle are divided (Fig. 5D). It is advisable to expose the entire nerve prior to dividing the branches to the sternocleidomastoid muscle.

The superior portion of the sternomastoid muscle is released from the mastoid tip, as in the radical neck dissection (see Fig. 4O). The digastric muscle is identified and soft tissue released from its inferior border to the eleventh cranial nerve (see Fig. 4R). The tissue of the superior compartment of the posterior triangle is dissected from the deep layer of the deep cervical fascia. The spinal accessory nerve is then retracted laterally, and the soft tissue in the apex of the posterior triangle is rotated underneath it (Fig. 5E). The nerve is thus positioned posteriorly and superiorly out of the operative field, and dissection of the neck can be continued.

Figure 5
Modified Neck Dissection; Preservation of Spinal Accessory Nerve

Plate 166

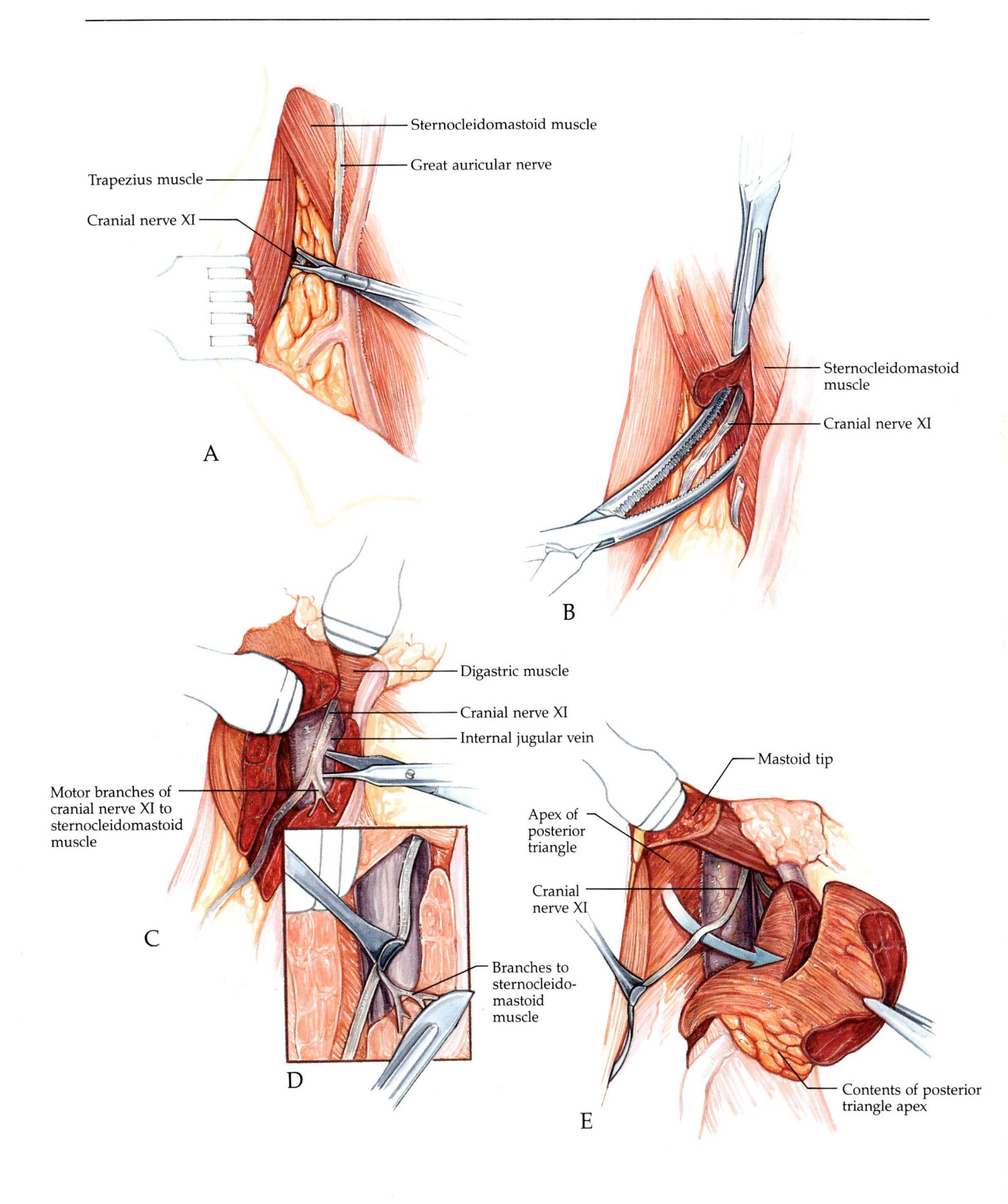

A
- Trapezius muscle
- Sternocleidomastoid muscle
- Great auricular nerve
- Cranial nerve XI

B
- Sternocleidomastoid muscle
- Cranial nerve XI

C
- Digastric muscle
- Cranial nerve XI
- Internal jugular vein
- Motor branches of cranial nerve XI to sternocleidomastoid muscle

D
- Branches to sternocleidomastoid muscle

E
- Mastoid tip
- Apex of posterior triangle
- Cranial nerve XI
- Contents of posterior triangle apex

401

TECHNIQUE FOR PRESERVATION OF THE INTERNAL JUGULAR VEIN. The jugular vein is usually sacrificed during this operation. In the circumstance in which clinically suspicious masses exist in both sides of the neck, it may be desirable to save the internal jugular vein on the side of least tumor burden. This can significantly reduce the risk of massive cerebrofacial edema produced by the sacrifice of both veins. The side chosen for preservation of the jugular vein is approached first. If it is not possible to save the vein, it may be advisable to attempt a similar procedure on the opposite side of the neck if the tumor permits.

The progress of the operation is the same as for the radical neck dissection, except that the internal jugular vein is identified carefully inferiorly and superiorly but *not* cross-clamped or ligated. The carotid arteries and the vagus, hypoglossal, and spinal accessory nerves are identified. Inferior and posterior dissection allows a visually controlled approach to the vein from behind. Instead of elevating the vein away from the carotid artery and vagus nerve, it is left intact with them. The connective tissue surrounding the vein is removed by either scissors or knife technique. Gentle handling and avoidance of undue traction on the vein are advised. Ligation of the common facial, inferior, middle, and superior thyroid veins is usually necessary. Venous spasm may develop and should be treated by application of a sponge saturated with 1 percent lidocaine (without epinephrine).

FUNCTIONAL NECK DISSECTION (BOCCA)

Patient positioning, sterile preparation, and draping are the same as for the radical neck dissection procedure. The incisions as outlined earlier may be utilized in the modified neck dissection. Skin flaps are again elevated in the subplatysmal plane to the clavicle, anterior border of the trapezius muscle, midline, and lower border of the mandible.

The spinal accessory nerve is identified in the posterior triangle and dissected free. The technique is outlined in the dissection and preservation of the spinal accessory nerve (see Fig. 5A). The dissection of the spinal accessory nerve at this point extends from the anterior border of the trapezius muscle to the posterior border of the sternocleidomastoid muscle. The nerve is completely freed up in its course through the posterior triangle. The fascia of the sternocleidomastoid muscle is then incised in the direction of the muscle fibers. This incision extends from the mastoid tip to the sternal and clavicular insertions. The fascia is then carefully peeled off the muscle belly. This is facilitated by placing clamps on the cut ends of the fascia and using these clamps for traction as the fascia is dissected from the muscle belly. The fascia is dissected in both an anterior and a posterior direction (Fig. 6A).

As the fascia is dissected in the anterior direction, the proximal end of the spinal accessory nerve may be identified as it enters the undersurface of the muscle belly. This is usually in the upper one-third of the muscle belly. Once the entire muscle belly is freed from its fascial containment, Army-Navy or Richardson retractors are used to elevate the

Cervical Lymphadenectomy

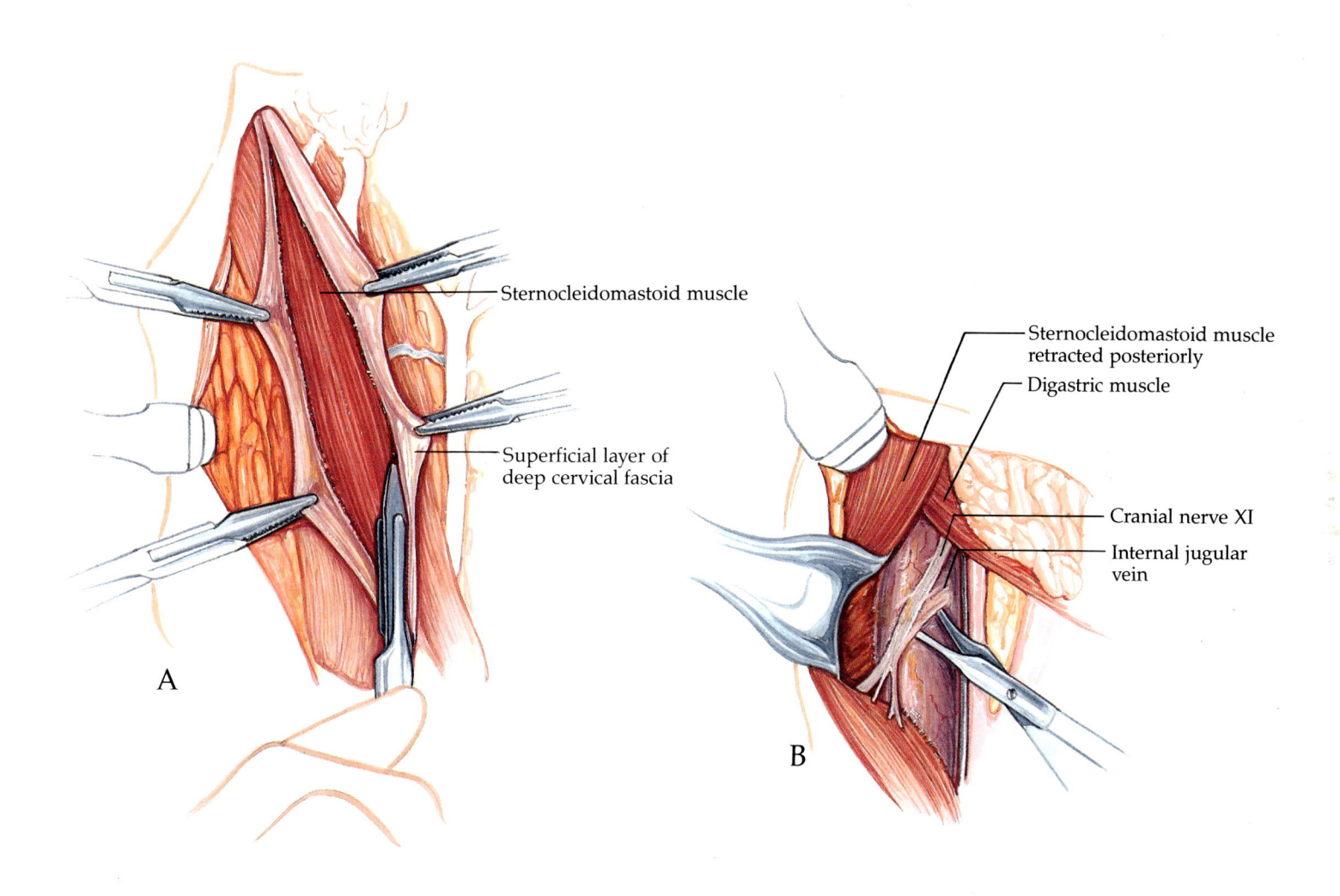

Plate 167
Figure 6
Functional Neck Dissection;
Development of Fascial Envelope

muscle belly posteriorly and laterally away from the node-bearing tissue of the neck. The proximal portion of the spinal accessory nerve is then dissected cephalad, up to the point at which it comes in close proximity to the jugular vein. The posterior belly of the digastric muscle is identified. The proximal portion of the spinal accessory nerve is completely dissected free, taking care to preserve the branches to the sternocleidomastoid muscle (Fig. 6B).

403

The fibrofatty tissue in the very apex of the posterior triangle lying underneath the upper end of the sternocleidomastoid muscle is freed from the area of the mastoid tip. Careful scissors dissection in this area allows identification of the deep layer of the deep cervical fascia. The apex of the posterior triangle is dissected off the deep layer of the deep cervical fascia, working toward the jugular vein and the spinal accessory nerve (Fig. 6C). Once this triangle of tissue is free, it is rolled underneath the nerve, and the nerve is retracted superiorly out of the surgical field (Fig. 6D).

The carotid sheath is identified in the lower portion of the neck. It is incised with the belly of a No. 10 blade or opened with Metzenbaum scissors (see Fig. 4H). This allows identification of the jugular vein, carotid artery, and vagus nerve (see Fig. 4I). The posterior belly of the omohyoid muscle is identified and dissected free from the surrounding fibrofatty tissue in the supraclavicular area.

As in the radical neck dissection operation, the fibrofatty tissue in the supraclavicular area is divided down to the deep layer of the deep cervical fascia. The phrenic nerve and brachial plexus are identified deep to the fascial layer (see Fig. 4L). This inferior dissection extends from the carotid sheath to the trapezius muscle.

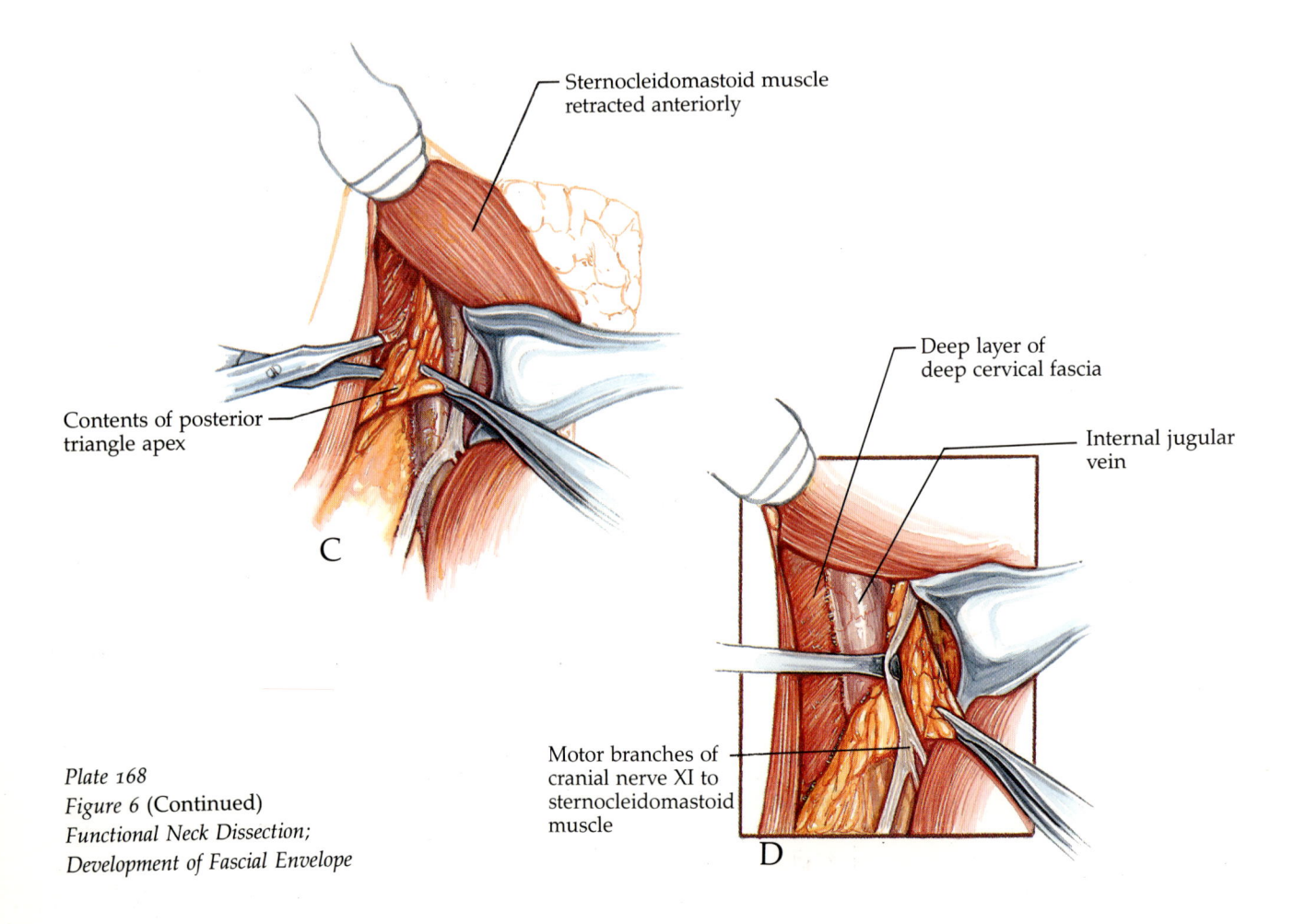

Plate 168
Figure 6 (Continued)
Functional Neck Dissection;
Development of Fascial Envelope

Cervical Lymphadenectomy

Cranial nerve XI
Internal jugular vein
Sensory branches of cervical plexus
Upper trunk of brachial plexus
Phrenic nerve
Contents of posterior triangle

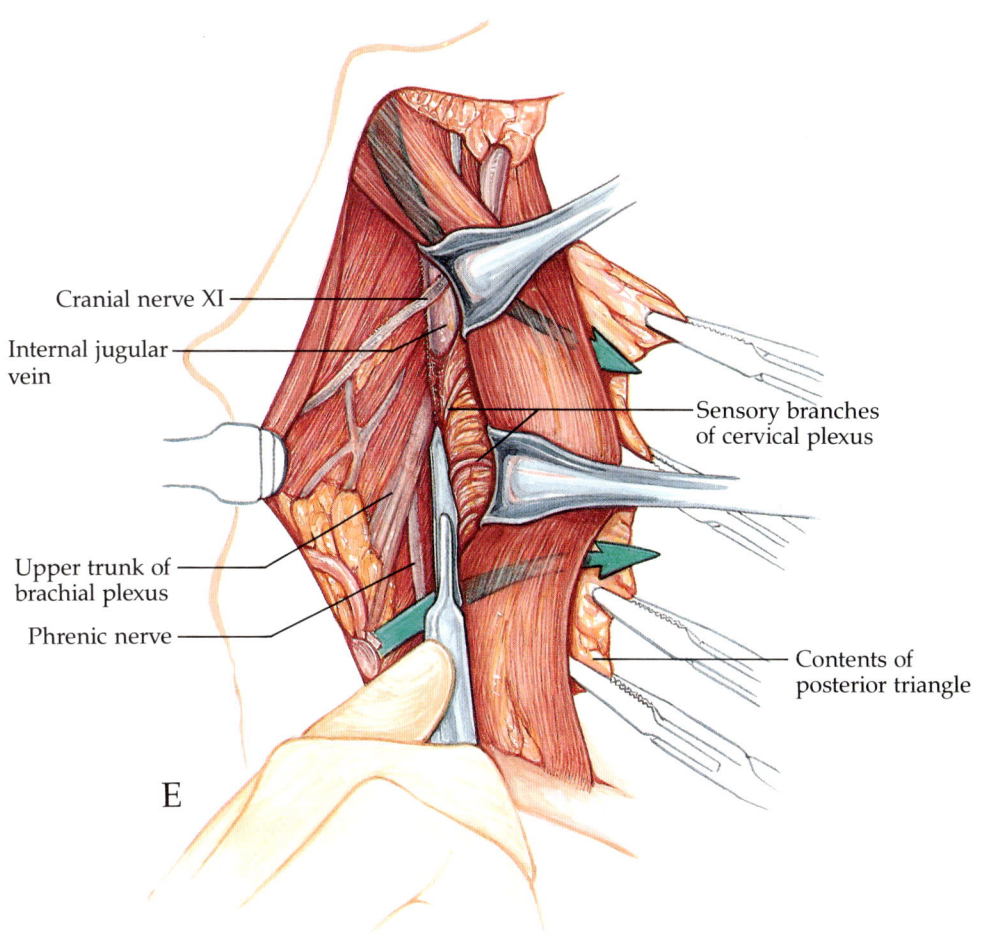

E

Plate 169
Figure 6 (Continued)
Functional Neck Dissection;
Removal of Carotid Sheath and Jugular Nodes

Kocher clamps are placed on the posterior aspect of the contents of the posterior triangle. The clamps are used for traction very much like they are in the radical neck dissection. Sharp knife dissection or dissection with Metzenbaum scissors beginning at the trapezius muscle is carried forward toward the carotid sheath. The deep margin of dissection is the deep layer of the deep cervical fascia. This fascia is preserved to prevent injury to the posterior or motor branches of the cervical plexus (see Fig. 4P). The belly of the sternocleidomastoid muscle is elevated off the neck using either Richardson or Army-Navy retractors.

The contents of the posterior triangle are then rolled underneath the belly of the sternocleidomastoid muscle (Fig. 6E). Continued sharp dissection anteriorly allows identification of the brachial plexus and phrenic nerves.

Cervical Lymphadenectomy

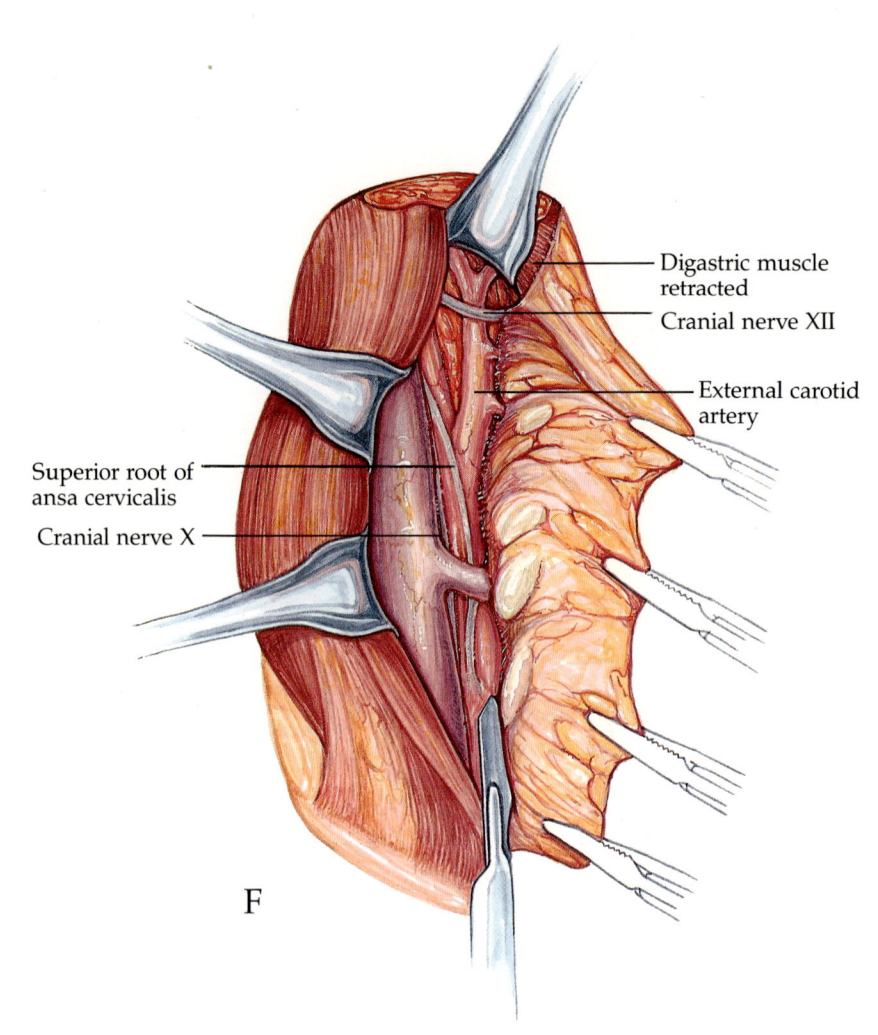

Plate 170
Figure 6 (Continued)
Functional Neck Dissection;
Removal of Carotid Sheath and Jugular Nodes

The anterior branches of the cervical plexus are divided as outlined in the radical neck dissection operation. The carotid sheath is incised on its posterior lateral extent using the belly of a No. 10 blade or Metzenbaum scissors. The contents of the neck are dissected off the jugular vein, carotid artery, and vagus nerve (Fig. 6F). The tributaries of the internal jugular vein are dissected free, clamped, divided, and tied as they are encountered. A tunnel is created on the lateral aspect of the posterior belly of the digastric muscle (see Fig. 4R). The tail of the parotid gland is divided lateral to this tunnel. The posterior facial vein is clamped, divided, and tied as it is encountered. The ansa hypoglossi may be preserved or it may be divided, depending on the conditions created by the primary tumor.

The remainder of the modified neck dissection for the dissection of the submandibular and submental triangles proceeds as outlined in the radical neck dissection procedure (see Figs. 4V through 4Y). If there is a low incidence of metastases to level I, dissection of level I may be omitted at this point. The remainder of the surgical steps and the postoperative considerations are identical to those for the radical neck dissection and have been outlined previously.

Cervical Lymphadenectomy

SUPRAOMOHYOID NECK DISSECTION

The preoperative considerations are identical to those outlined in the radical neck dissection section. Skin incisions and flap elevation techniques are also similar. It is not necessary to expose the posterior triangle.

Once the flaps are elevated, the fascia on the sternocleidomastoid muscle is incised from the mastoid tip to the sternal and clavicular insertions. Clamps are applied on the anterior aspect of this incision and used for anterior traction. The surgeon places a sponge on the belly of the sternocleidomastoid muscle and uses this to retract the muscle belly posteriorly. The fascia of the sternocleidomastoid muscle is dissected off the muscle belly with careful knife dissection. As the muscle belly is rolled posteriorly and the fascia is dissected anteriorly, the proximal portion of the spinal accessory nerve is seen to enter the undersurface of the muscle in its upper one-third (Fig. 7A). The nerve is then dissected free at its entrance into the muscle. Dissection medial to the muscle belly is continued posteriorly until the anterior branches of the cervical plexus are encountered. Remember that these branches divide from their roots and extend around the posterior portion of the sternocleidomastoid muscle.

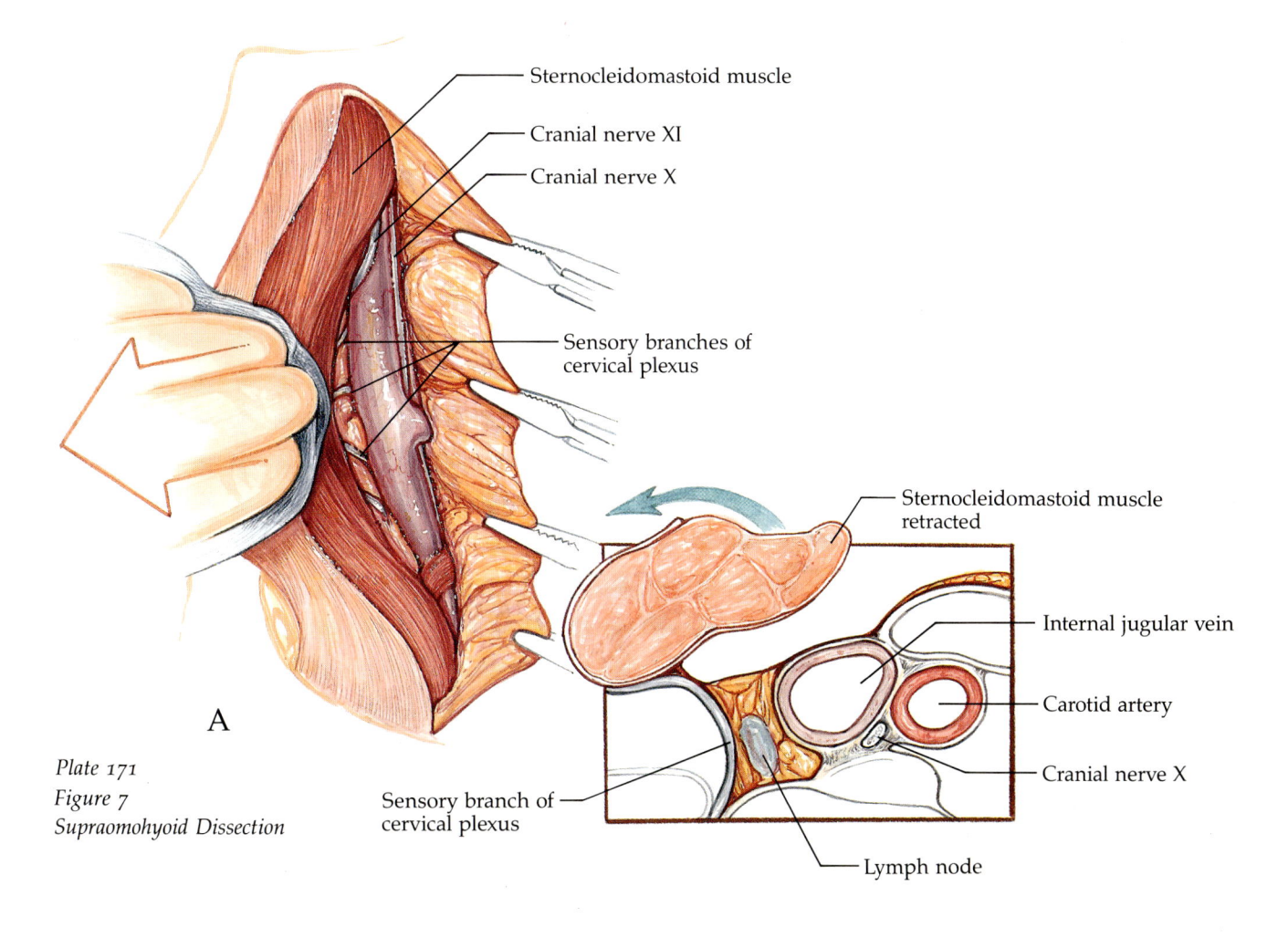

Plate 171
Figure 7
Supraomohyoid Dissection

The proximal portion of the spinal accessory nerve is dissected cephalad, up to the point where it comes in proximity to the jugular vein. The posterior belly of the digastric muscle is identified. A Richardson retractor is then placed underneath the posterior belly of the digastric muscle and a second is placed along the upper third of the sternocleidomastoid muscle. A small triangle of fibrofatty tissue lying above the spinal accessory nerve is then dissected off the deep layer of the deep cervical fascia and rolled underneath the nerve trunk (Fig. 7B).

The inferior margin of dissection is defined as the intermediate tendon of the omohyoid muscle. The structure is identified and dissected free from surrounding fibrofatty tissue. Richardson retractors are used to retract the belly of the sternocleidomastoid muscle posteriorly. Sharp dissection using scissors or a knife is used to cut through the fibrofatty tissue underlying the sternocleidomastoid muscle. This is done at the level of the anterior branches of the cervical plexus. This dissection is taken down to the deep layer of the deep cervical fascia. Fibrofatty tissue posterior to the jugular vein is divided along the line extending up the anterior branches of the cervical plexus. This goes from the clavicle to the previous dissection in the area of the spinal accessory nerve. Kocher clamps are placed on the fibrofatty tissue in the neck, and these are used to retract it anteriorly (Fig. 7C). Sharp dissection is used to divide the node-bearing tissue from the deep cervical fascia. The brachial plexus and phrenic nerves are identified below this fascial layer. This dissection is taken up to the carotid sheath. The carotid sheath is opened on its posterior lateral extent. If knife dissection is used, care is taken to use the belly of the knife blade. The node-bearing tissue in the jugular chain is dissected off the jugular vein, carotid artery, and vagus nerve (Fig. 7D). Tributaries to the jugular vein are clamped, divided, and tied as they are encountered. Superiorly the hypoglossal nerve is identified, and the ansa hypoglossi may be divided or preserved. The tail of the parotid gland is divided after creating a tunnel lateral to the posterior belly of the digastric muscle (see Fig. 4R).

The contents of the submandibular and submental triangles are removed, depending on the extent of the primary tumor. If the primary tumor has a low incidence of metastasis to these areas, these triangles may be left undisturbed. However, if a dissection is needed in these areas, it should proceed as outlined in the radical neck dissection procedure (see Figs. 4V through 4Y).

Postoperative Care

Prophylactic antibiotics are continued throughout the perioperative period. The wound suction catheters are placed on continuous wall suction at -100 mm. The output from the suction catheters is recorded on a daily basis. The catheters are removed individually as their output becomes less than 20 ml for a 24-hour period. The incisions are cleaned twice daily, and a light coating of antibacterial ointment is applied after each cleaning. Early ambulation is encouraged, generally on the first postoperative day. The diet may be advanced as tolerated beginning on the night of surgery, provided no suture lines are in the oral cavity or pharynx; otherwise, nasal tube feedings are begun on the first postoperative day. Sutures or

Plate 172

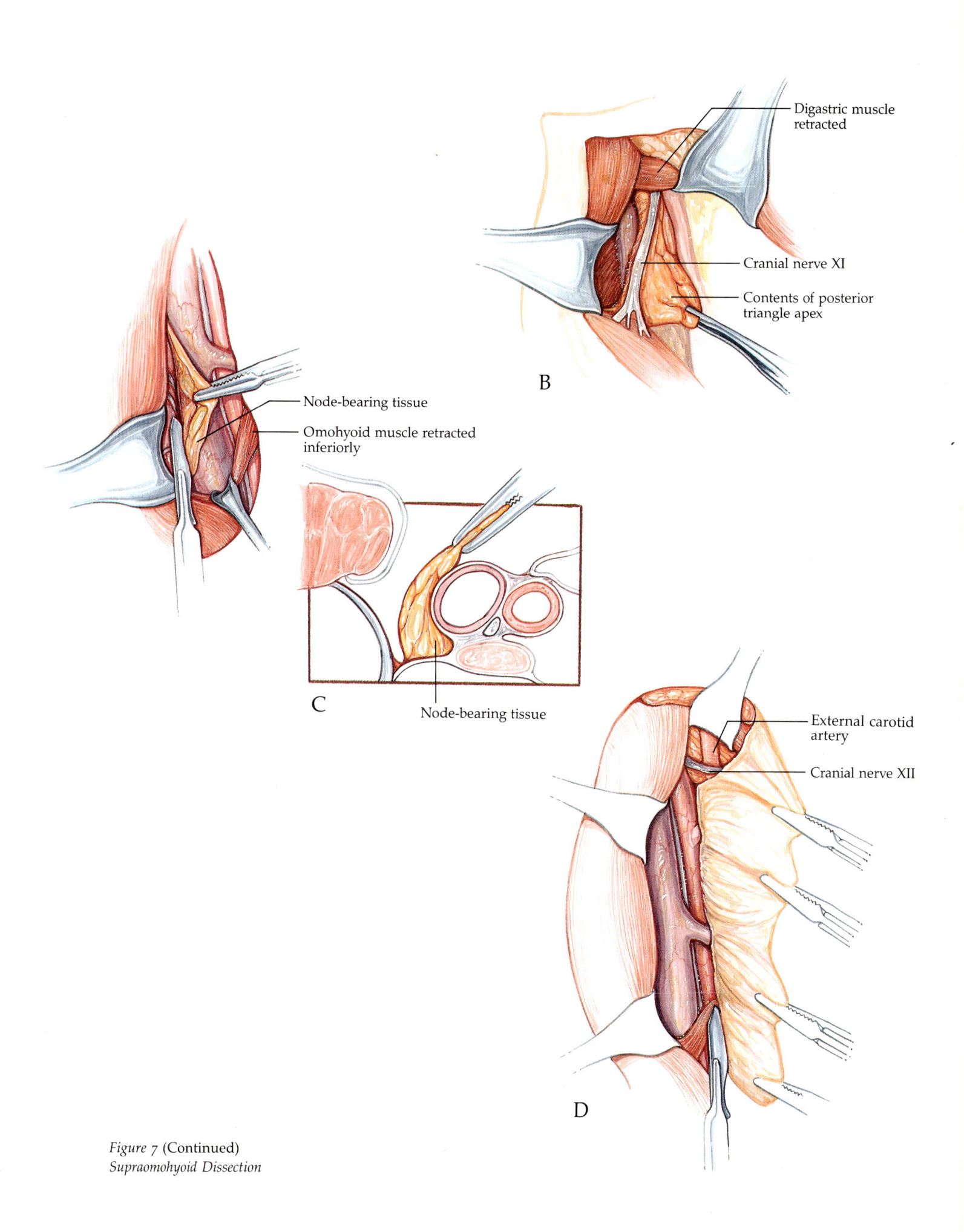

Digastric muscle retracted

Cranial nerve XI

Contents of posterior triangle apex

B

Node-bearing tissue
Omohyoid muscle retracted inferiorly

Node-bearing tissue

C

External carotid artery

Cranial nerve XII

D

Figure 7 (Continued)
Supraomohyoid Dissection

skin staples are removed on the seventh postoperative day if the patient has had no previous radiation therapy; if the patient has been irradiated, they should remain in until postoperative days 10 to 12.

Risks, Complications, and Sequelae

There are a number of risks, complications, and sequelae possible during or after cervical lymphadenectomy, as follows: (1) a visible scar on the neck; (2) wound infection (or fistula); (3) hemorrhage that may require transfusion or be life-threatening; (4) weakness in the lower lip as a result of injury to the marginal mandibular branch of the facial nerve; (5) injury to cranial nerves X, XI, or XII; (6) injury to the cervical sympathetics; (7) "shoulder syndrome," with pain and weakness in the shoulder caused by loss of trapezius muscle function; (8) numbness in the lower face, the ear, the neck, and the upper chest; (9) facial edema, generally transient; (10) injury to the thoracic duct or lymphatic channels with resultant chyle leak; (11) numbness and loss of taste in the anterior tongue on the side of the operation; (12) air embolism from uncontrolled venotomy in the jugular vein; (13) anesthetic complications; (14) perioperative death; (15) scar contracture resulting in a bandlike tightening in the neck; and (16) tumor recurrence.

Pearls and Pitfalls

Intubation with an armored tube prevents the tube from kinking under the drapes, and attaching the tube to the head drape prevents accidental extubation with movement of the head.

Careful attention to the platysma facilitates skin flap elevation. The platysma is deficient in the midline and over the lateral aspect of the posterior triangle.

Identification of the submandibular gland capsule and careful dissection of the superficial layer of the deep cervical fascia from the capsule help to avoid injury to the marginal branch of the facial nerve.

If a knife is used to divide the sternal and clavicular insertions of the sternocleidomastoid muscle, make certain that the rounded "belly" of the blade is used rather than the pointed tip. This helps to avoid inadvertent injury to the jugular vein.

The cut ends of the jugular vein should be doubly ligated.

Careful attention to the deep layer of the deep cervical fascia helps preserve the posterior (motor) branches to the levator scapulae and splenius capitis muscles. It also avoids injury to the brachial plexus and phrenic nerve.

Carefully clamp and tie the soft tissues between the phrenic and vagus nerves in the lower part of the neck. Failure to do so may result in a chyle leak. Both sides of the neck are at risk, not just the left side.

Adequate retraction of the posterior belly of the digastric muscle is essential for safe dissection of the upper end of the jugular vein.

Clamping and tying the lingual vein and veins draining the pharyngeal plexus must be done to avoid injury to the hypoglossal nerve.

The hypoglossal nerve lies in the floor of the submandibular triangle. Blind clamping in this area may result in injury.

Identify the lingual nerve and submandibular ganglion prior to dividing the submandibular duct. Otherwise, the duct may be confused for the nerve.

Stabilize suction catheters in the neck with absorbable sutures away from the carotid artery, jugular vein (if present), spinal accessory nerve, and suture lines in the oral cavity, pharynx, and skin.

Flat silicone-Silastic suction catheters are preferable for the following reasons: (1) flat drains decrease flap compromise, (2) large-caliber drains (10 mm) facilitate evacuation of blood and serum, (3) Silastic material tends to decrease the incidence of drain occlusion secondary to clotting, (4) such catheters provide constant negative pressure, and (5) they eliminate the need for pressure dressings.

Suggested Reading

Ballantyne AJ. Principles of surgical management of the pharyngeal walls. Cancer 1967; 20:663.

Beahrs OH. Surgical anatomy and technique of radical neck dissection. Surg Clin North Am 1977; 57:663.

Bocca E, Pignataro O, Sasaki CT. Functional neck dissection. Arch Otolaryngol 1980; 106:524.

Crile G. Excision of cancer of the head and neck with special reference to the plan of dissection based on 132 operations. JAMA 1906; 47:1780.

Feind CR. Head and neck. In: Haagensen CD, Feind CR, Herter FP, et al, eds. The lymphatics in cancer. Philadelphia: WB Saunders, 1972:60.

Fletcher GH. Elective irradiation of subclinical disease in cancers of the head and neck. Cancer 1972; 29:1450.

Lindberg RD. Distribution of cervical lymph node metastasis from squamous cell carcinoma of the upper respiratory and digestive tracts. Cancer 1972; 29:1446.

Martin H, Del Valle B, Ehrlich H, Cahan WG. Neck dissection. Cancer 1951; 4:441.

Sharpe DT. The pattern of lymph node metastasis in intraoral squamous cell carcinoma. Br J Plast Surg 1981; 34:97.

Tanner SB, Carter RL, Dalley UM, et al. The irradiated radical neck dissection in squamous carcinoma. Clin Otolaryngol 1980; 5:1.

INDEX

The letter "f" following a page number indicates a figure.

A

Abduction, 5f
 vocal cord, 5f, 6
Accessory nerve, cervical lymphadenectomy, 379
Adduction, 5f
 vocal cord, 4, 5f
Adenoma, parathyroid, 318, 319f, 320–321
Airway, 2
Airway obstruction, 49
 arytenoidectomy, 41
 nasal polypectomy, 104
 septoplasty, 109
 thyroglossal duct cyst excision, 373
Airway perforation, 67
Alveolar artery, superior, 210, 211f
Amyloidosis, 6
Anesthesia, laryngoscopy, 8, 16
Anterior ethmoid-middle meatal area, 80
Antral infection, postoperative, 207
Antrochoanal polyp, operative procedure, 106
Antrotomy, sublabial maxillary. See Caldwell-Luc procedure
Antrum neoplasm, maxillectomy, 276
Apnea technique, laryngoscopy, 16
Argon, hereditary hemorrhagic telangiectasia, 135
Artery. See specific name
Arytenoid, 4, 5f
 focal erythema, 6
Arytenoidectomy. See CO_2 laser arytenoidectomy
Asthma, nasal polypectomy, 104
Auricular composite graft, nasal reconstruction, 168–170, 169f, 171f
 auricular perichondrium, 171f
 closure, 171f
 elastic cartilage, 169f
 foil template, 169f
 nasal mucosa, 171f
 W-plasty release, 171f

B

Benign lesion, midfacial degloving sinus approach, 252
Bilobed flap, nasal reconstruction, 162, 163f
Biopsy
 fine needle aspiration. See Fine needle aspiration biopsy
 laryngoscopy, 18
Bleeding. See also Epistaxis
 mucosal origin, 100
Branchial apparatus, embryonic development, 358
Branchial cleft cyst. See First, second, and third branchial cleft cyst excision
Bronchoscopy
 diagnostic, 53–59
 anesthesia, 57f
 bite block, 55f, 57
 brush biopsy, 57f
 complications, 58
 forceps biopsy, 57f
 indications, 53
 nasal applicator, 50f
 operative steps, 54–56, 55f, 57f
 postoperative care, 56
 preoperative considerations, 53
 risks, 58
 sequelae, 58
 T-adapter, 55f
 foreign body removal. See Foreign body, bronchoscopic removal
Burn. See Caustic burn
Burrow's triangle, nasal reconstruction, 162, 163f

C

Caldwell-Luc procedure
 child, 208
 contraindications, 208
 incision, 202, 203f
 indications, 202
 maxillary antrotomy, 204, 204f
  infraorbital nerve, 204, 204f
 middle turbinate, 208
 nasal antrotomy
  ethmoid cells, 206, 206f
  infraorbital nerve, 204, 205f
  maxillary antrotomy, 206, 206f
  maxillary sinus ostium, 205, 205f
  transantral ethmoidectomy, 204–205, 205f, 206, 206f
 operative steps, 202–205, 203f–208f
 preoperative considerations, 202
 sublabial incision, 207
 with transantral ethmoidectomy, 202–208
  complications, 207
  postoperative care, 206
Cancer, laryngeal, 35
Carcinoma in situ, leukoplakia, 35
Caustic burn, esophagus. See Esophagus, caustic burn
Cerebrospinal fluid
 external ethmoidectomy, 220–222
 leak, transseptal hypophysectomy, 132
Cervical lymphadenectomy, 378–411. See also specific type
 accessory nerve, 379
 complications, 410
 indications, 378–379
 postoperative care, 408–410
 preoperative considerations, 379
 spinal accessory nerve, 379
Cheek advancement flap, nasal reconstruction, 168, 175f
Child
 Caldwell-Luc procedure, 208
 choanal atresia, 150–151, 158
 hyperparathyroidism, 321
Choanal atresia, 150–158
 associated malformations, 150
 atretic plate, 152, 153f, 154, 155f
 atretic plate resection, 154, 155f
 bilateral, 150
 bony septum, 152, 153f
 child, 150–151, 158

Choanal atresia (*Continued*)
  closure, 156, 157f
  complications, 156
  computed tomography, 151
  differential diagnosis, 150
  Dingman retractor, 154, 154f
  embryologic basis, 150
  endotracheal tube, 156, 157f
  greater palatine artery, 154, 155f
  hamulus, 154, 155f
  hard palate, 154, 155f, 156, 157f
  incisive foramen, 154, 154f
  indications, 150
  inferiorly based flap, 156, 157f
  mucoperiosteal flap, 152, 153f, 156, 157f
  nasopharyngeal mucosal membrane, 158
  operative steps, 152–156, 153f–155f, 157f
  palatal exposure, 154, 154f
  palatal incision closure, 156, 157f
  palatal mucoperiosteal flap, 154, 155f
  palate, 152, 153f
  postoperative care, 156
  preoperative considerations, 150–151
  radiographic evaluation, 151, 151f
  red rubber catheter, 156, 157f
  Rosen knife, 152, 153f
  sequelae, 156
  soft palate, 156, 157f
  speculum blade, 152, 153f
  stent, 156, 157f
  transnasal exposure, 150, 152, 153f
  transpalatal approach, 150–151
  W-shaped palatal incision, 154, 154f
CO_2 laser, telangiectasia, 135
CO_2 laser arytenoidectomy, 41–44
  arytenoid, 43f
  corniculate, 43f
  displaced cricoid lamina, 43f
  historical background, 41
  horizontal web, 43f
  indications, 41
  mucosal incision, 43f
  muscular attachment, 43f
  operative outcomes, 42
  operative steps, 42, 43f, 45f
  postoperative care, 44
  thermal injury, 44
  tracheotomy, 44
  transverse cordotomy, 42–43, 45f
  vertical web, 43f
CO_2 laser excision
  contact granuloma, 32
  cyst, 20–24
    complications, 24
    excessive tissue removal, 24
    indications, 20
    nonmalignant, 33
    operative steps, 20-24, 21f–23f
    postoperative care, 24
    preoperative considerations, 20
  infiltrative lesion, 33
  laryngeal web, 46–48
    false cord, 48f
    Jackson laryngeal dilator, 47f
    postoperative care, 48
    separated epithelium, 47f
    technique, 46–47, 47f–48f
    undersurface epithelium, 48f
    voice improvement, 48
    web, 48f
  malignant lesion, 35–39
    diagnostic objective, 36
  nodule, 20–24
    complications, 24
    excessive tissue removal, 24
    indications, 20
    operative steps, 20–24, 21f–23f
    postoperative care, 24
    preoperative considerations, 20
  polyp, 20–24
    benign lesion, 25-34
    complications, 24
    excessive tissue removal, 24
    false cord, 22, 22f
    incision, 22, 22f
    indications, 20
    mucosal incision, 21f
    operative steps, 20–24, 21f–23f
    polypoid swelling, 21f
    postoperative care, 24
    preoperative considerations, 20
    reattached epithelium, 22, 23f
    suction, 22, 23f
    ventricle, 22, 22f
  recurrent respiratory papillomatosis, 25–31
    atraumatic technique, 25
    cottonoid, 29f
    debulking forceps, 29f
    epithelial sealing, 29f
    exophytic lesion laser involution, 29f
    extralaryngotracheal sites, 30
    histologic confirmation, 25–26, 27f
    laser debulking, 29f
    papilloma, 29f
    suction, 29f
    technique, 26–30, 27f, 29f
    tracheobronchial lesion, 30
    treatment principles, 25–26
    ventilating bronchoscope, 30, 31f
  thermal injury, 33–34
Computed tomography, choanal atresia, 151
Concha bullosa, 98
  Blakesley straight forceps, 99f
  complications, 100
  intranasal scissors, 99f
  middle turbinate, 99f
  operative procedure, 98, 99f
  postoperative care, 98
  resected lateral half, 99f
  sequelae, 100
  sickle knife, 99f
Contact granuloma, 7
  CO_2 laser excision, 32
Converse scalping flap, nasal reconstruction, 182, 183f
  facial vessels, 182, 183f
  frontalis muscle, 182, 183f
  split-thickness skin graft, 182, 183f
    meshed, 182, 183f

Converse scalping flap, nasal
    reconstruction (*Continued*)
  superficial temporal vessels, 182, 183f
  supraorbital vessels, 182, 183f
  supratrochlear vessels, 182, 183f
Cordectomy, 38
  subtotal, 38, 39f
  total, 38, 39f
Cordotomy, transverse. *See* Transverse
    cordotomy
Corniculate, 5f
Cough, methylene blue to detect cause, 8
Cranial nerve VII palsy, 290
Craniotomy, pituitary adenoma, 121
Cricoarytenoid arthrodesis, 41
Cricoarytenoid joint fixation, 44
Cricoarytenoid muscle, 4
Cricoid, 5f
  retrograde tracheoscopic examination,
    13f
Cricoid lamina
  en face view, 19f
  tangential view, 19f
Croup, 6
Cyst. *See also specific type*
  CO_2 laser excision, 20–24. *See also* CO_2
    laser excision, cyst

D

Dental prosthesis, maxillectomy, 288
Dermoplasty, septal. *See* Septal
    dermoplasty
Dumbbell tumor, 347–348
Dysphonia plicae ventricularis, 4
Dysplasia, 35

E

Encephalocele, 107
Endophytic infiltration, 7
Endoscopic sphenoethmoidectomy, 88–97
  agger nasi cell, 93f
  anesthesia, 88, 89f
  angled spoon, 95f
  anterior ethmoidal artery, 93f
  carotid canal, 94f
  complications, 100
  ethmoid dome, 93f
  ethmoidal bulla, 90, 91f
  frontal sinus, 93f
    internal os, 93f
  ground lamella, 93f
  indications, 88
  infundibulotomy incision, 91f
  intranasal scissors, 95f
  lidocaine injection site, 89f
  maxillary ostium, 95f
  maxillary sinus ostium, 95f
  medial orbital wall, 95f
  middle meatal antrostomy, 94, 95f, 96f,
    97
  middle turbinate, 89f, 91f, 93f
    attachment, 95f
  operative steps, 88–97, 89f, 91f, 93f–96f
  posterior ethmoid cell, 93f
  preoperative considerations, 88
  septum, 89f, 91f
  sphenoid sinus, 94, 94f
  uncinate process, 89f, 95f
    resection, 91f
Endoscopy
  larynx. *See* Laryngoscopy
  nasal. *See* Nasal endoscopy
  repeat, 38
  sinus. *See* Maxillary sinuscopy *or*
    Sphenoid sinuscopy
Endotracheal tube, red rubber, 26, 27f
Epiglottis, 4
Epistaxis
  ethmoidal artery, 215
  hereditary hemorrhagic telangiectasia,
    135
  septoplasty, 109
  sphenopalatine artery, 209, 213–214
Erythroplakia, 7
Esophageal perforation, esophagoscopy,
    71
Esophageal tumor, esophagoscopy, 71
Esophagoscopy
  complications, 71
  diagnostic, 68–71
  esophageal perforation, 71
  esophageal tumor, 71
  foreign body removal. *See* Foreign
    body, esophagoscopic removal
  indications, 68
  operative steps, 68–70, 69f, 70f
  postoperative care, 68–70, 69f, 70f
  preoperative considerations, 68
  rigid, 68–70, 69f–70f
  risks, 71
  sequelae, 71
Esophagus, caustic burn, 75–77
  acids, 75
  basic substances, 75
  complications, 77
  cricopharyngeus, 76f
  deep, circumferential burn, 76f
  esophagectomy, 77
  flexible gastroscope, 75
  gastrectomy, 77
  gastroesophageal junction, 76f
  indications, 75
  Jesberg esophagoscope, 75
  left main bronchus, 76f
  operative steps, 75, 76f
  perforating burn, 76f
  postoperative care, 75
  preoperative considerations, 75
  reactive laryngeal edema, 76f
  risks, 77
  sequelae, 77
  sodium hydroxide, 75
  sodium hypochlorite, 77
  spotty, superficial burns, 76f
Ethmoid air cell, 268, 269f
Ethmoid air cell neoplasm, maxillectomy,
    276
Ethmoid foramen
  anterior, 218, 219f
  posterior, 218, 219f
Ethmoid sinus, external ethmoidectomy,
    218–222

Ethmoidal artery, epistaxis, 215
Ethmoidal artery ligation, 215–217
  anterior ethmoidal artery, 216, 216f
  complications, 217
  extraocular mobility, 217
  indications, 215
  operative steps, 215–216, 216f
  posterior ethmoidal artery, 216, 216f
  postoperative care, 217
  preoperative considerations, 215
  visual acuity, 217
Ethmoidectomy
  en bloc, with medial maxillectomy, 273–275, 275f
  external. *See* External ethmoidectomy
  frontal sinus-ethmoid complex. *See* Frontoethmoidectomy
  frontal sinus mucocele, 98
  medial maxillectomy, 268, 269f
  transantral, 206, 206f, 268
Ethmoidotomy, frontoethmoidectomy, 232
Exenteration. *See* Orbital exenteration
Exophytic proliferation, 7
External ethmoidectomy, 218–222
  advantages, 218
  anatomic relationships, 218, 219f, 221f
  anterior ethmoidal artery, 220, 221f
  cerebrospinal fluid, 220–222
  complications, 220
  incision, 218, 219f
  indications, 218
  lacrimal sac, 220, 221f
  M-plasty incision, 218, 219f
  medial canthal tendon, 218, 219f
  middle turbinate, 222
  operative steps, 218–220, 219f, 221f
  optic nerve, 220
  periorbita, 220, 221f
  postoperative care, 220
  suture tarsorrhaphy, 218, 219f
Eyelid, orbital exenteration, 296

F

Facial nerve, radical maxillectomy, 290
Facial pain, septoplasty, 109
False cord, 3f, 4
Fiberbronchoscopy
  anesthesia, 57f
  bite block, 55f, 57
  brush biopsy, 57f
  complications, 58
  forceps biopsy, 57f
  nasal applicator, 55f
  operative steps, 54–56, 55f, 57f
  postoperative care, 56
  risks, 58
  sequelae, 58
  T-adapter, 55f
Fiberoptic bronchoscope, foreign body, 62, 63f
Fiberoptic laryngoscopy, 10, 11f
Fiberoptic panendoscope, 68
Fibrous dysplasia, maxilla, midfacial degloving sinus approach, 252
Fine needle aspiration biopsy, 374–377
  complications, 376
  considerations, 374
  diagnostic accuracy, 376–377
  indications, 374
  operative steps, 374–376, 375f
  postoperative care, 376
Fine needle aspiration cytology, thyroid nodule, 305
First branchial cleft cyst excision, 343–346
  child, 343
  complications, 346
  cranial nerve VII, 344, 345f
  digastric muscle, 344, 345f
  external auditory canal, 344, 345f
  external opening, 344, 345f
  fistulous tract, 344, 346
  indications, 343
  operative steps, 343–344, 345f
  palpable tract, 344, 345f
  postoperative care, 346
  preoperative considerations, 343
  sternocleidomastoid muscle, 344, 345f
  stump inversion, 344, 345f
  work classification, 343
Flow-volume loop spirogram, 49
Foley catheter technique, foreign body, 73
Foreign body
  bronchoscopic removal
    bead forceps, 61f
    complications, 62
    double-action forceps, 60, 61f
    fenestrated forceps, 61f
    indications, 60
    Jackson-style forceps, 60, 61f
    microforceps, 62, 63f
    operative steps, 60–62, 61f, 63f
    optical forceps, 60–62, 63f
    postoperative care, 62
    preoperative considerations, 60
    risks, 62
    rotation forceps, 61f
    screw and nail forceps, 61f
    sequelae, 62
    side curved forceps, 61f
    tack and pin forceps, 61f
  esophagoscopic removal, 72–74
    complications, 73
    fluoroscopy, 74
    foreign body forceps, 73f
    indications, 72
    location, 72
    operative steps, 72, 73f
    postoperative care, 73
    preoperative considerations, 72
    sequelae, 73
    tooth guard, 73f
  fiberoptic bronchoscope, 62, 63f
  Foley catheter technique, 73
Foreign body forceps, 73f
Foreign body sensation, 20
Frey's syndrome, parotidectomy, 341, 342
Frontal recess dissection, 93
Frontal sinus, 81f
  mucociliary clearance, 229
Frontal sinus ablation, 247, 249f
  defect, 248, 249f
Frontal sinus mucocele
  complications, 100

Frontal sinus mucocele (*Continued*)
  ethmoidectomy, 98
  postoperative care, 98
  sequelae, 100
Frontal sinus trephination, 223-228
  complications, 226-228
  drainage, 226, 227f
  frontal bone, 224, 225f
  frontal sinus, 224, 225f
  frontal sinus mucosa, 224, 225f
  incisions, 224, 225f
  indications, 223
  irrigation, 224, 225f
  operative procedure, 224-226, 225f, 227f
  patient history, 223
  periosteum, 224, 225f
  postoperative care, 226
  preoperative considerations, 223
  sinus irrigation, 226, 227f
  subcutaneous tissue, 224, 225f
  suction, 224, 225f
  supraorbital nerve, 224, 225f
  supratrochlear nerve, 224, 225f
  trephination, 224, 225f
Frontal sinusitis, 88
  chronic, 237
  mucocele, 237
Frontoethmoidectomy, 229-236
  Blakesley forceps, 234, 235f
  complications, 236
  contraindications, 229
  diseased mucosa, 234, 235f
  ethmoid sinus, 234, 235f
  ethmoidotomy, 232
  frontal sinus recess, 234, 235f
  incisions, 230, 231f
  indications, 229
  lacrimal fossa, 230, 231f
  operative steps, 230-234
  osteoplastic flap, 233f, 234, 235f
  periosteal hinge, 230, 231f
  periosteal incision, 230, 231f
  periosteum, 233f
  postoperative care, 234-236
  preoperative considerations, 230
  reversible mucosa, 234, 235f
  supraorbital artery, 230, 231f
  supratrochlear artery, 230, 231f
Functional endoscopic sinus surgery
  advantages, 80
  defined, 80
Functional neck dissection, 402-406, 403f-406f
  brachial plexus, 405f
  carotid sheath artery, cranial nerve XII, 406f
  carotid sheath removal, 404-406, 405f-406f
    ansa cervicalis, 406f
    brachial plexus, 405f
    cervical plexus sensory branches, 405f
    cranial nerve X, 406f
    cranial nerve XI, 405f
    digastric muscle, 406f
    external carotid artery, 406f
    internal jugular vein, 405f
    phrenic nerve, 405f
    posterior triangle, 405f
  cervical plexus sensory branches, 405f
  complications, 410
  cranial nerve XI, 405f
  defined, 378
  facial envelope development, 402-404, 403f-404f
    cranial nerve XI, 403f, 404f
    deep cervical fascia, 403f, 404f
    digastric muscle, 403f
    internal jugular vein, 403f, 404f
    posterior triangle apex, 404f
    sternocleidomastoid muscle, 403f, 404f
  indications, 379
  internal jugular vein, 405f
  jugular node removal, 404-406, 405f-406f
    ansa cervicalis, 406f
    brachial plexus, 405f
    cervical plexus sensory branches, 405f
    cranial nerve X, 406f
    cranial nerve XI, 405f
    cranial nerve XII, 406f
    digastric muscle, 406f
    external carotid artery, 406f
    internal jugular vein, 405f
    phrenic nerve, 405f
    posterior triangle, 405f
  phrenic nerve, 405f
  posterior triangle, 405f
  postoperative care, 408-410
  preoperative considerations, 379
Fungal sinusitis, 98
  external ethmoidectomy, 220
  transseptal hypophysectomy, 121

G

Glabellar flap, nasal reconstruction, 166, 166f
  medial canthal ligament fixation, 166, 166f
Glossoepiglottic fold, median, 5f
Glottic band, 46
  synechial, 46
Glottic web
  anterior, 46, 47f
  horizontal posterior, 46
  posterior, 44
  types, 46
  vertical posterior, 46
Goiter, 306
Granular cell myoblastoma, 7
Granuloma, contact, 7, 32

H

Hardy retractor, complications, 132
Hematoma, 118
Hereditary hemorrhagic telangiectasia
  argon, 135
  epistaxis, 135
  Nd:YAG laser, 135
  septal dermoplasty, 135
    recurrence, 139

Hoarseness, 7, 20
Hyoid bone, thyroglossal duct, 364
Hypercalcemia, parathyroidectomy, 317
Hyperparathyroidism
    child, 321
    parathyroidectomy, 317
Hypocalcemia, thyroidectomy, 314
Hypoglossal nerve, thyroglossal duct cyst excision, 373
Hypophysectomy, transseptal. See Transseptal hypophysectomy

I

Incision, vestibulectomy, 37f
Indirect laryngoscopy, 2–8, 3f, 5f
Inferior turbinate, 81f
Infiltrative lesion, CO_2 laser excision, 33
Infraorbital artery, 210, 211f
Infraorbital nerve, 210, 211f
    anesthesia, 207
    Caldwell-Luc procedure, 204, 204f, 205f
    medial maxillectomy, 268
    midfacial degloving sinus approach, 259f
Infundibulotomy, 90, 91f
    incision, 91f
Interarytenoid muscle, 4, 5f
Intranasal ethmoidectomy, complications, 100
Intraoral mass, 348
    25
Inverted papilloma
    medial maxillectomy, 264
    midfacial degloving sinus approach, 252, 253

J

Juvenile angiofibroma, midfacial degloving sinus approach, 252, 253

K

KTP 532 laser, nasal polyp, 106

L

Lacrimal crest
    anterior, 218, 219f
    posterior, 218, 219f
Laryngeal asymmetry, 7
Laryngeal cancer, 35
Laryngeal cysts, nonmalignant, 33
Laryngeal mirror, 2, 4, 5f
Laryngeal nerve, recurrent, 304, 305f. See Recurrent laryngeal nerve
Laryngeal vestibule, 3f
Laryngeal web
    CO_2 laser excision, 46–48. See also CO_2 laser excision, laryngeal web
    types, 46
Laryngoscope
    adjusted position, 19f
    lateral placement, 15f
Laryngoscopy
    anesthesia, 8, 16
    apnea technique, 16
    biopsy, 18
    diagnostic, 2–13
    fiberoptic examination, 10, 11f
        indications, 10
        technique, 10, 11f
    indirect (mirror), 2–8, 3f, 5f
    operative, 14–19
        impaired vocal cord motion, 14
        indications, 14
        preoperative preparations, 14
        suspension apparatus, 17f
        technique, 14–18, 15f, 17f, 19f
    oxygenation, 16
    positioning, 8
    retrograde tracheoscopic examination, 12–13
        anesthesia, 12
        indications, 12
        technique, 12, 13f
    rigid telescopic, 9
        indications, 9
        technique, 9, 9f
    technique, 2–4, 3f
Larynx, posterior, focal erythema, 6
Laser. See specific type
Laser decortication, 36, 36f
    malignant lesion, 36, 36f
Lateral rhinotomy sinus approach, 270–272
    advantages, 270
    complications, 272
    incision, 270, 271f
    indications, 270
    infraorbital nerve, 270, 271f
    lacrimal sac, 270, 271f
    medial canthal ligament, 270, 271f
        repositioning, 272
    operative steps, 270, 271f
    piriform aperture incision extension, 270, 271f
    postoperative care, 272
    tarsorrhaphy, 270, 271f
Lesionectomy, defined, 38
Leukoplakia, 7, 36f
    carcinoma in situ, 35
    laryngeal cancer, 35
Lobectomy, thyroid. See Thyroid lobectomy
Lymphadenectomy, cervical. See Cervical lymphadenectomy

M

Malar eminence, maxillectomy, 288
Malignant lesion
    CO_2 laser excision, 35–39
        diagnostic objective, 36
        laser decortication, 36, 36f
        vestibulectomy, 36, 37f
Mandibulotomy, radical maxillectomy, 290
Maxilla, fibrous dysplasia, midfacial degloving sinus approach, 252
Maxillary antrotomy, Caldwell-Luc procedure, 204, 204f
    infraorbital nerve, 204, 204f

Maxillary artery
  internal, 210, 211f
    transantral ligation. *See* Transantral maxillary artery ligation
  sphenopalatine branch, 209
Maxillary sinus, 81f
  fungal disease, 98
    complications, 100
    postoperative care, 98
    sequelae, 100
Maxillary sinuscopy, 84
  complications, 100
  indications, 84
  technique, 84, 85f
Maxillary sinusitis, 88
Maxillectomy, 276–288. *See also* Medial maxillectomy; Radical maxillectomy
  anterior ethmoid foramina, 280, 281f
  anterior ethmoidal artery, 278, 279f
  antrum neoplasm, 276
  bipolar cautery, 278, 279f
  closure, 286, 287f
  complications, 286
  defect repair, 286, 287f
  dental prosthesis, 288
  ethmoid air cell neoplasm, 276
  first premolar extraction, 280, 280f, 282, 283f
  hamulus, 285f
  incision, 277, 277f
    modified Dieffenbach-Weber-Fergusson, 277, 277f
  indications, 276
  inferior orbital fissure, 280, 280f, 281f
  infraorbital foramen, 280, 280f
  infraorbital nerve stump, 278, 279f
  lacrimal duct transected, 278, 279f
  lacrimal fossa, 280, 281f
  lateral pterygoid plate, 285f
  malar eminence, 288
  malleable retractor, 278, 279f
  medial pterygoid plate, 285f
  nasomaxillary suture, 280, 281f
  operative steps, 277f, 277–286, 279f–281f, 283f, 285f, 287f
  optic canal, 280, 281f
  optic foramen, 280, 280f
  orbicularis oculi muscle, 278, 279f
  orbicularis oris fiber reanastomosis, 288
  orbital contents
    elevation, 278, 279f
    exposure, 278, 279f
    retraction, 280, 281f
  osteotomy, 280, 280f–281f
    palatal, 282, 283f, 285f
    posterior, 284, 285f
  palatal mucosal incisions, 282, 283f
  palatal prosthesis, 286, 287f
  periorbita, 278, 279f, 286, 287f
  periosteal incision, 278, 279f
  pie-crust perforations, 286, 287f
  piriform aperture, 282, 283f
  posterior ethmoid foramina, 280, 281f
  posterior ethmoidal artery, 278, 279f
  postoperative care, 286
  preoperative considerations, 276
  soft palate, 286, 287f
  specimen removal, 284, 285f
  split-thickness graft, 286, 287f
  suction, 280, 281f
  transected palate, 286, 287f
  zygoma, 280, 281f, 286, 287f
Meatal antrostomy, middle. *See* Middle meatal antrostomy
Meatal osteoplasty, middle. *See* Middle meatal osteoplasty
Medial maxillectomy, 264–269. *See also* Maxillectomy
  complications, 268
  electrocautery, 268
  with en bloc ethmoidectomy, 273–275
    ethmoid foramina, 274, 275f
    indications, 273
    lacrimal sac, 275
    operative steps, 274, 275f
    optic foramen, 274, 275f
    orbital fissure, 274, 275f
    preoperative considerations, 273
  ethmoidectomy, 268, 269f
  indications, 264
  infraorbital nerve, 268
  intranasal biopsy, 265
  inverted papilloma, 264
  myringotomy, 269
  operative steps, 265–268
  osteotomies, 266, 267f
  postoperative care, 268
  preoperative considerations, 264–265
  salivary gland neoplasm, 264
Medial orbital wall, identification, 101
Median forehead flap, nasal reconstruction, 174, 175f
  facial vessels, 174, 175f
  flap tip beveling, 174, 175f
  frontalis muscle, 174, 175f
  superficial defect, 174, 175f
  supraorbital vessels, 174, 175f
  supratrochlear vessels, 174, 175f
Methylene blue, 8
Middle meatal antrostomy, 94, 95f
  postoperative sponge placement, 96f
    backbiting forceps, 96f
    enlarged ostium, 96f
    forward cutting ring curet, 96f
    Merocel sponge, 96f
    middle turbinate, 96f
    silk suture, 96f, 97
Middle meatal osteoplasty, 94
Middle turbinate, 81f
Midfacial degloving sinus approach, 251–263
  anterior maxilla, 259f
  benign lesion, 252
  caudal septum, 259f
  columella, 259f
  complications, 262
  elevation, 258, 259f
  exposure, 258, 259f
  hyperplastic collagen deposition, 262
  indications, 252–253
  inferior turbinate, 259f
  infraorbital nerve, 259f

Midfacial degloving (*Continued*)
  infraorbital vessels, 259f
  inverted papilloma, 252, 253
  juvenile angiofibroma, 252, 253
  maxilla frontal process, 259f
  maxillary tunnel, 259f
  nasal incisions, 254, 255f
    caudal septal cartilage, 255f
    lower lateral cartilage, 255f
    nasal bone, 255f
    piriform margin, 255f
    upper lateral cartilage, 255f
  nasal tip, 259f
  nasal tunnel, 259f
  nasal vestibular narrowing, 263
  operative steps, 254–260
  oral incisions, 256, 257f
  paresthesia, 262
  piriform margin, 259f
  postoperative care, 260
  preoperative considerations, 253
  reflected bipedicle flap, 259f
  sinus approach
    closure, 260, 261f
    intercartilaginous suture, 260, 261f
    Keith needle, 260, 261f
    labial frenulum, 260, 261f
    nasal floor suture, 260, 261f
    nasal tip reposition key, 260, 261f
    piriform margin suture, 260, 261f
    transfixion suture, 260, 261f
  tissue adhesion, 259f
  upper lateral cartilage, 259f
  vs. external rhinoplasty, 262
Midline island forehead flap, nasal
    reconstruction, 172, 173f
  Burrow's triangle, 172, 173f
  skin island, 172, 173f
  subcutaneous pedicle, 172, 173f
  subcutaneous tunnel, 172, 173f
  supratrochlear vessels, 172, 173f
  wide undermining, 172, 173f
Midline transposition flap, nasal
    reconstruction, 166
Mirror laryngoscopy, 2–8, 3f, 5f
Modified neck dissection, 400–402, 401f
  complications, 410
  defined, 378
  indications, 379
  internal jugular vein preservation, 402
  postoperative care, 408–410
  preoperative considerations, 379
  spinal accessory nerve preservation,
      400, 401f
    cranial nerve XI, 401f
    cranial nerve XI motor branches, 401f
    digastric muscle, 401f
    great auricular nerve, 401f
    internal jugular vein, 401f
    mastoid tip, 401f
    posterior triangle apex, 401f
    sternocleidomastoid muscle, 401f
    trapezius muscle, 401f
Motion impairment, vocal cord, bilateral,
    41

Mucocele
  frontal sinusitis, 237
  transseptal hypophysectomy, 121
Mucociliary clearance, 80
  frontal sinus, 229
Multiple endocrine neoplasia syndrome,
    318, 321
Mylohyoid muscle, submandibular gland
    excision, 330
Myringotomy, medial maxillectomy, 269

N

Nasal antrotomy, Caldwell-Luc procedure
  ethmoid cells, 206, 206f
  infraorbital nerve, 204, 205f
  maxillary antrotomy, 206, 206f
  maxillary sinus ostium, 205, 205f
  transantral ethmoidectomy, 204–205,
      205f, 206, 206f
Nasal endoscopy, diagnostic, 80–83
  indications, 80
  limitations, 80
  middle turbinate, 81f
  technique, 81f, 82–83
  uncinate process, 81f
Nasal headache, septoplasty, 109
Nasal mucosa, vasoconstriction, 134
Nasal polyp, 104
  cause, 104
  KTP 532 laser, 106
  medical therapy, 104
  partial removal, 107
  recurrence, 107
  sites of origin, 104
  vs. encephalocele, 107
Nasal polypectomy, 104–107
  airway obstruction, 104
  anesthesia, 104–105, 107
  asthma, 104
  complications, 107
  indications, 104
  layered packing, 106f
  middle turbinate, 105f
  operative steps, 104–106, 105f, 106f
  polyp, 105f
  polyp remnant, 106f
  polyp stalk, 105f
  postoperative care, 107
  postoperative considerations, 104
  rhinorrhea, 104
  risks, 107
  sequelae, 107
  sinusitis, 104
  snare, 105f
  topical steroid, 107
  upbiting forceps, 106f
Nasal polyposis, external ethmoidectomy,
    220
Nasal prosthesis, 193–199
  advantages, 199
  casting, 196, 197
  extrinsic coloration, 198, 198f
  fabrication steps, 194–198
  fitting, 194

Nasal prosthesis (*Continued*)
　historical aspects, 193
　impression-taking techniques, 194, 195f
　indications, 193
　molding process, 196, 197f
　sculpting, 194
　vs. reconstructive surgery, 199
Nasal reconstruction, 160–186
　auricular composite graft, 168–170, 169f, 171f
　　auricular perichondrium, 171f
　　closure, 171f
　　elastic cartilage, 169f
　　foil template, 169f
　　nasal mucosa, 171f
　　W-plasty release, 171f
　bilobed flap, 162, 163f
　Burrow's triangle, 162, 163f
　cheek advancement flap, 168, 175f
　Converse scalping flap, 182, 183f
　　facial vessels, 182, 183f
　　frontalis muscle, 182, 183f
　　meshed split-thickness skin graft, 182, 183f
　　split-thickness skin graft, 182, 183f
　　superficial temporal vessels, 182, 183f
　　supraorbital vessels, 182, 183f
　　supratrochlear vessels, 182, 183f
　flap revision, 180, 181f
　full-thickness defect inner lining, 176, 177f
　　flap rotation, 176, 177f
　　full-thickness defect healed margin, 176, 177f
　　inner lining closure, 176, 177f
　　maxilla, 176, 177f
　　nasal dorsum, 176, 177f
　　nasal septum, 176, 177f
　　undermining, 176, 177f
　full-thickness defect outer lining, 176–178, 178f
　　cheek advancement flap, 178, 178f
　　flap tip, 178, 178f
　　median forehead flap, 178, 178f
　　vestibular margin, 178, 178f
　full-thickness defect primary closure, 178, 179f
　　banked cartilage, 178, 179f
　　cartilage graft, 178, 179f
　　split-thickness skin graft, 178, 179f
　　subcutaneous pocket, 178, 179f
　glabellar flap, 166, 166f
　　medial canthal ligament fixation, 166, 166f
　historical aspects, 160
　indications, 160
　large nasal defect regional flaps, 172–175
　local skin flaps, 161
　median forehead flap, 174, 175f
　　facial vessels, 174, 175f
　　flap debulking, 180f–181f
　　flap tip beveling, 174, 175f
　　frontalis muscle, 174, 175f
　　revision, 180, 180f, 181f
　　superficial defect, 174, 175f
　　supraorbital vessels, 174, 175f
　　supratrochlear vessels, 174, 175f
　midline island forehead flap, 172, 173f
　　Burrow's triangle, 172, 173f
　　skin island, 172, 173f
　　subcutaneous pedicle, 172, 173f
　　subcutaneous tunnel, 172, 173f
　　supratrochlear vessels, 172, 173f
　　wide undermining, 172, 173f
　midline transposition flap, 166
　nasal lining defect repair, 176–184
　nasal tip, 184, 185f
　nasolabial flap, 167f, 167–168, 168f
　　cheek advancement, 167–168, 168f
　　wide undermining, 167, 167f
　operative steps, 160–186
　pedicle flap revision, 180, 180f, 181f
　preoperative considerations, 160
　primary closure, 160–161
　rhomboid flap, 164, 165f
　　equilateral flap, 164, 165f
　　short axis, 164, 165f
　skin graft, 161
　support structure repair, 184–186
Nasal septal perforation
　closure. *See* Septal perforation closure
　etiology, 141
Nasal tip, nasal reconstruction, 184, 185f
Nasolabial flap, nasal reconstruction, 167–168, 167f, 168f
　cheek advancement, 167–168, 168f
　wide undermining, 167, 167f
Nd:YAG laser
　anesthesia, 67f
　bronchial use, 65–67
　　complications, 67
　　risks, 67
　　sequelae, 67
　hereditary hemorrhagic telangiectasia, 135
　laser fiber, 66f, 67f
　protective goggles, 67f
　suction, 67f
　swivel connector, 67f
　telescope, 67f
　tracheobronchial lesion, 65–67
　　complications, 67
　　indications, 65
　　operative steps, 65, 66f
　　postoperative care, 65
　　preoperative considerations, 65
　　risks, 67
　　sequelae, 67
Neck dissection. *See specific type*
Neck mass, 348, 358
Nerve. *See specific name*
Neurilemoma, 348
Nodule, 6. *See also* Polyp *and specific types*
　causes, 6
　CO_2 laser excision, 20–24. *See also* CO_2 laser excision, nodule
　organized, 24
Nose, 103–200
　endoscopy. *See* Nasal endoscopy

Nose (*Continued*)
  polyps. *See* Nasal polyp *or* Nasal polypectomy
  prosthesis. *See* Nasal prosthesis
  reconstruction. *See* Nasal reconstruction

O

Open tube esophagoscope, 68
Operative laryngoscopy. *See* Laryngoscopy, operative
Optic canal, 218, 219f
Optic nerve, external ethmoidectomy, 220
Oral antral fistula, 207
Orbit, tumor invading, 294f
Orbital exenteration, 292–296
  closure, 295, 295f
  complications, 296
  eyelid, 296
  incision, 294f, 294–295
  indications, 292
  ligation, 295, 295f
  modified Weber–Fergusson incision, 294f
  neurovascular pedicle, 295f
  neurovascular pedicle control, 294f, 294–295
  operative steps, 292–295, 293f–295f
  optic nerve, 294f
  perineural invasion, 296
  postoperative care, 296
  preoperative, 292
Orbital hematoma, 100
Orbital prosthesis, 297–302
  anterior mold, 301f
  casting, 297, 301f
  coloration, 300
  escape trough, 301f
  fabrication procedure, 297–302, 299f, 301f
  face cast, 301f
  globe, original position, 301f
  impression-taking techniques, 297
  indications, 297
  measurements for, 298, 299f
  molding, 298–300, 301f
  ocular, 299f, 301f
  orbit, 301f
  posterior mold, 301f
  registration dimples, 301f
  sculpting, 297–298
  silicone packing, 301f
  superior orbital rim, 299f
Osteoplastic frontal sinusectomy, 237–250
  bone flap elevation, 242, 243f
  closure, 246, 247f
  complications, 248–249
  fat graft, 246, 247f
  frontal sinus, 243f
  galea, 238, 239f
  grafting, 246, 247f
  incisions, 238, 239f
    brow, 238, 239f
    coronal, 238, 239f
    periosteal, 240, 241f
    reflected scalp, 240, 241f
    sinus outline, 240, 241f
    six-foot Caldwell view, 240, 241f
    template, 240, 241f
  indications, 237
  mucosal exenteration, 244, 245f
  nasofrontal duct, 245f
  operative steps, 238–248, 239f, 241f, 243f, 245f, 247f, 249f
  osteoplastic flap, 243f, 245f
  osteotomy, 242, 243f
  periosteum, 238, 239f
  postoperative care, 248
  preoperative considerations, 237
  Raney clip, 238, 239f
  scalp, 238, 239f
  skull, 238, 239f
Ostiomeatal complex, 80, 81f
Oxygenation, laryngoscopy, 16

P

Pain, septoplasty, 109
Palatine artery, descending, 210, 211f
Palatine nerve, descending, 210, 211f
Papilloma, 7
  excision, 25–31. *See also* Recurrent respiratory papillomatosis, CO_2 laser excision
Papillomatosis. *See* Recurrent respiratory papillomatosis
Paraganglioma, 348
Paranasal sinuses, 201–301
Parapharyngeal space, 347
Parapharyngeal space tumor, 347
  anatomy, 347–348, 351f
  excision, 347–355, 351f, 353f
Parathyroid adenoma, 318, 319f, 320–321
Parathyroid glands, 317
Parathyroidectomy, 317–321
  anatomic considerations, 317
  biopsy/resection technique, 318, 319f
  carotid bifurcation, 319f
  carotid sheath, 319f
  complications, 320
  hypercalcemia, 317
  hyperparathyroidism, 317
  indications, 317
  intrathyroidal, 319f
  localization studies, 321
  locations, 318, 319f
  operative steps, 317–320, 319f
  parathymic, 319f
  postoperative care, 320
  preoperative considerations, 317
  recurrent laryngeal nerve, 318, 320
  sternotomy, 321
  subclavicular, 319f
  superior mediastinum, 319f
  upper tracheoesophageal groove, 319f
Parotid duct stone, parotidectomy, 331
Parotid gland, 324
Parotid tumor, parotidectomy, 333f, 336, 338, 339f, 341
Parotidectomy, 331–342
  closure, 338, 339f
  complications, 340–341
  cranial nerve dissection, 336, 337f
  cranial nerve VII, 333f, 335f

Parotidectomy (*Continued*)
  cranial nerve visualization, 336, 337f
  deep lobe dissection, 338, 339f
  deep lobe parotid tumor, 339f
  digastric muscle, 333f, 335f
  duct, 333f, 339f
  facial nerve, 340
    graft, 338–340
    resection, 338–340
    retrograde dissection, 338
  fascical attachment, 335f
  Frey's syndrome, 341, 342
  great auricular nerve, 333f
  gustatory sweating, 341, 342
  incision, 332, 333f
  indications, 331
  masseter muscle, 333f, 339f
  nerve elevation, 339f
  operative steps, 332–340, 333f, 335f, 337f, 339f
  paralysis, 340
  parotid bridge, 335f
  parotid duct stone, 331
  parotid tail dissection, 332, 333f
  parotid tumor, 333f, 336, 338, 339f, 341
  posterior aspect mobilization, 334, 335f
  posterior facial vein, 333f, 339f
  postoperative care, 340
  preoperative considerations, 331–332
  salivary fistula, 340–341
  sialadenitis, 331
  sialocele formation, 340–341
  silicone drain, 339f
  sternocleidomastoid muscle, 333f, 339f
  sternocleidomastoid parotid fascia, 333f
  styloid process, 335f
  supraneural parotidectomy, 332–336, 333f, 335f, 337f
  total, 338, 339f
  tragal cartilage, 333f, 335f
Pedicle flap revision, nasal reconstruction, 180, 180f, 181f
Perforation. *See specific type*
Periorbita
  biopsy, 292, 293f
    orbicularis oculi muscle, 293f
    orbital septum, 293f
    periosteum, 293f
  evaluation, 292, 293f
  tumor involving, 293f
Petiole, 4, 5f
Pharyngeal space tumor, 347
  evaluation, 348–349
  pathology, 348
  signs, 348–349
  symptoms, 348–349
Pharyngeal space tumor excision, 347–355
  areolar tissue, 353f
  complications, 354
  cranial nerve, 354
  cranial nerve VII, 351f
  cranial nerve XI, 351f
  cranial nerve XII, 351f
  digastric muscle, 353f
  dissection, 352, 353f
  exposure, 350, 351f
  facial vein, 351f
  incision, 351f
  internal carotid artery, 351f
  internal jugular vein, 351f
  location, 350, 351f
  mandible, 351f, 353f
  mandibulotomy, 353f
  operative steps, 350–355
  parotid gland, 351f
  postoperative care, 354
  preoperative considerations, 349–350
  sternocleidomastoid muscle, 351f
  stylohyoid muscle, 353f
  superior constrictor muscle, 351f
Pharyngoepiglottic fold, lateral, 5f
Piriform sinus, 7–8
  medial wall bulge, 4
Pituitary adenoma
  craniotomy, 121
  transseptal hypophysectomy, 121
Polyp, 6. *See also* Nodule
  causes, 6
  CO_2 laser excision, 20–24. *See also* CO_2 laser excision, polyp
  nasal. *See* Nasal polyp
Polypectomy, nasal. *See* Nasal polypectomy
Polypoid degeneration, 20
Proptosis, 100
Prosthesis
  nasal. *See* Nasal prosthesis
  orbital. *See* Orbital prosthesis
Pterygomaxillary fossa, 210, 211f

R

Radical maxillectomy, 289–291. *See also* Maxillectomy
  complications, 290
  cranial nerve VII palsy, 290
  facial nerve, 290
  indications, 289
  inferior orbital fissure, 290, 291f
  lateral pterygoid plate, 290, 291f
  mandibulotomy, 290
  operative steps, 290, 291f
  optic canal, 290, 291f
  orbital floor resection, 290, 291f
  osteotomies, 290, 291f
  palatal osteotomy, 290, 291f
  pterygomaxillary fissure, 290, 291f
  pterygopalatine fossa dissection, 290, 291f
  soft palate resection, 290, 291f
  superior orbital fissure, 290, 291f
  tooth extraction, 290, 291f
  zygomatic buttress removal, 290, 291f
  zygomaticofrontal osteotomy, 290, 291f
Radical neck dissection
  anterior dissection, 393f–395f, 394
  clavicle, 383f
  closure, 398, 399f
  complications, 410
  cranial nerve VII, 383f
  deep cervical fascia, 383f
  defined, 378
  digastric tendon, 397f
  exposure, 382, 383f

Radical neck dissection (*Continued*)
  external jugular vein, 383f
  facial artery, 397f
  facial vein, 383f
  great auricular nerve, 383f
  hyoid bone, 383f
  incisions, 380, 381f
    anterior apron, 381f
    half-H, 381f
    McFee, 381f
    modified Schobinger, 381f
  indications, 378–379
  inferior dissection, 382–386, 383f, 387f
    clavicle, 387f
    internal jugular vein, 387f
    omohyoid muscle posterior belly, 387f
    phrenic nerve, 387f
    subclavian vein, 387f
    transverse cervical artery, 387f
  internal jugular vein inferior ligation, 384, 385f
    carotid artery, 384, 385f
    carotid sheath, 384, 385f
    cranial nerve X, 384, 385f
    omohyoid muscle posterior belly, 384, 385f
    sternocleidomastoid muscle, 384, 385f
    sternohyoid muscle, 384, 385f
  internal jugular vein superior ligation, 392, 393f, 394, 394f–395f
    cranial nerve X, 393f
    cranial nerve XI, 393f
    digastric muscle, 393f
    digastric muscle posterior belly, 393f
    great auricular nerve, 393f
    internal jugular vein, 393f
    mastoid tip, 393f
    parotid gland, 393f
    superior dissection, 394, 395f
  lingual nerve, 397f
  mandible, 383f
  masseter muscle, 383f
  mylohyoid muscle, 397f
  omohyoid muscle anterior belly, 383f
  operative steps, 380–399, 381f, 383f, 385f, 387f, 389f, 391f, 393f–395f, 397f, 399f
  parotid gland, 383f
  posterior dissection
    brachial plexus, 391f
    carotid artery, 391f
    cervical plexus motor branches, 391f
    cervical plexus sensory branches, 389f
    cranial nerve X, 391f
    cranial nerve XI, 389f
    internal jugular vein, 389f, 391f
    levator scapulae muscle, 389f, 391f
    omohyoid muscle posterior belly, 391f
    phrenic nerve, 389f
    scalenius anterior muscle, 391f
    scalenius capitis muscle, 391f
    scalenius medius muscle, 391f
    splenius capitis muscle, 389f
    sternocleidomastoid muscle, 389f
    trapezius muscle, 389f
  postganglionic fibers, 397f
  postoperative care, 408–410
  preoperative considerations, 379
  sternocleidomastoid muscle, 383f
  sternohyoid muscle, 383f
  submandibular duct, 397f
  submandibular ganglion, 397f
  submandibular gland, 383f, 397f
  submandibular triangle dissection, 396, 397f
  superficial anatomy, 382, 383f
  thyrohyoid muscle, 383f
  thyroid cartilage, 383f
  trapezius muscle, 383f
  trapezius muscle delineation, 388, 389f
    external jugular vein, 389f
    great auricular nerve, 389f
    mastoid tip, 389f
    parotid gland, 389f
    posterior dissection, 388–392
    sternocleidomastoid muscle, 389f
    trapezius muscle, 389f
Recurrent laryngeal nerve
  parathyroidectomy, 318, 320
  thyroidectomy, 316
Recurrent respiratory papillomatosis
  CO_2 laser excision, 25–31. *See also* CO_2 laser excision, recurrent respiratory papillomatosis
  human papillomavirus, 25
  systemic treatment, 25
Retrograde tracheoscopic examination, 12, 13f
Rhinectomy, 187–192
  closure, 190, 191f
  complications, 190
  cutaneous margins, 187
  hemostasis, 192
  incisions, 188, 189f
    anterior nasal spine, 188, 189f
    margin, 188, 189f
    nasal bone, 188, 189f
    periosteal incision, 188, 189f
    tumor, 188, 189f
  indications, 187
  inferior turbinate, 190, 191f
  middle turbinate, 190, 191f
  nasal bone, 190, 191f
  nasal mucosa, 190, 191f
  operative steps, 188–190, 189f, 191f
  postoperative care, 190
  preoperative considerations, 187
  prosthetic reconstruction, 192
  quadrangular cartilage, 190, 191f
  septal resection, 190, 191f
  sequelae, 190
  skin, 190, 191f
Rhinorrhea, nasal polypectomy, 104
Rhinotomy, lateral. *See* Lateral rhinotomy sinus approach
Rhomboid flap, nasal reconstruction, 164 165f
  equilateral flap, 164, 165f
  short axis, 164, 165f
Rigid telescopic laryngoscopy, 9, 9f
Round tumor, 347–348
  intraoral removal, 350

S

Salivary fistula, parotidectomy, 340–341
Salivary glands, 323–355. *See also specific glands*
  neoplasm, medial maxillectomy, 264
  tumor, 348
Sarcoidosis, 6
Second branchial cleft cyst, location, 358
Second branchial cleft cyst excision, 358–363
  anatomy, 358, 359f
  complications, 362
  cranial nerve IX, 360, 361f
  cranial nerve X, 360, 361f
  cranial nerve XI, 359f
  cranial nerve XII, 359f, 360, 361f
  digastric muscle, 360, 361f
  external carotid artery, 363f
  fistulous tract, 360, 361f, 363f
  fistulous tract location, 358
  incision, 359f, 360
  indications, 358
  internal carotid artery, 359f
  internal jugular vein, 360, 361f
  operative steps, 360–362, 361f, 363f
  postoperative care, 362
  preoperative considerations, 360
  sternocleidomastoid muscle, 360, 361f
  superior laryngeal nerve, 359f
  superior pharyngeal constrictor muscle, 363f
Segmental bronchus tumor, 67
Septal abscess, 118
Septal button, 142–144
Septal dermoplasty, 135–140
  columellar skin, 136, 137f
  columellar sutures, 138, 139f
  complications, 138–139
  curet, 136, 137
  exposed septal perichondrium, 136, 137
  hereditary hemorrhagic telangiectasia, 135
    recurrence, 139
  indications, 135
  middle turbinate, 136, 137f
  mucosal resection, 136, 137f, 138, 139f
  operative steps, 136–138, 137f, 139f
  optional alotomy, 136, 137f
  packing, 138, 139f
  postoperative care, 138
  preoperative considerations, 135
  sequelae, 138-139
  Silastic sheeting, 138, 139f
  skin graft, 138, 139f
  thrombin topical spray, 138, 140
Septal deviation, septoplasty, 109
Septal perforation closure, 141–149
  complications, 144
  contraindications, 141
  indications, 141
  preoperative considerations, 141
  septal button, 142–144
    complications, 144
    one-piece, 142f, 142–143
    operative steps, 142f, 142–143, 143f
    sequelae, 144
    two-piece, 143, 143f
  surgical closure, 145f, 145–149, 147f, 148f
    complications, 149
    conchal cartilage, 146, 147f
    conchal cartilage graft, 146, 147f
    incision, 145, 145f
    inferior subperiosteal tunnel, 145, 145f
    intact posterior perichondrium, 146, 147f
    mastoid periosteum, 146, 147f
    mucoperichondrial closure, 148f, 149
    mucosa, 145, 145f
    perichondrial incision, 145, 145f
    periosteum, 146, 147f
    postoperative care, 149
    relaxing incisions, 146, 147f
    sandwich graft, 146, 147f, 148f, 149
    septal flap elevation, 145, 145f
    septal mucoperiosteal flap, 145, 145f
    septal perforation, 145, 145f
    sequelae, 149
    Teflon, 148f, 149
Septoplasty, 109–120
  airway obstruction, 109
  anesthesia, 110, 111f
  anterior tunnel, 113f
  bone spur, 115f
  bony septum, 120
  cartilage release, 114, 115f
  cartilaginous deformity, 116, 117f
  caudal strip, 115f
  closure, 118, 119f
  complications, 118–120
  cribriform plate, 117f
  decussating fibers, 113f
  dorsal strip, 115f
  epistaxis, 109
  ethmoid bone perpendicular plate, 115f, 116f
  ethmoidal nerve, 111f
  exposure, 112, 113f
  facial pain, 109
  incisions, 110, 111f
  indications, 109
  inferior spur, 115f
  inferior tunnel, 113f
  inferior turbinate, 111f
  intracartilaginous elasticity, 117f
  maxillary crest, 115f
  membranous septum, 111f
  middle turbinate, 111f
  nasal deformity, 120
  nasal headache, 109
  nasal packing, 120
  nasal spine, 115f
  operative steps, 110–118, 111f, 113f, 115f–117f, 119f
  perichondrial incision, 111f
  perichondrium, 120
  piriform margin, 111f
  posterior septal resection, 116, 116f, 117f
  posterior tunnel, 113f

Septoplasty (*Continued*)
  postoperative care, 118
  preoperative considerations, 109
  quadrangular cartilage, 115f, 116f
  septal cartilage, 120
  septal deviation, 109, 117f
  septal morsalizer, 117f
  septal splint, 120
  sequelae, 118–120
  severe comminuted deformity, 117f
  sinusitis, 109
  sphenoid rostrum, 117f
  spur resection, 114, 115f
  subperichondrial infiltration, 111f
  superior tunnel, 113f
  vomer, 115f, 117f
Seventh cranial nerve palsy, radical maxillectomy, 290
Sialadenitis, parotidectomy, 331
Sialoadenitis, 324
Sialocele formation, parotidectomy, 340–341
Sialolithiasis, 324
Sialorrhea, 324
Sinus. *See specific type*
Sinusectomy. *See* Osteoplastic frontal sinusectomy
Sinuscopy
  maxillary. *See* Maxillary sinuscopy
  sphenoid. *See* Sphenoid sinuscopy
Sinusitis
  nasal polypectomy, 104
  purulent frontal, 223
  septoplasty, 109
  transseptal hypophysectomy, 121
Skin graft, nasal reconstruction, 161
Skull base, identification, 101
Speech pathologist, 20
Sphenoethmoidectomy, endoscopic. *See* Endoscopic sphenoethmoidectomy
Sphenoid cell, anterior wall, 94, 94f
Sphenoid sinus, location, 101
Sphenoid sinuscopy, 84
  carotid artery, 87f
  carotid canal, 87f
  indications, 84
  intersinus septa, 87f
  middle turbinate, 87f
  operative steps, 84–86, 87f
  optic canal, 87f
  optic nerve, 87f
  sella turcica, 87f
  septum, 87f
  sphenoid ostium, 87f
  sphenoid rostrum, 87f
  superior turbinate, 87f
Sphenopalatine artery, 210, 211f
  epistaxis, 209, 213–214
  transseptal hypophysectomy, 134
Sphenopalatine ganglion, 210, 211f
Spinal accessory nerve, cervical lymphadenectomy, 379
Stenosis
  anatomic composition, 49
  extent, 49
  severity, 49
  T-tube for, 49
Stent. *See* T-tube insertion
Sternotomy, parathyroidectomy, 321
Stiffness, 7
Stricture, caustic burn, 75, 77
Styloid musculature, 347
Styloid process, 347
Subglottic tumor, 19f
Subglottis, 3f
Sublabial maxillary antrotomy. *See* Caldwell-Luc procedure
Submandibular gland excision, 324–330
  anatomy, 326, 327f
  complications, 330
  digastric muscle, 326, 327f
  facial artery, 326, 327f
  hyoglossus muscle, 329f
  hypoglossal, 329f
  indications, 324
  lingual nerve, 329f
  mandibular border, 329f
  marginal mandibular nerve, 330
  mylohyoid muscle, 326, 327f, 329f, 330
  operative steps, 326–329
  postganglionic nerve fibers, 329f
  preoperative considerations, 325
  sialolith, 330
  submandibular ganglion, 329f
  submandibular mass, 326, 327f
  superficial exposure, 326, 327f
  unipolar cautery, 330
  Wharton's duct, 329f
Superior alveolar artery, 210, 211f
Superior orbital fissure, 218, 219f
Supraglottis, 4
Supraomohyoid neck dissection, 407f, 407–408, 409f
  carotid artery, 407f
  cervical plexus sensory branch, 407f
  complications, 410
  cranial nerve X, 407f
  cranial nerve XI, 407f, 409f
  cranial nerve XII, 409f
  defined, 378
  digastric muscle, 409f
  external carotid artery, 409f
  internal jugular vein, 407f
  lymph node, 407f
  node-bearing tissue, 409f
  omohyoid muscle, 409f
  posterior triangle apex, 409f
  postoperative care, 408–410
  preoperative considerations, 379
  sternocleidomastoid muscle, 407f
Suspension microlaryngoscopy, 20
Swallowing, 2
  fiberoptic laryngoscopy, 10
Synechial glottic band, 48

T

T-tube insertion, 49–52
  connecting silk suture, 51f
  indications, 49
  nasogastric tube, 51f
  operative steps, 49–50, 51f
  postoperative care, 50–52
  preoperative considerations, 49

T-tube insertion (*Continued*)
  tube design, 49
  Tucker retrograde esophageal bougie, 51f
Telangiectasia, CO_2 laser, 135
Telescopic laryngoscopy, 9, 9f
Thermal injury, CO_2 laser excision, 33–34
Third branchial cleft cyst, location, 358
Third branchial cleft cyst excision, 358–363
  anatomy, 358, 359f
  complications, 362
  cranial nerve IX, 360, 361f
  cranial nerve X, 360, 361f
  cranial nerve XI, 359f
  cranial nerve XII, 359f, 360, 361f
  digastric muscle, 360, 361f
  external carotid artery, 363f
  fistulous tract, 360, 361f, 363f
  fistulous tract location, 358
  incision, 359f, 360
  indications, 358
  internal carotid artery, 359f
  internal jugular vein, 360, 361f
  operative steps, 360–362, 361f, 363f
  postoperative care, 362
  preoperative considerations, 360
  sternocleidomastoid muscle, 360, 361f
  superior laryngeal nerve, 359f
  superior pharyngeal constrictor muscle, 363f
Third hand technique, 18, 19f
Throat
  competent, 2
  complete history, 2
Thrombin topical spray, septal dermoplasty, 138, 140
Thyroarytenoideus muscle, 3f
Thyroglossal duct, hyoid bone, 364
Thyroglossal duct cyst excision, 364–373
  airway obstruction, 373
  anatomy, 364, 365f
  central hyoid bone resection, 368, 369f
  closure, 372f, 373
  complications, 373
  cyst, 365f
  cyst mobilization, 366, 367f
  deep cervical fascia, 367f
  digastric muscle, 369f
  fistula, 365f
  fistulous tract, 365f
  foramen cecum, 365f
  hyoid bone, 365f
  hyoid bone body, 369f, 370, 371f
  hyoid bone lesser cornu, 369f
  hypoglossal nerve, 373
  hypopharyngeal mucosa, 372f
  incisions, 364, 365f
  indications, 364
  mylohyoid muscle, 369f, 372f
  operative steps, 364–373, 365f, 367f, 369f, 371f, 372f
  platysma, 367f
  postoperative care, 373
  preoperative considerations, 364
  pyramidal thyroid lobe attachment, 367f
  sites, 365f
  sternohyoid muscle, 367f, 369f, 372f
  suprahyoid tract resection, 370, 371f
  thyroid gland, 365f
  tongue, 365f
  tongue base, 371f
Thyrohyoid membrane, fullness, 4
Thyroid artery
  inferior, 304, 305f
  superior, 304, 305f
Thyroid gland, 303–316
  anatomy, 304, 305f
  removal. *See* Thyroidectomy
Thyroid lobectomy, 310, 311f
Thyroid nodule
  evaluation, 305, 306t
  fine needle aspiration cytology, 305
Thyroid papillary carcinoma, 373
Thyroid veins, 304, 305f
Thyroidea ima, 304
Thyroidectomy, 304–316
  anatomic considerations, 304
  anterior jugular vein, 308, 309f
  antithyroid medications, 306
  areolar tissue, 308, 309f
  bilateral vocal cord paralysis, 41
  carotid artery, 308, 309f, 312, 313f, 314, 315f
  closure, 314, 315f
  complications, 314
  cricothyroid muscle, 310, 311f
  flap elevation, 308, 308f
  hypocalcemia, 314
  incision, 314, 315f
  indications, 305
  inferior thyroid artery, 312, 313f, 314, 315f
  inferior thyroid vein, 310, 311f
  internal jugular vein, 314, 315f
  lateral gland mobilization, 308, 308f
  ligament of Berry, 312, 313f
  middle thyroid vein, 308, 309f
  operative steps, 306–314, 309f, 311f, 313f, 315f
  parathyroid gland, 312, 313f, 314, 315f
  platysma muscle, 308, 309f
  postoperative care, 314
  preoperative considerations, 305
  recurrent laryngeal nerve, 312, 313f, 314, 315f, 316
  sternocleidomastoid muscle, 314, 315f
  sternohyoid muscle, 308, 309f
  strap muscles, 310, 311f, 314, 315f
  subtotal, 312, 313f
  superficial cervical fascia, 308, 309f, 315f
  superior thyroid artery, 312, 313f
  thyroid carcinoma, 316
  thyroid gland, 308, 309f, 314, 315f
  thyroid gland upper pole, 310, 311f, 312, 313f
  thyroid isthmus, 310, 311f
  L-thyroxine, 316
  trachea, 312, 313f
L-Thyroxine, thyroidectomy, 316
Topical steroid, nasal polypectomy, 107
Tracheobronchial lesion, Nd:YAG laser excision, 65–67

Tracheobronchial lesion, Nd:YAG laser excision (*Continued*)
  complications, 67
  indications, 65
  operative steps, 65, 66f
  postoperative care, 65
  preoperative considerations, 65
  risks, 67
  sequelae, 67
Tracheoscopic laryngoscopy, retrograde, 12, 13f
Tracheostomy, retrograde tracheoscopy, 12, 13f
Tracheotomy, CO_2 laser arytenoidectomy, 44
Transantral ethmoidectomy, 268
  operative steps, 206, 206f
Transantral maxillary artery ligation, 209–214
  blunt hook, 212, 213f
  complications, 212
  descending palatine artery, 212, 213f
  indications, 210
  infraorbital nerve, 210, 211f
  internal maxillary artery, 212, 213f
  internal maxillary artery dissection, 212, 213f
  maxillary mucosal flap, 210, 211f
  operative steps, 210, 211f, 213f
  palatine bone orbital process, 210, 211f
  periosteum cruciate incision, 212, 213f
  posterior ostectomy, 210, 211f
  postoperative care, 212
  preoperative considerations, 210
  pterygomaxillary fossa approach, 210, 211f
  sphenopalatine artery, 212, 213f
  surgical anatomy, 210, 211f
  timing, 212–214
Transseptal hypophysectomy, 121–134
  anterior nasal spine, 123f, 132, 133f
  bone graft, 132, 133f
  bony cartilaginous junction, 125f
  bony septum resection, 126, 127f
  cartilaginous nasal septum, 123f, 132, 133f
  cerebrospinal fluid leak, 132
  closure, 132, 133f
  complications, 132–133
  cruciate incision, 130, 131f
  displaced septal cartilage, 127f
  ethmoid perpendicular plate, 127f
  ethmoid perpendicular plate attachment, 128, 129f
  fat graft, 132, 133f
  fungal sinusitis, 121
  Hardy retractor, 128, 129f
  incisions, 122, 123f
  indications, 121
  inferior rim, 123f
  inferior tunnels, 125f
  initial mucosal incision, 134
  intersphenoid septum, 128, 129f
  mucocele, 121
  mucoperichondrial flap, 132, 133f
  nasal submucosal tunnels, 124, 125f
  operative steps, 122–132, 123f, 125f, 127f, 129f, 131f, 133f
  pituitary adenoma, 121, 128, 129f
  postoperative care, 132
  preoperative considerations, 121
  ring curet, 130, 131f
  septal cartilage, 127f
  sequelae, 132
  Silastic septal splint, 132, 133f
  sinusitis, 121
  special mucosal tunnel, 125f
  sphenoid obliteration, 132, 133f
  sphenoid ostium, 128, 129f
  sphenopalatine artery, 134
  sphenotomy, 128, 129f
  suction dissection, 130, 131f
  vasoconstriction, 134
  vomer, 127f
Transverse cordotomy
  contracting arytenoidectomy defect, 45f
  enlarged posterior aperture, 45f
  improved airway, 45f
  indications, 44
  vocal cord retraction, 45f
Trephination, frontal sinus. *See* Frontal sinus trephination
True cord, 3f, 4–8
  inferomedial pink swelling, 6
  lesion
    hidden portion, 37f
    vestibulectomy, 39f
    visible, 37f
  normal, 4–8
Tumor. *See specific type*
Turbinate. *See specific type*

U

Ulcer, 7
Uncinate process, 81f
Upper airway obstruction, fiberoptic laryngoscopy, 10

V

Vagus nerve, 304
Vallecula, 7–8
Vein. *See specific name*
Ventricle, 3f
Vestibulectomy, 22
  incision, 37f
  malignant lesion, 36, 37f
  true cord lesion, 39f
Vidian artery, 210, 211f
Vidian nerve, 210, 211f
Vocal abuse, 20
Vocal cord
  abduction, 5f, 6
  adduction, 4, 5f
  epithelium, 21f, 21–22
  false. *See* False cord
  imperfect apposition, 4–6
  induration-fibrosis, 41, 44
  motion impairment, 6, 8
    bilateral, laser procedures, 41–44, 43f, 45f
  palpation, 16

Vocal cord (*Continued*)
  paralysis. *See* Vocal cord, motion impairment
  stripping, 24
  swelling, 6
  true. *See* True cord
  undersurface, retrograde tracheoscopic examination, 13f

Vocalization, 2
Voice counseling, 20
Voice quality, 24

W

Web, laryngeal. *See* Laryngeal web
Wedge cordectomy, 42–43, 45f